Tumors of the Central Nervous System

Tumors of the Central Nervous System
Volume 1

For other titles published in this series, go to
www.springer.com/series/8812

Tumors of the Central Nervous System
Volume 1

Tumors of the Central Nervous System

Gliomas: Glioblastoma (Part 1)

Edited by

M.A. Hayat
Distinguished Professor
Department of Biological Sciences,
Kean University, Union, NJ, USA

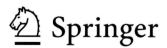 Springer

Editor
M.A. Hayat
Department of Biological Sciences
Kean University
Union, NJ, USA
ehayat@kean.edu

ISBN 978-94-007-0343-8   e-ISBN 978-94-007-0344-5
DOI 10.1007/978-94-007-0344-5
Springer Dordrecht Heidelberg London New York

Library of Congress Control Number: 2011923069

Printed on acid-free paper

Springer is part of Springer Science+Business Media (www.springer.com)

Although touched by technology, surgical pathology always has been, and remains, an art. Surgical pathologists, like all artists, depict in their artwork (surgical pathology reports) their interactions with nature: emotions, observations, and knowledge are all integrated. The resulting artwork is a poor record of complex phenomena.

Richard J. Reed MD

Preface

It is recognized that scientific journals not only provide current information but also facilitate exchange of information, resulting in rapid progress. In this endeavor, the main role of scientific books is to present current information in more detail after careful additional evaluation of the investigational results, especially those of new or relatively new methods and their potential toxic side-effects.

Although subjects of diagnosis, drug development, therapy and its assessment, and prognosis of tumors of the central nervous system, cancer recurrence, and resistance to chemotherapy are scattered in a vast number of journals and books, there is need of combining these subjects in single volumes. An attempt will be made to accomplish this goal in the projected six-volume series of handbooks.

In the era of cost-effectiveness, my opinion may be a minority perspective, but it needs to be recognized that the potential for false-positive or false-negative interpretation on the basis of a single laboratory test in clinical pathology does exist. Interobservor or intraobservor variability in the interpretation of results in pathology is not uncommon. Interpretive differences often are related to the relative importance of the criteria being used.

Generally, no test always performs perfectly. Although there is no perfect remedy to this problem, standardized classifications with written definitions and guidelines will help. Standardization of methods to achieve objectivity is imperative in this effort. The validity of a test should be based on the careful, objective interpretation of the tomographic images, photo-micrographs, and other tests. The interpretation of the results should be explicit rather than implicit. To achieve an accurate diagnosis and correct prognosis, the use of molecular criteria and targeted medicine is important. Equally important are the translation of molecular genetics into clinical practice and evidence-based therapy. Translation of medicine from the laboratory to clinical application needs to be carefully expedited. Indeed, molecular medicine has arrived.

An attempt has been made to achieve the above-mentioned goals in the present, first volume of this series of handbooks, *Tumors of the Central Nervous System*. The volume presents almost all aspects of Gliomas: Glioblastoma tumors. The volume discusses specifically details of relevant molecular genetics, diagnosis (using, for example, biomarkers, immunohistochemistry, and imaging techniques), therapies (including targeted therapy, resection, chemotherapy and cannabinoids, immunotherapy, hormonal therapy, anti-VEGF therapy, combination of bevacizumab and irinotecan as well as bortezomib and celecoxib, cyclosporine, interleukin-6, interferone, heparin, oncolytic adenovirus, chemovirotherapy, and radiotherapy). A constructive evaluation of commonly used methods for primary and secondary cancer initiation, progression, relapse, and metastasis is presented. The toxic side-effects of treatments are pointed out. Also are included prognostic factors and crucial role played by cancer stem cells in malignancy. Risk of cancer survivors developing other cancers is pointed out.

There exists a tremendous, urgent demand by the public and the scientific community to address to cancer prevention, diagnosis, treatment, and hopefully cures. This volume was written by 150 oncologists representing 17 countries. Their practical experience highlights their writings which should build and further the endeavors of the readers in this important area of disease. The volume provides unique, individual, practical knowledge based on the vast practical experience of the authors. The text is divided into subheadings for the convenience of the readers. It is my hope that the most up-to-date information contained in this volume will assist the readers in reaching to a more complete understanding of globally relevant cancer syndromes. I am also hoping that this information will help the practicing readers in their clinical work. I am grateful to the contributors for their promptness in accepting my suggestions. I respect their dedication and diligent work in sharing their invaluable knowledge with the public through this volume.

I am thankful to Dr. Dawood Farahi and Dr. Kristie Reilly for recognizing the importance of scholarship (research, writing, and publishing) in an institution of higher education and providing resources for completing this project.

Union, New Jersey   M.A. Hayat
July 19, 2010

Contents

Contents of Volume 2

Contributors

Mohamed Abdouh Maisonneuve- Rosemont Hospital, Montreal, QC H1T2M4, Canada; Department of Ophthalmology, University of Montreal, Montreal, QC H1T2M4, Canada, abdouhm2009@gmail.com

George A. Alexiou Department of Neurosurgery, Children's Hospital "Agia Sofia", Athens, Attikis, Greece, alexiougrg@yahoo.gr

Marta M. Alonso Department of Neuro-Oncology, University of Texas M.D. Anderson Cancer Center, Houston, TX, USA, mmalonso@unav.es

Oliver Bähr Dr. Senckenberg Institute of Neurooncology, University Cancer Center, Goethe University Hospital Frankfurt, Frankfurt, Germany, Oliver.baehr@med.uni-frankfurt.de

Adriana Bajetto Laboratory of Pharmacology, Department of Oncology, Biology and Genetics, University of Genova, Genova, Italy, adriana.bajetto@unige.it

Federica Barbieri Laboratory of Pharmacology, Department of Oncology, Biology and Genetics, University of Genova, Genova, Italy, federica.barbieri@unige.it

Ana M.O. Battastini Departmento de Bioquimica, Universidade Federal do Rio Grande do Sul, Porto Alegre, RS, Brazil, abattastini@gmail.com

Patrick D. Beauchesne Neuro-Oncologie/Neurologie, CHU de Nancy, CO N°34, Hospital Central, Nancy, France, beaupatt@orange.fr

Marie E. Beckner Department of Neurology, Louisiana State University Health Sciences Center School of Medicine in Shreveport, Shreveport, LA, USA, mbeckner@sprynet.com

Christoph P. Beier Department of Neurology, RWTH Aachen, Medical School, Aachen, Germany, Christoph.beier@gmx.de

Dagmar Beier Department of Neurology, RWTH Aachen, Medical School, Aachen, Germany, dbeier@ukaachen.de

Mitchel S. Berger Department of Neurological Surgery, Brain Tumor Research Center, University of California San Francisco, San Francisco, CA, USA, bergerm@neurosurg.ucsf.edu

Andressa Bernardi   Departmento de Bioquimica, Universidade Federal do Rio Grande do Sul, Porto Alegre, RS, Brazil, andressabernardi@yahoo.com.br

Gilbert Bernier   Maisonneuve- Rosemont Hospital, Montreal, QC, Canada; Department of Ophthalmology, University of Montreal, Montreal, QC, Canada, gbernier.hmr@ssss.gouv.qc.ca

A. Berretta   Department of Medicine, Italian National Research Council, Institute of Neurological Sciences, Section of Catania, Catania, Italy, antonioberretta@libero.it

Ayhan Bilir   Istanbul Faculty of Medicine, Department of Histology and Embryology, Istanbul University, Istanbul, Turkey, aybilir@gmail.com; bilira@istanbul.edu.tr

Atle Bjornerud   The Interventional Centre, Rikshospitalet, Oslo University Hospital, Oslo, Norway, atle.bjornerud@oslo-universitetssykehus.no

Elizandra Braganhol   Departmento de Bioquimica, Universidade Federal do Rio Grande do Sul, Porto Alegre, RS, Brazil, elizandra.braganhol@ufrgs.br

Luis F. Callado   Departments of Pharmacology, Centro de Investigación Biomédica en Red de Salud Mental, CIBERSAM, Spain, lf.callado@ehu.es

Angélica R. Cappellari   Departmento de Bioquimica, Universidade Federal do Rio Grande do Sul, Porto Alegre, RS, Brazil, angelica_cappellari@yahoo.com.br

M.V. Catania   Department of Medicine, Italian National Research Council, Institute of Neurological Sciences, Section of Catania, Catania, Italy, m.catania@isn.cnr.it

Jenghwa Chang   Department of Radiation Oncology, New York University Medical Center, New York, NY, USA, jec2046@med.cornell.edu

Kevin S. Chen   Duke Brain Tumor Immunotherapy Program, Division of Neurosurgery, Department of Surgery, Duke University Medical Center, Durham, NC, USA, kevin.s.chen@duke.edu

William K.C. Cheung   Department of Chemistry, The University of Hong Kong, Hong Kong, China, ckchun@hkusua.hku.hk

Rati Chkheidze   Institute of Medical and Applied Biophysics, Ivane Javakhisvili Tbilisi State University, Tbilisi, Republic of Georgia, dr_chkheidze@yahoo.com

Bryan D. Choi   Duke Brain Tumor Immunotherapy Program, Division of Neurosurgery, Department of Surgery, Duke University Medical Center, Durham, NC, USA, bryan.choi@duke.edu

Giorgio Corte   Department of Translational Oncology, National Institute for Cancer Research (IST), Genova, Italy, giorgio.corte@unige.it

S. D'Antoni   Department of Medicine, Italian National Research Council, Institute of Neurological Sciences, Section of Catania, Catania, Italy, simonadantoni@yahooh.it

Antonio Daga   Department of Translational Oncology, National Institute for Cancer Research (IST), Genova, Italy, antonio.daga@istge.it

Maame Dankwah-Quansah Department of Neurology, Memorial Sloan-Kettering Cancer Center, New York, NY, USA, doonbugs@hotmail.com

Stacy A. Decker Department of Neuroscience, University of Minnesota Medical School, Minneapolis, MN, USA, Decke120@umn.edu

John F. de Groot Department of Neuro-Oncology, Cancer Center, The University of Texas M.D. Anderson, Houstan, TX, USA, jdegroot@mdanderson.org

P. Dell'Albani Department of Medicine, Italian National Research Council, Institute of Neurological Sciences, Section of Catania, Catania, Italy, p.dellalbani@isn.cnr.it

Kyrre E. Emblem The Interventional Centre, Rikshospitalet, Oslo University Hospital, Oslo, Norway, kyrre.eeg.emblem@oslo-universitetssykehus.no

Mine Erguven Department of Biochemistry, Faculty of Medicine, Yeni Yüzyil University, Istanbul, Turkey, mine.erguven@gmail.com; mine.erguven@yeniyuzyil.edu.tr

Sabrina Facchino Maisonneuve-Rosemont Hospital, Montreal, QC, Canada; Department of Ophthalmology, University of Montreal, Montreal, QC, Canada, sabrina.facchino@gmail.com

Talal M. Fael Al-Mayhani Department of Clinical Neuroscience, Cambridge Center for Brain Repair, E. D. Adrian Building, Forvie Site, Robinson Way, Cambridge, UK, mtf31@cam.ac.uk

Roberto E. Favoni Department of Translational Oncology, National Institute for Cancer Research (IST), Genova, Italy, roberto.favoni@istge.it

Sherise D. Ferguson Brain Tumor Center, University of Chicago, Chicago, IL, USA, sherise@uchicago.edu

Tullio Florio Laboratory of Pharmacology, Department of Oncology, Biology and Genetics, University of Genova, 16132 Genova, Italy, Tullio.florio@unige.it

Kostas N. Fountas Department of Neurosurgery, University Hospital of Larisa, School of Medicine, University of Thessaly, Larisa, Greece, fountas@med.uth.gr

Wen-Mei Fu College of Medicine, Pharmacological Institute, National Taiwan University, Taipei, Taiwan, wenmei@ntu.edu.tw

Juan Fueyo Department of Neuro-Oncology, University of Texas M.D. Anderson Cancer Center, Houston, TX, USA, jfueyo@mdanderson.org

Oliver Ganslandt Department of Neurosurgery, University of Erlangen-Nuremberg, Erlangen, Germany, ganslandt@nch.imed.uni-erlangen.de

Jesús M. Garibi Departments of Surgery, University of the Basque Country, Leioa, Bizkaia, Spain; Neurosurgery Service, Cruces Hospital, Barakaldo, Bizkaia, Spain, amuriza27@hotmail.com

Monica Gatti Laboratory of Pharmacology, Department of Oncology, Biology and Genetics, University of Genova, Genova, Italy, monica.gatti@unige.it

Candelaria Gomez-Manzano Department of Neuro-Oncology, University of
Texas M.D. Anderson Cancer Center, Houston, TX, USA,
cmanzano@mdanderson.org

Marc-Eric Halatsch Department of Neurosurgery, University of Ulm School of
Medicine, Ulm, Germany, marc-eric.halatsch@uniklinik-ulm.de

M.A. Hayat Department of Biological Sciences, Kean University, Union, NJ,
USA, ehayat@kean.edu

Tur-Fu Huang College of Medicine, Pharmacological Institute, National Taiwan
University, Taipei, Taiwan, turfu@ntu.edu.tw

Ivo J. Huijbers The Netherlands Cancer Institute, Amsterdam, CX, The
Netherlands, i.hujibers@nki.nl

Clare M. Isacke The Netherlands Cancer Institute, Amsterdam, CX, The
Netherlands, clare.isacke@icr.ac.uk

Randy L. Jensen Department of Neurosurgery, University of Utah, Salt Lake
City, UT, USA, randy.jensen@hsc.utah.edu

Dorota Jesionek-Kupnicka Department of Pathology, Chair of Oncology,
Medical University of Lodz, Lodz, Poland, kupidor@poczta.onet.pl

Eftychia Z. Kapsalaki Department of Neurosurgery, School of Medicine,
University Hospital of Larisa, University of Thessaly, Larisa, Greece,
ekapsal@med.uth.gr

Georg Karpel-Massler Department of Neurosurgery, University of Ulm School
of Medicine, Ulm, Germany, georg.karpel@uniklinik-ulm.de

Kikuya Kato Research Institute, Osaka Medical Center for Cancer and
Cardiovascular Diseases, Osaka, Japan, katou-ki@mc.pref.osaka.jp

Ralf Ketter Department of Neurosurgery/Neurooncology, Saarland University,
Homburg, Germany, Ralf.ketter@uks.eu

Justin Kranzler Brain Tumor Center, University of Chicago, Chicago, IL, USA

Hsiang-Fu Kung Stanley Ho Centre for Emerging Infectious Diseases and State
Key Laboratory in Oncology in South China, The Chinese University of Hong
Kong, Shatin, Hong Kong, China, hkung@cuhk.edu.hk

Michael J. LaRiviere Brain Tumor Center, University of Chicago, Chicago, IL,
USA, mlariviere@surgery.bsd.uchicago.edu

Maciej S. Lesniak Brain Tumor Center, University of Chicago, Chicago, IL,
USA, mlesniak@surgery.bsd.uchicago.edu

Ying Li Department of Chemistry, The University of Hong Kong, Hong Kong,
China, liyinglynn@hotmail.com

Pawel P. Liberski Department of Molecular Pathology and Neuropathology, Chair
of Oncology, Medical University of Lodz, Lodz, Poland, ppliber@csk.am.lodz.pl

Marie C. Lin Brain Tumor Centre and Division of Neurosurgery, Department of
Surgery, The Chinese University of Hong Kong, Shatin, Hong Kong, China,
mcllin@surgery.cuhk.edu.hk

Nassir Mansour   Brain Tumor Center, University of Chicago, Chicago, IL, USA, nassir.mansour@uchospitals.edu

Olga Martinho   School of Health Sciences, Life and Health Sciences Research Institute, University of Minho, Braga, Portugal, olgamartinho@ecsaude.uminho.pt

Tetsuo Mashima   Division of Molecular Biotherapy, Cancer Chemotherapy Center, Japanese Foundation for Cancer Research, Tokyo, Japan, tmashima@jfcr.or.jp

J. Javier Meana   Departments of Pharmacology, Centro de Investigación Biomédica en Red de Salud Mental, CIBERSAM, Spain, javier.meana@ehu.es

Ashwatha Narayana   Department of Radiation Oncology, New York University Medical Center, New York, NY, USA, ashwatha.narayana@nyumc.org

Samuel S. Ng   School of Biological Sciences, The University of Hong Kong, Hong Kong, China, ssmng@hku.hk

Mary L. Nordberg   School of Medicine and Feist-Weiller Cancer Center, Louisiana State University School of Medicine, Shreveport, LA, USA, MLower@lsuhsc.edu

John R. Ohlfest   Department of Neurosurgery, University of Minnesota Medical School, Minneapolis, MN, USA, Ohlfe001@umn.edu

Antonio M. Omuro   Department of Neurology, Memorial Sloan-Kettering Cancer Center, New York, NY, USA, omuroa@mskcc.org

Richa Pandey   Department of Neuro-Oncology, Cancer Center, The University of Texas M.D. Anderson, Houstan, TX, USA

Rahima Patel   Brain Tumour North West, Faculty of Science, University of Central Lancashire, Preston, UK, RPatel@picr.man.ac.uk

Alessandra Pattarozzi   Laboratory of Pharmacology, Department of Oncology, Biology and Genetics, University of Genova, Genova, Italy, alpat25@hotmail.com

R. Pellitteri   Department of Medicine, Italian National Research Council, Institute of Neurological Sciences, Section of Catania, Catania, Italy, r.pellitteri@isn.cnr.it

Ian F. Pollack   Department of Neurosurgery, Children's Hospital of Pittsburgh, University of Pittsburgh Brain Tumor Center, University of Pittsburgh School of Medicine, Pittsburgh, PA, USA, ian.pollack@chp.edu

Carola Porcile   Laboratory of Pharmacology, Department of Oncology, Biology and Genetics, University of Genova, Genova, Italy, carola.porcile@unige.it

Neofytos Prodromou   Department of Neurosurgery, Children's Hospital "Agia Sofia", Athens, Attikis, Greece, neurosurg@paidon-agiasofia.gr

Rui Manuel Reis   School of Health Sciences, Life and Health Sciences Research Institute, University of Minho, Braga, Portugal; Molecular Oncology Research Center, Barretos Cancer Hospital, Barretos, S. Paulo, Brazil, rreis@ecsaude.uminho.pt

John H. Sampson Duke Brain Tumor Immunotherapy Program, Division of Neurosurgery, Department of Surgery, Duke University,Medical Center, Durham, NC, USA, john.sampson@duke.edu

Nader Sanai Department of Neurological Surgery, Barrow Neurological Institute, Phoenix, AZ, USA, nader.sanai@bnaneuro.net

Axel H. Schönthal Keck School of Medicine, University of Southern California, Los Angeles, CA, USA, schonthal@usc.edu

Hiroyuki Seimiya Division of Molecular Biotherapy, Cancer Chemotherapy Center, Japanese Foundation for Cancer Research, Tokyo, Japan, hseimiya@jfcr.or.jp

Amal Shervington Brain Tumour North West, Faculty of Science, University of Central Lancashire, Preston, UK, aashervington@googlemail.com

Leroy Shervington Brain Tumour North West, Faculty of Science, University of Central Lancashire, Preston, UK, lashervington@uclan.ac.uk

Markus D. Siegelin Department of Pathology and Cell Biology, Columbia University College of Physicians and Surgeons, New York, NY, USA, msiegelin@t-online.de

Yasemin Siegelin Department of Pathology and Cell Biology, Columbia University College of Physicians and Surgeons, New York, NY, USA, ysiegelin@gmail.com

Nicole Simonavicius The Netherlands Cancer Institute, Amsterdam, The Netherlands

A. Stadlbauer Department of Neurosurgery, University of Erlangen-Nuremberg, Erlangen, Germany

Alexander H. Stegh Department of Neurology, The Robert H. Lurie Comprehensive Cancer Center, The Brain Tumor Institute, Northwestern University, Chicago, IL, USA, a-stegh@northwestern.edu

Joachim P. Steinbach Dr. Senckenberg Institute of Neurooncology, University Cancer Center, Goethe University Hospital Frankfurt, Frankfurt, Germany, joachim.steinbach@med.uni-frankfurt.de

Yasuo Sugita Department of Pathology, Kurume University School of Medicine, Kurume, Fukuoka, Japan, sugita_yasuo@med.kurume-u.ac.jp

Nikhil G. Thaker Departments of Neurosurgery, Pharmacology and Chemical Biology, Children's Hospital of Pittsburgh, University of Pittsburgh School of Medicine, University of Medicine and Dentistry of New Jersey, New Jersey Medical School, Lyndhurst, NJ, USA, thakerng@umdnj.edu

Kyriaki Theodorou Department of Medical Physics, School of Medicine, University Hospital of Larisa, University of Thessaly, Larisa, Greece, ktheodor@med.uth.gr

E.M. Tricarichi Department of Medicine, Italian National Research Council, Institute of Neurological Sciences, Section of Catania, Catania, Italy, elisa.tricarichi@gmail.com

Ioannis Tsougos Department of Medical Physics, School of Medicine, University Hospital of Larisa, University of Thessaly, Larisa, Greece, tsougos@med.uth.gr

Matthew A. Tyler Brain Tumor Center, University of Chicago, Chicago, IL, USA

Ilya V. Ulasov Brain Tumor Center, University of Chicago, Chicago, IL, USA, iulasov@surgery.bsd.uchicago.edu

Steffi Urbschat Department of Neurosurgery/Neurooncology, Saarland University, Homburg, Germany, Steffi.Urbschat@uks.eu

Colin Watts Cambridge Centre for Brain Repair, Department of Clinical Neuroscience, E. D. Adrian Building, Forvie Site, Robinson Way, Cambridge, cw209@cam.ac.uk

Silke Wemmert Department of Neurosurgery/Neurooncology, Saarland University, Homburg, Germany, Silke.Wemmert@uks.eu

Márcia R. Wink Departamento de Ciências Fisiológicas, UFCSPA, Porto Alegre, RS, Brasil, marciawink@yahoo.com.br

Roberto Würth Laboratory of Pharmacology, Department of Oncology, Biology and Genetics, University of Genova, Genova, Italy, roberto.wurth@unige.it

Ming-Tao Yang College of Medicine, Pharmacological Institute, National Taiwan University, Taipei, Taiwan, d93443002@ntu.edu.tw

Izabela Zawlik Department of Molecular Pathology and Neuropathology, Chair of Oncology, Medical University of Lodz, Lodz, Poland, Izazawlik@yahoo.com

Part I
Introduction

Chapter 1

Introduction

M.A. Hayat

Keywords Gliomas · CNS · Astrocytomas · Genetics · Mutation · Temozolomide

Gliomas

Gliomas are the most common tumors accounting for 49% of all primary brain tumors and ~2% of all new cases of cancer in the United States. Approximately, 18,000 new gliomas are diagnosed each year in the United States and >60% belong to the most malignant grade IV glioblastomas. Most of these tumors are untreatable, and patients survive as an average of <12 months, and 16,000 will die of this disease during this time despite 30 years of intensive efforts to find an effective chemotherapy. Even lower grade astrocytomas frequently progress toward a higher grade and hence carry a similarly dismal prognosis. Gliomas are not common neoplasms, for their incidence ranges from 5 to 10 per 100,000 people, although their frequency is slightly increasing. As mentioned earlier, the majority of the CNS tumors are malignant gliomas and their high mortality rate leads this relatively infrequent malignancy into the third and fourth leading cause of cancer-related death among 15- and 54-year old men and women, respectively. In fact, malignant gliomas arise in individuals of any age, but are more common in older persons, with a peak in incidence during the sixth and seventh decades of life.

A glioma is a type of neoplasm that starts in the brain or spine. The name glioma is appropriate because it arises from glial cells. Gliomas are the most frequent tumors of the CNS, especially in the brain. Numerous classification systems are in use. Gliomas are classified based on the cell origin, grade, and location. Based on the cell type, they are classified below (http://en.wikipedia.org/wiki/Glioma):

Ependymomas:	ependymal cells
Astrocytomas:	astrocytes
Oligodendrogliomas:	oligodendrocytes
Mixed gliomas:	cells from different types of glia

Classification based on the grading system (increased cellular density, nuclear atypias, mitosis, vascular proliferation, and necrosis) is given below.

Low-grade:	gliomas are well-differentiated (non-anaplastic)
High-grade:	gliomas are undifferentiated (anaplastic)

Classification based on the location is given below. Gliomas can be classified according to whether they are above or below a membrane in the brain called the tentorium that separates the cerebrum (above) from the cerebellum (below).

Supratentorial:	above the tentorium (in the cerebrum), mostly in adults (70%).
Infratentorial:	below the tentorium (in the cerebellum), mostly in children (70%).

M.A. Hayat (✉)
Department of Biological Sciences, Kean University, Union, NJ, USA
e-mail: ehayat@kean.edu

M.A. Hayat (ed.), *Tumors of the Central Nervous System, Volume 1*, DOI 10.1007/978-94-007-0344-5_1, © Springer Science+Business Media B.V. 2011

Glioblastoma Multiforme

Glioblastoma multiforme is the most frequent primary brain tumor in adults, and accounts for most of the 18,500 primary brain tumor cases diagnosed each year in the United States. Based on standard histopathologic grading, >40% of the CNS tumors are WHO grade IV glioblastoma that accounts for >50% of all malignant gliomas. The incidence of this tumor in the United States is ~2.36 cases/100,000 persons. Glioblastoma is one of the most devastating human cancers because of its rapid growing nature, infiltrating growth, resistance to radiotherapy and chemotherapy, and rapid progression from diagnosis to death. It is a rapidly fatal tumor, and most patients succumb to this disease within 12–18 months from the time of diagnosis. Without therapy, patients die within 4 months, while median survival of those receiving optimal, aggressive treatments, such as surgery, radiation, and chemotherapy, is ~15 months. Despite aggressive management, glioblastoma invariably recurs and prognosis remains dismal, with a median survival of only 3–5 months at recurrence. In fact, this primary brain tumor is virtually incurable despite advances in neurosurgical instrumentation and adjuvant therapies. These statistics clearly show that glioblastoma is among the most aggressive neoplasms. Novel, targeted therapeutic approaches are needed, which are discussed in other chapters.

Glioblastoma tumors display extensive morphological and molecular heterogeneity, and thus may reflect their origin from different population of astrocytes, and possibly from oligodendrocytic and ependymal cell lineages. Glioblastomas, however, consist mainly of undifferentiated anaplastic cells of astrocytic origin, which exhibit marked nuclear pleomorphism, necrosis, and vascular endothelial proliferation. These tumor cells are arranged radially with respect to the necrotic region, and occur most frequently in the cerebrum of adults. Giant cell glioblastoma is a histologic form with large often multinucleated, unusual tumor cells.

The highly invasive nature of glioblastoma makes surgical resection rarely curative. In addition, these invading cell types are more resistant to radiation and chemotherapy. Glioblastoma cells invade initially as single cells, and travel along white matter tracts and blood vessel walls, and through the subpial glial space. Some of these cells travel long distances and do not generally invade through blood vessel walls and/or

bone. Glioblastomas rarely metastasize outside the brain. This invasive behavior differs from that shown by other cancer cells that metastasize to the brain. Moreover, the latter invading cells are more delineated from the surrounding brain tissue, subsequently invade short distances as groups of cells, and invade through blood vessel walls and/or bone.

Glioblastoma can be classified into primary type and secondary type. Although these two types develop through mutations of different genetic pathways (see below), both behave in a clinically indistinguishable manner and the survival rates are also similar. Primary glioblastoma shows amplification of the epidermal growth factor receptor (EGFR), accompanied by deletions in the *INK4a* gene with loss of p14 and p16. These tumors also show marked amplification of the loss of heterozygosity (LOH) on chromosome 10 (10q), PTEN mutation, deletion of *CDKN2A* and *MDM2* genes. Primary glioblastomas, in addition, are thought to show overexpression of the G protein coupled receptor 26 (GPR26) (Carter et al., 2009). This biomarker could be a suppressor of primary glioblastoma development. Additional studies are required using larger number of samples to confirm these results.

On the other hand, secondary glioblastoma frequently acquires mutations within the tumor suppressor protein p53 (*p53*) (Dai and Holland, 2001). Such mutations allow the accumulation of additional aberrations, resulting in the progression of malignancy from low-grade astrocytoma to high-grade glioblastoma, but rarely in the development of primary glioblastoma. Secondary glioblastomas also show overexpression of PDGF and PDGF receptors.

Molecular Genetics

Complex biology and molecular heterogeneity of these tumors have made it difficult to develop effective therapy. Recent studies have focused on deciphering the molecular biology of gliomas. These studies indicate that multiple chromosomal abnormalities, receptor anomalies, and oncogene and tumor suppressor dysregulation are characteristics of high-grade gliomas (Maher et al., 2001).

Genetic studies demonstrate that primary or de novo giloblastomas typically are found in older patients with alterations in the EGFR but without *TP53* mutations, while secondary glioblastomas tend to arise from gradual progression of lower-grade lesions with primarily *TP53* mutations but without changes in the EGFR. More recent microarray studies indicate that the glioblastoma tumor genotype corresponds with survival phenotype, and that expression data can be used to classify these tumors in genomic subgroups with phenotypic significance (Marko et al., 2008). In this study, 43 genes code for proteins that may be functionally significant in the molecular genetics of glioblastomas. This information can be used to assign unknown tumors into genotypic subgroups that associate directly with the survival phenotypes. Although these and other related findings are beginning to contribute to decisions regarding patient management, their translation into clinically relevant context has been difficult. Thus, a persistent gulf exists between glioblastoma research and treatment of this disease.

In the past, cytogenetic studies of human gliomas have implicated a gain of chromosome 7p and loss of chromosome 10q as important markers of glioblastoma. Other genetic studies have identified EGFR (HER-1) as the gene most frequently increased in gene dosage as a result of the 7p gain, whereas 10q deletions target phosphatase and tensin homolog (*PTEN*) gene. Both EGFR and PTEN control the activation state of the Ras-Raf-mitogen activated protein kinase (MAPK) and phosphoinositol–3–Akt pathways that control cell proliferation, growth, and apoptosis in glioblastoma (McLendon et al., 2007). *PTEN* is a tumor suppressor gene located on the long arm of chromosome 10 at 10q23, and in its mutated form is most common in solid cancers, while EGFR protein is overexpressed not only in brain tumors but also in many other cancer types.

Both *EGFR* and *PTEN* mutations also cause aberrant activation of the phosphoinositide – 3 – kinase pathway. This pathway activates multiple down-stream kinases, including protein kinase C type 1 (PKC1) (Ohgaki and Kleihues, 2007). A recent study demonstrates that PKC_1 is activated in glioblastoma because of aberrant upstream P13K signaling. Repression of RhoB is a key downstream event in PKC_1 signaling, leading to enhanced cell motility (Baldwin et al., 2008). This repression by PKC_1 also provides a mechanism for down regulation of RhoB in glioblastoma and the PKC_1– mediated loss of actin stress fibers. In the light of this information, PKC_1 should be evaluated further as a potential drug target for glioblastoma therapy.

Glioblastoma Stem Cells

Glioblastoma tumors were among the first solid tumor in which stem cell-like features (cancer stem cells) were identified. Such cells constitute a subpopulation of tumor cells that later differentiate into progenitor – like tumor cells or differentiated tumor cells. Biological properties of cancer stem cells are one of the reasons for the failure of chemotherapy in long-term survival of glioblastoma patients. It is known that a number of tumor types overexpress multidrug resistance proteins that protect them against cytotoxic drugs that are able to kill proginator and differentiated cells. As a result, cancer stem cells give rise to recurrent tumors. A recent study has shown that temozolomide preferentially eliminates glioblastoma cancer stem cells and prolongs the survival of patients (Beier et al., 2008). This drug spares more differentiated tumor cells.

However, the relevant question is whether chemoresistance of glioblastoma stem cells is due to reduced drug uptake or due to drug efflux. An in vitro study indicates that neither of these two alternatives are fully applicable to answer this question (Eramo et al., 2006). According to this study, drug resistance by glioblastoma stem cells depends on abnormalities of apoptotic pathways such as over-expression of anti-apoptotic factors or silencing of key death effectors. In other words, altered expression of apoptosis – related proteins may render normal neural stem cells or glioblastoma stem cells strongly resistant to death receptor ligands and inflammatory cytokines. More extensive studies are required to fully understand the mechanisms of chemoresistance by glioblastoma stem cells.

Kang and Kang (2007) and Kang et al. (in this volume) have developed a dissociated cell system for fascilitating identification and characterization of cancer stem-like cell subpopulations in glioblastoma, which showed resistance to 1,3-bis(2-chloroethyl)-1-nitrosourea (BCNU, Carmustine) chemotherapy. (This drug is the most commonly used pharmacological agent in chemotherapy of glioblastoma following surgery and radiation therapy). This and other similar studies clearly indicate that glioblastoma contains subpopulations of cells with intrinsic resistance to therapy, which can repopulate the tumor after treatment. The identification of the cell types involved in drug resistance phenomenon is critical in improving the therapeutic outcome of glioblastoma and better anticancer strategies.

Treatment

The choice of treatment for malignant gliomas, including glioblastoma, should depend on various factors such as age of the patient, the volume and localizations of the mass (tumor), and the quality of life considerations. Therapeutic alternatives include chemotherapy, total resection, subtotal resection with postoperative radiotherapy, cyst aspiration and/or biopsy followed by radiotherapy. A number of therapeutic agents, including temozolomide, nitrosoureas, procarbazine, etopside, irinotecan, and platinum analogs, are being used for treating recurrent gliomas, but responses are usually transient (Padros et al., 2006). Treatment of drug resistant glioma with imatinib mesylate and chlorimipramine is described by Bilir and Erguven in this volume.

There has been increasing hope that temozolomide (an alkylating agent) is efficacious against malignant gliomas, as this agent has shown activity in the treatment of newly diagnosed and recurrent gliomas (Stupp et al., 2005). Temozolomide, in addition, is relatively well-tolerated. However, the treatment with this drug, like other chemotherapeutic agents, is resisted by gliomas. A known factor responsible for the resistance is methylguanine – O^6 – methyltransferase (MGMT) expression. Clinical trials have demonstrated that promoter hypermethylation of the MGMT gene and low level expression of this protein are associated with an enhanced response to alkylating agents (Sasai et al., 2008). Thus, MGMT is a molecular marker for patients with glioblastoma (Hegi et al., 2004). For additional information, see page... and the chapter by Beir and Beir in this volume.

Recently, encouraging results were obtained by using liposomal peglyated doxorubicin (PEG-DOX) in patients with glioblastoma (Glas et al., 2007). This drug shows moderate efficacy against this malignancy within and outside clinical studies. Telozolomide is an alkylating drug, while PRG-DOX is non–alkylating. PEG-DOX can be used in combination with telozolomide to achieve a synergistic efficacy. However, additional studies are needed to recommend using PEG-DOX.

Another point of view is that comparatively, ionizing radiation is the most effective therapy for glioblastoma (WHO grade IV glioma); however, this therapy, as pointed out earlier, remains only palliative because of radioresistance. Although the mechanisms responsible for this resistance have not been fully elucidated, some evidence is available indicating that cancer stem cells contribute to glioblastoma radioresistance through preferential activation of the DNA damage checkpoint response and an increase in DNA repair capacity. Recent studies show that CD133 (Prominin-1) – expressing glioma cells survive ionizing radiation in increased proportions compared with most tumor cells that lack CD133 (Bao et al., 2006). Thus, targeting DNA damage checkpoint response in cancer stem cells may overcome the radioresistance, and offer a therapeutic model for malignant brain cancers.

Glioblastomas present as diffuse tumors with invasion in normal brain frequently recur or progress after radiation as focal masses, suggesting that only a fraction of tumor cells is responsible for regrowth. It has been accepted that glioblastomas contain a small number of cancer stem cells that have the capacity to self-renew and are essential for the continuous outgrowth of the tumor. These cancer stem cells are highly tumorigenic, while the more differentiated glia-like cells, which form the majority of cells in glioblastoma tumors, are only poorly tumorigenic.

In the light of limited effectiveness of temozolomide or radiotherapy alone against glioblastoma, the temozolomide-radiotherapy paradigm is considered by some workers to be the best therapy for this disease. Optimal treatment of patients with newly diagnosed glioblastoma consists of the use of this drug concurrently with radiotherapy and adjuvantly thereafter. Radiotherapy is applied at the dosage of 75 mg/m^2/day for 42 consecutive days, followed by 6 adjuvant cycles of this drug at a dosage of 150–200 mg/m^2/day for 5 consecutive days.

Antivascular EGF therapy is another approach being used against malignant gliomas. This approach is based on the realization that rapidly dividing glioma cells require adequate oxygen and nutrient delivery through coopting existing blood vessels and the formation of new vessels (angiogenesis). The delivery of these substances can be reduced or stopped by treating the patients with antivascular growth factor human monoclonal antibody bevacizumab (de Goot and Yung, 2008). According to these authors, the use of this antibody, in combination with irinotecan, can significantly improve the 6-month prognostic progression-free survival of patients with malignant gliomas. However, the impact of cytotoxic chemotherapy on the efficacy of the antibody remains to be answered.

Reactive oxygen species (ROS) are mediators of various cell signaling pathways. Nox family NADH oxidases are a major source of ROS production in various cell types, which play a crucial role in many physiological and pathological processes. NOX4 is prominently expressed in various neuroepithelial tumors, and its expression is critical for neoplastic proliferation. Shono et al. (2008) have demonstrated that the expression levels of NOX4 mRNA were significantly higher in glioblastoma (WHO IV) than those in other astrocytomas (WHO II and III). They also indicated that specific knockdown of NOX4 expression with RNA interference resulted in cell growth inhibition and enhanced induction of apoptosis by chemotherapeutic agents, such as cisplatin, in glioma cell lines. In the light of this information, development of treatments targeting NOX4 in human malignant gliomas should be explored. The delivery of oncolytic adenovirus into intracranial glioma is discussed by Kanzler et al. in this volume

In conclusion, the therapeutic failure in glioblastoma patients is, in part, attributable to the highly diffuse invasiveness of these tumors. The difficulties in detecting and destroying (excising) such tumors are related to the migration of single glioma cells within healthy brain tissue at large distances from the main primary tumor. Such disseminated cancer cells escape cytoreductice surgery and radiotherapy.

Temozolomide

Temozolomide (TMZ) is the most commonly used chemotherapeutic drug for newly diagnosed glioblastoma and recurrent gliomas. It is a DNA – alkylating agent, and is usually well-tolerated depending on the dosage. Sensitivity to this drug is correlated with the

hypermethylation of the 0^6 – methylguanine – DNA – alkyltransferase promoter glioma cells. This reaction leads to the absence of AGAT DNA repair protein that repairs the 0^6 – methylguanine adduct created by TMZ (Hegi et al., 2006). In other words, TMZ achieves its cytotoxic effect mainly by methylating the 0^6 position of guanine. This adduct is removed with the DNA repair protein 0^6 – methylguanine – DNA – methyltransferase (MGMT) that is expressed in a subgroup of glioblastoma. MGMT is a repair enzyme that removes promutagenic 0^6 – methylguanine adducts in DNA to protect cells from acquisition of G:C $\longrightarrow$ A:T mutations. As expected, TMZ is most effective against tumors lacking MGMT expression due to a methylated MGMT promoter.

TMZ also exerts antitumor effects by impairing angiogenic processes. In vitro and in vivo studies have shown antiangiogenic activity by TMZ even when it is used alone (Mathieu et al., 2008). The efficacy of TMZ can be further enhanced by combining this treatment with bevacizumab. This antibody also has an antiangiogenic effect although with a different mechanism of action. Antiangiogenic compounds also increase the therapeutic benefits of radiotherapy (Nieder et al., 2006). A phase 2 pilot study of bevacizumab in combination with TMZ and regional radiotherapy for the treatment of patients with newly diagnosed glioblastoma recently reported that toxicities were acceptable to continue enrollment, and a preliminary analysis of efficacy showed encouraging mean progression-free survival (Lia et al., 2008).

Temozolomide is often prescribed five times for a 28 day regimen, at a dose of 150–200 mg/m^2 (Neyns et al., 2008). This treatment depletes AGAT activity in peripheral blood mononuclear cells and may improve the antitumor activity. Daily dosing for 6 weeks during radiation therapy has become the standard care for newly diagnosed glioblastoma. This regimen is thought to have low acute toxicity, in terms of causing thrombocytopenia and neuropenia, no cumulative toxicity, and not associated with an increased incidence of secondary malignancies, such as treatment – related myelodysplastic syndrome, acute leukemia, or aplastic anemia.

Although TMZ significantly increases the proportion of patients surviving for ~2 years, longer survival is still rare. Caution is warranted in the use of dose-dense regimens of TMZ for extended periods of time because of its immunosuppression effect. TMZ is a potentially carcinogenic alkylating drug and thus poses the risk for secondary malignancies. Temozolomide-based chemotherapy for glioblastoma is discussed by Beier and Beier in this volume.

References

Baldwin RM, Parolin DAE, Lorimer IAJ (2008) Regulation of glioblastoma cell invasion by PKC and rhob. Oncogene 27:3587–3595

Bao S, Wu Q, McLendon RE, Hao Y, Shi Q, Hjelmedland AB, Dewhirst MW, Bigner DD, Rich JN (2006) Glioma stem cells promote radioresistance by preferential activation of DNA damage response. Nature 444:756–760

Beier D, Rohrl S, Pillai DR, Schwarz S, Kunz-Schughart LA, Leukel P, Proescholdt M, Brawanski A, Bogdahn U, Trampe-Kieslich A, Giebel B, Wischhusen J, Reifenberger G, Hau P, Beirer CP (2008) Temozolomide preferentially depletes cancer stem cells in glioblastoma. Cancer Res 14:5706–5715

Carter AN, Cole CL, Playle AG, Ramsay EJ, Shervington AA (2009) GPR26: a marker for primary glioblastoma?. Mol Cell Probes 22:133–137

Dai C, Holland EC (2001) Glioma models. Biochem Biophys Acta 1551:M19–M27

de Goot JF, Yung WK (2008) Bevacizumab and irinotecan in the treatment of recurrent malignant gliomas. Cancer J 14:279–285

Eramo A, Ricci-Vitiani L, Zeuner A, Pallini R, Lotti F, Sette G, Pilozzi E, Larocca LM, Peschle C, De Maria R (2006) Chemotherapy resistance of glioblastoma stem cells. Cell Death Differ 13:1238–1241

Glas M, Koch H, Hirschman B, Jauch T, Steinbrecher A, Herrlinger U, Bagdahn U, Hau P (2007) Pegylated liposomal doxorubicin in recurrent malignant glioma: analysis of a case series. Oncology 72:302–307

Hegi ME, Diserens AC, Godard S, Dietrich PY, Regli L, Ostermann S, Otten P, VanMelle G, de Tribolet N, Stupp R (2004) Clinical trial substantiates the predictive value of 0-6-methylguanine-DNA methyl-transferase promoter methylation in glioblastoma patients treated with tomozolomide. Clin Cancer Res 10:1871–1874

Hegi B, Diserens AC, Gorila T, Hamou F, de Tribolet N, Weller M, Kros JM, Hainfellner JA, Mason W, Mariani L, Bromberg JE, Hau P, Mirimanoff RO, Cairncross JG, Janzer RC, Stupp R (2006) MGMT gene silencing and benefits from temozolomide in glioblastoma. N Engl J Med 352:997–2005

Kang M-K, Kang S-K (2007) Tumorigenesis of chemotherapeutic drug- resistant cancer stem- like cells in brain glioma. Stem Cells Develop 16:837–847

Lia A, Filka E, McGibbon B, Nghiemphu Pl, Graham C, Yong WH, Mischel P, Liau LM, Bergsneider M, Pope W, Selch M, Cloughesy T (2008) Phase II pilot study of bevacizumab in combination with temozolomide and regional radiation therapy for up-front treatment of patients with newly diagnosed glioblastoma multiforme: interim analysis of safety and tolerability. Int J Radiat Oncol Biol Phys 71:1372–1380

Maher EA, Furnari FB, Bachoo M, Rowitch DH, Louis DN, Cavenee WK, DePinho RA (2001) Malignant glioma: genetics and biology of a grave matter. Genes Develop 15:1311–1333

Marko NF, Toms SA, Barnett GH, Weil R (2008) Genomic expression patterns distinguish long-term glioblastoma survivors: a preliminary feasibility. Genomics 91:395–406

Mathieu V, De Neve N, Le Mercier M, Dewelle J, Gaussin J-F, Dehoux M, Kiss R, Lefranc F (2008) Combining bevacizumab with temozolomide increases the antitumor efficacy of temozolomide in a human glioblatoma orthotopic xenograft model. Neoplasia 10:1383–1392

McLendon RE, Turner K, Perkinsen K, Rich J (2007) Second messenger systems in human gliomas. Arch Pathol Lab Med 131:1585–1590

Neyns B, Cordera S, Joosens E, Nader P (2008) Non-hodgkin's lymphoma in patients with glioma-treated with temozolomide. J Clin Oncol:4518–4519

Nieder C, Wiedenmann N, Andratschke N, Molls M (2006) Current status of angiogenesis inhibitors combined with radiation therapy. Cancer Treat Rev 32:348–364

Ohgaki H, Kleihues P (2007) Genetic pathways to primary and secondary glioblastomas. Am J Pathol 170:1445–1453

Padros MD, Lamberton K, Yung WK, Jaeckle K, Robins HI, Mehta M, Fine HA, Wen PY, Cloughesy T, Chang S, Nicholas MK, Schiff D, Greenberg H, Junck K, Fink K, Kuhn J (2006) A phase 2 trial of irinotecan (CPT-11) in patients with recurrent malignant glioma: a North American Brain Tumor Consortium study. Neuro Oncol 8: 189–193

Sasai K, Nodagashira M, Nishihara H, Aoyanagi E, Wang L, Katoh M, Murata J, Ozaki Y, Ito T, Fujimoto S, Kaneko S, Nagashima K, Tamaka S (2008) Careful exclusion of non-neoplastic brain components is required for an appropriate evaluation of O^6-methylguanine-DNA methyltransferase status in glioma: relationship between immunohistochemistry and methylation analysis. Am J Surg Pathol

Shono T, Yokoyama N, Uesaka T, Kuroda J, Takeya R, Yamasaki T, Amano T, Mizoguchi M, Suzuki SO, Niiro H, Miyamoto K, Akashi K, Iwaki T, Sumimoto H, Sasaki T (2008) Enhanced expression of NADPH oxidase NOX4 in human gliomas and its roles in cell proliferation and survival. Int J Cancer 123:787–792

Stupp R, Mason WP, van den Bent MJ, Weller M, Fischer B, Taphoorn MJB, Belanger K, Brandes AA, Marosi C, Bogdahn U, Curschmann J, Janzer RC, Ludwin SK, Gorlia T, Allgeier A, Lacombe D, Cairncross G, Eisenhauer E, Mirimanoff RO (2005) Radiotherapy plus concomitant adjuvant temozolomide for glioblastoma. N Engl J Med 352:987–996

Chapter 2

Molecular Classification of Gliomas

Kikuya Kato

Abstract Molecular markers have been intensively explored to overcome the limitations in the histopathological diagnosis of gliomas. Gene expression profiling, i.e., genome wide analysis of gene expression, has given rise to new molecular classification schemes. In particular, diagnostic systems for differential diagnosis of anaplastic oligodendroglioma and glioblastoma, or for prediction of prognosis for displastic astrocytoma, anaplastic astrocytoma, anaplastic oligodendroglioma and glioblastoma have been constructed through studies employing machine learning. Classification by gene expression profiling has also revealed molecular classes with distinct biological characteristics not detected by histopathology. The promoter methylation of the O^6-methylguanine methyltransferase gene has been reported as prognostic as well as predictive for alkylating agents such as temozolomide in glioblastoma. Partly due to technical difficulties in detection of methylation with PCR, the results of studies are not necessarily consistent. However, a recent study with bisulfite sequencing revealed good prognostic ability, which promises future clinical application. Among other molecular markers, 1p-/19q- has been established as a prognostic factor in oligodendroglial tumors, and is being used as a diagnostic test in several institutes. *IDH1* and *EGFR* are being explored for differentiation of primary and secondary glioblastoma, and as a possible predictive factor for molecular targeted drugs, respectively. Adequate prospective studies will help evaluate the ability of the above classification schemes as diagnostics tests to support histopathological diagnoses.

Keywords Gene expression profiling · MGMT promoter methylation · 1p-/19q- · IDH1

Introduction

Risk assessment is an important clinical aspect for malignant tumors, including gliomas. Invasion and metastasis are significant features of malignant tumors, and a stage classification system has been invented to simplify the interpretation of complicated pathological information from certain tumors, such as gastrointestinal cancers. However, gliomas are macroscopically less complicated, are restricted to the brain, and do not require any simplification of the pathologic information. Because the histology of a glioma is informative for assessing the malignant potential of gliomas, histological classification, especially grade classification, is critical for predicting prognosis. Currently, the standard for classifying tumors of the central nervous system is the 2007 version of the WHO classification standard (Louis et al., 2007).

However, the standard grade classification system is limited in diagnostic accuracy, and there is a wide range in the prognosis even within the same grade. Diagnosis depends on individual pathologists, and the results are often not concordant among multiple pathologists (Coons et al., 1997). Therefore, it is desirable to have more objective diagnostic systems.

Recent developments in anti-cancer drug research have resulted in a new type of diagnostic approach that is often called "personalized medicine." The goal of personalized medicine is the selection of patients

K. Kato (✉)
Research Institute, Osaka Medical Center for Cancer and Cardiovascular Diseases, Osaka 537-8511, Japan
e-mail: katou-ki@mc.pref.osaka.jp

M.A. Hayat (ed.), *Tumors of the Central Nervous System, Volume 1*, DOI 10.1007/978-94-007-0344-5_2, © Springer Science+Business Media B.V. 2011

with particular molecular diagnoses for treatment with a specific anti-cancer drug. Temozolomide (Temodar) is an imidazotetrazine-based second-generation alkylating agent, the leading compound in a new class of chemotherapeutic agents, and is now a standard for post-operative adjuvant chemotherapy for glioblastoma (Stupp et al., 2005). It has been shown that the methylation status of the O^6-methylguanine methyltransferase (*MGMT*) gene promoter is strongly correlated with the efficacy of temozolomide (Hegi et al., 2005). If a methylation assay could be established as a diagnostic test, then oncologists may quickly and effectively identify patients who may benefit from treatment with temozolomide. Some molecular-targeted drugs, such as trastuzumab or gefitinib, are already used for patients who undergo routine diagnostic tests that involve selection based on aberrations of target genes; the selection process allows for the treatment of patients who will successfully respond to the therapy. Because most anti-cancer drugs in the pharmaceutical pipeline are molecular targeted, personalized medicine will definitely be important for the treatment of gliomas as well.

Several molecular changes in gliomas have been extensively studied for possible clinical applications. In this review, I will focus on two topics: gene expression profiling and *MGMT* promoter methylation. Several studies have indicated a strong correlation between gene expression patterns and the malignant potential of gliomas. In addition, *MGMT* promoter methylation has also been extensively studied. Additional molecular markers, such as 1p-/19q-, *EGFR*, and *IDH1*, will also be discussed in the last part of this review.

Gene Expression Profiling: General Introduction

Gene expression profiling is the genome-wide analysis of gene expression, i.e., the simultaneous measurement of the gene expression level of thousands of genes or ideally, all the genes in the genome. Technological advancements such as DNA microarrays have been essential for gene expression profiling. After the introduction of DNA microarrays, researchers have applied this technology to cancer diagnostics. One example of the success in using this approach is the ability to predict prognosis for breast cancer patients: van't Veer

and colleagues found a strong correlation between gene expression patterns and the malignant potential of breast cancer (van't Veer et al., 2002). This work led to the development of MammaPrint, a microarray-based diagnostic system that assists in the decision-making process of whether to treat the patient with adjuvant therapy.

Gene expression profiling studies are characterized by the need for specific statistical techniques to handle the high volume of data. Aside from developing diagnostic systems, many studies have focused on the biological aspects of gene expression profiles. For this purpose, statistical approaches that are categorized as "class discovery" or "unsupervised feature extraction" have been used. The most popular technique is cluster analysis (Eisen et al., 1998), which creates groups of genes or samples based on similarities found in the gene expression profiles. In this type of analysis, the biological characteristics of each group are deduced from gene function and clinical information. However, because the classification obtained by class discovery is not necessarily correlated with outcomes or clinical parameters, many studies have performed class discovery mainly with genes known to be correlated with clinical outcomes. This approach enables easy accessibility to biological discussions and often maintains a correlation with clinical parameters. However, such classification has not been optimized to function as a diagnostic test. As discussed previously (Dupuy and Simon, 2007), class discovery is not the method of choice to construct a diagnostic system.

To construct a diagnostic system, different statistical approaches categorized as "supervised prediction" are used. Supervised prediction was originally developed in the field of machine learning. First, diagnostic genes that are correlated with a specific outcome, such as survival, are selected. Then, a classification algorithm is constructed to calculate a single diagnostic score from the expression values of the diagnostic genes (Dupuy and Simon, 2007). The main feature of this type of diagnostic system is the requirement of such an algorithm. Conventional molecular diagnostic tests usually use the level of a molecular marker as a diagnostic score, without requiring a complicated algorithm. Considering this feature, the Food and Drug Administration (FDA) created a new category of diagnostic tests known as "in vitro diagnostic multivariate index assays" (IVDMIA). MammaPrint is the first IVDMIA cleared by the FDA.

To date, only a few molecular classifiers based on gene expression profiling have been established as diagnostic tests, and the FDA has only cleared two assays as IVDMIAs: Agendia's MammaPrint and Pathwork Diagnostics' Tissue of Origin. Several factors block such molecular classifiers from practical use. First, the method is technically demanding. Although DNA microarrays are now an established laboratory tool, the quality control issues for using DNA microarrays as diagnostic tests can be quite difficult to overcome. Secondly, a molecular classifier needs a calculation algorithm, which is often a "black box" for clinicians. The difficult concept of the algorithm constitutes a psychological hurdle for clinicians to accept as part of the diagnostic routine. Thirdly, a new diagnostic test must have apparent advantages over existing methods. For example, in gastrointestinal cancer, the stage classification is dominant, and most prognostic factors, including the gene expression profile, are too weak for practical use. The first two barriers against using DNA microarrays for diagnostic purposes are more easily overcome, but the third point is critical and is the main reason for why there are not more established diagnostic tests using these new technologies.

New Classes of Gliomas Deduced from Gene Expression Profiling

There have been a number of studies examining the gene expression profiles of gliomas. The representative studies are summarized in Table 2.1. Each study used different statistical approaches, and they focused either on characterizing the biological properties or on constructing a diagnostic system.

Gene expression profiling has been used to characterize the biological features distinguishing glioma subgroups. Early studies focused on the biological characterization of existing histopathological classes (Godard et al., 2003; Shai et al., 2003). The first study (Godard et al., 2003) compared the gene expression profile of low-grade astrocytomas, secondary glioblastomas derived from low-grade astrocytomas, and primary glioblastomas. The study found increased expression of angiogenesis-related genes (e.g., *VEGF*, *fms-related tyrosine kinase 1*) and *IGFBP2* in primary glioblastomas. However, clinicians are mainly interested in whether there are novel molecular classes

of gliomas to improve their current clinical practice. From their viewpoint, the three-class model proposed by a different study may refine the current histopathological classification (Phillips et al., 2006). In this study, the authors selected 105 genes correlated with survival and constructed a three-class model based on hierarchical cluster analysis. Then, they refined the model with 35 genes that were representative for the three classes, designated as proneural (*PN*), proliferative (*Prolif*), and mesenchymal (*Mes*). A three-dimensional plot of these classes is shown in Fig. 2.1.

In Phillips et al., the researchers focused on biological characterization rather than the development of a diagnostic test. The *PN* class had markedly longer survival than the *Prolif* and *Mes* classes. The reproducibility of the three-class model and its correlation with survival were confirmed using external datasets. Most anaplastic astrocyotomas were classified as *PN*, but glioblastomas were classified as *PN*, *Prolif*, or *Mes*. The *Prolif* and *Mes* classes were subtypes with poor prognosis and had unique gene expression characteristics: *Prolif* glioblastomas highly expressed markers for proliferation, such as *PCNA* and *topoisomerase II α (TOP2A)*, and *Mes* glioblastomas highly expressed angiogenesis markers, including *VEGF*, *flt1/VEGFR1*, and *kdr/VEGFR2*, and the endothelial marker *PECAM1*. Previously, elevated expression of angiogenesis-related genes was observed in primary glioblastomas with poor prognosis (Godard et al., 2003). The model by Phillips et al. suggested that the elevated expression of angiogenesis-related genes was restricted to a subpopulation of glioblastomas with poor prognosis. In addition, genes related to neural stem cells were highly expressed by glioblastomas in the *Prolif* and *Mes* classes. In contrast, the *PN* class was characterized by the elevated expression of genes related to neuroblasts or developing neurons, such as *OLIG2*, *MAP2*, *DCX*, *ENC1 (NeuN)*, *ERBB4*, and *GAD2*. It should be noted that the *PN* cases were separated by two different prognostic groups using grade classification, suggesting that the three-class model leaves room for improving prognosis prediction.

Class discovery has usually been performed using genes selected based on investigator-driven criteria. A recent study used all genes for cluster analysis and identified seven clusters that were designated "intrinsic subtypes" (Gravendeel et al., 2009). All of the clusters contained tumors with various histological subtypes and had different prognostic characteristics. The main

Table 2.1 Representative studies of molecular classification based on gene expression profiling

	Godard et al. (2003)	Nutt et al. (2003)	Freije et al. (2004)	Phillips et al. (2006)	Shirahata et al. (2009)	Gravendeel et al. (2009)
Tumor	Low grade astrocytoma Primary and secondary glioblastoma	Anaplastic oligo-dendroglioma Glioblastoma	Anaplastic astrocytoma Glioblastoma	Anaplastic astrocytoma Glioblastoma	Diffuse astrocytoma anaplastic Oligodendroglioma Anaplastic astrocytoma Glioblastoma	Pilocytic astrocytoma Oligodendroglioma II, III Oligoastrocytoma II, III Astrocytoma II, III Glioblastoma
Number of tumors	51	50	74	115	152	276
Analysis technique	Filter array (1176 genes)	Affymetrix U95Av2	Affymetrix HG-U133A/B	Affymetrix HG-U133A/B	ATAC-PCR (3546 genes)	Affymetrix HU133 Plus 2.0
Statistics	Unsupervised Intermediate[a]	Supervised	Supervised Intermediate	Intermediate	Supervised Intermediate	Unsupervised
Gene selection criteria	NA	Histological class	Overall survival	Overall survival	Progression-free survival	NA
Outcome	Biological observation	Predictor of histological classes and prognosis (20)	Four-class model related to prognosis (595)	Three-class model related to prognosis (35)	Prognosis predictor (58)	Seven-class model
Validation	Test set	Cross-validation Test set	Cross-validation Test set External data sets	Test set External data sets	Cross-validation Test set External data sets	External data sets
Comparison with other clinical parameters	NA	No	(Yes)[b]	No	Yes	No

NA: not applied.

"Intermediate (statistics)" denotes unsupervised analysis with selected genes.

"Predictor" denotes a molecular classifier using a single score calculated by a specific algorithm.

Figure inside parenthesis indicates the number of diagnostic genes.

[a]Supervised approach was only used for confirmation of the class model.

[b]Comparison was only performed with the entire data matrix, not with the class model.

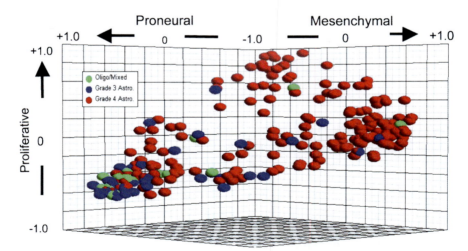

Fig. 2.1 Three-dimensional graphical representation of the three classes of gliomas designated as proneural (*PN*), proliferative (*Prolif*), and mesenchymal (*Mes*) (Phillips et al., 2006). The position occupied by each point represents the similarity (Spearman *r*) between an individual sample and each of the three centroids, defined by the k-means clustering of the reference (MDA) sample set. Nearly all grade III tumors with astrocytic (*blue*) or oligodendroglial (*green*) morphology are most similar to the *PN* centroid, while the population of grade IV tumors (*red*) is more evenly divided according to the similarity to the centroids

conceptual problem with this study is the questionable appropriateness to use all genes for cluster analysis. At first glance, the cluster analysis using all genes, without any particular selection criteria, could build groups unbiased to any biological factors, such as malignancy. However, it is important to note that the weight of each gene in producing the phenotypes of gliomas should not be considered to be equal. Genes have different functional importance, and the question remains as to whether the use of all genes equally for grouping the tumors is appropriate. In addition to this problem, the study's "intrinsic subtypes" are too complicated for practical use.

Usually the aim of unsupervised feature extraction from gene expression is class discovery or tumor grouping. In another recent study, the correlation between gene expression and the biological characteristics of gliomas was described as axes in a plane generated following principal component analysis (Shirahata et al., 2009) (Fig. 2.2). Phenotypes change gradually along these axes. From the distribution of histological subtypes of gliomas, two axes, i.e., grade axis and oligo axis were deduced. From the correlation between gene expression and prognosis, the prognosis axis was deduced. This discovery is the basis for the supervised prediction of prognosis shown below.

Constructionn of Diagnostic Systems for the Prediction of Prognosis

There have been two examples of diagnostic system construction (Nutt et al., 2003; Shirahata et al., 2009). Nutt et al. constructed a classifier to separate anaplastic oligodendroglioma and glioblastoma. Histological diagnosis is often difficult for non-classic types of these gliomas. The authors of the study selected genes that were differentially expressed between the classic anaplastic oligodendroglioma and glioblastoma, constructed a molecular classifier, and applied it to the non-classic types. While the molecular classifier separated the types into two prognostic groups, the histological diagnosis did not separate the types into such groups. Shirahata et al. constructed a prognosis predictor for gliomas ranging from grade II to IV. The diagnostic score, called the PC1 score, correlated with

the progression-free survival of all types of analyzed gliomas, and the score classified glioblastomas into two groups with different prognoses.

Both methods described here used a standard machine-learning procedure. In the first step, the diagnostic genes were selected. These were genes that were differentially expressed between anaplastic oligodendroglioma and glioblastoma (Nutt et al., 2003) or those correlated with progression-free survival (Shirahata et al., 2009). In the second step, the classifiers were constructed with the selected genes using algorithms such as the K-nearest neighbor or a linear classifier deduced by supervised principal component analysis. In the third step, the performance of the classifiers was evaluated by cross-validation, changing the parameter (K of K-nearest neighbor) or the number of diagnostic genes. Cross-validation is a statistical technique that assesses how the results of a statistical analysis will generalize to an independent data set. One round of cross-validation involves partitioning a sample of data into complementary subsets, performing the analysis on one subset (called the learning or training set), and validating the analysis on the other subset (called the validation set or test set). To reduce variability, multiple rounds of cross-validation are performed using different partitions, and the validation results are averaged over the rounds. During this process, the optimum number of the parameter or diagnostic genes was determined (20 in the Nutt et al. study; 58 in the Shirahata et al. study). Finally, the classifiers were confirmed using the test set. The entire process is summarized in Fig. 2.3.

Both studies described here suggested the possibility of diagnostic systems that exceed the utility of current histopathological diagnostic procedures. The diagnostic system of Nutt et al. was a binary classifier for anaplastic oligodendroglioma and glioblastoma. The diagnostic system of Shirahata et al. was more general, spanning from grade II to IV. In addition, the latter diagnostic system was based on a diagnostic score, enabling the quantitative evaluation of the prognosis. In a previous study from the same authors, a diagnostic system for the differential diagnosis of anaplastic oligodendroglioma and glioblastoma was constructed (Shirahata et al., 2007). A considerable proportion of the diagnostic genes for this classifier were the same as those used in the diagnostic system in their second study (Shirahata et al., 2009). This suggests

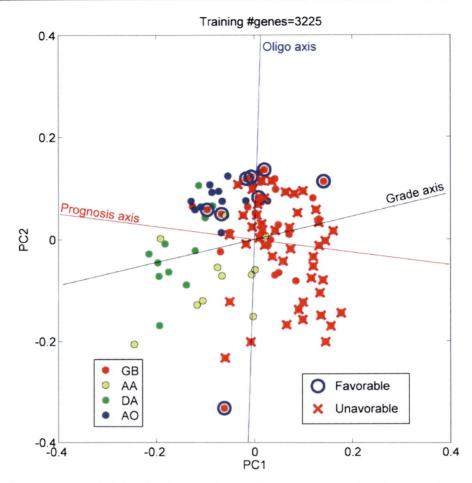

Fig. 2.2 Principal component analysis based on the expression of 3,225 genes in 110 gliomas in the training set (Shirahata et al., 2009). The *circles* indicate tumor samples, with the different colors representing histological classes. GB, AA, DA, and AO are abbreviations for glioblastoma, anaplastic astrocytoma, diffuse astrocytoma, and anaplastic oligodendroglioma, respectively. GB samples with PFS of 2 years or longer (favorable) are circled in *blue*, and those with an OS shorter than 2 years (unfavorable) are marked with a *red* x

that the diagnostic system for anaplastic oligodendroglioma and glioblastoma might be extended for use in classifying other gliomas.

A new prognostic factor must be evaluated against other existing prognostic factors using multivariate Cox analysis. The PC1 score was a better prognostic factor compared to the grade classification (III vs. IV) (Shirahata et al., 2009). In predicting the overall survival of patients with glioblastoma, the PC1 score was as good as extent of resection, a known strong prognostic factor.

Studies using the class discovery process also evaluated the relationship between the new models and patients' outcomes. However, the clinical analyses in these studies were mostly limited to Kaplan-Meier analyses. One study did perform a multivariate Cox analysis, although the analysis was performed using only the preliminary model based on using all genes for the partitioning (Freije et al., 2004).

O⁶-Methylguanine Methyltransferase Promoter Methylation

O^6-methylguanine methyltransferase (MGMT), a repair enzyme, removes methylguanine from damaged DNA. This enzyme has two different roles related to cancer. Because MGMT is a repair enzyme, its inactivation plays a role in the development of cancer

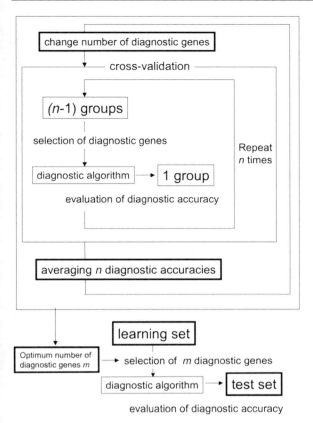

Fig. 2.3 Construction of a diagnostic system based on supervised prediction (Shirahata et al., 2009). The learning set is first divided into *n* groups. After setting the number of diagnostic genes, cross-validation is performed. Diagnostic accuracy is determined by averaging the results of *n* trials. By changing the parameter or the number of diagnostic genes, an optimum number (*m*) is determined through repeating this process. Finally, *m* diagnostic genes are selected from the entire learning set, and the diagnostic algorithm is evaluated with the test set

caused by environmental carcinogens. In addition, the inactivation of MGMT may help promote the action of an alkylating agent commonly used as a type of anti-cancer drug. Alkylating agents are some of the most widely used anti-cancer drugs for gliomas and have long been used for adjuvant therapy. The methylation of the *MGMT* promoter was a predictive factor for the efficacy of the alkylating agent carmustine (1,3-bis(2-chloroethyl)-1-nitrosourea or BCNU) (Esteller et al., 2000). Adjuvant therapy with temozolomide, a new alkylating agent, in the treatment of glioblastoma was found to give a survival benefit compared to radiation therapy alone (Stupp et al., 2005). In an accompanying paper, the *MGMT* promoter methylation status was evaluated (Hegi et al., 2005). Promoter

methylation was suggested to be a prognostic factor, because methylation-positive patients had better survival compared to methylation-negative patients. In addition, there was no additional benefit in terms of survival in methylation-negative patients treated with temozolomide. In contrast, methylation-positive patients experienced a significant increase in survival, suggesting that *MGMT* promoter methylation was predictive for the efficacy of temozolomide. Adjuvant therapy using temozolomide is now the standard treatment for glioblastoma.

Because the use of adjuvant therapy without temozolomide is considered unethical, it is not possible to confirm that *MGMT* promoter methylation is the predictive factor for the efficacy of alkylating agents in prospective studies. Therefore, research has focused on whether *MGMT* promoter methylation is a sufficient prognostic indicator for clinical application. Several reports have presented contradictory results, as summarized previously (Park et al., 2009). In addition, the protein and mRNA expression of *MGMT* did not correlate with the frequency of promoter methylation (Preusser et al., 2008). Despite large efforts, *MGMT* promoter methylation has not been established as a diagnostic test. The methylation assay is technically difficult, which is one of the reasons why promoter methylation has not been established as diagnostic test.

Technical Considerations of the Methylation Assay

Promoter methylation occurs in CpG islands, the genomic areas upstream of exons. At the methylation site, the cytosine of CpG is modified to become 5-methylcytosine. One method to detect methylation is the use of methylation-sensitive and -insensitive restriction enzymes. After digestion with each of these enzymes, the fragments containing the restriction enzyme sites are amplified by PCR with appropriate primers. The methylated fragment is determined from the amplified product of the fragment that was digested with the methylation-sensitive enzyme. One caveat of this technique is that it depends on specific recognition sites for methylation-sensitive and -insensitive enzymes.

When DNA is treated with bisulfite, cytosine is converted to thymidine, while methylcytosine is not modified. A series of techniques have been invented using bisulfite-treated genomic DNA. In a combined bisulfite restriction analysis (COBRA) (Xiong and Laird, 1997), bisulfite-treated genomic DNA is digested by a restriction enzyme that recognizes and cuts only methylated DNA, and the fragments are amplified by PCR. The fragments from methylated DNA and unmethylated DNA have different sizes, and the relative ratio of methylated to unmethylated DNA is estimated from the ratio of digested products. COBRA enables the quantification of methylation, but the method requires specific enzymes that recognize the methylated sites of genomic DNA.

Another method is methylation-specific PCR (MSP), which uses PCR primers that bind to methylation sites (Hegi et al., 2005). These primers are designed to be complementary to bisulfite-treated genomic DNA. Due to the sequence specificity of the primers, amplification is expected to occur only with methylated DNA. In MSP, amplification products are detected using gel electrophoresis. An advanced version of MSP utilizes real-time PCR (Vlassenbroeck et al., 2008) and is often called quantitative methylation-specific PCR (QMSP). Real-time PCR is performed either with or without a TaqMan probe. A potential benefit of the QMSP assay is that a TaqMan probe can be designed to be sequence-specific for a particular methylation site. However, QMSP performed without a TaqMan probe uses SyberGreen for detection and does not have the same benefit.

It should be noted that the sequence specificity of the primers and probes is not perfect. Because of the incomplete elimination of residual amplification of unmethylated DNA, quantification of methylated DNA is not accurate. In addition, all PCR-based assays detect only methylation sites within the primer and probe regions and cannot detect other sites.

The sequencing of bisulfite-treated DNA is currently the only method to completely detect methylation sites. Tumors are usually comprised of a mixture of methylation-positive and -negative cells. This intratumor heterogeneity is a common feature of human tumors, so it is exceptionally rare for all cells in one tumor to be methylation-positive. Pyrosequencing can detect sequences from both methylation-positive and -negative cells (Colella et al., 2003). In pyrosequencing, each nucleotide is individually examined at each base position, enabling semiquantitative analysis of the nucleotides. Therefore, pyrosequencing

can resolve the intratumor methylation heterogeneity. Alternatively, the Sanger method can be used to sequence multiple clones of a PCR product and can yield similar information.

The most popular techniques used for detecting *MGMT* promoter methylation are MSP and QMSP. However, as mentioned above, they have potential technical problems. The results of MSP and QMSP should be validated with results of bisulfite sequencing, because bisulfite sequencing enables the complete description of the methylation status. COBRA, pyrosequencing, and ion pair reverse-phase high-performance liquid chromatography (SIRPH) have been compared to bisulfite sequencing of multiple clones (Mikeska et al., 2007). SIRPH is a sequencing technique that detects a single nucleotide next to a primer. The results of pyrosequencing and SIRPH were significantly correlated, but the results from COBRA were significantly different from the results obtained from the bisulfite sequencing of multiple clones. Although none of these studies compared their results with results from MSP or QMSP, these studies suggest that the results with PCR-based techniques possibly differ from the results obtained using methods that are able to detect the actual methylation status.

Recent work has demonstrated a correlation between *MGMT* promoter methylation detected by pyrosequencing and outcomes of glioblastoma patients (Dunn et al., 2009). This is strong evidence in support of promoter methylation as a prognostic factor. More studies, especially prospective studies, using pyrosequencing are necessary to provide additional evidence demonstrating that promoter methylation is a reliable prognostic factor.

1p-/19q-

The loss of both the short arm of chromosome 1 (1p-) and the long arm of chromosome 19 (19q-), usually denoted as 1p-/19q-, was found to be predictive of a better response to chemoradiation and longer survival (Cairncross et al., 1998). This finding has been confirmed in prospective studies (Cairncross et al., 2006), and now recognized as the most promising prognostic factor among oligodendroglial tumors. Another study suggested that the presence of classic oligodendroglioma histology was predictive of 1p-/19q- (Smith et al., 2000), although 1p-/19q- sometimes appeared in other histological types as well. Due to difficulty in the histopathological diagnosis of oligodendroglial tumors, it may be practical to consider 1p-/19q- as a prognostic factor irrespective of oligodendroglial or astrocytic appearance.

The detection of 1p-/19q- is done using in situ hybridization or loss of heterozygosity (LOH) analysis. Although both assays are not necessarily robust, and some results are difficult to interpret, 1p-/19q- has already been established as a diagnostic test by several institutes, and large scale prospective studies are ongoing under stratification of 1p/19q status.

Epidermal Growth Factor Receptor

Gliomas are often accompanied by genetic aberrations in epidermal growth factor receptor (*EGFR*). *EGFR* amplification and over-expression appear in about 50% of glioblastomas (Brandes et al., 2008), and the *EGFR* locus in glioblastoma often displays structural rearrangements. The most common form is EGFRvIII, which lacks a part of the extracellular receptor domain (Wong et al., 1992). Although these genetic aberrations undoubtedly contribute to malignant transformation, their prognostic value is unknown.

Several drugs targeting EGFR have been developed. Erlotinib and gefitinib, small molecule inhibitors, bind to intracellular domains of EGFR and are used in the treatment of non-small cell lung cancer (NSCLC). Gefitinib is effective only in NSCLC patients who have somatic mutations in the kinase domain of EGFR (Lynch et al., 2004). Frequent genetic aberrations in *EGFR* occur in glioblastomas, and clinical trials using gefitinib or erlotinib have been performed. As reviewed previously (Brandes et al., 2008), the results of these trials were contradictory: three prospective studies with biomarkers (*EGFR* genetic aberrations) reported negative findings, whereas two retrospective studies suggested positive effects in glioblastomas that had specific molecular characteristics. These characteristics may involve EGFR or molecules downstream of the EGFR signal transduction pathway. A well-designed clinical trial with a large number of patients will be required to examine the true performance of these small molecule inhibitors.

Isocytrate Dehydrogenase 1 (NADP+) (IDH1)

The *IDH1* somatic mutation in glioblastomas was discovered during a sequencing analysis of coding regions from 20,661 genes (Parsons et al., 2008). Subsequent studies revealed that low-grade astrocytomas, oligodendrogliomas, oligoastrocytomas, and secondary glioblastomas frequently carry the mutation (Watanabe et al., 2009; Yan et al., 2009). In contrast, very few studies detected the mutation in primary glioblastomas (Watanabe et al., 2009). Therefore, the *IDH1* mutation has been regarded as a marker that discriminates primary from secondary glioblastoma. It has been reported to be a good prognostic factor of anaplastic gliomas (Wick et al., 2009), but additional evidence is required to further explore the mutation and its value as a prognostic factor.

Conclusions

The expectation for a molecular classification of gliomas comes from the limitations in current diagnostic procedures. In particular, histopathological diagnoses provide classifications that are often clinically inadequate due to the diversity of tumors that fall within the same class. The molecular markers described here are good candidates that may be developed to support the current diagnostic scheme. The direct benefit of a new classification scheme is the accurate risk assessment involved in therapeutic decision-making. For example, in grade II and III patients, the optimal timing of radiation therapy is still controversial (van den Bent et al., 2005; Wick et al., 2009). The precise risk assessment, including prediction of possible malignant transformation, may be useful for the decision on the timing. Patients of this category could receive benefit from the molecular classification scheme by gene expression profiling (Shirahata et al., 2009) in addition to 1p-/19q-.

Another important application is "personalized medicine," i.e., therapeutic decision making based on molecular markers, especially for adjuvant chemotherapy. The effect of *MGMT* promoter methylation on the efficacy of temozolomide is the representative example. However, as described above, because temozolomide is now the standard treatment for all glioblastoma patients, it is currently not possible to prospectively confirm the effect of *MGMT* promoter methylation by clinical trials with and without temozolomide.

Recently, bevacizumab (Avastin) is emerging as a possible treatment option for the adjuvant therapy of glioblastoma, being confirmed by a large-scale clinical trial. Because of complications such as hemorrhage and vascular thromboembolism (Friedman et al., 2009), selection of patients based on gene expression profiles would be beneficial. Gene expression profiling studies have demonstrated that specific classes exhibited increased expression of angiogenesis-related genes; these specific classes may be the poor prognosis group (Shirahata et al., 2009) or the *Mes* class (Phillips et al., 2006). Observations suggest that these classes may be more sensitive to bevacizumab than other classes.

The technical difficulties of gene expression profiling and the assays measuring DNA methylation are substantial hurdles to establishing them as diagnostic tests. While gene expression profiling has been successful in breast cancer (e.g., MammaPrint and Oncotype-DX), the methylation assay has not been successfully used. In principle, however, these technical problems can be resolved. Adequate prospective studies will evaluate the ability of these methods to be diagnostics tests to support histopathological diagnoses.

Acknowledgment The author thanks Dr Mitsuaki Shirahata for critical reading of the manuscript.

References

Brandes AA, Franceschi E, Tosoni A, Hegi ME, Stupp R (2008) Epidermal growth factor receptor inhibitors in neuro-oncology: hopes and disappointments. Clin Cancer Res 14(4):957–960

Cairncross G, Berkey B, Shaw E, Jenkins R, Scheithauer B, Brachman D, Buckner J, Fink K, Souhami L, Laperierre N, Mehta M, Curran W (2006) Phase III trial of chemotherapy plus radiotherapy compared with radiotherapy alone for pure and mixed anaplastic oligodendroglioma: intergroup radiation therapy oncology group trial 9402. J Clin Oncol 24(18):2707–2714

Cairncross JG, Ueki K, Zlatescu MC, Lisle DK, Finkelstein DM, Hammond RR, Silver JS, Stark PC, Macdonald DR, Ino Y, Ramsay DA, Louis DN (1998) Specific genetic predictors of chemotherapeutic response and survival in patients with anaplastic oligodendrogliomas. J Natl Cancer Inst 90(19):1473–1479

Colella S, Shen L, Baggerly KA, Issa JP, Krahe R (2003) Sensitive and quantitative universal pyrosequencing methylation analysis of CpG sites. Biotechniques 35(1): 146–150

Coons SW, Johnson PC, Scheithauer BW, Yates AJ, Pearl DK (1997) Improving diagnostic accuracy and interobserver concordance in the classification and grading of primary gliomas. Cancer 79(7):1381–1393

Dunn J, Baborie A, Alam F, Joyce K, Moxham M, Sibson R, Crooks D, Husband D, Shenoy A, Brodbelt A, Wong H, Liloglou T, Haylock B, Walker C (2009) Extent of MGMT promoter methylation correlates with outcome in glioblastomas given temozolomide and radiotherapy. Br J Cancer 101(1):124–131

Dupuy A, Simon RM (2007) Critical review of published microarray studies for cancer outcome and guidelines on statistical analysis and reporting. J Natl Cancer Inst 99(2):147–157

Eisen MB, Spellman PT, Brown PO, Botstein D (1998) Cluster analysis and display of genome-wide expression patterns. Proc Natl Acad Sci USA 95(25):14863–14868

Esteller M, Garcia-Foncillas J, Andion E, Goodman SN, Hidalgo OF, Vanaclocha V, Baylin SB, Herman JG (2000) Inactivation of the DNA-repair gene MGMT and the clinical response of gliomas to alkylating agents. N Engl J Med 343(19):1350–1354

Freije WA, Castro-Vargas FE, Fang Z, Horvath S, Cloughesy T, Liau LM, Mischel PS, Nelson SF (2004) Gene expression profiling of gliomas strongly predicts survival. Cancer Res 64(18):6503–6510

Friedman HS, Prados MD, Wen PY, Mikkelsen T, Schiff D, Abrey LE, Yung WK, Paleologos N, Nicholas MK, Jensen R, Vredenburgh J, Huang J, Zheng M, Cloughesy T (2009) Bevacizumab alone and in combination with irinotecan in recurrent glioblastoma. J Clin Oncol 27(28): 4733–4740

Godard S, Getz G, Delorenzi M, Farmer P, Kobayashi H, Desbaillets I, Nozaki M, Diserens AC, Hamou MF, Dietrich PY, Regli L, Janzer RC, Bucher P, Stupp R, de Tribolet N, Domany E, Hegi ME (2003) Classification of human astrocytic gliomas on the basis of gene expression: a correlated group of genes with angiogenic activity emerges as a strong predictor of subtypes. Cancer Res 63(20): 6613–6625

Gravendeel LA, Kouwenhoven MC, Gevaert O, de Rooi JJ, Stubbs AP, Duijm JE, Daemen A, Bleeker FE, Bralten LB, Kloosterhof NK, De Moor B, Eilers PH, van der Spek PJ, Kros JM, Sillevis Smitt PA, van den Bent MJ, French PJ (2009) Intrinsic gene expression profiles of gliomas are a better predictor of survival than histology. Cancer Res 69(23):9065–9072

Hegi ME, Diserens AC, Gorlia T, Hamou MF, de Tribolet N, Weller M, Kros JM, Hainfellner JA, Mason W, Mariani L, Bromberg JE, Hau P, Mirimanoff RO, Cairncross JG, Janzer RC, Stupp R (2005) MGMT gene silencing and benefit from temozolomide in glioblastoma. N Engl J Med 352(10): 997–1003

Louis DN, Ohgaki H, Wiestler OD, Cavenee WK, Burger PC, Jouvet A, Scheithauer BW, Kleihues P (2007) The 2007 WHO classification of tumours of the central nervous system. Acta Neuropathol 114(2):97–109

Lynch TJ, Bell DW, Sordella R, Gurubhagavatula S, Okimoto RA, Brannigan BW, Harris PL, Haserlat SM, Supko JG, Haluska FG, Louis DN, Christiani DC, Settleman J, Haber DA (2004) Activating mutations in the epidermal growth factor receptor underlying responsiveness of non-small-cell lung cancer to gefitinib. N Engl J Med 350(21):2129–2139

Mikeska T, Bock C, El-Maarri O, Hubner A, Ehrentraut D, Schramm J, Felsberg J, Kahl P, Buttner R, Pietsch T, Waha A (2007) Optimization of quantitative MGMT promoter methylation analysis using pyrosequencing and combined bisulfite restriction analysis. J Mol Diagn 9(3):368–381

Nutt CL, Mani DR, Betensky RA, Tamayo P, Cairncross JG, Ladd C, Pohl U, Hartmann C, McLaughlin ME, Batchelor TT, Black PM, von Deimling A, Pomeroy SL, Golub TR, Louis DN (2003) Gene expression-based classification of malignant gliomas correlates better with survival than histological classification. Cancer Res 63(7):1602–1607

Park CK, Park SH, Lee SH, Kim CY, Kim DW, Paek SH, Kim DG, Heo DS, Kim IH, Jung HW (2009) Methylation status of the MGMT gene promoter fails to predict the clinical outcome of glioblastoma patients treated with ACNU plus cisplatin. Neuropathology 29(4):443–449

Parsons DW, Jones S, Zhang X, Lin JC, Leary RJ, Angenendt P, Mankoo P, Carter H, Siu IM, Gallia GL, Olivi A, McLendon R, Rasheed BA, Keir S, Nikolskaya T, Nikolsky Y, Busam DA, Tekleab H, Diaz LA Jr., Hartigan J, Smith DR, Strausberg RL, Marie SK, Shinjo SM, Yan H, Riggins GJ, Bigner DD, Karchin R, Papadopoulos N, Parmigiani G, Vogelstein B, Velculescu VE, Kinzler KW (2008) An integrated genomic analysis of human glioblastoma multiforme. Science 321(5897):1807–1812

Phillips HS, Kharbanda S, Chen R, Forrest WF, Soriano RH, Wu TD, Misra A, Nigro JM, Colman H, Soroceanu L, Williams PM, Modrusan Z, Feuerstein BG, Aldape K (2006) Molecular subclasses of high-grade glioma predict prognosis, delineate a pattern of disease progression, and resemble stages in neurogenesis. Cancer Cell 9(3):157–173

Preusser M, Charles Janzer R, Felsberg J, Reifenberger G, Hamou MF, Diserens AC, Stupp R, Gorlia T, Marosi C, Heinzl H, Hainfellner JA, Hegi M (2008) Anti-O6-methylguanine-methyltransferase (MGMT) immunohistochemistry in glioblastoma multiforme: observer variability and lack of association with patient survival impede its use as clinical biomarker. Brain Pathol 18(4):520–532

Shai R, Shi T, Kremen TJ, Horvath S, Liau LM, Cloughesy TF, Mischel PS, Nelson SF (2003) Gene expression profiling identifies molecular subtypes of gliomas. Oncogene 22(31):4918–4923

Shirahata M, Iwao-Koizumi K, Saito S, Ueno N, Oda M, Hashimoto N, Takahashi JA, Kato K (2007) Gene expression-based molecular diagnostic system for malignant gliomas is superior to histological diagnosis. Clin Cancer Res 13(24):7341–7356

Shirahata M, Oba S, Iwao-Koizumi K, Saito S, Ueno N, Oda M, Hashimoto N, Ishii S, Takahashi JA, Kato K (2009) Using gene expression profiling to identify a prognostic molecular spectrum in gliomas. Cancer Sci 100(1):165–172

Smith JS, Perry A, Borell TJ, Lee HK, O'Fallon J, Hosek SM, Kimmel D, Yates A, Burger PC, Scheithauer BW, Jenkins RB (2000) Alterations of chromosome arms 1p and 19q as predictors of survival in oligodendrogliomas, astrocytomas, and mixed oligoastrocytomas. J Clin Oncol 18(3):636–645

Stupp R, Mason WP, van den Bent MJ, Weller M, Fisher B, Taphoorn MJ, Belanger K, Brandes AA, Marosi C, Bogdahn U, Curschmann J, Janzer RC, Ludwin SK, Gorlia T, Allgeier A, Lacombe D, Cairncross JG, Eisenhauer E, Mirimanoff RO (2005) Radiotherapy plus concomitant and adjuvant temozolomide for glioblastoma. N Engl J Med 352(10):987–996

van den Bent MJ, Afra D, de Witte O, Ben Hassel M, Schraub S, Hoang-Xuan K, Malmstrom PO, Collette L, Pierart M, Mirimanoff R, Karim AB (2005) Long-term efficacy of early versus delayed radiotherapy for low-grade astrocytoma and oligodendroglioma in adults: the EORTC 22845 randomised trial. Lancet 366(9490):985–990

van't Veer LJ, Dai H, van de Vijver MJ, He YD, Hart AA, Mao M, Peterse HL, van der Kooy K, Marton MJ, Witteveen AT, Schreiber GJ, Kerkhoven RM, Roberts C, Linsley PS, Bernards R, Friend SH (2002) Gene expression profiling predicts clinical outcome of breast cancer. Nature 415(6871):530–536

Vlassenbroeck I, Califice S, Diserens AC, Migliavacca E, Straub J, Di Stefano I, Moreau F, Hamou MF, Renard I, Delorenzi M, Flamion B, DiGuiseppi J, Bierau K, Hegi ME (2008) Validation of real-time methylation-specific PCR to determine O6-methylguanine-DNA methyltransferase gene promoter methylation in glioma. J Mol Diagn 10(4):332–337

Watanabe T, Nobusawa S, Kleihues P, Ohgaki H (2009) IDH1 mutations are early events in the development of astrocytomas and oligodendrogliomas. Am J Pathol 174(4):1149–1153

Wick W, Hartmann C, Engel C, Stoffels M, Felsberg J, Stockhammer F, Sabel MC, Koeppen S, Ketter R, Meyermann R, Rapp M, Meisner C, Kortmann RD, Pietsch T, Wiestler OD, Ernemann U, Bamberg M, Reifenberger G, von Deimling A, Weller M (2009) NOA-04 randomized phase III trial of sequential radiochemotherapy of anaplastic glioma with procarbazine, lomustine, and vincristine or temozolomide. J Clin Oncol 27(35):5874–5880

Wong AJ, Ruppert JM, Bigner SH, Grzeschik CH, Humphrey PA, Bigner DS, Vogelstein B (1992) Structural alterations of the epidermal growth factor receptor gene in human gliomas. Proc Natl Acad Sci USA 89(7):2965–2969

Xiong Z, Laird PW (1997) COBRA: a sensitive and quantitative DNA methylation assay. Nucleic Acids Res 25(12):2532–2534

Yan H, Parsons DW, Jin G, McLendon R, Rasheed BA, Yuan W, Kos I, Batinic-Haberle I, Jones S, Riggins GJ, Friedman H, Friedman A, Reardon D, Herndon J, Kinzler KW, Velculescu VE, Vogelstein B, Bigner DD (2009) IDH1 and IDH2 mutations in gliomas. N Engl J Med 360(8):765–773

Chapter 3

Glioblastoma: Endosialin Marker for Pericytes

Nicole Simonavicius, Clare M. Isacke, and Ivo J. Huijbers

Abstract Glioblastoma multiforme (GBM) is characterized by extensive microvascular proliferations. This abnormal vasculature is a potential target for anti-angiogenic therapy. Here, we describe the current literature on a novel target for antibody-based therapy, endosialin (CD248/TEM1). This type I transmembrane protein is often observed in the tumor vasculature of GBM patients, but absent in normal, mature vessels of the brain. We describe the protein structure, regulation of expression and potential function of endosialin, and pay particular attention to the cell type distribution of endosialin in GBM vasculature, which we identified to be limited to pericytes.

Keywords Glioblastoma · Endosialin · Marker · Pericytes · Antibody · Vasculature

Introduction

Glioblastoma multiforme (GBM) is the most common and most aggressive type of primary brain tumor in humans with an incidence of 2–5 cases per 100,000 people in Europe and North America (Brown et al., 2009; Dobec-Meic et al., 2006). GBM belongs to the group of astrocytic tumors, a morphologically diverse set of malignancies graded by the World Health Organization (WHO) on the basis of their histology (Louis et al., 2007). Like lower grade astrocytic tumors, i.e., diffuse astrocytoma (grade II) and anaplastic astrocytoma (grade III), GBM (grade IV) shows cytological atypia, anaplasia and mitotic activity. In addition, GBM displays extensive microvascular proliferations and/or necrosis. The median survival of patients with GBM is low, between 12 and 15 months (Stupp et al., 2009). Standard treatment is surgical resection and radiotherapy combined with chemotherapy. The limited impact of these treatments on patient survival has revealed the need for additional treatment strategies. One of the most promising approaches is targeting the abnormal tumor vasculature seen in GBMs. Recently, bevacizumab (avastin), a humanized monoclonal antibody targeting vascular endothelial growth factor (VEGF), has been granted accelerated approval by the U.S. Food and Drug Administration as a single agent treatment for GBM patients with progressive disease following prior therapy (Cohen et al., 2009). Additional targets for anti-angiogenic treatment could be invaluable to further improve treatment. Here, we describe the data we and others have generated on a novel marker for tumor vasculature in GBM, endosialin.

Identification of Endosialin

The newly formed vasculature in malignant disease differs from normal stable blood vessels. Several studies have been conducted to identify genes differentially expressed in tumor endothelium as compared to their normal counterpart (Madden et al., 2004; Parker et al., 2004; St Croix et al., 2000). In these studies, endothelial cells were isolated from both normal and tumor tissues using antibody-coated beads in a series of negative and positive selection steps. The messenger RNA isolated from these cells was profiled using

I.J. Huijbers (✉)
The Netherlands Cancer Institute, Amsterdam, CX 1066
The Netherlands
e-mail: i.hujibers@nki.nl

M.A. Hayat (ed.), *Tumors of the Central Nervous System, Volume 1*,
DOI 10.1007/978-94-007-0344-5_3, © Springer Science+Business Media B.V. 2011

the Serial Analysis of Gene Expression (SAGE) technique, which provides a global unbiased, quantitative determination of the transcriptome (Velculescu et al., 1995). In a pioneering study by St. Croix et al. (2000), an expressed sequence tag (EST) with similarity to thrombomodulin was identified as the most highly upregulated gene transcript in endothelial cells isolated from colon carcinoma as compared to endothelial cells isolated from neighboring tissue and given the name Tumor Endothelial Marker 1 or TEM1. Subsequently, it was demonstrated that TEM1 was the transmembrane protein endosialin (Christian et al., 2001) recognized by the FB5 monoclonal antibody (mAb) (Rettig et al., 1992). In a similar SAGE screen on gliomas, endosialin ESTs were also highly represented in the transcriptome of endothelial cells derived from gliomas as compared to that of endothelial cells derived from non-neoplastic brain tissue (Madden et al., 2004). A possible explanation for the enhanced expression of endosialin in the vasculature in GBM might be related to the hypoxic conditions often observed in these tumors (Oliver et al., 2009). Indeed, cell lines cultured under low oxygen conditions showed an increase in endosialin expression. Subsequent promoter analysis revealed that the human endosialin promoter has several hypoxia-responsive elements that are directly and indirectly responsive to increased hypoxia-inducible transcription factors, HIF-1 and HIF-2 (Ohradanova et al., 2008). The preferential expression of endosialin in angiogenic vasculature in tumors raised interest in this molecule as a potential target for antibody-based immunotherapy and warranted a closer evaluation of the expression and function of the endosialin protein.

Endosialin Protein

Endosialin is a type I transmembrane glycoprotein. The extracellular proportion consists of a C-type lectin-like domain, a sushi/complement control protein (CCP) domain, three epidermal growth factor (EGF) repeats and a serine/threonine rich mucin-like stalk (Fig. 3.1). The later provides for multiple attachment points of O-linked oligosaccharides (Christian et al., 2001; MacFadyen et al., 2005; Rettig et al., 1992). The core protein of endosialin is 80 kDa, and the mature form of the protein after extensive glycosylation is 175 kDa. The cytoplasmic domain of

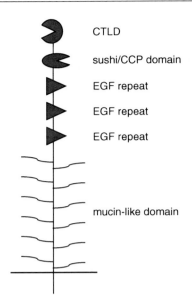

Fig. 3.1 Schematic representation of the endosialin protein. Endosialin is a single-pass transmembrane glycoprotein. The extracellular proportion of endosialin consists of a C-type lectin-like domain, a sushi/complement control protein (CCP) domain, three epidermal growth factor (EGF) repeats and a serine/threonine rich mucin-like stalk. This stalk provides for multiple attachment points of O-linked oligosaccharides

endosialin is only 51 amino acids and has no apparent signaling motifs. Sequence analysis and conservation of domain structure has placed endosialin in a family of proteins together with CD93 (the complement receptor C1qRp), CD141 (thrombomodulin) (Christian et al., 2001) and C-type lectin domain family 14, member A (CLec14A) (NCBI Reference Sequence: NM_175060).

Endosialin Expression in the Angiogenic Vasculature

Expression of endosialin in embryonic tissue is observed in two main compartments, stromal fibroblasts and the developing vasculature (MacFadyen et al., 2007; Rupp et al., 2006). The expression is dynamically regulated and is downregulated during development. For example, in the developing brain, endosialin is exclusively observed on the developing vessels but little or no endosialin is seen in the mature, normal brain vasculature. As initially revealed by SAGE analysis, during tumorigenesis endosialin is strongly upregulated in the angiogenic vasculature of a large number of different tumor types, such as those of the brain, colon, skin and breast (Brady et al., 2004; Carson-Walter et al., 2001; Huber et al., 2006; MacFadyen et al., 2005, 2007; Rettig et al., 1992). Controversy still exists as to whether in the tumor vasculature endosialin is expressed by endothelial cells or by the intimately associated perivascular cells, i.e., pericytes. To form a better picture of which cell type expresses endosialin a closer look at the literature is required.

P1h12 Antibody

In the initial SAGE screen undertaken by St. Croix et al. (2000), endothelial cells were isolated with beads coated with the anti-endothelial mAb, P1H12. Two reports contested the cell specificity of this antibody. By double immunofluorescent labeling on cryosections of colon and breast carcinoma with a CD31 antibody and the P1H12 antibody, MacFadyen et al. (2005) demonstrated that expression of CD146, the target of the P1H12 mAb, was not restricted to endothelial cells but could also be seen in cells closely associated with the endothelial cells. Later it was confirmed that perivascular cells expressed low levels of CD146, as pericytes isolated from human fetal brain showed weak, but appreciable, expression of CD146 as analyzed by flow cytometry using the P1H12 mAb (Bagley et al., 2008b). The lack of specificity of P1H12 needs to be taken into account when considering these SAGE results as the reported differential expression of endosialin in tumor versus normal vasculature could represent upregulated expression of endosialin on endothelial cells, pericytes or both.

Endosialin Expression in Mesenchymal Cells

Expression of endosialin has been observed by antibody detection and real-time PCR (RT-PCR) in a variety of cell lines such as pericytes, fibroblasts, smooth muscle cells and mesenchymal stem cells (Christian et al., 2008; MacFadyen et al., 2005; Rettig et al., 1992; Simonavicius et al., 2008). These cells all share a common mesenchymal origin. Cultured endothelial cells lacked expression of endosialin, even when stimulated by numerous activating growth factors (Carson-Walter et al., 2009; MacFadyen et al., 2005). Two

exceptions have been reported. First, human dermal microvascular endothelial cells (HMVEC) cultured on a collagen-rich substrate mimicking the basement membrane of blood vessels (Matrigel), showed a marked induction of endosialin expression as measured by RT-PCR (Carson-Walter et al., 2009). Second, VE-cadherin positive endothelial precursor cells isolated from bone marrow or stage III ovarian carcinomas showed increased expression of endosialin as compared to normal human umbilical vein endothelial cells (HUVEC) again measured by RT-PCR (Bagley et al., 2008b; Conejo-Garcia et al., 2005). Unfortunately, both these studies failed to relate this relative increase in expression to other endosialin-positive cell types, therefore it is difficult to appreciate their absolute levels of endosialin. In general, studies with cultured cells indicate that endosialin is predominantly expressed by cells from mesenchymal origin and can only be detected in endothelial cells under specific conditions using very sensitive detection methods.

Endosialin: A Marker for Pericytes

As a rule, the most informative way to determine the cell type distribution of a protein in vivo is by using specific antibodies to stain tissue sections. For endosialin numerous antibodies have been generated, either commercially or by individual research groups (Bagley et al., 2008a; Brady et al., 2004; MacFadyen et al., 2005; Marty et al., 2006; Rettig et al., 1992; Rupp et al., 2006). These antibodies have been used to address the issue as to whether endosialin is expressed by pericytes or endothelial cells. Several strategies have been employed each with their own limitations. Classical immunohistochemistry on formalin-fixed paraffin embedded (FFPE) specimens has been used in several studies. This technique typically depends on detection of the primary antibody by a biotinylated secondary antibody followed by an avidin-biotin-peroxidase complex and development with a soluble chromogenic substrate. The technique is very robust and reliable and can be scored easily. Its weakness is that it only stains one protein at a time and it has a limited resolution due to precipitation of the chromogenic substrate. Two studies used this approach on a panel of astrocytic tumors with their in-house generated rabbit polyclonal antibodies (Brady et al., 2004; Carson-Walter et al., 2009). In the largest study on 275 cases, endosialin expression was observed in 82% of grade II, 80% of grade III and 78% of GBM (grade IV). The expression level in GBM varied from weak in 46.7% of cases to moderate/strong in 31.8% of cases (Carson-Walter et al., 2009). Both studies reported expression of endosialin exclusively in the tumor vasculature, but both realized the limitations of the immunohistochemical approach that precluded the ability to distinguish between expression on endothelial cells and/or pericytes. To resolve the issue, immunofluorescence labeling was employed. This technique has the capability for labeling of multiple targets and is of higher resolution due to the fluorophores being directly conjugated to the antibody. The disadvantage is that frozen tissue sections are used which in general have poor tissue morphology. Using this approach, Brady et al. (2004) reported that in GBM endosialin expression co-localized with both the pericyte marker alpha-smooth muscle actin (αSMA) and the endothelial marker CD31. Unfortunately, the limited quality of the presented images makes this observation difficult to assess.

To obtain a definitive answer on the cell type distribution of endosialin our laboratory developed an optimized method for high resolution immunofluorescence labeling of FFPE tissues (Robertson et al., 2008). This technique overcomes the specific problems seen in the other two methods allowing for high-resolution confocal imaging of multiple targets on high quality tissue sections. For these studies, we employed our anti-endosialin mAb B1/35, which had been verified for its specificity towards endosialin in western blots, immunohistochemistry and immunofluorescence (MacFadyen et al., 2005; Simonavicius et al., 2008). A small panel of GBMs was double-labeled for endosialin and the endothelial marker CD34. In all of the samples examined, no overlap between these two markers was detected (Fig. 3.2a). In contrast, double-labeling for endosialin and pericyte marker αSMA resulted in a very clear colocalization of expression, showing that endosialin was exclusively and abundantly expressed by pericytes in GBM (Fig. 3.2b) (Simonavicius et al., 2008). These observations were consistent with data obtained by Virgintino et al. (2007) using the B1/35 antibody where they performed double immunofluorescent labeling on briefly fixed embryonic brain tissue cut into thick 20 μm slices. Clear co-localization of endosialin and pericyte marker NG2 was observed, whereas no overlap was

observed with endothelial markers, CD31 and GLUT1. Additional labeling showed that endosialin-positive pericytes were embedded in collagen IV containing basement membrane (Virgintino et al., 2007). Based on these observations, we conclude that endosialin expression in embryonic brain and in gliomas is restricted to pericytes and that extreme care needs to be taken when analyzing protein distribution in the vascular compartment due to the intimate association of endothelial cells and pericytes.

Endosialin Function on Pericytes

The function of endosialin in angiogenesis under normal and pathological circumstances remains elusive. Endosialin-null mice have been generated. These mice developed normally, were fertile and had physiological wound healing (Nanda et al., 2006). However, abdominal implantation of colorectal cancer cells led to reduced tumor growth, invasiveness and metastasis as compared to wild-type mice. The tumors in the endosialin-null mice displayed increased numbers of small vessels as compared to the controls and reduced numbers of medium and large vessels (Nanda et al., 2006). Endosialin-null mice were also subjected to GBM xenograft experiments by intracranial injection with U87MG glioma cells. In contrast to colorectal tumors, no difference in survival time or tumor volume was observed between endosialin knockout and wild type mice, however the same increase in microvessels was observed in the endosialin-null mice (Carson-Walter et al., 2009). This increase was not related to loss of pericytes as both groups reported similar pericyte coverage in both wild-type and knockout xenografts. Alternatively, the increase in microvessels might be related to an impaired functionality of pericytes. In vitro studies revealed that loss of endosialin leads to a reduced ability of pericytes to form tubes in an in vitro tube formation assay reflecting a defect in early angiogenesis (Bagley et al., 2008a). Pericytes are known to extend long cytoplasmic processes on the abluminal surface of the endothelial cells, making tight contacts that are important for blood vessel stabilization, remodeling, and function (Allt and Lawrenson, 2001; Armulik et al., 2005). Experimental data indicates that endosialin does not interact directly with endothelial cells, but that it acts as an adhesion molecule that binds to extracellular matrix components

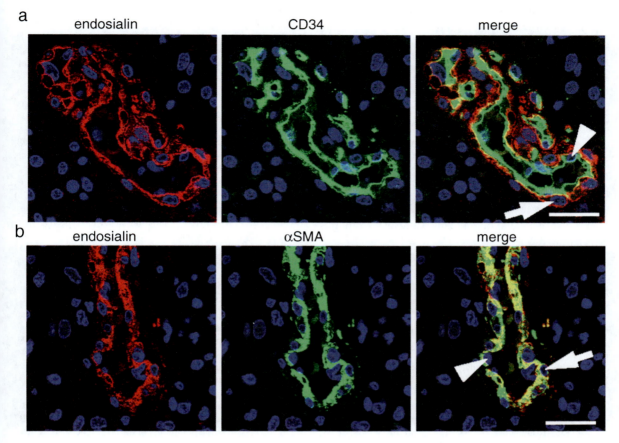

Fig. 3.2 Distribution of endosialin on tumor-associated vessels in GBM. Formalin-fixed paraffin-embedded sections of a GBM were costained with (**a**) anti-endosialin mAb B1/35 (*red*) and anti-CD34 (*green*) or (**b**) anti-endosialin mAb B1/35 (*red*) and anti-α-smooth muscle actin (αSMA, *green*). Nuclei were counterstained with DAPI (*blue*). *Arrowheads* indicate endothelial cells. *Arrows* indicate pericytes. Scale bar, 25 μm

deposited into the basement membrane of vessels, such as fibronectin I and collagen IV (Tomkowicz et al., 2007). The reduced adhesion of endosialin-null pericytes to these ligands might prevent optimal contact between pericyte and endothelial cells, which in turn could lead to a less tight control in the formation of new blood vessels.

Endosialin as a Target for Therapeutic Antibodies

Anti-angiogenic therapy targeting the vascular endothelial growth factor (VEGF)-mediated proangiogenic signaling pathways has resulted in demonstrable clinical benefit in various cancers, however after an initial response tumors often progress resulting in limited survival advantage (Ellis and

Hicklin, 2008). Several modes of resistance to antiangiogenic therapy have been described (Bergers and Hanahan, 2008). In one, it is postulated that tumor vessels are protected from VEGF-signaling inhibition by their tight coverage with pericytes. Therefore, targeting both endothelial cells and pericytes could provide additional therapeutic benefits. Indeed, mice suffering from pancreatic cancer responded beneficially to a combination treatment of VEGF inhibitor SU5416 and an inhibitor of the platelet-derived growth factor receptor (PDGFR) signaling in pericytes (Bergers et al., 2003). In this light, endosialin could be an additional promising target for pericyte-directed therapy as it is specifically upregulated in tumor vasculature (Teicher, 2007). Several biotechnology companies are currently pursuing this. Morphotek Inc. has started a phase I clinical trial with their MORAb-004 antibody targeting endosialin (Tomkowicz et al.,

2007). This study is however not aimed at targeting tumor vasculature, but solid tumors expressing endosialin, as it has been shown that various sarcomas and malignant fibrous histocytomas often express the endosialin protein (Dolznig et al., 2005; Rouleau et al., 2008). Genzyme Cooperation also proposes to target sarcomas with their anti-endosialin antibody bound to an immunotoxin (Rouleau et al., 2008). The use of an anti-endosialin antibody to target tumor vasculature is still in its early stages. In GBM an additional hurdle to overcome is that the antibody has to pass the blood brain barrier, however it is apparent that targeting the abnormal and extensive vasculature in GBM could be highly beneficial to patients suffering from this devastating disease.

References

Allt G, Lawrenson JG (2001) Pericytes: cell biology and pathology. Cells Tissues Organs 169:1–11

Armulik A, Abramsson A, Betsholtz C (2005) Endothelial/pericyte interactions. Circ Res 97:512–523

Bagley RG, Honma N, Weber W, Boutin P, Rouleau C, Shankara S, Kataoka S, Ishida I, Roberts BL, Teicher BA (2008a) Endosialin/TEM 1/CD248 is a pericyte marker of embryonic and tumor neovascularization. Microvasc Res 76:180–188

Bagley RG, Rouleau C, St Martin T, Boutin P, Weber W, Ruzek M, Honma N, Nacht M, Shankara S, Kataoka S, Ishida I, Roberts BL, Teicher BA (2008b) Human endothelial precursor cells express tumor endothelial marker 1/endosialin/CD248. Mol Cancer Ther 7:2536–2546

Bergers G, Hanahan D (2008) Modes of resistance to anti-angiogenic therapy. Nat Rev Cancer 8:592–603

Bergers G, Song S, Meyer-Morse N, Bergsland E, Hanahan D (2003) Benefits of targeting both pericytes and endothelial cells in the tumor vasculature with kinase inhibitors. J Clin Invest 111:1287–1295

Brady J, Neal J, Sadakar N, Gasque P (2004) Human endosialin (tumor endothelial marker 1) is abundantly expressed in highly malignant and invasive brain tumors. J Neuropathol Exp Neurol 63:1274–1283

Brown M, Schrot R, Bauer K, Letendre D (2009) Incidence of first primary central nervous system tumors in california, 2001–2005. J Neurooncol 94:249–261

Carson-Walter EB, Watkins DN, Nanda A, Vogelstein B, Kinzler KW, St Croix B (2001) Cell surface tumor endothelial markers are conserved in mice and humans. Cancer Res 61:6649–6655

Carson-Walter EB, Winans BN, Whiteman MC, Liu Y, Jarvela S, Haapasalo H, Tyler BM, Huso DL, Johnson MD, Walter KA (2009) Characterization of TEM1/endosialin in human and murine brain tumors. BMC Cancer 9:417

Christian S, Ahorn H, Koehler A, Eisenhaber F, Rodi HP, Garin-Chesa P, Park JE, Rettig WJ, Lenter MC (2001) Molecular cloning and characterization of endosialin, a C-type lectin-like cell surface receptor of tumor endothelium. J Biol Chem 276:7408–7414

Christian S, Winkler R, Helfrich I, Boos AM, Besemfelder E, Schadendorf D, Augustin HG (2008) Endosialin (tem1) is a marker of tumor-associated myofibroblasts and tumor vessel-associated mural cells. Am J Pathol 172:486–494

Cohen MH, Shen YL, Keegan P, Pazdur R (2009) FDA drug approval summary: bevacizumab (avastin) as treatment of recurrent glioblastoma multiforme. Oncologist 14:1131–1138

Conejo-Garcia JR, Buckanovich RJ, Benencia F, Courreges MC, Rubin SC, Carroll RG, Coukos G (2005) Vascular leukocytes contribute to tumor vascularization. Blood 105:679–681

Dobec-Meic B, Pikija S, Cvetko D, Trkulja V, Pazanin L, Kudelic N, Rotim K, Pavlicek I, Kostanjevec AR (2006) Intracranial tumors in adult population of the varazdin county (croatia) 1996–2004: a population-based retrospective incidence study. J Neurooncol 78:303–310

Dolznig H, Schweifer N, Puri C, Kraut N, Rettig WJ, Kerjaschki D, Garin-Chesa P (2005) Characterization of cancer stroma markers: in silico analysis of an mrna expression database for fibroblast activation protein and endosialin. Cancer Immun 5:10

Ellis LM, Hicklin DJ (2008) VEGF-targeted therapy: mechanisms of anti-tumour activity. Nat Rev Cancer 8:579–591

Huber MA, Kraut N, Schweifer N, Dolznig H, Peter RU, Schubert RD, Scharffetter-Kochanek K, Pehamberger H, Garin-Chesa P (2006) Expression of stromal cell markers in distinct compartments of human skin cancers. J Cutan Pathol 33:145–155

Louis DN, Ohgaki H, Wiestler OD, Cavenee WK, Burger PC, Jouvet A, Scheithauer BW, Kleihues P (2007) The 2007 WHO classification of tumours of the central nervous system. Acta Neuropathol 114:97–109

MacFadyen JR, Haworth O, Roberston D, Hardie D, Webster MT, Morris HR, Panico M, Sutton-Smith M, Dell A, van der Geer P, Wienke D, Buckley CD, Isacke CM (2005) Endosialin (TEM1, CD248) is a marker of stromal fibroblasts and is not selectively expressed on tumour endothelium. FEBS Lett 579:2569–2575

MacFadyen J, Savage K, Wienke D, Isacke CM (2007) Endosialin is expressed on stromal fibroblasts and CNS pericytes in mouse embryos and is downregulated during development. Gene Expr Patterns 7:363–369

Madden SL, Cook BP, Nacht M, Weber WD, Callahan MR, Jiang Y, Dufault MR, Zhang X, Zhang W, Walter-Yohrling J, Rouleau C, Akmaev VR, Wang CJ, Cao X, St Martin TB, Roberts BL, Teicher BA, Klinger KW, Stan RV, Lucey B, Carson-Walter EB, Laterra J, Walter KA (2004) Vascular gene expression in nonneoplastic and malignant brain. Am J Pathol 165:601–608

Marty C, Langer-Machova Z, Sigrist S, Schott H, Schwendener RA, Ballmer-Hofer K (2006) Isolation and characterization of a scfv antibody specific for tumor endothelial marker 1 (TEM1), a new reagent for targeted tumor therapy. Cancer Lett 235:298–308

Nanda A, Karim B, Peng Z, Liu G, Qiu W, Gan C, Vogelstein B, St Croix B, Kinzler KW, Huso DL (2006) Tumor endothelial marker 1 (tem1) functions in the growth and progression of abdominal tumors. Proc Natl Acad Sci USA 103: 3351–3356

Ohradanova A, Gradin K, Barathova M, Zatovicova M, Holotnakova T, Kopacek J, Parkkila S, Poellinger L, Pastorekova S, Pastorek J (2008) Hypoxia upregulates expression of human endosialin gene via hypoxia-inducible factor 2. Br J Cancer 99:1348–1356

Oliver L, Olivier C, Marhuenda FB, Campone M, Vallette FM (2009) Hypoxia and the malignant glioma microenvironment: regulation and implications for therapy. Curr Mol Pharmacol 2:263–284

Parker BS, Argani P, Cook BP, Liangfeng H, Chartrand SD, Zhang M, Saha S, Bardelli A, Jiang Y, St Martin TB, Nacht M, Teicher BA, Klinger KW, Sukumar S, Madden SL (2004) Alterations in vascular gene expression in invasive breast carcinoma. Cancer Res 64:7857–7866

Rettig WJ, Garin-Chesa P, Healey JH, Su SL, Jaffe EA, Old LJ (1992) Identification of endosialin, a cell surface glycoprotein of vascular endothelial cells in human cancer. Proc Natl Acad Sci USA 89:10832–10836

Robertson D, Savage K, Reis-Filho JS, Isacke CM (2008) Multiple immunofluorescence labelling of formalin-fixed paraffin-embedded (FFPE) tissue. BMC Cell Biol 9:13

Rouleau C, Curiel M, Weber W, Smale R, Kurtzberg L, Mascarello J, Berger C, Wallar G, Bagley R, Honma N, Hasegawa K, Ishida I, Kataoka S, Thurberg BL, Mehraein K, Horten B, Miller G, Teicher BA (2008) Endosialin protein expression and therapeutic target potential in human solid tumors: sarcoma versus carcinoma. Clin Cancer Res 14:7223–7236

Rupp C, Dolznig H, Puri C, Sommergruber W, Kerjaschki D, Rettig WJ, Garin-Chesa P (2006) Mouse endosialin, a C-type lectin-like cell surface receptor: expression during embryonic development and induction in experimental cancer neoangiogenesis. Cancer Immun 6:10

Simonavicius N, Robertson D, Bax DA, Jones C, Huijbers IJ, Isacke CM (2008) Endosialin (CD248) is a marker of tumor-associated pericytes in high-grade glioma. Mod Pathol 21:308–315

St Croix B, Rago C, Velculescu V, Traverso G, Romans KE, Montgomery E, Lal A, Riggins GJ, Lengauer C, Vogelstein B, Kinzler KW (2000) Genes expressed in human tumor endothelium. Science 289:1197–1202

Stupp R, Hegi ME, Mason WP, van den Bent MJ, Taphoorn MJ, Janzer RC, Ludwin SK, Allgeier A, Fisher B, Belanger K, Hau P, Brandes AA, Gijtenbeek J, Marosi C, Vecht CJ, Mokhtari K, Wesseling P, Villa S, Eisenhauer E, Gorlia T, Weller M, Lacombe D, Cairncross JG, Mirimanoff RO (2009) Effects of radiotherapy with concomitant and adjuvant temozolomide versus radiotherapy alone on survival in glioblastoma in a randomised phase III study: 5-year analysis of the EORTC-NCIC trial. Lancet Oncol 10:459–466

Teicher BA (2007) Newer vascular targets: endosialin (review). Int J Oncol 30:305–312

Tomkowicz B, Rybinski K, Foley B, Ebel W, Kline B, Routhier E, Sass P, Nicolaides NC, Grasso L, Zhou Y (2007) Interaction of endosialin/TEM1 with extracellular matrix proteins mediates cell adhesion and migration. Proc Natl Acad Sci USA 104:17965–17970

Velculescu VE, Zhang L, Vogelstein B, Kinzler KW (1995) Serial analysis of gene expression. Science 270:484–487

Virgintino D, Girolamo F, Errede M, Capobianco C, Robertson D, Stallcup WB, Perris R, Roncali L (2007) An intimate interplay between precocious, migrating pericytes and endothelial cells governs human fetal brain angiogenesis. Angiogenesis 10:35–45

Chapter 4

Glioma Grading Using Cerebral Blood Volume Heterogeneity

Kyrre E. Emblem and Atle Bjornerud

Keywords Glioma grading · MR imaging · Blood volume · Histogram · DSC (dynamic susceptibility contrast) imaging

Introduction

Treatment of tumors of the central nervous system (CNS) constitutes a considerable challenge in spite of important advances in surgery, radiotherapy and chemotherapy. The majority of malignant brain tumors make up a heterogeneous group of vascular neoplasms known as gliomas. According to the 2008 Central Brain Tumor Registry of the United States, gliomas account for 36% of all brain tumors and 81% of all malignant brain tumors. Using the World Health Organization (WHO) criteria, the conventional method for diagnosing glioma patients is based on histopathological evaluation of tissue samples from surgery. Here, gliomas are graded according to the degree of malignancy (I-IV) of which grades I-II represent *low-grade* gliomas, whereas grades III-IV represent *high-grade* gliomas. Although survival estimates show large variations, relative survival rates correlate well with glioma grade. Less than 4% of patients diagnosed with a grade IV glioblastoma survive 5 years after initial diagnosis whereas 50% of patients diagnosed with low-grade fibrillary astrocytomas and 70% diagnosed

with oligodendrogliomas survive 5 years. Given that long-term prognosis is highly correlated to glioma grade, correct tumor grading is critical in order to ensure optimal treatment planning. Furthermore, accurate non-invasive glioma characterization is important for the life-long follow-up of patients after partial or full tumor resection, and may also become increasingly important to evaluate response to new treatment regimes. Current invasive grading procedures are inherently limited by sampling errors associated with stereotactic biopsy techniques and suboptimal resection due to tumor inaccessibility. Compared to open tumor resection, a study by Woodworth et al. (2005) showed that biopsy accuracy of frameless and frame-based stereotaxis was 89 and 69%, respectively. The study also showed that the results of a biopsy sample from a large tumor volume (>50 cm^3) were 8-fold less likely to coincide with the results from open surgery compared to in a small tumor volume. Furthermore, repeated invasive procedures to follow tumor growth and treatment response is not a common approach. With this in mind, efforts have been made to develop non-invasive diagnostic methods for assessment of tumor malignancy. Of these, based on its high level of soft tissue contrast, magnetic resonance (MR) is the imaging modality of choice to characterize brain tumors prior to, during and after treatment. The conventional procedure for MR imaging in glioma patients is based on administration of a gadolinium-based, MR compatible contrast agent. High malignancy is commonly (but not always) associated with disruption or increased permeability of the blood brain barrier which is seen as regions of increased signal intensity in the MR images acquired after contrast administration. The degree of contrast enhancement is, however, a relatively poor indicator of tumor grade and an unreliable

K.E. Emblem (✉)
The Interventional Centre, Rikshospitalet, Oslo University Hospital, N-0027 Oslo, Norway
e-mail: kyrre.eeg.emblem@oslo-universitetssykehus.no

M.A. Hayat (ed.), *Tumors of the Central Nervous System, Volume 1*,
DOI 10.1007/978-94-007-0344-5_4, © Springer Science+Business Media B.V. 2011

marker for separating tumor recurrence from necrosis induced by radiation because the two conditions may show similar contrast agent uptake characteristics. For assessment of treatment response after surgery, radiation therapy or anti-angiogenic treatment, tumor size is currently regarded as the MR imaging criterion with the highest prognostic value. Accurate assessment of tumor size from structural MR images is challenging and associated with some inherent limitations. Also, correct tumor delineation on MR images may prove a formidable challenge for several reasons. It is well known that malignant tumor infiltration extends beyond the MR visible tumor margins. Moreover, MR visible components of both untreated and recurrent gliomas may convey complex, heterogeneous signal intensities, making exact definition of tumor volumes and assessment of longitudinal volume change, challenging. To address these limitations, rapid MR imaging sequences measuring such *functional* tumor characteristics as tissue blood flow, blood volume, and water diffusion have been introduced. Among these, perfusion MR imaging show promise through direct assessment of tumor angiogenesis, tissue viability and tumor malignancy. While contrast agent uptake is restricted to brain tumors with disrupted or absent blood-brain-barriers, MR perfusion imaging provides functional information in all vascular brain tissues. From this, parameters such as blood volume and blood flow can be derived, usually by injection of a MR contrast agent. During the last couple of decades, tremendous progress has been made with respect to MR perfusion imaging techniques and post-processing routines. As a result, several studies have shown a stronger correlation between MR perfusion metrics and glioma grade compared to conventional contrast enhanced MR imaging findings. Also, MR perfusion images have been shown to aid stereotactic biopsy by identifying the most malignant areas of the tumor. Current MR perfusion based glioma grading techniques do, however, suffer from significant user-dependence and inter-institutional variations which indicates that these techniques may not provide the required robustness for a non-invasive alternative to biopsy. To correct these variations, new MR-perfusion based methods assessing blood volume heterogeneity have recently been reported, and this chapter will address the utility of MR perfusion imaging in glioma grading with focus on state-of-the-art methods for addressing the shortcomings mentioned above.

Magnetic Resonance Perfusion Parameters in Glioma Imaging

MR perfusion imaging is a collective term describing methods for assessing tissue blood flow or perfusion related parameters from MR imaging. These methods are based on the basic concept that the temporal effect of a blood *tracer* (a contrast agent) on the MR image signal intensity in a given tissue type can be related to tissue perfusion, blood volume or both. Although completely non-invasive tracers exist as demonstrated by Williams et al. (1992) among others, this chapter will focus on MR perfusion imaging by intravenous administration of a MR imaging contrast agent. The contrast agent alters the biophysical properties of tissue, thereby, increasing the so-called proton relaxation rates which result in a local signal change in the tissues where the contrast agent is distributed. If the tracer is administered as a rapid, intravenous bolus injection and the effect in the brain is monitored with sufficient temporal resolution (typically 1-sec intervals), the resulting change in the MR image intensity as a function of time can be related to relevant functional information. In general, it is assumed that there is a well-defined relationship between the observed signal change in the MR images due to the presence of the contrast agent and the tissue concentration of the contrast agent. A central concept to all perfusion imaging is the so-called *central volume principle* stating that the blood volume of a given tissue is equal to the blood flow into the tissue multiplied by the mean transit time (MTT) of the blood tracer passing through the tissue. The theory of deriving functional information from the observed effect of this tracer is historically referred to as *tracer kinetic modeling* of which the theoretical foundations were developed already by Meier and Zierler (1954). The use of MR perfusion imaging in brain tumor patients, however, was first reported by Edelman et al. (1990). In their study, areas of strongly enhanced tumor regions during the bolus inflow and a rapid, but incomplete washout effect was observed in five of six patients suggesting a method that might provide useful information in assessing tumor vascularity.

Glioma grading from MR perfusion imaging is usually based on assessment of cerebral blood volume (CBV). The CBV parameter is defined as the total volume of blood per volume brain tissue (e.g., a volume element (voxel) in the MR image) and is measured in milliliters of blood per 100 g of brain tissue (ml/100 g). Quantitative assessment of CBV is difficult in MRI because it requires accurate knowledge of the arterial blood flow, dose-response of the contrast agent, tissue density, and large/small vessel hematocrit values. Relative CBV can, however, be measured directly as the area under the signal intensity curve (after conversion to relative contrast agent concentration) generated from the bolus passage. Measurement of (cerebral blood flow (CBF) (in units of ml/100 g/min) is more complex because it requires that the tissue response of the contrast agent injection must be corrected for variations in the shape of the bolus as it enters the tissue of interest. Several methods have been developed to address this problem which may at least enable estimation of a CBF index comparable between individuals and between scans acquired at different times in the same individual. Qualitative versus quantitative perfusion assessment will be addressed in more detail later in the chapter. The MTT parameter is a measure of the average transit time (in seconds) of the tracer through the capillary structure of the tissue. An elevated MTT is associated with a *mismatch* between CBF and CBV (typically reduced CBF without corresponding decrease in CBV). Although multiple approaches exist, MTT can be estimated according to the central volume principle, which states that MTT = CBV/CBF. Despite their widespread use in stroke imaging, there has been less focus on assessment of CBF and MTT as predictors for glioma grade. Hence, the focus of this review will be on measurement of cerebral blood volume. It should be noted, however, that reports by Shin et al. (2002) and Hakyemez et al. (2005) suggest that CBF correlates well with both CBV and glioma grade. For a number of pathophysiologic reasons, Law et al. (2006) showed that MTT does not appear to correlate with glioma grade. Finally, direct assessment of the capillary permeability of the contrast agent has also shown to be a promising method in glioma grading. In this type of permeability analysis, the rate of contrast agent leakage from the intravascular to the extracellular space of the tumor is measured from the dynamic MR signal response following a bolus contrast agent injection. Using a two-compartment tissue model, the rate of leakage between the two compartments can be assessed in addition to estimations of the relative volume of the extravascular-extracellular space as shown by Tofts

and Kermode (1991). The correlation between permeability and pathologic grade was first shown in patients by Roberts et al. (2000).

Magnetic Resonance Perfusion Techniques

There are two main techniques for contrast enhanced MR perfusion imaging; so-called T1- and T2- or T2*-weighted perfusion imaging. The notation T1- and T2-weighting refers to which proton relaxation effect the MR image is made sensitive to. T1-weighted imaging is most sensitive to variations in so-called *spin-lattice* (T1) relaxation, whereas T2/T2*-weighted imaging is most sensitive to variations in *spin-spin* (T2) relaxation and variations in magnetic *susceptibility* (T2*). The susceptibility effects induced by gadolinium based contrast agents are especially dominant in the brain due to the intravascular distribution of the agents, causing large local variations in the magnetic field in the vicinity of the capillaries and consequent signal loss in T2*-weighted images. All gadolinium-based MR contrast agents induce enhancements in both T1- and T2/T2* proton relaxation and the effect of the agent on the MR signal intensity depends on whether the acquisition is made T1- or T2/T2* sensitive. In a T1-weighted acquisition, the MR signal intensity increases dynamically as a function of local contrast agent concentration, whereas in a T2/T2*-weighted acquisition the signal intensity decreases as a function of contrast agent concentration. When applied to dynamic MR perfusion analysis, T1-weighted imaging is commonly referred to as dynamic contrast enhanced (DCE) imaging whereas T2/T2* weighted imaging is referred to as dynamic susceptibility contrast (DSC) imaging.

There are certain advantages and disadvantages of both T1-weighted and T2/T2*-weighted perfusion imaging. The main advantage of T1-weighted perfusion imaging is that T1-weighting can be obtained with sufficient temporal resolution using "conventional" MR imaging techniques that are inherently insensitive to unwanted susceptibility effects. Image distortion and artificial signal loss can therefore to a large extent be avoided. In T2/T2* weighted imaging so-called echo-planar imaging (EPI) techniques must be used in order to obtain good T2/T2* sensitivity with sufficient temporal resolution. The EPI technique is inherently sensitive to T2/T2* effects of the contrast agent, but is also very sensitive to unwanted susceptibility effects present in the brain (due to local variations in magnetic susceptibility), which cause signal loss and image distortion, especially in brain regions close to air-filled cavities. There are also major differences in the spatial extent of the respective relaxation effects. The T1-relaxation is primarily a local effect which requires the water protons to come in direct contact with the paramagnetic centre of the contrast agent in order to be affected (i.e., induce T1-relaxation). Because all MR contrast agents are confined to the intravascular space in the brain, T1-enhancement is restricted to the intravascular volume in the absence of contrast agent extravasation. The sensitivity of the method in terms of the achievable dynamic MR signal change is, therefore, limited by the low blood volume in normal brain tissue. T2* effects, on the other hand, are long reaching and as such also affect a large proportion of the extravascular water protons in the brain, resulting in a much larger dynamic MR signal change relative to T1-weighted imaging techniques. T1-effects do, however, become much larger in the event of extravascular leakage secondary to tumor pathology, and T1-weighted imaging is therefore the preferred technique for estimation of tumor induced changes in capillary permeability. Permeability estimation typically requires images to be acquired over a period of several minutes in order for appreciable leakage effects to be detected. In contrast, CBV from DSC imaging can be measured from just the first passage of the contrast agent through the tissue (of the order of 1 min acquisition time). A further issue with DSC imaging is that the kinetic models used to derive CBV values assume the tracer to be confined to the intravascular space. Hence, in areas of extravascular leakage this assumption is no longer valid resulting in errors in the CBV estimation. The situation is further complicated by the unpredictable relaxation effects which dominate once the contrast agent extravasates. Depending on exact sequence parameters and probably also local extravascular concentration, the resulting relaxation effect may be predominant T1- or T2/T2*- dependent. As shown in a review by Covarrubias et al. (2004), numerous methods exist for correction of contrast agent extravasation in DSC imaging. One approach is to administer a small contrast bolus prior to the standard bolus injection in order to "saturate" possible T1-induced relaxation effects caused by extravascular

leakage. Alternative methods exist which are based on pure post-processing, either by fitting the dynamic curve to a predefined function which is "forced" to return to its expected baseline level or to account for the leakage by using a kinetic model similar to the one used in DCE imaging.

As mentioned earlier, DSC imaging is based on the very rapid EPI acquisition. Two different types of EPI sequences have been applied in DSC imaging; either based on a spin echo (SE-EPI) readout or a gradient echo (GRE-EPI) readout. Here, SE and GRE refer to two different methods used for encoding the MR signal, and a SE based sequence is less sensitive to T2* effects compared to a GRE based sequence. A potential advantage of the SE-EPI sequence is a more selective sensitivity to relaxation effects occurring at a capillary level, with reduced sensitivity to large vessel relaxation effects compared to GRE-EPI sequences. The disadvantage of SE-GRE is, however, reduced overall sensitivity to the susceptibility induced T2*relaxation effect, thereby giving a smaller dynamic MR signal response to the contrast bolus compared to when a GRE-EPI sequence is used. One could, therefore, speculate that the SE-EPI approach better reflects *true* tumor pathophysiology compared to GRE-EPI due to increased sensitivity to capillary relaxation effects. However, it has been reported by Schmainda et al. (2004) and Sugahara et al. (2001) that GRE-EPI based DSC imaging provides a stronger correlation between glioma grade and tumor CBV compared to when SE-EPI sequences are used. Also, using GRE-EPI sequences may aid in the differentiation between infiltrating vessels and true tumor CBV elevation as shown by Aronen and Perkio (2002). In this chapter, focus will be on glioma grading using GRE-EPI acquisition.

Quantitative Versus Qualitative Magnetic Resonance Perfusion

Estimation of quantitative perfusion metrics from dynamic MRI is challenging because the exact relationship between contrast agent concentration and corresponding MR signal change is generally not known. It is, however, possible to estimate perfusion indices which can be compared on an inter-patient basis by assuming the dose-response to be the same in all individuals (and also for all MR scanners used). With this assumption, perfusion values can be estimated by comparing the dynamic signal MR response in the tissue of interest to the response in the artery feeding the tissue known as the arterial input function (AIF). The effect of the AIF on the tissue response can then be accounted for using a mathematical technique called *deconvolution*. When the tissue response is deconvolved with the AIF one can estimate what the response would be like for an "ideal" AIF in the form of a spike input with negligible duration (i.e., no contrast agent dispersion taking place between site of injection and tissue of interest). The corresponding tissue response to such a spike input is called the *residue function*, and it describes how much the bolus is dispersed as it passes through the capillary bed of the tissue. Both blood flow and MTT can be estimated quantitatively from the residue function. Although a detailed deduction of the mathematics behind the tracer kinetic fundamentals is beyond the scope of this review, the most common deconvolution routine of the tissue response curves (dynamic curves for all pixels) is based on the mathematical method known as singular value deconvolution (SVD). This approach was first proposed for this purpose by Ostergaard et al. (1996). It should be noted that the final output is semi-quantitative perfusion values only, as absolute quantification requires exact knowledge about tissue density and large/small vessel hematocrit values as well as the exact relaxation properties of the contrast agent used. Also, all contrast agent based MR perfusion imaging assumes a linear relationship between the measured MR signal change and the underlying contrast agent concentration, which is not entirely correct. Still, if properly defined, approximate quantitative perfusion values may be obtained allowing comparison of perfusion data obtained in different patients or at different time-points in the same patient.

Quantitative assessment of capillary permeability metrics in DCE imaging requires similar type of mathematical deconvolution and AIF definition and also requires the dose-response of the contrast agent to be known. Quantitative assessment of permeability parameters in glioma patients have been attempted in DCE imaging as shown by Roberts et al. (2000), but there has been little focus on similar quantitative perfusion assessments in DSC imaging for glioma characterization. This is probably because high diagnostic accuracy values are obtained even using qualitative methods, and also because qualitative analysis is much easier to implement in a clinical setting. However, as

reported by Law et al. (2006), quantitative values may also correspond to glioma grade.

The alternative to quantitative perfusion values are *relative* or *qualitative* measurements. In this approach, the analysis can be performed without definition of an AIF resulting in great simplification of the postprocessing routine. An example of such is relative CBV (rCBV) values, where the rCBV value in a given voxel is simply a measure of the area under the signal intensity curve. To provide meaningful values comparable between patients, the rCBV value in a given voxel must be related to reference rCBV values from other brain regions. Although numerous notations exist, the complete distribution of rCBV values in a particular image slice is often referred to as a *relative CBV map*. By normalizing the rCBV values in a given voxel to a reference rCBV value or area, normalized rCBV values between patients can be compared. The majority of literature on glioma grading from DSC imaging are related to rCBV measurements and will be the focus of this review.

Use of Cerebral Blood Volume in Current Glioma Grading Methods

MR perfusion sequences are now incorporated in the clinical MR protocols of several hospitals with a comprehensive MR imaging program. Although still relatively new, and the subject of much research and debate, the added value of glioma grading from MR perfusion to conventional MR imaging is promising. Especially the rCBV parameter has been shown to provide a much higher correlation to glioma malignancy than conventional MRI, and may also aid in the selection of the optimal biopsy site as suggested by Lev et al. (2004). In addition, as new anti-angiogenic cancer drugs are developed, this measure can potentially be used to assess treatment effects as suggested by Cha et al. (2000). Current DSC imaging methods for differentiating high-grade gliomas from low-grade are based on measuring the ratio ($rCBV_{max}$) between the most elevated rCBV area within the glioma and a rCBV value in unaffected, reference tissue. This method is often referred to as the *hot-spot method* and the $rCBV_{max}$ parameter shows a strong correlation to glioma grade, as high-grade gliomas tend to have higher $rCBV_{max}$ values than low-grade gliomas. Aronen et al. (1994), Knopp et al. (1999), and Hakyemez et al. (2005) reported 3–4 times higher mean $rCBV_{max}$ values in high-grade gliomas compared to low-grade. In a similar study, Law et al. (2003) obtained sensitivity and specificity values of 95.0 and 57.5%, respectively, when using the hot-spot method to differentiate between high- and low-grade gliomas in 160 patients. Recently, Law et al. (2008) also reported that the hot-spot method may predict median time to tumor progression in glioma patients independent of pathologic findings. In their study, tumor progression was defined as a decline in neurologic status or an increase in tumor size of more than 25% on MR images. The results showed that patients with a $rCBV_{max}$ value of <1.75 had a median time to tumor progression of 3585 days whereas patients with a $rCBV_{max}$ value of >1.75 had a median time to tumor progression of 265 days.

Although the hot-spot method shows promise, some challenges remain. Separating glioma regions with high rCBV values from similar rCBV values in vessels is difficult and reliable results may only be obtained by experienced operators with good anatomical knowledge. Thus, the hot-spot method is relatively user-dependent and regions-of-interests (ROIs) are typically identified by a neuroradiologist. Similarly, the few voxels that constitute the glioma ROI are inherently prone to image noise and other sources of spurious pixel values (e.g. spikes introduced by the algorithms used to generate the rCBV maps). Furthermore, the choice of unaffected reference tissue is somewhat challenging. Typically, a contra-lateral, white matter value in the same slice as the glioma ROI is selected. This is based on the assumption that most gliomas are located in white matter. It should be noted however, that slightly different approaches exist such as reported by Law et al. (2007b) in which a reference, contra-lateral white matter region was selected for lesions in the white matter, whereas a contra-lateral gray matter value was selected for lesions in the gray matter. Nevertheless, because the rCBV values in the gray matter of a healthy individual is approximately twice as high as rCBV values in white matter, correct selection of reference tissue may be critical. Incorrect selection of reference rCBV values might result in either under- or overestimation of $rCBV_{max}$ values, whereas a patients specific selection of gray- or white-matter reference tissue is highly subjective. This problem however, may be avoided by using quantitative MR perfusion values at the cost of

more complex post-processing routines as discussed above. Finally, as shown by Lev et al. (2004) and Cha et al. (2005), oligodendroglial tumors (oligodendrogliomas and oligoastrocytomas) tend to show high $rCBV_{max}$ values irrespective of glioma grade. A reason for this might be that most oligodendroglial tumors are located in cortical areas and have direct involvement with grey matter as shown by Cha et al. (2005). Also, as suggested by Jenkinson et al. (2006) and Law et al. (2007a), the higher oligodendroglial tumor vascularity may be associated with loss of heterozygosity (LOH) on the short arm of chromosome 1 (1p) and the long arm of chromosome 19 (19q), seen in 40–90% of oligodendroglial tumors. Cut-off $rCBV_{max}$ values between glioma grades may thus be harder to establish if oligodendroglial tumors are included. Because oligodendroglial tumors constitute ~10% of all gliomas, it would represent a major limitation to the hot-spot method if these tumors had to be characterized by other diagnostic means.

The Histogram Analysis Method

To address some of the shortcomings of the hot-spot method mentioned above, a different approach to glioma grading from DSC imaging has recently been proposed in studies by Law et al. (2007b) and Emblem et al. (2008a). Instead of measuring a single $rCBV_{max}$ value, it has been suggested that assessing the complete distribution of glioma rCBV values from either a single MR image slice or the complete glioma volume may provide a more robust estimate of tumor neovascularity. This is done under the hypothesis that the distribution of rCBV values is somehow related to tumor malignancy. In general, as described in reviews by Folkerth (2004) and Jain et al. (2007), histopathology has shown that low-grade gliomas tend to incorporate preexisting vessels, whereas high-grade gliomas no longer can rely on this vascular supply and consequently develop new vessels. Tumor angiogenesis with vessel tortuosity, apoptosis and necrotic tumor components will result in reduced tissue homogeneity. With this in mind, the rCBV distribution in a high-grade glioma should convey a more heterogeneous spectrum of rCBV values than a low-grade glioma, and that a measure of rCBV heterogeneity should correspond to glioma grade. To date, the quantity of this heterogeneity has been assessed through histogram analysis, and the method is thus referred to as the histogram method.

A number of approaches to glioma grading from histogram analysis have been proposed. For all methods, the resulting histogram is divided into a predefined number of histogram bins and normalized by dividing each histogram bin frequency value by the total number of pixels in the glioma ROI. The reason for this normalization is to account for inter-patient variations in tumor size, ensuring that the area under the normalized histogram is always equal to one. Another advantage of normalizing the rCBV histogram distribution is that the heterogeneity is then inversely proportional to the peak height of the normalized distribution. Examples of histogram "signatures" for glioma grades I-IV are shown in Fig. 4.1. Moreover, the shape of the normalized rCBV histogram distribution for a specific glioma is fixed even though the rCBV values are in arbitrary units. Thus, the histogram method can in theory be independent of reference tissue. The hot-spot method, however, is critically dependent on correct selection of reference tissue because the determination of $rCBV_{max}$ is based on this parameter alone.

In a study by Law et al. (2007b) in 92 patients (excluding juvenile pilocytic astrocytomas and oligodendroglial tumors), normalized rCBV values (related to a reference rCBV value from unaffected tissue) from a single glioma ROI was assessed. An ellipsoid ROI was drawn around the maximum tumor diameter on a single MR image regardless of glioma heterogeneity or radiological suggestions, and glioma margins were defined as, if present, the total contrast-enhancing lesion or hyperintense abnormality as seen on the T2 images. A similar study was performed by Young et al. (2007) in the same patient material. Here, both normalized rCBV values and quantitative CBV and CBF values were included. Also, two additional tumor regions were assessed; (1) a six-pixel wide peritumoral glioma region was selected around and not including the previously described glioma region, (2) every single pixel from every single slice of the MR perfusion acquisition was included. In both studies, the resulting histograms were divided into 40 equally-spaced histogram bins and a total of 14 different histogram parameters were compared; (1) mean histogram value, (2) median value, (3) standard deviation, (4) mean of the top 50% percentile of the histogram, (5) standard deviation of the top 50% percentile, (6) mean of the top 25% percentile of the histogram, (7) standard deviation

of the top 25% percentile, (8) mean of the top 10% percentile of the histogram, (9) standard deviation of the top 10% percentile, (10) histogram skewness, (11) histogram kurtosis, (12) histogram peak height, (13) peak position of the histogram and (14) area under the histogram curve within one standard deviation.

Using Spearman Rank correlation tests, the results in both studies showed that measures of histogram means and standard deviations from normalized rCBV values were similar to the hot-spot method (R = 0.680–0.740) using peritumoral glioma ROIs and glioma ROIs from a single slice. In addition, the same histogram metrics detected high-grade gliomas with significantly higher specificity (~96%) than the hot-spot method (~80%) at similar sensitivity (~95%). Although no direct assessment of inter- and intraobserver variability was performed, the authors suggested that the histogram method is more user-independent for grading gliomas compared to the hot-spot method due to simpler definition of glioma ROI. In turn, the histogram method may, therefore, provide a more robust method for life-long monitoring of treatment response from angiogenetic inhibitors which require low observer variability.

Emblem et al. (2008a) used a somewhat different approach for selecting the glioma rCBV values used in the histogram analysis. Based on 53 patients (glioma grades I-IV), four neuroradiologists independently defined glioma ROIs in every MR image slice with presence of tumor tissue. Here, as described by Schmainda et al. (2004), care was taken to avoid areas of necrosis, edema or non-tumor macrovessels evident on the post-contrast T1-weighted images. Signal hyper-intensities thought to represent tumor tissue, as seen on the T2-weighted images were used to define the outermost tumor margin, and areas of contrast enhancement seen on the post-contrast T1-weighted images were always included. From this, glioma grade and inter-observer reproducibility were assessed using the peak height of the normalized histogram distribution and the optimal number of histogram bins resulting in the highest diagnostic accuracy was iteratively derived. The results showed that using ~100 bins resulted in the highest diagnostic accuracy. Furthermore, at similar specificity (~83%), the sensitivity of the histogram method was higher for all observers (90%) compared to the reference hot-spot method (55–76%). The most important result from this study, however, was that the interobserver agreement

Fig. 4.1 (**a**) *Top* to *bottom*;
axial T2-weighted MR
images, axial post-contrast
T1-weighted MR images and
axial rCBV maps of patients
diagnosed with (*left* to *right*);
WHO grade I pilocytic
astrocytoma (female, 10
years), WHO grade II diffuse
astrocytoma (male, 54 years),
WHO grade III anaplastic
astrocytoma (male, 59 years)
and WHO grade IV
glioblastoma (female, 64
years). Contrast enhancement
and cystic components are
typically seen in patients with
grade I and IV gliomas and in
some patients with grades II
and III. Note the increased
rCBV values in the tumor area
with increasing glioma grade.
Also, compared to the
homogenous contrast
enhancement rim typically
seen in grade IV gliomas, MR
perfusion may aid in selecting
the most optimal target for a
biopsy (*yellow arrow*). (**b**)
Corresponding normalized
histogram signatures of the
complete distribution of
normalized CBV values from
the tumor area of all MR
images with visible tumor
tissue. Generally, a higher
histogram peak height and a
narrow histogram width are
observed in low-grade
gliomas (WHO grade I-II)
compared to high-grade
gliomas (WHO grades III-IV).
[Emblem et al., unpublished
data]

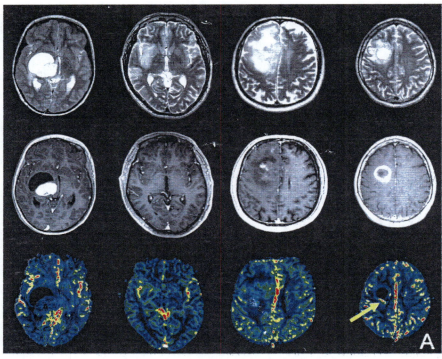

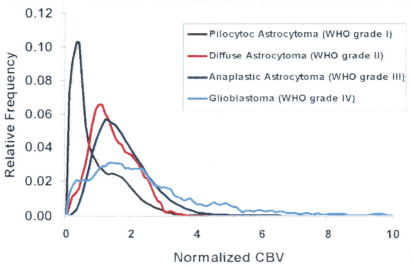

between the four observers for the histogram method
was almost perfect (Fleiss-kappa = 0.923). Even
though glioma ROI definitions between the four
observers showed large variations, this result suggested
that potential imperfect glioma delineation was relatively unimportant when using the histogram method.
This is an attractive feature, as optimal operational definition of tumor volume is considered difficult because

gliomas are infiltrating tumors with indistinct borders beyond the conventional radiographic margins as
shown by Price et al. (2006). Examples of variations
between manually defined tumor areas and corresponding histogram signatures are shown in Fig. 4.2.
Also, the large number of pixels included in the
glioma ROI may limit to the influence of rCBV values
from blood vessels erroneously included in the tumor

Fig. 4.2 (**a**) Axial T2-weighted MR images of a patient with a WHO grade III anaplastic astrocytoma (male, 59 years), also shown in Fig. 4.1. The histogram analysis is based on normalized CBV values from the complete tumor area which can be assessed using either a manual or automatic tumor identification approach. Even though the tumor area as defined by two experienced neuroradiologist (white and red ROIs) may vary, the resulting histogram signatures are almost identical as shown in (**b**). [Emblem et al., unpublished data]

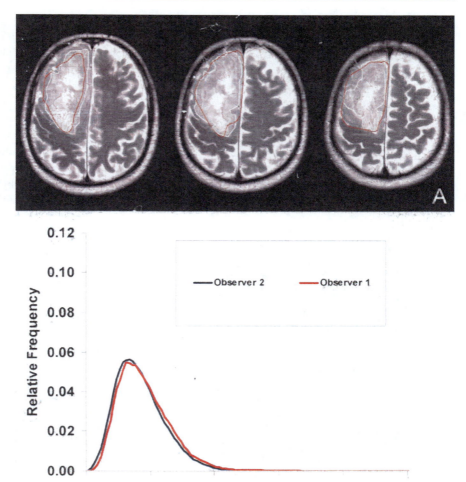

ROI. A challenge with the histogram method was that the observers reported using longer analysis time per patient for the histogram method compared to the hotspot method. The reason for this was that the tumor volume had to be identified in every slice. However, the methods were considered equally difficult to perform. With the continuous progress in advanced routines for post-processing segmentation of tumors from anatomical MR images, an automated method for total volume identification may further improve the utility of the histogram analysis method. An example of such was reported by Clark et al. (1998), showing that a tumor segmentation method based on multispectral analysis of multiple MR images conveyed good correspondence to radiologist-labeled "ground truth" tumor volumes.

The result of a similar multispectral MR image analysis of a glioma patient is shown in Fig. 4.3.

Histogram Analysis of Oligodendroglial Tumors

The histogram analysis method has also been used to differentiate between low-grade oligodendroglial tumors *with* or *without* loss of LOH on 1p/19q. In concordance with the higher $rCBV_{max}$ values observed in low-grade oligodendrogliomas with LOH on 1p/19q, a study by Emblem et al. (2008b) reported that low-grade oligodendrogliomas with LOH on 1p/19q conveyed a more heterogeneous distribution of rCBV

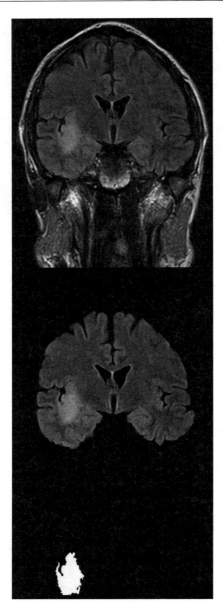

Fig. 4.3 *Top*; coronal MR image using the so-called FLAIR technique. An important feature of the FLAIR technique is that the glioma area is easily identified as high intensity areas compared to normal appearing brain tissue and fluids (*dark*). From this, automatic segmentation of multiple MR image classes (T2-weighted, T1-weighted, FLAIR, etc.) can be applied to remove non-brain pixels (*middle*) and to identify the tumor area (*Bottom*). As the histogram analysis method is relatively insensitive to variations in tumor area definitions, an automatic method for whole tumor area identification may readily be implemented in the post-processing routine thereby further improving the utility of a histogram based glioma grading method. [Emblem et al., unpublished data]

values compared to low-grade oligodendrogliomas without LOH on 1p/19q. However, in their study, no significant difference between low-grade oligodendroglial tumors and low-grade diffuse astrocytomas was observed. When grading a glioma as either high-grade or low-grade, this lack of difference between low-grade glioma subtypes can be attractive because a glioma grading method aiming at optimal differentiation between high- and low-grade gliomas should have minimal variations within each grade. Also, the histogram method was able to identify 6 low-grade oligodendroglial tumors *without* LOH on 1p/19q from 17 other low-grade glioma types and 29 high-grade glioma types with a sensitivity of 100% and a specificity of 91%. This result suggests that tumors which exhibit the most homogenous distributions of rCBV values in a population of patients with astrocytic and oligodendroglial tumors have a high probability of being low-grade oligodendroglial tumors without LOH on 1p/19q. As shown by Smith et al. (2000), patients diagnosed with low-grade oligodendroglial tumors *with* LOH on 1p/19q are expected to respond more favorably to radiation treatment and have prolonged survival rates compared to patients *without* LOH on 1p/19q. Consequently, a diagnostic method able to detect low-grade oligodendroglial tumors *without* LOH on 1p/19q is desirable as these patients may require more aggressive surgery.

Histogram Analysis of Dynamic Susceptibility Contrast Time Series

The spatial heterogeneity of perfusion values from DSC imaging has also been assessed by Slotboom et al. (2008). In their study, histogram signatures of gliomas and healthy tissue were assessed by deriving DSC *difference images* between the first baseline DSC image prior to the bolus passage and the remaining DSC images during the bolus passage. Here, the DSC difference images were divided into four time intervals; the baseline period, the bolus inflow period, outflow period and recirculation period. Using intensity values from manually selected or semi-automatically segmented ROIs in well-perfused tumor areas and healthy, contra-lateral tissue areas, a histogram analysis approach was applied to assess time-dependent histogram center-positions and histogram widths. This was done under the hypothesis that the change in perfusion heterogeneity as a function of time is related to glioma grade. The results suggested that the histogram width parameter, in particular, could discriminate between glioma tissue and healthy tissue and between glioma grades II, III, and IV. The most significant differences were observed when using DSC difference images from the outflow and recirculation period. This is in compliance with the results of Law et al. (2007b) and Emblem et al. (2008a) as the intensity difference between baseline values and the recirculation phase is correlated to the cerebral blood volume (in the absence of extravascular contrast agent leakage). An attractive feature of this method is that the histogram analysis approach is not dependent on the selection of a reference tissue. In general, although the method may be prone to suboptimal ROI selections and DSC imaging artifacts described in this review, the work by Slotboom et al. (2008) support the hypothesis that tumor heterogeneity as seen on MR perfusion images is related to tumor grade and viability.

Prospective Glioma Grading from Histogram Analysis

An attractive potential of any diagnostic method is the ability to use prior knowledge from previous patients to predict status or outcome of new patients or to compare MR images of a single patient from different examination dates. However, the use of predictive modeling in glioma grading from DSC imaging has not received much attention. A reason for this may be that current grading methods rely on threshold values between patient groups that are difficult to generalize into an accurate predictive model. As shown in numerous studies using the hot-spot method from DSC imaging, current threshold values show large variations. Even though all studies reported threshold values that significantly separated high-grade from low-grade gliomas, Hakyemez et al. (2005) reported an optimal threshold value of 1.98 for the $rCBV_{max}$ value. Shin et al. (2002) however, reported an optimal threshold value of 2.93, whereas Emblem et al. (2008a) reported optimal threshold values of 3.75–5.58. In the latter, it was also shown that the threshold value was dependent on the operator. From this, it can be concluded that the usefulness of a proposed threshold value in the literature also requires some prior knowledge about the specific

study. In addition to operator variations, the optimal threshold value may be dependent on several site-specific parameters including contrast agent properties and dose, imaging technique, and post-processing routines. Consequently, optimal threshold value may need to be determined specifically at each site, which complicates comparison of data between sites and also places restrictions on future modification of any model sensitive parameters.

As suggested by Emblem et al. (2008c), the histogram analysis method may provide a more attractive starting point for predictive modeling because each new case is described by the normalized histogram signature curve of the rCBV distribution within the glioma volume. By using this signature curve rather than a single threshold, a more robust base for prediction is created, which can readily be compared to a database of histologically confirmed gliomas with signatures representative for each glioma grade. In this study, a predicative model was created with the aid of a generalized linear classification algorithm known as *Support Vector Machines* (SVM). As described by Boser et al. (1992), the SVM model creates a separating *hyperplane*, a higher-dimensional generalization, so that it optimally discriminates between two or more classes such as glioma grade. During an iterative minimization procedure, the hyperplane is tuned so that the SVM model generalization error is minimized; thus, achieving an optimal separation between the glioma grades. In general, the SVM model as presented by Emblem et al. (2008c) is derived from existing histogram signatures in patients with known histology and applied on new signatures from new patients with unknown histology. After surgery, the histological result and corresponding histogram signature are added to the SVM model database and a new, updated SVM hyperplane is created. The result of this is a dynamic, continuously updated SVM model that improves with increasing data size. One potential feature of the SVM model is that multiple channels of information can be included in addition to the histogram signatures. In addition to MR perfusion parameters such as CBV, CBF and K^{trans}, a standard MR imaging protocol in patients suspected of a glioma may consist of conventional MR imaging, MR diffusion imaging and MR spectroscopy all with diagnostic parameters that can be included in the analysis. Finally, in addition to prediction of glioma grade, a predictive model can be used to establish a base for longitudinal monitoring of time to tumor progression in recurrent and untreated low-grade gliomas. With life-long assessment of tumor status from consequent MR examinations, a similar predictive model encompassing the whole battery of structural and functional MR image metrics may provide a powerful tool for individual patient care.

In conclusion, the infiltrative and aggressive nature of most intraaxial brain tumors make these neoplasms a formidable challenge to treatment. Both accurate preoperative assessment of tumor location and function as well as lifelong monitoring of postoperative tumor recurrence and growth are important. The added value of MR imaging in the diagnosis of glioma patients is unquestioned for providing excellent anatomical and functional tumor information. Since the early 1990's, considerable progress has been made within the field of MR perfusion imaging with respect to MR sequence development and post-processing routines. With focus on cost-benefit and cost-effectiveness in the medical workflow, fast user-friendly diagnostic methods are becoming increasingly accessible with potential for improved efficacy. One of these methods, analysis of cerebral blood volume heterogeneity, is the focus of this chapter. This method is based on the hypothesis that blood volume heterogeneity is related to vascular proliferation secondary to tumor malignancy. Although several approaches have been proposed, the general methodology is based on a quantitative histogram analysis of the distribution of cerebral blood volume values in the tumor area. While the selection of multiple, small region-of-interests in the tumor area is inherently prone to user-bias, the large number of pixels included in the whole-tumor histogram analysis results in a protocol relatively insensitive to suboptimal tumor area selection. The histogram approach may, therefore, be less dependent on expert users, and more amenable to automatic tumor segmentation approaches. A potential gain of this is that the histogram analysis methods described in this review can readily be implemented in clinical routine; thereby, providing fully automated methods for pre- and post-operative monitoring of glioma patients. This method may also have an important role in the evaluation of therapy response due to its user-independence and reproducibility. Also, the complete distribution of blood volume values in terms of a histogram signature provides a strong measure for comparing MR perfusion metrics from different patients and examination

dates. From this, large databases of histogram signatures can form the basis for predictive models. In conclusion, methods for glioma characterization from histogram analysis of blood volume heterogeneity have been proposed in several recent articles. Current experiences suggest that this approach provides objective measures for tumor vascularity and malignancy with minimal user-bias, providing an important step towards a fully automated MR-based glioma characterization regime.

Acknowledgments The authors thank John K Hald, Division for Diagnostics and Intervention, Rikshospitalet, Oslo University Hospital, N-0027 Oslo, Norway

References

Aronen HJ, Gazit IE, Louis DN, Buchbinder BR, Pardo FS, Weisskoff RM, Harsh GR, Cosgrove GR, Halpern EF, Hochberg FH, Rosen BR (1994) Cerebral blood volume maps of gliomas: comparison with tumor grade and histologic findings. Radiology 191:41–51

Aronen HJ, Perkio J (2002) Dynamic susceptibility contrast MRI of gliomas. Neuroimaging Clin N Am 12:501–523

Boser BE, Guyon IM, Vapnik VN 1992. A training algorithm for optimal margin classifiers. In: Proceedings of the 5th annual workshop on computational learning theory, Pittsburgh, USA, pp 144–152

Cha S, Knopp EA, Johnson G, Litt A, Glass J, Gruber ML, Lu S, Zagzag D (2000) Dynamic contrast-enhanced T2-weighted MR imaging of recurrent malignant gliomas treated with thalidomide and carboplatin. AJNR Am J Neuroradiol 21:881–890

Cha S, Tihan T, Crawford F, Fischbein NJ, Chang S, Bollen A, Nelson SJ, Prados M, Berger MS, Dillon WP (2005) Differentiation of low-grade oligodendrogliomas from low-grade astrocytomas by using quantitative blood-volume measurements derived from dynamic susceptibility contrast-enhanced MR imaging. AJNR Am J Neuroradiol 26:266–273

Clark MC, Hall LO, Goldgof DB, Velthuizen R, Murtagh FR, Silbiger MS (1998) Automatic tumor segmentation using knowledge-based techniques. IEEE Trans Med Imag 17:187–201

Covarrubias DJ, Rosen BR, Lev MH (2004) Dynamic magnetic resonance perfusion imaging of brain tumors. Oncologist 9:528–537

Edelman RR, Mattle HP, Atkinson DJ, Hill T, Finn JP, Mayman C, Ronthal M, Hoogewoud HM, Kleefield J (1990) Cerebral blood flow: assessment with dynamic contrast-enhanced T2*-weighted MR imaging At 1.5 T. Radiology 176: 211–220

Emblem KE, Nedregaard B, Nome T, Due-Tonnessen P, Hald JK, Scheie D, Borota OC, Cvancarova M, Bjornerud A (2008a) Glioma grading by using histogram analysis of blood volume heterogeneity from MR-derived cerebral blood volume maps. Radiology 247:808–817

Emblem KE, Scheie D, Due-Tonnessen P, Nedregaard B, Nome T, Hald JK, Beiske K, Meling TR, Bjornerud A (2008b) Histogram analysis of MR imaging-derived cerebral blood volume maps: combined glioma grading and identification of low-grade oligodendroglial subtypes. AJNR Am J Neuroradiol 29:1664–1670

Emblem KE, Zoellner FG, Tennoe B, Nedregaard B, Nome T, Due-Tonnessen P, Hald JK, Scheie D, Bjornerud A (2008c) Predictive modeling in glioma grading from MR perfusion images using support vector machines. Magn Reson Med 60:945–952

Folkerth RD (2004) Histologic measures of angiogenesis in human primary brain tumors. Cancer Treat Res 117:79–95

Hakyemez B, Erdogan C, Ercan I, Ergin N, Uysal S, Atahan S (2005) High-grade and low-grade gliomas: differentiation by using perfusion MR imaging. Clin Radiol 60:493–502

Jain RK, di Tomaso E, Duda DG, Loeffler JS, Sorensen AG, Batchelor TT (2007) Angiogenesis in brain tumours. Nat Rev Neurosci 8:610–622

Jenkinson MD, Smith TS, Joyce KA, Fildes D, Broome J, du Plessis DG, Haylock B, Husband DJ, Warnke PC, Walker C (2006) Cerebral blood volume, genotype and chemosensitivity in oligodendroglial tumours. Neuroradiology 48:703–713

Knopp EA, Cha S, Johnson G, Mazumdar A, Golfinos JG, Zagzag D, Miller DC, Kelly PJ, Kricheff II (1999) Glial neoplasms: dynamic contrast-enhanced T2*-weighted MR imaging. Radiology 211:791–798

Law M, Brodsky JE, Babb J, Rosenblum M, Miller DC, Zagzag D, Gruber ML, Johnson G (2007a) High cerebral blood volume in human gliomas predicts deletion of chromosome 1p: preliminary results of molecular studies in gliomas with elevated perfusion. J Magn Reson Imag 25:1113–1119

Law M, Yang S, Wang H, Babb JS, Johnson G, Cha S, Knopp EA, Zagzag D (2003) Glioma grading: sensitivity, specificity, and predictive values of perfusion MR imaging and proton MR spectroscopic imaging compared with conventional MR imaging. AJNR Am J Neuroradiol 24:1989–1998

Law M, Young RJ, Babb JS, Peccerelli N, Chheang S, Gruber ML, Miller DC, Golfinos JG, Zagzag D, Johnson G (2008) Gliomas: predicting time to progression or survival with cerebral blood volume measurements at dynamic susceptibility-weighted contrast-enhanced perfusion MR imaging. Radiology 247:490–498

Law M, Young R, Babb J, Pollack E, Johnson G (2007b) Histogram analysis versus region of interest analysis of dynamic susceptibility contrast perfusion MR imaging data in the grading of cerebral gliomas. AJNR Am J Neuroradiol 28:761–766

Law M, Young R, Babb J, Rad M, Sasaki T, Zagzag D, Johnson G (2006) Comparing perfusion metrics obtained from a single compartment versus pharmacokinetic modeling methods using dynamic susceptibility contrast-enhanced perfusion MR imaging with glioma grade. AJNR Am J Neuroradiol 27:1975–1982

Lev MH, Ozsunar Y, Henson JW, Rasheed AA, Barest GD, Harsh GR, Fitzek MM, Chiocca EA, Rabinov JD, Csavoy AN, Rosen BR, Hochberg FH, Schaefer PW, Gonzalez RG (2004) Glial tumor grading and outcome prediction using dynamic spin-echo MR susceptibility mapping

compared with conventional contrast-enhanced MR: confounding effect of elevated rCBV of oligodendrogliomas [corrected]. AJNR Am J Neuroradiol 25:214–221

Meier P, Zierler KL (1954) On the theory of the indicator-dilution method for measurement of blood flow and volume. J Appl Physiol 6:731–744

Ostergaard L, Weisskoff RM, Chesler DA, Gyldensted C, Rosen BR (1996) High resolution measurement of cerebral blood flow using intravascular tracer bolus passages. Part I: mathematical approach and statistical analysis. Magn Reson Med 36:715–725

Price SJ, Jena R, Burnet NG, Hutchinson PJ, Dean AF, Pena A, Pickard JD, Carpenter TA, Gillard JH (2006) Improved delineation of glioma margins and regions of infiltration with the use of diffusion tensor imaging: an image-guided biopsy study. AJNR Am J Neuroradiol 27:1969–1974

Roberts HC, Roberts TP, Brasch RC, Dillon WP (2000) Quantitative measurement of microvascular permeability in human brain tumors achieved using dynamic contrast-enhanced MR imaging: correlation with histologic grade. AJNR Am J Neuroradiol 21:891–899

Schmainda KM, Rand SD, Joseph AM, Lund R, Ward BD, Pathak AP, Ulmer JL, Badruddoja MA, Krouwer HG (2004) Characterization of a first-pass gradient-echo spin-echo method to predict brain tumor grade and angiogenesis. AJNR Am J Neuroradiol 25:1524–1532

Shin JH, Lee HK, Kwun BD, Kim JS, Kang W, Choi CG, Suh DC (2002) Using relative cerebral blood flow and volume to evaluate the histopathologic grade of cerebral gliomas: preliminary results. AJNR Am J Roentgenol 179:783–789

Slotboom J, Schaer R, Ozdoba C, Reinert M, Vajtai I, El-Koussy M, Kiefer C, Zbinden M, Schroth G, Wiest R (2008) A novel method for analyzing DSCE-images with an application to tumor grading. Invest Radiol 43:843–853

Smith JS, Perry A, Borell TJ, Lee HK, O'Fallon J, Hosek SM, Kimmel D, Yates A, Burger PC, Scheithauer BW, Jenkins RB (2000) Alterations of chromosome arms 1p and 19q as predictors of survival in oligodendrogliomas, astrocytomas, and mixed oligoastrocytomas. J Clin Oncol 18:636–645

Sugahara T, Korogi Y, Kochi M, Ushio Y, Takahashi M (2001) Perfusion-sensitive MR imaging of gliomas: comparison between gradient-echo and spin-echo echo-planar imaging techniques. AJNR Am J Neuroradiol 22:1306–1315

Tofts PS, Kermode AG (1991) Measurement of the blood-brain barrier permeability and leakage space using dynamic MR imaging. 1. Fundamental concepts. Magn Reson Med 17:357–367

Williams DS, Detre JA, Leigh JS, Koretsky AP (1992) Magnetic resonance imaging of perfusion using spin inversion of arterial water. Proc Natl Acad Sci USA 89:212–216

Woodworth G, McGirt MJ, Samdani A, Garonzik I, Olivi A, Weingart JD (2005) Accuracy of frameless and frame-based image-guided stereotactic brain biopsy in the diagnosis of glioma: comparison of biopsy and open resection specimen. Neurol Res 27:358–362

Young R, Babb J, Law M, Pollack E, Johnson G (2007) Comparison of region-of-interest analysis with three different histogram analysis methods in the determination of perfusion metrics in patients with brain gliomas. J Magn Reson Imag 26:1053–1063

Chapter 5

The Role of Ectonucleotidases in Glioma Cell Proliferation

Elizandra Braganhol, Andressa Bernardi, Angélica R. Cappellari, Márcia R. Wink, and Ana M.O. Battastini

Abstract Glioma invasion is a multifactorial process consisting of numerous genetic and physiological alterations, which affect glioma cell interactions with neurons, glia, and vascular cells. Purinergic signaling is emerging as an important component to give invasive potential to glioma cells. Specific purinergic receptor subtypes have been implicated in a variety of biological effects, including proliferation, differentiation, trophic actions and immune/inflammatory responses. Signaling events induced by extracellular nucleotides are controlled by the action of ectonucleotidases. These enzymes operate in concert for the complete nucleotide hydrolysis to nucleoside and represent a powerful manner to control the effects mediated by extracellular purines. It was demonstrated that glioma cell lines have altered extracellular ATP, ADP and AMP catabolism, presenting low rates of extracellular ATP hydrolysis and high rates of extracellular AMP hydrolysis when compared to astrocytes. Therefore, the ATP released by tumor adjacent cells, often damaged by growing tumors or due to ongoing inflammation together with the low glioma ability to hydrolyze extracellular ATP could result in powerful purinergic receptor activation, which in turn modulates glioma cell proliferation and neuronal toxicity. In addition, the high expression and activity of ecto-5′-NT/CD73 in glioma cells and the extracellular adenosine generation could also be involved in the immunosupression process, angiogenesis and glioma invasion. These alterations could have important consequences in the activation of purinergic receptors and modulate events related to glioma advance. Although more studies are necessary, the ectonucleotidases may be considered as new molecular markers of gliomas and future target for pharmacological or gene therapy.

Keywords Ectonucleotidases · Gliomas · Purinergic signaling

Introduction

Malignant gliomas are the most common primary brain tumors and have characteristics similar to those of glial cells. These tumors account for >70% of all neoplasms of the central nervous system (CNS) and vary considerably in morphology, location, genetic alterations, and response to therapy.

The brain tumor classification system organized by World Health Organization (WHO) divides the gliomas in four types based on their malignancy, invasive characteristics, and necrosis development: Pilocytic astrocytoma (grade I) present low malignance grade and occurs frequently in children and adults; low grade astrocytoma (grade II) present the capacity to infiltrate diffusely into cerebral parenchyma; anaplastic astrocytoma (grade III) is constituted by fibrilar astrocytes and could progress rapidly to glioblastoma and finally, glioblastoma multiforme (grade IV), the most common and malignant brain tumor (Kleihues et al., 2002).

Glioblastomas are relatively resistant to therapeutic strategies and patients have a median survival after first diagnosis of only ~12 months. Although systemic metastases of malignant gliomas are relatively rare, the highly infiltrative nature exhibited by these tumors is

A.M.O. Battastini (✉)
Departmento de Bioquimica, Universidade Federal do Rio Grande do Sul, Porto Alegre, RS, Brazil
e-mail: abattastini@gmail.com

M.A. Hayat (ed.), *Tumors of the Central Nervous System, Volume 1*,
DOI 10.1007/978-94-007-0344-5_5, © Springer Science+Business Media B.V. 2011

the main cause of treatment failure and high recurrence rates (Stupp et al., 2007).

Among the phenotypic characteristics associated with malignant gliomas are rapid growth, intratumoral necrosis and hypoxia, abundant microvascular proliferation, blood-brain barrier breakdown, edema, and perivascular infiltration of glioma cells. Proliferative changes in the blood vessels and in the vasculature associated with the altered expression of adhesion molecules also contribute to the invasive potential of glioma cells and have been target of intense investigation (Wong et al., 2009).

Investigations have been contributed for identifying the molecular origin of gliomas. Glioma cells present characteristics similar to stem cells, such as high motility, blood vase association, immature antigenic phenotype expression and activation of growth and proliferation signaling pathways (Sanai et al., 2005).

Recent studies suggest that increased on nestin and CD133 expression, markers for multipotential neuroephitelial stem cells, correlates with histological malignancy grade and clinical outcome (Maderna et al., 2007; Strojnik et al., 2007). In addition to neoplastic and cancer stem cells, immune cells comprise the glioma microenvironment and appear to be associated with tumor progression (Watters et al., 2005).

Glioma invasion is a multifactorial process consisting of numerous genetic and physiological alterations, which affect glioma cell interactions with neurons, glia, and vascular cells in the CNS. Among the cellular alterations that impart to glioma cells invasive potential, purinergic signaling is emerging as an important component. ATP is recognized as a mitogenic factor that could induce glioma cell proliferation. Hence, the substantial decrease in ATP/ADP hydrolysis and the high AMP hydrolysis observed in glioma cells lead us to suggest that alterations in the ectonucleotidases pathway may represent an important mechanism associated with malignant transformation of glioma cell lines.

Purinergic Signaling

Purines represent an important and ubiquitous class of extracellular molecules that have a key role in neurotransmission and neuromodulation by activating specific purinergic receptors. Purinergic mechanisms and specific receptor subtypes have been implicated in a variety of biological effects, including proliferation, differentiation, trophic actions, immune/inflammatory responses, and neuronal development (Burnstock, 2008). In addition, the involvement of purinergic signaling and a proposed role of ATP in different cancers have been revised (White and Burnstcok, 2006).

Presently, 15 subtypes of P2 receptors and 4 subtypes of P1 receptors have been cloned and classified (Burnstock, 2008). Purinoceptors are functionally classified as: 1) metabotropic: G-protein coupled receptors, that include the P1 (A_1, A_2A, A_2B, A_3) and P2Y ($P2Y_{1, 2, 4, 6, 11-14}$); 2) ionotropic: ionic channel couple receptors, which are included in the P2X ($P2X_{1-7}$) (Abbracchio et al., 2006).

The P2Y subtypes differ in their selectivity toward adenine (ATP, ADP) and uracil nucleotides (UTP, UDP), while all P2X receptors are activated by ATP. The P2Y receptor stimulation is usually associated with phospholipase C (PLC), leading to the formation of inositol phosphates (and/or modulation of adenylyl cyclase), resulting in increased of Ca^{2+} release from intracellular stores. P2Y receptors can be coupled to functionally distinct G proteins and, in addition, they can associate as homo- or hetero-oligomers; hence, providing the possibility of different functions and agonist-specific signaling (Abbracchio et al., 2006). P2X receptors are nonselective cation channels. Under physiological conditions, P2X receptor activation will result in Na+ and Ca^{2+} influx and K^+ efflux across the cell membrane, which leads to depolarization of the plasma membrane, causing firing of action potentials. The $P2X_7$ receptor differs in that, in addition to functioning like other P2X receptors, when exposed at high concentration or for a long period to ATP, its cation channel can be converted to a large nonselective transmembrane pore that allows the passage of not only cations but also small molecules up to 900 Da in size (Abbracchio et al., 2006).

The adenosine P1 purinoceptors (A_1, A_2A, A_2B, A_3) can be differentiated by distinct affinity to agonist/antagonist interaction and by distinct activation of G protein coupled signaling pathways (Abbracchio et al., 2006). A_1 receptors act by inhibiting adenylyl cyclase, phospholipase C (PLC), and phospholipase A_2 (PLA_2) pathways resulting in the inhibition of excitatory neurotransmission. A_2 receptors are stimulatory G-protein coupled, its activation result in cAMP intracellular increase and consequent excitatory neurotransmission stimulus. A_3 receptors stimulate ERK 1/2 phosphorilation in human astrocytes and in microglial cells. The P1 receptor stimulation is associated with a variety of responses, including cardioprotective and neuroprotective effects, inhibition of inflammatory reaction, modulation of platelet aggregation, and regulation of tumorigenesis (Fredholm et al., 2005). Additionally, adenosine could act as a proliferative factor for glioma cells (Morrone et al., 2003; Spychala, 2000). The nucleotide receptor-mediated cell communication is controlled by ectonucleotidases, which hydrolyze extracellular nucleotides to respective nucleosides, as described below.

Ectonucleotidases

Signalling events induced by extracellular nucleotides are controlled by the action of ectonucleotidases, which includes ectonucleoside pyrophosphatase/phosphodiesterases (E-NPPases), ectonucleoside triphosphate diphosphohydrolases (E-NTPDases) and ecto-5′-nucleotidase/CD73 (Robson et al., 2006; Zimmermann, 2001). These enzymes operate in concert with the complete nucleotide hydrolysis (e.g., ATP) to nucleoside (e.g., adenosine) and represent a powerful tool to control the effects mediated by extracellular purines.

The family of ectonucleotide pyrophosphatase/phosphodiesterases (ENPPs) consists of seven structurally-related ectoenzymes that are located at the cell surface, either expressed as transmembrane proteins or as secreted enzymes. They hydrolyze pyrophosphate or phosphodiester bonds in a variety of extracellular compounds, including nucleotides, lysophospholipids and choline phosphate esters. They have a broad substrate specificity that may reflect their roles in various physiological and biochemical processes, including modulation of purinergic receptor, regulation of extracellular pyrophosphate levels, nucleotide recycling and cell motility (Goding et al., 2003).

E-NTPDase family, previously classified as E-type ATPases, is a class of ectoenzymes characterized by their capacity to hydrolyze nucleoside tri- and diphosphates, strict dependence upon divalent cations and insensitivity to the classical inhibitors of the P-, F-, and V-type ATPases (Plesner, 1995). In mammals, at least eight related and homologous enzymes sharing five apyrase conserved regions (ACRs), named NTDPase1 to 8, have been cloned and characterized: NTPDase1 (CD39, ATPDase, ecto-apyrase or ecto-ATP diphosphohydrolase), NTPDase2 (CD39L1, ecto-ATPase),

NTPDase3 (CD39L3, HB6), NTPDase4 (UDPase, LALP70), NTPDase5 (CD39L4, ER-UDPAse, PCPH), NTPDase6 (CD39L2), NTPDase7 (LALP1), and NTPDase8 (Robson et al., 2006; Zimmermann, 2001). NTPDase1-3 and 8 share common membrane topography with two transmembrane domains at the N- and C terminus and a catalytic site facing the extracellular compartment. These NTPDase members differ regarding the preferences for nucleotides as substrates. While NTPDase1 hydrolyses nucleoside tri- and diphosphates almost equally well, NTPDase3 and 8 reveal a clear preference for ATP over ADP, and the NTPDase2 presents a high preference for nucleoside triphosphates, which justifies its identification as an ecto-ATPase. As a result, the action of NTPDase1 produces almost directly AMP with minor amounts of free ADP in the extracellular space. This functional property implicates the participation of this enzyme in the control of activation of specific P2Y-receptors for nucleoside triphosphates. Otherwise, ADP is transiently produced by the action of NTPDase2, which implicates the generation of agonist for nucleoside diphosphate-sensitive receptors such as platelet $P2Y_1$ and $P2Y_{12}$ receptors (Robson et al., 2006).

NTPDases4–7 have an intracellular localization such as the Golgi apparatus and endoplasmic reticulum. NTPDase5 and NTPDase6 lack the C terminal transmembrane domain and are also expressed in the plasma membrane or as secreted enzymes with specificity for the hydrolysis of nucleoside diphosphates (Robson et al., 2006).

The nucleotide hydrolysis is terminated by the action of ecto-5′-nucleotidase/CD73 (ecto-5′-NT/CD73; EC 3.1.3.5), which hydrolyzes extracellular nucleoside monophosphates to their respective nucleosides, with AMP being considered the major physiological substrate and also the best characterized extracellular source of adenosine. Ecto-5′-NT/CD73 is a homodimer linked to the plasma membrane through a glycosylphosphatidylinositol lipid anchor with its catalytic site exposed to the extracellular space. It contains zinc firmly bound to the protein structure, which is necessary for enzyme catalysis and ATP and ADP are known competitive inhibitors (Zimmermann, 1992). It colocalizes with the detergent-resistant and glycolipid-rich membrane subdomain, called the lipid raft, which are important for controlling signal transduction and membrane trafficking (Matsuoka and Ohkubo, 2004). Other non-enzymatic functions are assigned to this enzyme, for example, as inductor of intracellular signaling pathways and mediation of cell–cell or cell – extracellular matrix interactions. In addition, a role for the ecto-5′-NT/CD73 as a proliferative factor involves in the control of cell growth, maturation and differentiation processes (references in Bavaresco et al., 2008). The final product of AMP hydrolysis, adenosine, can be uptaken or converted to inosine by the action of ecto-adenosine deaminase (ADA; EC 3.5.4.4), which is another ectoenzyme, not included in the ectonucleotidase family but is also involved in purine salvage pathway (Robson et al., 2006).

Ectonucleotidases and Gliomas

As started earlier, gliomas are the most malignant of the primary brain tumors and are almost always fatal. The transformation of a normal cell to a malignant tumor is a multifactorial process. This process, in addition, modulates in gene expression that controls cell proliferation and differentiation; it requires specific conditions that provide a physiological support to tumor development. Accumulating evidence suggests that the purinergic signaling is involved in the growth and progression of glioma. First, it was demonstrated that glioma cell lines have altered extracellular ATP, ADP and AMP catabolism, presenting low rates of extracellular ATP hydrolysis and high rates of extracellular AMP hydrolysis when compared to astrocytes (Wink et al., 2003). Secondly, the influence of these adenine nucleotides on proliferation induction in human glioma cell lines was demonstrated (Morrone et al., 2003). Finally, glioma cells present a clear resistance to cell death induced by cytotoxic concentrations of ATP when compared with normal brain tissue (Morrone et al., 2005). Therefore, the ATP released by tumor adjacent cells, often damaged by growing tumors or due to ongoing inflammation together with the low glioma ability to hydrolyze extracellular ATP, could result in powerful purinergic receptor activation, which in turn modulates glioma cell proliferation and neuronal toxicity. In addition, the high expression and activity of ecto-5′-NT/CD73 in glioma cells and the extracellular adenosine, generation could also be involved in the process of immunosupression, angiogenesis and glioma invasion. Based on these results, our group hypothesizes that alterations in the extracellular ATP metabolism could be a malignant

characteristic of glioma cells and a line of investigation was developed in order to better understand the participation of ectonuleotidases on glioma invasion.

Studies from our laboratory showed that the coinjection of apyrase (NTDPase1; low ATPAse: ADPase ratio) to glioma cells resulted in a decrease in tumor size. Pathological analysis demonstrated lack of some important malignant characteristics, typical of the glioblastomas in the tumors coinjected with apyrase. Note among these is the reduction of the mitotic index and VEGF expression in the rats treated with apyrase, indicating that ATP has an important role in glioma proliferation and angiogenesis in vivo. Considering that the injection of apyrase was done only at the moment of implantation, the effect of ATP depletion is important probably at the implantation and initial growth of the glioma. This could be of therapeutic interest, because the application of apyrase in the surgical resection cavity could be helpful in reducing the initial growth of invaded tumor (Morrone et al., 2006).

In a further study, we have shown that the overexpression of NTPDase2, (high ATPase/ADPase ratio) in rat C6 glioma cells promoted a dramatic increase of tumor growth and malignant characteristics in vivo. Additionally, a sizable platelet sequestration in the tumor area and an increase in angiogenesis and inflammatory response were observed. The treatment with clopidogrel, a $P2Y_{12}$ antagonist that prevents the platelet activation by ADP, decreased these parameters to control levels. These data suggest that the ADP derived from NTPDase2 activity stimulates platelet migration to the tumor area and that NTPDase2, by regulating angiogenesis and inflammation, seems to play an important role in tumor progression (Braganhol et al., 2009). Interestingly, the contradictory results obtained by using NTPDase1 or NTPDase2 as ATP scavengers in an in vivo glioma model revealed additional complexities in the interactions between tumor, immune cells, and purines. These results also reinforce the importance of the overlapping of NTPDases expression commonly found in different cells, such as astrocytes (Wink et al., 2006), in the maintenance of extracellular nucleotide levels, and in the purinergic receptor activation control.

Other potential ectoenzymes that hydrolyzes ATP to AMP, the ENPPase family, were also considered as potential effectors involved in the molecular basis of gliomas. For example, NPP2 and NPP3 are related to increased tumor motility and invasion (Goding et al.,

2003). The presence of a nucleotide pyrophosphatase (E-NPPase) on the plasma membrane of rat C6 glioma has been demonstrated and further studied by Grobben et al. (1999) collaborators. Based on these studies, they proposed that E-NPPase has a modulatory effect on purinoceptor-mediated signalling in C6 glioma cell cultures.

The involvement of ecto-5′-NT/CD73 on glioma development has also been the object of interest. Early (Ludwig et al., 1999) as well recent studies describe this enzyme as a key protein for glioma growth. There is considerable evidence in support of a positive correlation between the expression of ecto-5′-NT/CD73 and nitric oxide synthase and epidermal growth factor receptor, and important prognostic factor for high rate tumor recurrence in glioblastomas, and still, the ecto-5′-NT/CD73 showed a role as adhesion molecule and has been proposed a function for it as tumor invasiveness promoter in human glioblastoma (Spychala, 2000). Studies from our laboratory showed that glioma cells have increased ecto-5′-NT/CD73 activity when

compared to normal astrocytes in culture (Wink et al., 2003), and that increasing confluence and culture times lead to increase in the expression and in the specific activity of ecto-5′-NT/CD73. In accordance with the importance of ecto-5′-NT/CD73 and adenosine in tumor promotion, the treatment with APCP (α,β-methilene ADP), a synthetic inhibitor of this enzyme, and AMP significantly reduced glioma cell proliferation. Although the exact mechanism of AMP cytotoxicity on glioma cells remains to be elucidated, these data support the notion that the increase of ecto-5′-NT/CD73 expression is important in the brain tumor development for different reasons: (1) as adhesion molecule per se; (2) as extracellular source of adenosine, a well known proliferative an angiogenesis inductor; and (3) as scavenger of extracellular AMP, a toxic molecule for glioma cells (Bavaresco et al., 2008).

Several factors have been described to regulate the expression of ecto-5′-NT/CD73 and for this reason may represent a potentially useful agent

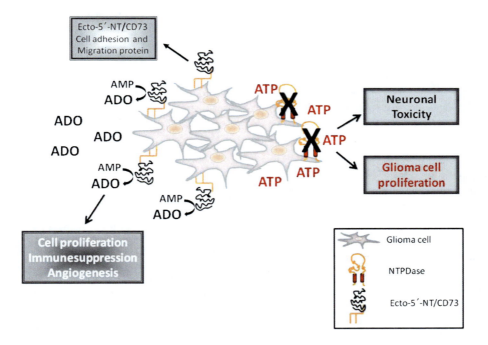

Fig. 5.1 Possible pathways connecting alterations in the ectonucleotidase expression and glioma advance. Gliomas exhibit an inversion in the extracellular nucleotide metabolism when compared to astrocytes in culture, hydrolyzing poorly the ATP and highly the AMP. This pattern of enzymatic activity may favor the accumulation of extracellular ATP and adenosine in the tumor milieu, inducing cell proliferation, angiogenesis and immunesuppression. Conversely, ATP could induce neuronal cell death, increasing the extracellular ATP pool and further facilitating the tumor invasion. Finally, the high expression of ecto-5′-NT/CD73, an adhesion and migration cell related protein, may mediate the interactions between tumor cells and tumor cell-ECM, essential for glioma progression

for glioma chemoprevention or adjuvant therapy. Quercetin has been reported to have an inhibitory effect on ecto-5′-NT/CD73 activity and mRNA expression in U138MG glioma cell line, which was correlated to inhibition of glioma cell proliferation (Braganhol et al., 2007). It has also been found that dexamethasone and indomethacin, two important anti-inflammatory drugs showed stimulatory effects on expression and activity of ecto-5′-NT/CD73 in C6 and U138MG glioma cell lines while they inhibit glioma cell proliferation (Bavaresco et al., 2007; Bernardi et al., 2007). We suggested that the increase in ecto-5′-NT/CD73 activity could result in a higher adenosine production, which could be involved in glioma cell death, probably via the adenosine A_3 receptor (Bernardi et al., 2007).

The inversion of extracellular nucleotide metabolism exhibited by gliomas, when compared to astrocytes in culture, may result in disruption of purinergic receptor activation. A variety of studies have proposed participation of P2 and P1 receptors in tumorigenesis. P2 receptors have been found in different kinds of human tumors and cell lineages, targeting cell proliferation, differentiation and apoptosis (White and Burnstcok, 2006). In addition, P1 receptors could modulate cell protection and proliferation pathways (A_1, A_2 and A_3), as well as apoptosis (A_3) (Spychala, 2000). More specifically in gliomas, the involvement of $P2X_7$ in the resistance to citotoxicity of ATP has been reported (Morrone et al., 2005), while the P1 receptors inhibit the paclitaxel-induced apoptosis and stimulate the VEGF expression in response to hypoxia (Merighi et al., 2006; 2007). Hence, alterations in the purinergic signaling, including purinergic receptors and enzymes, may be important participants in the pathology of gliomas.

In conclusion, the information presented here, supports the idea that alterations in the activity and expression of ectonucleotidases are involved in the glioma progression. The low expression of NTPDases together with the high expression of ecto-5′-NT/CD73 seem to favor the ATP and adenosine accumulation in the extracellular milieu. These alterations could have important consequences in the activation of purinergic receptors and modulate events related to tumor advance, as described here (Fig. 5.1). Although addition studies are needed to determine whether the altered nucleotide hydrolysis pattern is the cause or consequence of malignant transformation, the ectonucleotidases may be considered as new molecular markers of gliomas and future target for pharmacological or gene therapy.

Acknowledgements We thank Luci Bavaresco, MsC. Departamento de Bioquímica, ICBS; Dr. Guido Lenz, Departamento de Biofísica, I.B., UFRGS; Maria Isabel A. Edelweiss, Departamento de Patologia, HCPA, UFRGS; Fernanda B. Morrone, Faculdade de Farmácia, PUCRS, Porto Alegre, RS, Brasil and Dr. Simon C. Robson, Beth Israel Deaconess Medical Center, Harvard University, Boston, MA, USA for their collaboration and advice. We acknowledge the Brazilian Funding Agencies: CNPq, FIPE-HCPA and FAPERGS for the financial support.

References

Abbracchio MP, Burnstock G, Boeynaems JM, Barnard EA, Boyer JL, Kennedy C, Knight GE, Fumagalli M, Gachet C, Jacobson KA, Weisman GA (2006) International union of pharmacology LVIII: update on the P2Y g protein-coupled nucleotide receptors: from molecular mechanisms and pathophysiology to therapy. Pharmacol Rev 58:281–341

Bavaresco L, Bernardi A, Braganhol E, Cappellari AR, Rockenbach L, Farias PF, Wink MR, Cañedo AD, Battastini AMO (2008) The role of ecto-5′-nucleotidase in glioma cell line proliferation. Mol Cell Biochem 319(1–2):61–68

Bavaresco L, Bernardi A, Braganhol E, Wink MR, Battastini AMO (2007) Dexamethasone inhibits proliferation and stimulates ecto-5′-nucleotidase/CD73 activity in C6 rat glioma cell line. J Neurooncol 84:1–8

Bernardi A, Bavaresco L, Wink M, Silva MC, Delgado-Cañedo A, Lenz G, Battastini AMO (2007) Indomethacin stimulates activity and expression of ecto-5′-nucleotidase/CD73 in glioma cell lines. Eur J Pharmacol 569:8–15

Braganhol E, Morrone FB, Bernardi A, Huppes D, Meurer L, Edelweiss MIA, Lenz G, Wink MR, Robson SC, Battastini AMO (2009) Selective ntpdase2 expression modulates in vivo rat glioma growth. Cancer Sci 100:1434–1442

Braganhol E, Tamajusuku A, Bernardi A, Wink M, Battastini AMO (2007) Ecto-5′-nucleotidase/CD73 inhibition by quercetin in the human U138MG glioma cell line. Biochim Biophys Acta 1770:1352–1359

Burnstock G (2008) Purinergic signalling and disorders of the central nervous system. Nat Rev Drug Discov 7(7):575–590

Fredholm BB, Chen JF, Masino SA, Vaugeois JM (2005) Actions of adenosine at its receptors in the CNS: insights from knockouts and drugs. Annu Rev Pharmacol Toxicol 45:385–412

Goding JW, Grobben B, Slegers H (2003) Physiological and pathophysiological functions of the ectonucleotide pyrophosphatase/phosphodiesterase family. Biochim Biophys Acta 1638:1–19

Grobben B, Anciaux K, Roymans D, Stefan C, Bollen M, Esmans EL, Slegers H (1999) An ectonucleotide pyrophosphatase is one of the main enzymes involved in the extracellular metabolism of ATP in rat C6 glioma. J Neurochem 72:826–834

Kleihues P, Louis DN, Scheithauer BW, Rorke LB, Reifenberger G, Burger PC, Cavenee WK (2002) The WHO classification of tumors of the nervous system. J Neuropathol Exp Neurol 61:215–225

Ludwig HC, Rausch S, Schallock K, Markakis E (1999) Expression of CD73 (ecto-5′-nucleotidase) in 165 glioblastomas by immunohistochemestry and electronmicroscopic histochemistry. Anticancer Res 19:1747–1752

Maderna E, Salmaggi A, Calatozzolo C, Limido L, Pollo B (2007) Nestin, pdgfrbeta, CXCL12 and VEGF in glioma patients: different profiles of (pro-angiogenic) molecule expression are related with tumor grade and May provide prognostic information. Cancer Biol Ther 6(7):1018–1024

Matsuoka I, Ohkubo S (2004) ATP- and adenosine-mediated signaling in the central nervous system: adenosine receptor activation by ATP through rapid and localized generation of adenosine by ectonucleotidases. J Pharmacol Sci 94:95–99

Merighi S, Benini A, Mirandola P, Gessi S, Varani K, Leung E, Maclennan S, Baraldi PG, Borea PA (2007) Hypoxia inhibits paclitaxel-induced apoptosis through adenosine-mediated phosphorylation of bad in glioblastoma cells. Mol Pharmacol 72(1):162–172

Merighi S, Benini A, Mirandola P,, Gessi S, Varani K, Leung E, Maclennan S, Borea PA (2006) Adenosine modulates vascular endothelial growth factor expression via hypoxia-inducible factor-1 in human glioblastoma cells. Biochem Pharmacol 72(1):19–31

Morrone FB, Horn AP, Stella J, Spiller F, Srkis JJF, Salbego C, Lenz G, Battastini AMO (2005) Increased resistance of glioma cell lines to extracellular ATP cytotoxicity. J Neurooncol 71:135–140

Morrone FB, Jacques-Silva MC, Horn AP, Bernardi A, Schwartsmann G, Rodnight R, Lenz G (2003) Extracellular nucleotides and nucleosides induce proliferation and increase nucleoside transport in human glioma cell lines. J Neurooncol 64:211–218

Morrone FB, Oliveira DL, Gamermann PW, Stella J, Wofchuk S, Wink MR, Meurer L, Edelweiss MIA, Lenz G, Battastini AMO (2006) Involvement of extracellular ATP on the glioblastoma growth in a rat glioma model. BMC Cancer 6:226–236

Plesner L (1995) Ecto-atpases: identities and functions. Int Rev Cytol 158:141–214

Robson SC, Sévigny J, Zimmermann H (2006) The E-ntpdase family of ectonucleotidases: structure function relationships and phatophysiological significance. Purinergic Signal 2:409–430

Sanai N, Alvarez-Buylla A, Berger MS (2005) Neural stem cells and the origin of gliomas. N Engl J Med 353(8):811–822

Spychala J (2000) Tumor-promoting functions of adenosine. Pharmacol Ther 87:161–173

Strojnik T, Rosland GV, Sakariassen PO, Kavalar R, Lah T (2007) Neural stem cell markers, nestin and musashi proteins, in the progression of human glioma: correlation of nestin with prognosis of patient survival. Surg Neurol 68:133–143

Stupp R, Hegi ME, Gilbert M,R,, Chakravarti A (2007) Chemoradiotherapy in malignant glioma: standard of care and future directions. J Clin Oncol 25:4127–4136

Watters JJ, Schartner JM, Badie B (2005) Microglia function in brain tumors. J Neurosci Res 81(3):447–455

White N, Burnstcok G (2006) P2 receptors and cancer. Trends Pharmacol Sci 27(4):211–217

Wink MR, Braganhol E, Tamajusuku ASK, Lenz G, Zerbini LF, Libermann TA, Sèvigny J, Battastini AMO, Robson SC (2006) Nucleoside triphosphate diphosphohydrolase-(ntpdase2/CD39L1) is the dominant ectonucleotidase expressed by rat astrocytes. Neuroscience 138:421–432

Wink MR, Lenz G, Braganhol E, Tamajusuku ASK, Schwartsmann G, Sarkis JJF, Battastini AMO (2003) Altered extracellular ATP, ADP and AMP catabolism in glioma cell lines. Cancer Lett 198:211–218

Wong ML, Prawira A, Kaye AH, Hovens CM (2009) Tumour angiogenesis: its mechanism and therapeutic implications in malignant gliomas. J Clin Neurosci 16:1119–1130

Zimmermann H (1992) 5′-Nucleotidase: molecular structure and functional aspects. Biochem. J. 285:345–365

Zimmermann H (2001) Ectonucleotidases: some developments and a note on nomenclature. Drug Dev Res 52:44–56

Chapter 6

Gliomas: Role of Monoamine Oxidase B in Diagnosis

Luis F. Callado, Jesús M. Garibi, and J. Javier Meana

Abstract Glioma is the most common type of brain tumour in humans. These tumours account for high morbidity and mortality because therapies are largely ineffective. A higher histologic grade of the glioma corresponds to increasing malignancy and reduced survival of the patient. Therefore, tumour classification and grading represent key factors for patient management. However, current grading schemes are still limited by subjective histological criteria. In this context, the enhancement in the glial content of the brain that appears during gliosis has been linked to increases in monoamine oxidase B (MAO-B) activity. In consequence, we decided to assess the hypothesis that MAO-B activity may be also increased in human glial tumours. Thus, we quantified MAO-B activity in membranes of low-grade astrocytomas (WHO grade I-II; $n = 3$), anaplastic astrocytomas (WHO grade III; $n = 6$), glioblastoma multiformes (WHO grade IV; $n = 11$), meningiomas ($n = 12$) and non-pathological human brains ($n = 15$) by [^{14}C]PEA oxidation. MAO-B activity was significantly greater in glioblastoma multiformes than in postmortem control brains ($p < 0.01$) or meningiomas ($p < 0.001$). There were no significant differences in MAO-B activity between glioblastoma multiformes (WHO grade IV $n = 11$) and anaplastic astrocytomas (WHO grade III; $n = 6$) or low-grade astrocytomas (WHO grade I-II, $n = 3$). In conclusion, our results demonstrate a significant and selective increase in MAO-B activity in human gliomas when compared with meningiomas or non-tumoural tissue. These results suggest that the quantification of MAO-B activity may be a useful diagnostic tool for differentiating glial tumours from other types of brain tumours or surrounding normal brain tissue.

Keywords Glioma · Human brain · Monoamine oxidase B

Introduction

Gliomas constitute the most frequent group of malignant primary brain neoplasm in humans and one of the most aggressive forms of cancer. These brain tumours span a wide range of neoplasms with distinct clinical, histopathological, and genetic features. The World Health Organization classified gliomas into 4 distinct grades based on histological features of cellularity, nuclear morphology, mitotic activity and vascular proliferation. This system is based primarily on semisubjective observations by conventional light microscopy as well as immunohistochemical reactions. In this classification, a higher histologic grade corresponds to a less differentiated phenotype and to increasing malignancy. The median survival of patients with grade III gliomas is approximately 3 years, whereas it is only 9–12 months for grade IV glioblastoma multiformes. The mechanisms that underlie this correlation between higher histologic grade and poor prognosis are still unknown. Nevertheless, all grades of glial tumours are characterized by inappropriate proliferation, infiltration into surrounding normal brain tissue and disruption of normal brain functions.

Currently available therapies (surgery, radiotherapy, and chemotherapy), have failed to significantly improve the prognosis of patients with glial tumours.

L.F. Callado (✉)
Departments of Pharmacology, Centro de Investigación Biomédica en Red de Salud Mental, CIBERSAM, Spain
e-mail: lf.callado@ehu.es

M.A. Hayat (ed.), *Tumors of the Central Nervous System, Volume 1*,
DOI 10.1007/978-94-007-0344-5_6, © Springer Science+Business Media B.V. 2011

Surgery is in many cases only able to relieve symptoms by decompressing the brain. On the other hand, despite radiotherapy and chemotherapy increase survival of the patient, the recurrence of the tumour is virtually inevitable.

A key question in establishing individualized treatment protocols and predicting prognosis is the combination of histopathologic and imaging information (Burnet et al., 2007). Thus, accurate histopathological diagnosis is a first crucial prerequisite for patient treatment. However, the current morphological classification of glial brain tumours remains unsatisfactory, not only by the subjectivity of the histologic criteria but also by the diagnostic discrepancies among neuropathologists (Behin et al., 2003; Coons et al., 1997). In consequence, clinically relevant diagnostic mistakes take place in a substantial number of glial tumours biopsy cases, affecting immediate patient care decisions. An incorrect diagnosis may result in inadequate therapy for a high grade tumour or, worse, harmfully aggressive treatment for a low grade glioma (Coons et al., 1997). It is therefore essential to identify new molecular and biological markers for the diagnosis and grading of gliomas. Therefore, identifying biologically relevant markers that are associated with tumour but not normal tissue can not only improve diagnosis and prognosis of the patient, but can also guide individualized treatment and hopefully result in significant improvement in patient survival.

The enzyme Monoamine oxidase (MAO, EC 1.4.3.4) catalyses the oxidative deamination of monoamines as serotonin, histamine, dopamine or noradrenaline. The reaction produces hydrogen peroxide, a source of hydroxyl radicals. MAO exists in two forms: MAO-A and MAO-B that are encoded by different genes located on the X chromosome and share 70% amino acid identity. These isoenzymes differ in their sensitivities to the inhibitors clorgyline and deprenyl, and by their substrate specificities (Youdim et al., 2006). Both isoenzymes are mainly located in the inner side of the mitochondrial outer membrane, although a small proportion of each isoform is associated with the microsomal fraction. MAO is present in most mammalian tissues but the proportion of both isoenzymes is different in each specific tissue.

The MAO-B is the predominant subtype in the human brain (Stenström et al., 1987), where it is mainly localized in glial cells (Westlund et al., 1988). MAO-B appears later during brain development, but its density increases dramatically after birth. MAO-B activity in human brain has been described to increase with age both in postmortem tissue (Saura et al., 1997) as well as in living subjects (Fowler et al., 1997). This increase has been attributed to the compartmentalization of MAO-B within glial cells, and to the proliferation of these glial cells that appears during the normal ageing process. Similarly, increased MAO-B activity has also been reported in the brains of patients with neurodegenerative disorders such as Alzheimer's and Huntington's diseases (Mann et al., 1986; Oreland and Gottfries, 1986; Saura et al., 1994; Sherif et al., 1992). These data suggest a parallel relationship between elevation of brain MAO-B activity, and increased vulnerability to age-related neurological degenerative diseases. Furthermore, this increase in MAO-B activity has been also linked to gliosis involving reactive astrocytes (Nakamura et al., 1990; Oreland and Gottfries, 1986).

The aim of our study was to evaluate the activity of the MAO-B in human glial tumours (Gabilondo et al., 2008). Our hypothesis was that as MAO-B is mainly located in glial cells its activity must be increased in glial tumours when compared with non-tumoral brain. This increase in MAO-B activity may be used as a diagnostic tool for differentiating glial tumours from surrounding normal brain tissue or even from other types of non-glial brain tumours.

Mao-B Assays (Methodology)

Brain Samples

We collected small pieces of brain tissue containing tumour at the time of craniotomy for tumour resection at the Neurosurgery Service of Cruces Hospital (Bizkaia, Spain). These samples were immediately stored at −70°C until binding assays were performed. A second sample from each patient was also taken for diagnosis performed by neuropathologists and in accordance with the International Classification of CNS tumours drafted under the auspices of the World Health Organization (WHO). The tumours were diagnosed as low-grade astrocytoma (WHO grade I-II; $n = 3$), anaplastic astrocytoma (WHO grade III; $n = 6$), glioblastoma multiforme (WHO grade IV; $n = 11$) or meningioma ($n = 12$).

Human brain samples used as controls were obtained at autopsy in the Instituto Vasco de Medicina Legal (Bilbao, Spain) from 15 subjects without a history of neurophatological or psychiatric disorders and who had died suddenly, mainly in car accidents. Toxicological screening was negative for all these subjects and brain samples were histologically determined as normal. The frontal cortex of each subject was dissected at the time of necropsy, stored at −70°C until assay and encoded in order to protect the identity of the subject. The time interval between death and autopsy (post-mortem delay at 4°C) was 35.6 ± 4.8 h. Sample collection was performed in accordance with approved protocols of the Instituto Vasco de Medicina Legal (Bilbao, Spain) for post-mortem human studies.

All tissue samples were collected following protocols approved by the Human Studies Committee of each of the institutions involved. Informed consent was obtained from each surgical subject.

There were no significant differences in either male/female ratio or in age between the different experimental groups. The age mean for the different groups was as follows: 54 ± 3 years for control brains, 54 ± 3 years for glioblastomas, 55 ± 3 years for meningiomas, 39 ± 8 years for low-grade astrocytomas and 49 ± 7 years for anaplastic astrocytomas.

Membrane Preparation and MAO-B Assays

Tumour containing samples were carefully dissected in order to isolate the abnormal tissue. Tissue samples of each subject (~ 200 mg) were thawed and homogenized in 5 ml of ice-cold Tris-sucrose buffer (5 mM Tris-HCl, 250 mM sucrose, EDTA 5 mM, pH 7.4). The crude homogenate was centrifuged at $1,100 \times g$ (4°C) for 10 min and the supernatant was recentrifuged at $40,000 \times g$ (4°C) for 10 min. The resultant pellet was washed twice in 2 ml of incubation buffer (50 mM Tris-HCl, pH 7.5) and recentrifuged in similar conditions. The final pellet was resuspended in an appropriate volume of incubation buffer for MAO-B assays. Final protein content was 1.42 ± 0.11 mg/ml for control brain ($n = 15$), 0.84 ± 0.15 mg/ml for glioblastomas ($n = 11$), 0.76 ± 0.12 mg/ml for meningiomas ($n = 12$), 1.18 ± 0.39 mg/ml for low-grade astrocytomas ($n = 3$) and 1.26 ± 0.20 mg/ml for anaplastic astrocytomas ($n = 6$). Protein content was determined with the Bio-Rad Protein Assay Kit (Bio-Rad, Munich, Germany) using bovine albumin as standard.

MAO-B activity was assessed by a radioenzymatic method (Fowler and Tipton, 1981) in which radiolabelled β-[ethyl-1-^{14}C]phenylethylamine HCl ([^{14}C]PEA) was used as the substrate (specific activity 41.8 mCi/mmol). Briefly, 50 μl of the membrane suspension were preincubated with 150 μl potassium phosphate buffer (50 mM; pH 7.2) at 37°C for 5 min. Then the enzymatic reaction was started by adding 25 μl of the substrate solution (180 μM). Following a 4 min incubation period at 37°C, the reaction was stopped with 100 μl citric acid (2 M) and the oxidation products were extracted into 2 ml ethyl acetate at −20°C. Finally, 1 ml from the ethyl acetate phase from each tissue sample was transferred on to a vial containing 10 ml of Optiphase Hisafe II cocktail (Packard) and its radioactivity level was quantified by liquid scintillation spectrometry (Packard model 2200CA). Non-specific activity of MAO-B was considered as that obtained in the presence of deprenyl (3 μM). The non-specific activity was determined in every sample and consequently subtracted from the total activity in order to obtain the specific MAO-B activity. The results are expressed as pmol PEA min^{-1} mg^{-1} protein.

Statistical Analyses

Values are expressed as means ± standard error of the mean (S.E.M.). One-way analysis of variance (ANOVA) with post hoc application of the Tukeys' multiple comparison test as well as t-test were used for statistical evaluation. Level of significance was established at $p < 0.05$.

Mao-B Activity in Human Gliomas

Typically, MAO-A is inhibited by low concentrations of clorgiline and catalyses mainly the oxidation of serotonin. Conversely, MAO-B is inhibited by low concentrations of deprenyl and is active towards benzylamine and 2-phenylethylamine (Youdim et al., 2006). In order to determine the degree of selectivity of the radioenzymatic assay with [^{14}C]PEA for the A and B isoforms of MAO, inhibition experiments were performed in control ($n = 3$) and glioblastoma samples ($n = 3$) with the MAO selective irreversible inhibitors clorgyline and deprenyl ($10^{-12} – 10^{-3}$ M). MAO activity, defined as [^{14}C]PEA oxidation, was sensitive to inhibition by nanomolar concentrations of the MAO-B selective inhibitor deprenyl. This effect was similar in control brain membranes (IC$_{50}$= 5.56 ± 1.14 nM, n = 3) and glioblastomas (IC$_{50}$= 5.20 ± 1.21 nM, n = 3). Conversely, the MAO-A selective inhibitor clorgyline only inhibited MAO activity at high micromolar concentrations (IC$_{50}$= 10.72 ± 1.19 μM, n = 3; and 9.88 ± 1.20 μM, n = 3, for control brain and glioblastoma membranes, respectively). These results confirmed the selectivity of the assay for determining MAO-B activity in our brain samples (Gabilondo et al., 2008).

The next step was to evaluate the activity of the MAO-B in membranes of human glial and non-glial tumours as well as in non-tumoral control brain. The activity of MAO-B was significantly greater in membranes of glioblastoma multiformes (2834 ± 930 pmol min^{-1} mg^{-1} protein; n = 11) than in postmortem control brains (692 ± 93 pmol min^{-1} mg^{-1} protein; n =15; p < 0.01) or meningiomas (205 ± 72 pmol min^{-1} mg^{-1} protein; n = 12; p < 0.001) (Fig 6.1). This significance did not change when an ANCOVA with age as the controlled variable was performed (F[2,31] = 7.53; p < 0.001). Conversely, MAO-B activity in membranes of meningiomas was significantly lower than in control brains (p < 0.01, t-test,).

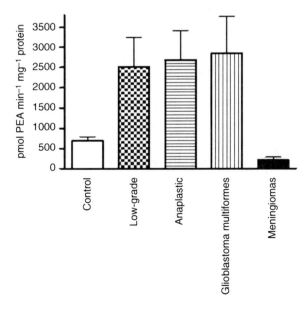

Fig. 6.1 Specific MAO-B activity in membranes of low-grade astrocytomas (n = 3), anaplastic astrocytomas (n = 6), glioblastoma multiformes (n = 11), meningiomas (n = 12) or postmortem non-tumoural control brain tissue (n = 15). Each bar represents the mean ± SEM

There were no significant differences in MAO-B activity between glioblastoma multiformes (2834 ± 930 pmol min^{-1} mg^{-1} protein; n = 11) and low-grade astrocytomas (2506 ± 739 pmol min^{-1} mg^{-1} protein; n = 3) or anaplastic astrocytomas (2676 ± 744 pmol min^{-1} mg^{-1} g protein; n = 6) (Fig 6.1). These results confirmed that the increase in MAO-B activity was selective for all types of glial-tumours (Gabilondo et al., 2008).

There are numerous evidences about increases in MAO-B activity with age. As expected, in our samples there was a significant correlation between MAO-B activity and age in membranes from non-tumoral control brains (r = 0.59, p = 0.02, n = 15). However, this correlation disappeared in glioblastoma multiformes (r = 0.34, p = 0.29, n = 11) and meningiomas (r = 0.095, p = 0.76, n = 12). On the other hand, there was not a significant correlation between MAO-B activity and post-mortem delay in membranes from non-tumoral control brains (r = 0.284, p = 0.31, n = 15).

Discussion

Several authors support the need for biologically relevant markers associated with tumour but not non-tumoral tissue that could improve the actual diagnosis of brain glial tumours. The results of our study demonstrate a significant increase in MAO-B activity in human glial tumours when compared with non-pathological brain tissue or with other non-glial intracranial tumours such as meningiomas. Additionally, our data show a statistical non-significant trend to the existence of a correlation between increase in MAO-B activity and the grade of malignancy of the different types of glial tumours (Fig. 6.1).

Similar increases in MAO-B activity have been described during normal ageing process (Saura et al., 1997) and in the brain of patients suffering neurodegenerative diseases (Mann et al., 1986; Oreland and Gottfries, 1986; Saura et al., 1994; Sherif et al., 1992). The increase in MAO-B activity during the ageing process or in neurodegenerative diseases has been usually regarded as a result of a proliferative reaction of glial cells, rich in MAO-B, secondary to neuronal loss. This would be consistent with the results of our study because gliomas originate from the neoplastic transformation and proliferation of different types of neuroglial cells. Furthermore, it has been described that reactive astrocytes linked to gliosis process are richer in MAO-B than "normal" glial cells (Ekblom et al., 1994). Thus, increased MAO-B activity in gliomas may be due to an increased number of astrocytes as well as an increased content of MAO-B in reactive astrocytes.

Conversely, a decrease in MAO activity in other non-glial tumours has been reported (Odegaard et al., 1986). Moreover, Lizcano et al. (1991) observed that in induced rat breast cancer an increasing degree of malignancy was associated with an increase in MAO-A activity but a decrease in MAO-B activity. This data could explain the decrease in MAO-B activity observed in meningiomas when compared to glioblastoma multiformes in the present study. In addition, the decrease in MAO-B activity in meningiomas when compared with non-tumoral control brain could be explained by the fact that the control brain samples contain a mixture of cell types, some of them very rich in MAO-B (e.g. astrocytes), whereas the meningioma samples consist mainly of one cell type present which seems to have a low MAO-B content.

Some amine oxidases have been involved in cancer growth inhibition because of the higher content in tumour cells of biogenic amines compared to non-tumoral cells. However, the oxidation products of biogenic amines could be also carcinogenic. A putative patophysiological role of MAO-B activity in human gliomas is yet to be determined. MAO-B activity appears to be the most significant contributor to hydrogen peroxide production in glioma cells (Mazzio and Soliman, 2005). It has been suggested that an increased MAO-B activity could produce more hydrogen peroxide, and this product could contribute to neuronal degeneration (Cohen, 1986). Moreover, hydrogen peroxide can degrade different cellular components by reacting with free iron to produce highly reactive hydroxyl radicals that induce DNA damage (Fahn and Cohen, 1992). These alterations could contribute to the development and progression of human gliomas.

One of the points to bear in mind is the PEA selectivity as a MAO-B substrate. Glia from the human brain has been described to contain both MAO-A and MAO-B activity (Riederer et al., 1987). Nevertheless, the ratio of MAO-B enzymatic activity versus MAO-A activity was 7.5:1 in glial cells in the human frontal cortex (Riederer et al., 1987). In this way, it has been reported a considerable MAO-A component of PEA oxidation at high concentrations (Galva et al., 1995). However, the MAO activity measured in our experiments was relatively insensitive to the MAO-A selective inhibitor clorgyline. In the same way, other authors did not detect MAO-A activity in the astrocytes of post-mortem brain (Nakamura et al., 1990). These data could reflect the fact that glial MAO-A activity in the post-mortem human brain is under the detectable range of the methods used to detect MAO-B enzymatic activity.

On the other hand, the semicarbazide-sensitive amine oxidase, an enzyme that is present in brain vessels, also shows an important sensitivity to PEA (Elliot et al., 1989). Nevertheless, the activity of this enzyme remains after pre-treatment with the MAO-B selective inhibitor deprenyl (Lyles and Chalmers, 1992; Obata and Yamanaka, 2000). In our experiments, MAO activity was completely abolished with low concentrations of deprenyl, ruling out an important contribution of semicarbazide-sensitive amine oxidase to our effect.

Tobacco smokers have an average of 40% lower brain MAO-B values than non-smokers. The degree of MAO-B inhibition is quite variable between subjects, ranging from 17 to 67% (Fowler et al., 2002). This reduction in MAO-B activity in smokers occurs gradually and requires chronic tobacco smoke exposure (Fowler et al., 2002). In our study, the percentage of tobacco smokers was similar in the different groups assessed. Thus, smoking can also be discarded as a potential factor directly related to the differences in MAO-B activity reported between glial tumours and the other tissues.

Another possible bias could be related to the effect of the pharmacological treatment administered to the patients before tumour was excised. In our Health Service, dexamethasone, and occasionally phenytoine, are administered to patients with brain tumours before neurosurgery. It has been reported that dexamethasone is able to elicit a dose-dependent increase of MAO-B activity in cultured astrocytes (Carlo et al., 1996). Conversely, chronic treatment with dexamethasone and corticosterone produced a significant decrease of MAO-B activity in the rat hypothalamus (Cvijic et al., 1995). In the same way, whereas aged rats given dexamethasone showed an increase in MAO-B activity (Slotkin et al., 1998), in vivo treatment of young rats with dexamethasone produces overall decreases in total brain MAO activity (Veals et al., 1977). Nevertheless, in our samples the same pharmacological treatment was used in gliomas and meningiomas. Thus, the opposite changes in MAO-B activity described for both types of tumours suggest that despite drug treatment is a potential modifying factor it is not probably the main reason for the alterations described in our study.

In many glioma patients the invasive procedure of surgical biopsy is performed in an attempt to delineate a diagnosis that could help to define patient treatment. In this clinical situation, it is important to ensure that a correct histopathologic grading of the tumour is made. Currently, there are significant problems with reproducibility and interobserver variability when classifying and grading primary gliomas according to histopathological and immunohistochemical criteria (Coons et al., 1997). Moreover, analysed samples are not necessarily representative because regional tumour heterogeneity may lead to sampling errors and misclassification (Behin et al., 2003). Many of the errors might not change patient survival but could affect the decision for the type of treatment to apply and even the prognosis of the disease. In this situation, all the research efforts to find new biological markers that could clarify the classification and grading of human glial tumours are absolutely crucial.

In this context, the application of positron emission tomography (PET) has proven useful for grading and prognosis of brain tumours (Spence et al., 2002). In addition, MAO-B activity can be localised and quantified in the living human brain using PET and radiotracers labelled with ^{11}C (Bench et al., 1991; Lammertsma et al., 1991), and this methodology has been adapted for the determination of gliosis in neurodegenerative diseases and epilepsy (Bergstrom et al., 1998). By demonstrating a significantly increased MAO-B activity in glial tumours when compared with normal tissue or non-glial tumours, our findings provide evidence to support the feasibility of using PET evaluation of MAO-B activity as an improved method for the diagnosis of gliomas.

In conclusion, the results of our study demonstrate a significant and selective increase in MAO-B activity in human gliomas when compared with meningiomas or non-tumoural tissue. Thus, the quantification of MAO-B activity in the living human brain by PET might be a useful tool for differentiating gliomas from other types of brain tumours and non-pathological tissue. New studies are needed in order to clarify is this marker could be also used to establish a clinical

relevant grading between the different types of glial tumours.

Acknowledgements This work was supported by grants from FIS (PI 03/0498), Plan Nacional sobre Drogas (PI 2006I045), Gobierno Vasco (IT-199-07), and the Instituto de Salud Carlos III, Centro de Investigación Biomédica en Red de Salud Mental, CIBERSAM.

We thank staff members of the Instituto Vasco de Medicina Legal, and the Neurosurgery Service of the Cruces Hospital for their cooperation.

References

Behin A, Hoang-Xuan K, Carpentier AF, Delattre JY (2003) Primary brain tumours in adults. Lancet 361:323–331

Bench CJ, Price GW, Lamertsma AA, Cremer CJ, Luthra SK, Turton D, Dolan RJ, Kettler R, Dingemanse J, Da Prada M, Biziere K, McClelland GR, Jamieson VL, Wood ND, Frackowiak RSJ (1991) Measurement of human cerebral monoamine oxidase type B (MAO-B) activity with positron emission tomography (PET): a dose ranging study with the reversible inhibitor Ro 19-6327. Eur J Clin Pharmacol 40:169–173

Bergstrom M, Kumlien E, Lilja A, Tyrefors N, Westerberg G, Langstrom B (1998) Temporal lobe epilepsy visualized with PET with ^{11}C-L-deuterium-deprenyl: analysis of kinetic data. Acta Neurol Scand 98:224–231

Burnet NG, Lynch AG, Jefferies SJ, Price SJ, Jones PH, Antoun NM, Xuereb JH, Pohl U (2007) High grade glioma: imaging combined with pathological grade defines management and predicts prognosis. Radiother Oncol 85:371–378

Carlo P, Violani E, Del Rio M, Olasmaa M, Santagati S, Maggi A, Picotti GB (1996) Monoamine oxidase B expression is selectively regulated by dexamethasone in cultured rat astrocytes. Brain Res 711:175–183

Cohen G (1986) Monoamine oxidase, hydrogen peroxide, and parkinson's disease. Adv Neurol 45:119–125

Coons SW, Johnson PC, Scheithauer BW, Yates AL, Pearl DK (1997) Improving diagnostic accuracy and interobserver concordance in the classification and grading of primary gliomas. Cancer 79:1381–1393

Cvijic G, Radojicic R, Djordjevic J, Davidovic V (1995) The effect of glucocorticoids on the activity of monoamine oxidase, cooper-zinc superoxide dismutase and catalase in the rat hypothalamus. Funct Neurol 10:175–181

Ekblom J, Jossan SS, Oreland L, Walum E, Aquilonius S-M (1994) Reactive gliosis and monoamine oxidase B. J Neural Transm 41:253–258

Elliot J, Callingham BA, Sharman DF (1989) Semicarbazide-sensitive amine oxidase (SSAO) of the rat aorta. Interactions with some naturally occurring amines and their structural analogues. Biochem Pharmacol 38:1507–1515

Fahn S, Cohen G (1992) The oxidant stress hypothesis in parkinson's disease: evidence supporting it. Ann Neurol 32:804–812

Fowler JS, Logan J, Volkow ND, Wang G-J, Macgregor R, Ding Y-S (2002) Monoamine oxidase: radiotracer development and human studies. Methods 27:263–277

Fowler CJ, Tipton KF (1981) Concentration dependence of the oxidation of tyramine by the two forms of rat liver mitochondrial monoamine oxidase. Biochem Pharmacol 30:3329–3332

Fowler JS, Volkow ND, Wang G-J, Logan J, Pappas N, Shea C, Macgregor R (1997) Age-related increases in bran monoamine oxidase B in living healthy human subjects. Neurobiol Aging 18:431–435

Gabilondo AM, Hostalot C, Garibi JM, Meana JJ, Callado LF (2008) Monoamine oxidase B activity is increased in human gliomas. Neurochem Int 52: 230–234

Galva MD, Bondiolotti GP, Olasmaa M, Picotti GB (1995) Effect of aging on lazabemide binding, monoamine oxidase activity and monoamine metabolites in human frontal cortex. J Neural Transm 101:83–94

Lammertsma AA, Bench CJ, Price GW, Cremer CJ, Luthra SK, Turton D, Wood ND, Frackowiak RSJ (1991) Measurement of cerebral monoamine oxidase B activity using L-[^{11}C]deprenyl and dynamic positron emission tomography. J Cereb Blood F Met 11:545–556

Lizcano JM, Escrich E, Ribalta T, Muntané J, Unzeta M (1991) Amine oxidase activities in rat breast cancer induced experimentally with 7,12-dimethylbenz(α)anthracene. Biochem Pharmacol 42:263–269

Lyles GA, Chalmers J (1992) The metabolism of aminoacetone to methylglyoxal by semicarbazide-sensitive amine oxidase in human umbilical artery. Biochem Pharmacol 43:1409–1414

Mann JJ, Kaplan RD, Bird ED (1986) Elevated postmortem monoamine oxidase B activity in the caudate nucleus in huntington's disease compared to schizophrenics and controls. J Neural Transm 65:277–283

Mazzio EA, Soliman KFA (2005) Glioma cell antioxidant capacity relative to reactive oxygen species produced by dopamine. J Appl Toxicol 24:99–106

Nakamura S, Kawamata T, Akiguchi I, Kameyama M, Nakamura N, Kimura H (1990) Expression of monoamine oxidase B activity in astrocytes of senile plaques. Acta Neuropathol 80:419–425

Obata T, Yamanaka Y (2000) Inhibition of monkey brain semicarbazide-sensitive amine oxidase by various antidepressants. Neurosci Lett 286:131–133

Odegaard S, Borkje B, Skagen DW, Laerum OD, Schrumpf E (1986) Enzyme activities in human gastric cancer and polyps. Scand J Gastroenterol 21:1250–1256

Oreland L, Gottfries CG (1986) Brain and brain monoamine oxidase in aging and in dementia of Alzheimer's type. Prog Neuro-Psychopharmacol Biol Psychiatry 10:533–540

Riederer P, Konradi C, Schay V, Kienzl E, Birkmayer J, Danielczyk W, Sofic E, Youdim MB (1987) Localization of MAO-a and MAO-b in human brain: a step in understanding the therapeutic action of L-deprenyl. Adv Neurol 45:111–118

Saura J, Andrés N, Andrade C, Ojuel J, Eriksson K, Mahy N (1997) Biphasic and region-specific MAO-b response to aging in normal human brain. Neurobiol Aging 18:497–507

Saura J, Luque JM, Cesura AM, Da Prada M, Chan-Palay V, Huber G, Löffler J, Richards JG (1994) Increased monoamine oxidase B activity in plaque-associated astrocytes of Alzheimer brains revealed by quantitative enzyme radioautography. Neuroscience 62:15–30

Sherif F, Gottfries CG, Alafuzoff I, Oreland L (1992) Brain gamma-aminobutyrate aminotransferase (GABA-T) and monoamine oxidase (MAO) in patients with Alzheimer's disease. J Neural Transm 4:227–240

Slotkin TA, Seidler FJ, Ritchie JC (1998) Effects of aging and glucocorticoid treatment on monoamine oxidase subtypes in rat cerebral cortex: therapeutic implications. Brain Res Bull 47:345–348

Spence AM, Muzi M, Krohn KA (2002) Molecular imaging of regional brain tumor biology. J Cell Biochem 87:25–35

Stenström A, Hardy J, Oreland L (1987) Intra- and extra-dopamine-synaptosomal localization of monoamine oxidase in striatal homogenates from four species. Biochem Pharmacol 36:2931–2935

Veals JW, Korduba CB, Symchowicz S (1977) Effect of dexamethasone on monoamine oxidase inhibition by iproniazid in rat brain. Eur J Pharmacol 41:291–299

Westlund KN, Denney RM, Rose RM, Abell CW (1988) Localization of distinct monoamine oxidase a and monoamine oxidase B cell populations in human brainstem. Neuroscience 25:439–456

Youdim MBH, Edmondson D, Tipton KF (2006) The therapeutic potential of monoamine oxidase inhibitors. Nat Neurosci 7:295–309

Chapter 7

Glioma: Role of Integrin in Pathogenesis and Therapy

Ming-Tao Yang, Tur-Fu Huang, and Wen-Mei Fu

Abstract Despite the current standard treatments including surgical resection, radiation therapy and chemotherapy for maliganat gliomas, the survival of these patients remains dismal. More effective therapies are urgently needed to be developed. Integrins affect multiple normal and abnormal CNS functions, including neural development, synaptogenesis, angiogenesis and inflammation. The up-regulation of integrins, focal adhesion complexes and extracellular matrix of laminin, vitronectin and osteopontin in malignant gliomas provides new insights for glioma therapy. There are three major functions of integrins in gliomas including tumor survival and proliferation, tumor invasion and metastasis, and tumor angiogenesis. In addition, the integrin-dependent regulation of hypoxic responses also modulates the tumor radiosensitivity. There are several integrin-targeted anticancer drugs in clinical trial. Furthermore, combination therapy in gliomas with disintegrin and radiotherapy is also available in clinical trial. In conclusion, integrins and cell-matrix adhesion complexes regulate cell proliferation, survival, invasion, migration, angiogenesis and radiosensitivity. To improve the overall survival rate of malignant gliomas, integrin-targeted therapy is a promising adjunctive therapy to standard therapy with surgery, radiotherapy and temozolomide.

Keywords Glioma · Integrin · Extracellular matrix

Introduction

The worldwide incidence rate of primary brain and central nervous system (CNS) tumors, age-adjusted using the world standard population, is 0.6–10.2 per 100,000 person-years in males and 0.7–8.3 per 100,000 person-years in females (Curado et al., 2007). Gliomas account for 33% of all primary brain and CNS tumors, while anaplastic astrocytoma and glioblastoma, WHO grade III and IV (so called malignant gliomas), account for 60% of all gliomas. Despite the current standard treatments including surgical resection, radiation therapy and chemotherapy for maliganat gliomas, the survival of these patients remains dismal, with a median survival of 2–3 years for patients with anaplastic astrocytoma and 9–12 months for patients with glioblastoma (Desjardins et al., 2009). More effective therapies for these patients are thus needed.

Integrins are a family of heterodimeric, transmembrane receptors, composed of α subunit and β subunit. In mammals, 18 α and 8 β subunits have been found and combine to form 24 specific heterodimers, sensing various extracellular matrix ligands (e.g. fibronectin, laminin, vitronectin etc.) and regulated by intracellular adaptor and signaling proteins (e.g. talin, kindlins, vinculin, paxillin etc.) (Moser et al., 2009). Extracellar matrix ligands, integrins and intracellular adaptor proteins constitute cell-matrix adhesion complexes (CMACs) and influence many major cellular functions, including cell proliferation, survival, migration, invasion and angiogenesis (Lock et al., 2008; Silva et al., 2008).

Integrins affect multiple normal and abnormal CNS functions, including neural development, synaptogenesis, angiogenesis and inflammation (Milner and

W.-M. Fu (✉)
College of Medicine, Pharmacological Institute, National Taiwan University, Taipei, Taiwan
e-mail: wenmei@ntu.edu.tw

Campbell, 2002b). During CNS development, neuronal migration is an important step. Inhibition of β1 integrins perturbs neuronal migration during CNS development. On the aspect of synaptogenesis, expression of β3 integrins produces robust changes in the abundance and composition of synaptic AMPARs without affecting dendritic spine structure (Cingolani et al., 2008). In addition, RGD peptides (integrin inhibitors) and antibodies against β3 integrin subunit activity-dependently reduce glutamate release and a switch in the subunit composition of synaptic NMDA receptors, and time-dependently reverse long-term potentiation (Chavis and Westbrook, 2001). During CNS angiogenesis, β1 integrin expression is upregulated, and β1 integrins are expressed predominantly by endothelial cells lining blood vessels in adult CNS (Milner and Campbell, 2002a). Rapid loss of microvascular expression of β1 integrins can reflect the neuronal injury (Tagaya et al., 2001). In addition to β1 integrins, αvβ3 is highly expressed in actively sprouting vessels and considered as a therapeutic target for diseases characterized by neovascularization (Silva et al., 2008). Another function of integrins in CNS is involved inflammation. Expression of integrins (e.g. β1, β2, αv, Mac-1, lymphocyte function-associated antigen (LFA) -1) is upregulated following microglial activation in multiple sclerosis and Alzheimer's disease lesions, both in vitro and in vivo (Milner and Campbell, 2002b).

Expression of integrins in gliomas has also been demonstrated. All vestibular schwannomas and most ependymomas demonstrate strong αvβ3 expression, while oligodendrogliomas, medulloblastomas, and pilocytic astrocytomas demonstrate variable expression. Expression of αvβ3 integrin in gliomas correlates with tumor grade, higher in primary glioblastoma than in low-grade gliomas. The αvβ3 integrin is expressed in both glial tumor cells and endothelial cells (Schnell et al., 2008). In addition, expression of integrin β1 and phosphorylated focal adhesion kinase (FAK) is upregulated by receptor tyrosine kinase Tie2 in malignant gliomas (Lee et al., 2006). Comparison of adhesion molecules between glioblastoma and normal brain tissue by immunohistochemistry, inter-cellular adhesion molecule-1 (ICAM-1; ligand for LFA-1) and LFA-3 are the most distinctive markers for glioblatoma (Gingras et al., 1995). The up-regulation of integrins and focal adhesion complexes provides new insights for the highly infiltrative phenotype of malignant gliomas.

Tumor Survival and Proliferation

Many kinds of integrins are reported to be involved in the tumor growth of glioma. Glioblastomas overexpress integrin α6β1 and its main ligand laminin (Gingras et al., 1995). Enhancement of α6β1 expression in U87 cell line develops more voluminous tumors in nude mice and has a marked increase in vascularization of tumors (Delamarre et al., 2009). Overexpression of α6β1 in U87 cell line in vitro also shows an increased proliferation and reduced apoptosis. On the other hand, primary human medulloblastomas and D283 medulloblastoma cells demonstrate an increased expression of α9 and β1. Blockade of α9 and β1 integrins by antibodies or disintegrins decreases tumor survival and adhesion to leptomeninges, which is rescued by adding tenascin, a ligand for integrin α9β1. This proliferation and survival effect is mediated by the activation of MAPK pathway in a growth factor deficient environment (Fiorilli et al., 2008). Furthermore, α9β1 integrin also induces nerve growth factor (NGF) expression in glioblastoma cell lines, and blockade of α9β1 inhibits NGF-induced proliferation of glioblastoma cells (Brown et al., 2008). Medulloblastoma growth is inhibited by the blockade of matrix metalloproteinase (MMP)–9, which sequentially activates β1 integrin, ERK, and NF-κB (Bhoopathi et al., 2008). It has also been reported that α5β1 integrin inhibitor, JSM6427, reduces growth of GL261 glioma cells inoculated in mouse brains, and microglia attenuation is involved in this tumor inhibitory effect (Färber et al., 2008). Another specific α5β1 integrin inhibitor, SJ749, reduces proliferation and clonogenicity of human astrocytoma cells, depending on the level of α5β1 expression (Maglott et al., 2006). In summary, the role of β1 integrin in tumor proliferation and survival is well established. Various subtypes of α integrins are also involved in tumor growth.

Tumor Invasion and Metastasis

One characteristic phenotype of malignant gliomas is to infiltrate surrounding normal brain tissue. Three processes contribute to this tumor invasion: (1) detach and migrate forward (2) adhere via local and self-produced extracellular matrix (3) degrade the local/surrounding extracellular matrix in order to clear a path for further invasion (D'Abaco and Kaye, 2007). As mentioned above and well known, CMACs, composed of extracellular matrix, integrins and intracellular adaptor proteins, play a major role in cellular detachment and migration. α3- and α5-laminins, found in basement membrane of brain vasculature, selectively promote glioma cell migration, which is inhibited by pretreatment with blocking antibodies to α3β1 integrin (Kawataki et al., 2007). Degradation of surrounding extracellular matrix requires a number of proteases (e.g. matrix metalloproteases), and many evidences also show that integrins influence the proteolysis of extracellular matrix. For example, angiopoietin 2 induces the expression of matrix metalloprotease-2 in human glioma cells through αvβ1 integrin, focal adhesion kinase, ERK and JNK-mediated signaling pathway (Hu et al., 2006).

Osteopontin and vitronectin expression correlates with the malignancy grade and is overexpressed in many stages of cancer progression. Gliomas-derived vitronectin can protect tumor cells from apoptotic death. In addition, Jang et al. (2006) reported that osteopontin expression was over 20-fold in tumoral brain tissue compared to normal tissue. Lamour et al. (2010) found that selective osteopontin knockdown inhibited tumor growth and also decreased the motility and migration of U87-MG and U373-MG cells. These results indicate that both osteopontin and vitronectin are attractive targets for invasion inhibition. One of the main common receptor for osteopontin and vitronectin is integrin αvβ3. We have previously found that snake venom disintegrin inhibits the adhesion, migration and invasion of tumor cells (Yang et al., 2005). Therefore, integrin is a good target for the development of inhibitor for tumor metastasis.

Tumor Angiogenesis

Endothelial cells and pericytes both express a subset of mammalian integrins including: the fibronectin receptors, α4β1, α5β1; the collagen receptors, α1β1, α2β1; the laminin receptors, α3β1, α6β1, and α6β4; and the osteopontin receptor, α9β1 and αvβ3 (Silva et al., 2008). The vitronectin receptors, αvβ3 and αvβ5, are expressed by activated endothelial cells, and αvβ3 is also expressed on glial cells (Silva

et al., 2008). In addition, αvβ3 is overexpressed in high-grade gliomas (Schnell et al., 2008). Therefore, it is reasonable to target integrins for the inhibition of tumor angiogenesis and tumor growth. For example, the collagen type IV cleavage fragment tumstatin and its active subfragment T3 binding to αvβ3 integrin inhibit FAK/PI3K/Akt/mTOR pathway and trigger apoptosis in endothelial cells, and then reduce angiogenesis. The active subfragment T3 also shows a direct αvβ3-dependent growth-inhibitory action in glioma cells in vitro and in vivo (Kawaguchi et al., 2006). Unfortunately, inhibitors of these integrins (e.g. αvβ3/αvβ5 inhibitors) suppressing tumor growth in certain pre-clinical models failed to produce significant results in the majority of clinical trials. One explanation to this contradictory effect is that integrin inhibitor at low concentration (e.g. cilengitide) may paradoxically enhance tumor growth and angiogenesis by up-regulating vascular endothelial growth factor receptor-2 expression (Reynolds et al., 2009). Another consideration is the host integrin expression. Although glioma cells implanted in β3 wild-type mice show greater vessel density than in β3 knock-out mice, the tumor size in wild-type animals is not larger than that in β3 knock-out animals. The anti-tumor effect derived from tumor necrosis factor α-secreting, apoptosis-inducing macrophages in wild-type mice limits tumor growth (Kanamori et al., 2006). Therefore, intracranial microenvironment of glioma should be considered when the anti-integrin therapy is applied.

Other Pathogenic Mechanisms

In addition to the regulation of tumor proliferation, survival and angiogenesis, integrins also affect gliomas in other aspects. Hypoxia induces the recruitment of αvβ3 and αvβ5 integrins to the cell membranes of glioblastoma cells, thereby activating the FAK (Skuli et al., 2009). Inhibition of αvβ3 and αvβ5 integrins with their specific inhibitors or with siRNA decreases the hypoxia-inducible factor 1α level through FAK, GTPase RhoB, GSK3-β pathway. This integrin-dependent regulation of hypoxic response also modulates the tumor radiosensitivity. Silencing αvβ3 and αvβ5 integrins with their specific siRNAs or treatment with αv integrin inhibitor cilengitide significantly amplifies the effects of radiation in glioma (Mikkelsen et al., 2009).

Targeting Integrins in Glioma Therapy

The prognosis of malignant gliomas under currently available surgery and radiotherapy is still miserable. Therefore, more effective therapies, e.g. molecular targeted therapies, are desperately needed. The molecular targeted therapies available for glioma nowadays are summarized in Table 7.1. $\alpha v\beta 3/\alpha v\beta 5$ integrin is also one possible target. Temozolomide (TMZ), a DNA methylator, is now a standard adjunctive chemotherapy and FDA-approved first-line chemotherapy for fresh glioblastoma multifome (GBM) (Villano et al., 2009). The five-year analysis of the EORTC-NCIC

trial in newly diagnosed GBM shows overall survival is 27.2% (95% CI 22.2–32.5) at 2 years, 16.0% (12.0–20.6) at 3 years, 12.1% (8.5–16.4) at 4 years, and 9.8% (6.4–14.0) at 5 years with concomitant TMZ and radiotherapy, versus 10.9% (7.6–14.8), 4.4% (2.4–7.2), 3.0% (1.4–5.7), and 1.9% (0.6–4.4) with radiotherapy alone (hazard ratio 0.6, 95% CI 0.5–0.7; $p<0.0001$) (Stupp et al., 2009). Methylation of the methyl-guanine methyl transferase (MGMT) promoter is the strongest predictor for outcome and benefit from TMZ chemotherapy. Although TMZ's beneficial role in glioma treatment is proved, the poor survival rate still calls for exploring more effective interventions.

Table 7.1 Clinical trials of new molecular targeted therapies in malignant gliomas (updated in December 2009)

Drug	Mechanism	Trials in malignant gliomas	Status
Temozolomide (Temodal®)	DNA methylator	Phase IV, montherapy/combination therapy, fresh GBM/brain tumors	Recruiting
Bevacizumab (Avastin®)	monoclonal antibody to VEGF-A	Phase III, adjunctive with temozolomide and radiotherapy, freshBGM	Recruiting
Vatalanib (PTK787/ZK222584)	Inhibitor of VEGFRs	Phase I/II, adjunctive with temozolomide or lomustine, recurrent GBM	Completed
		Phase I/II, adjunctive with temozolomide and radiotherapy, fresh GBM	Active
Gefinitib (Iressa®)	Inhibit the tyrosine kinase activity of EGFR	Phase II, monotherapy, fresh/recurrent GBM	Completed
Erlotinib (Tarceva®)	Inhibit EGFR-specific tyrosine phosphorylation	Phase II, monotherapy, recurrent malignant gliomas	Completed
Imatinib mesylate (Gleevec®)	Kinase inhibitor of PDGFR	Phase III, adjunctive with hydroxyurea, recurrent malignant gliomas	Completed
Tipifarnib (Zarnestra®)	Inhibitor of RAS	Phase II, monotherapy, fresh/recurrent malignant gliomas	Completed
Temsirolimus (CCI-779)	Inhibitor of mTOR	Phase II, monotherapy, fresh/recurrent malignant gliomas	Completed
Enzastaurin (LY317615)	Serine/threonine kinase inhibitor targeting PKC	Phase III, monotherapy, recurrent GBM	Completed
Cilengitide (EMD121974)	Inhibitor of $\alpha v\beta 3$ and $\alpha v\beta 5$ integrin receptors	Phase III, combination therapy, fresh GBM	Recruiting
Vandetanib (Zactima®)	Dual inhibitor of EGFR/VEGFR-2	Phase II, monotherapy, fresh/recurrent malignant gliomas	Recruiting
Sunitinib malate (Sutent®)	Inhibitor of VEGFR-2, PDGFR, c-KIT, etc.	Phase II, monotherapy, fresh/recurrent malignant gliomas	Recruiting

Currently available integrin-targeted anticancer therapies include vitaxin/abergin (targeting αvβ3, for melanoma, solid tumors, colorectal cancers), cilengitide (targeting αvβ3, for solid tumors, lymphoma, gliomas, glioblastomas), volociximab/ATN 161 (targeting α5β1, for solid tumors), and E 7820 (targeting α2β1, for lymphoma, colorectal cancer) (Silva et al., 2008).

Cilengitide, a cyclic RGD peptide, competitively binds αvβ3 and αvβ5 integrin receptors (Smith, 2003). The drug suppressed the growth of GBM and medulloblastoma cell lines implanted orthotopically in nude mice. Randomized phase II study of cilengitide in GBM at first recurrence shows no significant toxicities under regimen of 500 or 2000 mg intravenously twice weekly (Reardon et al., 2008). Antitumor activity is observed in both treatment cohorts but trended more favorably among patients treated with 2000 mg, including a 6-month progression-free survival of 15% and a median overall survival of 9.9 months. In addition, cilengitide shows synergistic effect with radiotherapy in an orthotopic rat glioma xenograft model (Mikkelsen et al., 2009). Phase III clinical trial of combination therapy with cilengitide and radiotherapy is on going.

Abegrin (MEDI-522 or Vitaxin), which is a humanized monoclonal antibody against human integrin αvβ3, is currently in phase II clinical trials for the treatment of melanoma, solid tumors, and colorectal cancer. Integrin αvβ3-targeted radioimmunotherapy with ^{90}Y-labeled Abegrin reduced tumor volume in subcutaneous human glioblastoma xenograft model (Veeravagu et al., 2008). Therefore, ^{90}Y-labeled Abegrin may be a promising choice in regional glioma therapy.

In conclusion, integrins and cell-matrix adhesion complexes regulate cell proliferation, survival, invasion, migration, angiogenesis and radiosensitivity. To improve the overall survival rate of malignant gliomas, integrin-targeted therapy is a promising adjunctive therapy to standard therapy with surgery, radiotherapy and temozolomide. So far, there are two successfully developed and commercially available disintegrin products targeting αIIbβ3 integrin of platelet, Tirofiban (Aggrastat, Merck) and Eptifibatide (Integrilin, COR Therapeutics), which are used for preventing restenosis of coronary vessels after percutaneous transluminal coronary angioplasty (PTCA). Therefore, it is promising to develop specific disintegrins for glioma therapy.

References

Bhoopathi P, Chetty C, Kunigal S, Vanamala SK, Rao JS, Lakka SS (2008) Blockade of tumor growth Due To matrix metalloproteinase-9 inhibition is mediated by sequential activation of beta1-integrin, ERK, and NF-kappab. J Biol Chem 283:1545–1552

Brown MC, Staniszewska I, Lazarovici P, Tuszynski GP, Del Valle L, Marcinkiewicz C (2008) Regulatory effect of nerve growth factor in α9β1 integrin-dependent progression of glioblastoma. Neurooncol 10:968–980

Chavis P, Westbrook G (2001) Integrins mediate functional pre- and postsynaptic maturation at a hippocampal synapse. Nature 411:317–321

Cingolani LA, Thalhammer A, Yu LMY, Catalano M, Ramos T, Colicos MA, Goda Y (2008) Activity-dependent regulation of synaptic AMPA receptor composition and abundance by β3 integrins. Neuron 58:749–762

Curado MP, Edwards B, Shin HR, Storm H, Ferlay J, Heanue M, Boyle P (2007) Cancer incidence in five continents, vol IX. International Agency for Research on Cancer, Lyon, France

Delamarre E, Taboubi S, Mathieu S, Berenguer C, Rigot V, Lissitzky J-C, Figarella-Branger D, Ouafik LH, Luis J (2009) Expression of integrin α6β1 enhances tumorigenesis in glioma cells. Am J Pathol 175:844–855

Desjardins A, Reardon DA, Vredenburgh JJ (2009) Current available therapies and future directions in the treatment of malignant gliomas. Biologics 3:15–25

D'Abaco GM, Kaye AH (2007) Integrins: molecular determinants of glioma invasion. J Clin Neurosci 14:1041–1048

Fiorilli P, Partridge D, Staniszewska I, Wang JY, Grabacka M, So K, Marcinkiewicz C, Reiss K, Khalili K, Croul SE (2008) Integrins mediate adhesion of medulloblastoma cells to tenascin and activate pathways associated with survival and proliferation. Lab Invest 88:1143–1156

Färber K, Synowitz M, Zahn G, Vossmeyer D, Stragies R, van Rooijen N, Kettenmann H (2008) An α5β1 integrin inhibitor attenuates glioma growth. Mol Cell Neurosci 39:579–585

Gingras M-c, Roussel E, Bruner JM, Branch CD, Moser rP (1995) Comparison of cell adhesion molecule expression between glioblastoma multiforme and autologous normal brain tissue. J Neuroimmunol 57:143–153

Hu B, Jarzynka MJ, Guo P, Imanishi Y, Schlaepfer DD, Cheng S-Y (2006) Angiopoietin 2 induces glioma cell invasion by stimulating matrix metalloprotease 2 expression through the αVβ1 integrin and focal adhesion kinase signaling pathway. Cancer Res 66:775–783

Jang T, Savarese T, Low HP, Kim S, Vogel H, Lapointe D, Duong T, Litofsky NS, Weimann JM, Ross AH, Recht L (2006) Osteopontin expression in intratumoral astrocytes marks tumor progression in gliomas induced by prenatal exposure to N-ethyl-N-nitrosourea. Am J Pathol 168:1676–1685

Kanamori M, Kawaguchi T, Berger MS, Pieper RO (2006) Intracranial microenvironment reveals independent opposing functions of host αVβ3 expression on glioma growth and angiogenesis. J Biol Chem 281:37256–37264

Kawaguchi T, Yamashita Y, Kanamori M, Endersby R, Bankiewicz KS, Baker SJ, Bergers G, Pieper RO (2006) The PTEN/akt pathway dictates the direct αVβ3-dependent growth-inhibitory action of an active fragment of tumstatin in glioma cells *in vitro* and *in vivo*. Cancer Res 66 11331–11340

Kawataki T, Yamane T, Naganuma H, Rousselle P, Andurén I, Tryggvason K, Patarroyo M (2007) Laminin isoforms and their integrin receptors in glioma cell migration and invasiveness: evidence for a role of α5-laminin(S) and α3β1 integrin. Exp Cell Res 313:3819–3831

Lamour V, Le Mercier M, Lefranc F, Hagedorn M, Javerzat S, Bikfalvi A, Kiss R, Castronovo V, Bellahcène A (2010) Selective osteopontin knockdown exerts anti-tumoral activity in a human glioblastoma model. Int J Cancer 126:1797–1805

Lee OH, Xu J, Fueyo J, Fuller GN, Aldape KD, Alonso MM, Piao Y, Liu TJ, Lang FF, Bekele BN, Gomez-Manzano C (2006) Expression of the receptor tyrosine kinase tie2 in neoplastic glial cells is associated with integrin beta1-dependent adhesion to the extracellular matrix. Mol Cancer Res 4:915–926

Lock JG, Wehrle-Haller B, Strömblad S (2008) Cell-matrix adhesion complexes: master control machinery of cell migration. Semin Cancer Biol 18:65–76

Maglott A, Bartik P, Cosgun S, Klotz P, Ronde P, Fuhrmann G, Takeda K, Martin S, Dontenwill M (2006) The small α5β1 integrin antagonist, SJ749, reduces proliferation and clonogenicity of human astrocytoma cells. Cancer Res 66:6002–6007

Mikkelsen T, Brodie C, Finniss S, Berens ME, Rennert JL, Nelson K, Lemke N, Brown SL, Hahn D, Neuteboom B, Goodman SL (2009) Radiation sensitization of glioblastoma by cilengitide has unanticipated schedule-dependency. Int J Cancer 124:2719–2727

Milner R, Campbell IL (2002a) Developmental regulation of [beta]1 integrins during angiogenesis in the central nervous system. Mol. Cell Neurosci 20:616–626

Milner R, Campbell IL (2002b) The integrin family of cell adhesion molecules has multiple functions within the CNS. J Neurosci Res 69:286–291

Moser M, Legate KR, Zent R, Fassler R (2009) The tail of integrins, talin, and kindlins. Science 324:895–899

Reardon DA, Fink KL, Mikkelsen T, Cloughesy TF, O'Neill A, Plotkin S, Glantz M, Ravin P, Raizer JJ, Rich KM, Schiff D, Shapiro WR, Burdette-Radoux S, Dropcho EJ, Wittemer SM, Nippgen J, Picard M, Nabors LB (2008) Randomized phase II study of cilengitide, an integrin-targeting arginine-glycine-aspartic acid peptide, in recurrent glioblastoma multiforme. J Clin Oncol 26:5610–5617

Reynolds AR, Hart IR, Watson AR, Welti JC, Silva RG, Robinson SD, Da Violante G, Gourlaouen M, Salih M, Jones MC, Jones DT, Saunders G, Kostourou V, Perron-Sierra F, Norman JC, Tucker GC, Hodivala-Dilke KM (2009) Stimulation of tumor growth and angiogenesis by low concentrations of RGD-mimetic integrin inhibitors. Nat Med 15:392–400

Schnell O, Krebs B, Wagner E, Romagna A, Beer AJ, Grau SJ, Thon N, Goetz C, Kretzschmar HA, Tonn J-C, Goldbrunner RH (2008) Expression of integrin αVβ3 in gliomas correlates with tumor grade and is not restricted to tumor vasculature. Brain Pathol 18:378–386

Silva R, D'Amico G, Hodivala-Dilke KM, Reynolds LE (2008) Integrins: the keys to unlocking angiogenesis. Arterioscler Thromb Vasc Biol 28:1703–1713

Skuli N, Monferran S, Delmas C, Favre G, Bonnet J, Toulas C, Cohen-Jonathan Moyal E (2009) αVβ3/αVβ5 integrins-FAK-rhob: a novel pathway for hypoxia regulation in glioblastoma. Cancer Res 69:3308–3316

Smith JW (2003) Cilengitide Merck. Curr Opin Invest Drugs 4:741–745

Stupp R, Hegi ME, Mason WP, van den Bent MJ, Taphoorn MJB, Janzer RC, Ludwin SK, Allgeier A, Fisher B, Belanger K, Hau P, Brandes AA, Gijtenbeek J, Marosi C, Vecht CJ, Mokhtari K, Wesseling P, Villa S, Eisenhauer E, Gorlia T, Weller M, Lacombe D, Cairncross JG, Mirimanoff R-O (2009) Effects of radiotherapy with concomitant and adjuvant temozolomide versus radiotherapy alone on survival in glioblastoma in a randomised phase III study: 5-year analysis of the EORTC-NCIC trial. Lancet Oncol 10:459–466

Tagaya M, Haring H-P, Stuiver I, Wagner S, Abumiya T, Lucero J, Lee P, Copeland BR, Seiffert D, del Zoppo GJ (2001) Rapid loss of microvascular integrin expression during focal brain ischemia reflects neuron injury. J Cereb Blood Flow Metab 21:835–846

Veeravagu A, Liu Z, Niu G, Chen K, Jia B, Cai W, Jin C, Hsu AR, Connolly AJ, Tse V, Wang F, Chen X (2008) Integrin αVβ3-targeted radioimmunotherapy of glioblastoma multiforme. Clin Cancer Res 14:7330–7339

Villano J, Seery T, Bressler L (2009) Temozolomide in malignant gliomas: current use and future targets. Cancer Chemother Pharmacol 64:647–655

Yang RS, Tang CH, Chuang WJ, Huang TH, Peng HC, Huang TF, Fu WM (2005) Inhibition of tumor formation by snake venom disintegrin. Toxicon 45:661–669

Chapter 8

Proton Magnetic Resonance Spectroscopy in Intracranial Gliomas

Eftychia Z. Kapsalaki, Ioannis Tsougos, Kyriaki Theodorou, and Kostas N. Fountas

Abstract   Recent MRI advances have focused on the development and application of molecular and physiological imaging capabilities. One of these relatively new MRI methods, Magnetic Resonance Spectroscopy (MRS) reflects the continuing evolution from purely anatomic to physiological and molecular imaging of the brain. Magnetic Resonance Spectroscopy yields images of the distribution and concentration of naturally occurring molecules such as N-acetyl aspartate (NAA) (one of the most abundant amino acids in the brain), choline (Cho) (a key constituent of cell membranes), lactate (Lac) (a reflection of anaerobic metabolism) and Creatines (Cr). It has been suggested that the sum of Cr and Phosphocreatine is relatively constant in the human brain, and for this reason Cr is often used as a reference signal, and it is a common practice for metabolite ratios to be expressed as a ratio relative to Cr. However, with the development of quantitative analysis techniques, it is clear that total Cr is not constant, both in different brain regions and in pathological processes, so the assumption of Cr as a reference signal should be used with caution. It is well known that gliomas represent the most common type of primary intracranial tumors. The establishment of an accurate diagnosis, the preoperative evaluation of tumor metabolism and the obtaining information regarding tumor histological grade, may increase the efficacy of the currently employed treatments and eventually improve the overall clinical outcome in gliomas cases. Magnetic Resonance Spectroscopy may substantially improve the non-invasive categorization of human brain tumors, especially gliomas. The utilization of MRS (coupled to conventional MRI techniques) in the evaluation of tumors provides greater information concerning tumor activity and metabolism. In addition, it may provide valuable information regarding the tumor response to the employed treatments.

Keywords Choline · Creatine · Glioma · Lipids · MR spectroscopy · N-acetyl-aspartate

Introduction

Magnetic Resonance Imaging (MRI) is considered the method of choice for the identification and the evaluation of brain tumors. The MR characteristics of brain tumors depend on their consistency and their histopathology. The role of MRI in the evaluation of patients with intracranial masses is to identify the lesion, provide a differential diagnosis and contribute to the selection process of the best therapeutic approach for these patients. Since many brain tumors have similar imaging characteristics, advanced MR techniques have been introduced and may further attribute to the differential diagnosis of these lesions. Such techniques include Diffusion Weighted Imaging (DWI), fractional anisotropy and tractography (DTI), perfusion weighted Imaging (pWI), and Magnetic Resonance Spectroscopy (MRS). Use of these advanced methodologies in the preoperative evaluation of gliomas, may significantly narrow the differential diagnosis and minimize the possibility

K.N. Fountas (✉)
Department of Neurosurgery, University Hospital of Larisa,
School of Medicine, University of Thessaly, Larisa, Greece
email:fountas@med.uth.gr

of misdiagnosis, particularly in the cases of ring enhancing lesions. In addition, the establishment of an accurate diagnosis may clarify some occasionally perplexing issues, regarding the best surgical planning for these patients.

It is well known that gliomas represent the majority of primary intracranial brain tumors. They may be circumscribed (WHO I), or diffuse and infiltrative (WHO II-IV). The degree of malignancy increases as pyrinokinesias and mitotic activity increase, and necrosis and neovascularization develop in these lesions. Preoperative imaging evaluation needs to provide accurate information regarding the extent of the lesion, which is better identified after contrast administration, but also to detect the presence of any neoplastic cells in the peritumoral edema. In a large number of cases, infiltrative gliomas are characterized by a remarkable heterogeneity and significantly varying stages of malignancy in different areas of the same tumor. The employment of advanced MR imaging, using DWI, pWI and MRS, may accurately identify the areas of highest malignancy in a tumor, and thus navigate the surgeon to the most aggressive area of this tumor. Moreover, MRS provides information regarding tumors' biochemical profile, by measuring specific metabolite concentrations and their ratios, and thus may potentially predict their histological grade.

Furthermore, identification of the presence of tumor cells in the peritumoral edema, contributes to a more aggressive surgical resection, and a more efficient post operative radiation planning. In addition, the question of postsurgical radiation necrosis and/or interstitial brachytherapy associated necrosis versus tumor recurrence constitutes a puzzling issue in the management of patients with surgically resected gliomas. Magnetic Resonance Spectroscopy combined with pWI may be useful, particularly in those cases that these two methodologies provide concordant results.

In this chapter, we provide a brief overview of the MRS general principles, a brief description of the necessary hardware and software for performing MRS and its technical limitations. We outline the usually recognized metabolites in normal brain and other pathological conditions, we describe the most frequently used metabolic ratios in clinical practice, we analyze the spectral characteristics of gliomas, and we also refer to the future directions of MRS.

General Principles of Magnetic Resonance Spectroscopy

Proton Magnetic Resonance Spectroscopy (also Hydrogen^{-1} MRS, or H^1 MRS) is the application of nuclear magnetic resonance with respect to Hydrogen-1 nuclei within the molecules of a substance. Since the atomic number of hydrogen is 1, a positive hydrogen ion (H$^+$) has no electrons and corresponds to a bare nucleus with one proton. Regarding clinical applications, water is the biggest source of protons in the human body, therefore, allows the application of brain H^1 MRS.

Magnetic Resonance Spectroscopy depends on the chemical shift theory, which corresponds to a change in the resonance frequency of the nuclei within the molecules, according to their chemical bonds. The presence of an electron cloud constitutes an electronic shield, which slightly lowers the static magnetic field to which the nucleus would normally be subjected. Thus, same nuclei will resonate in different frequencies, according to which molecular group they belong to, as they experience this different "shielding effect". This resonance frequency difference (chemical shift) is expressed as parts per million or ppm, a value that is independent of the amplitude of the magnetic field. Thus, the value of the chemical shift provides information about the molecular group carrying the hydrogen nuclei, and therefore provides differentiation among several metabolites.

Therefore, within a certain region of interest, ideally a voxel of at least 8 cm^3, it is possible to gather information on these molecular groups and present it as a spectrum. In this spectrum, the x-axis (oriented from right to left) represents the precession frequency, which differentiates the identity of a certain compound. On the other hand, the intensity on the y-axis can be used to quantify the amount of a substance, although this is a matter of great dispute and includes serious risks that should be taken into account. To obtain reliable absolute concentrations, one has to consider potential complicating factors, with respect to both the data acquisition method and the data processing method. For example, relaxation effects in data acquisition can be either corrected or eliminated, whereas data fitting is complicated by factors such as the contribution of macromolecules (Jansen et al., 2006).

Peaks of several molecular groups on the spectrum are also called resonances. Some metabolites do not have simple resonances, but may be split into two (called doublet), three (triplet) or even more sub-peaks. As spins can be considered to be small magnets, they interact with the main magnetic field, thus the degree of interaction, known as spin-spin coupling, causes a peak to split into more than one sub peaks. The frequency separation of each peak and the clear representation of its characteristics depends on the field strength, on the magnetic field homogeneity, the degree of chemical shift, the samples' chemical composition, and on the digital resolution i.e. the precision with which the signal is sampled.

At low fields with a poor shim, the peaks tend to overlap and that causes difficulty in interpreting and in measuring peak heights. In proton MRS (H^1MRS), the water signal must be suppressed, as it is much greater than the signal from other H^1 containing compounds and it has overlapping spectroscopic peaks. The reference frequency used, set at zero ppm, is that of the standard tetra-methyl silane $Si-(CH_3)_4$, which has a single proton resonance due to its a completely symmetrical molecule. It should be mentioned here, that above 4 ppm the spectrum becomes unreliable, since the suppression of the water peak at 4.7 ppm tends to destroy the neighbouring portions of the spectrum.

Proton MRS Apparatus

In-vivo H^1MRS uses MRI apparatus that is virtually identical to that used in routine imaging, but nevertheless requires:

- A sufficiently strong and very homogenous magnetic field (at least 1.5 T), to distinguish resonance peaks, shimming ideally less than 0.5 ppm over the central 20 cm Diameter of a Spherical Volume (DSV).
- Specific sequences for spectroscopic signal acquisition. There are two types of H^1MRS: Single Voxel Spectroscopy (SVS), which receives the spectrum from a single voxel only, and Chemical Shift Imaging (CSI), which measures spectra in a single dimension projection (1D), on a two dimension slice (2D), or a three dimensional volume (3D)

- Adapted data processing software, and
- An adapted radiofrequency system (in the resonance frequency of the studied nucleus).

Single-Voxel (SV) Spectroscopy

In SV spectroscopy, the signal is received from a volume limited to a single voxel. This acquisition is fairly fast (1–5 min) and a spectrum is easily obtained. It is performed in three steps. Initially, the suppression of the water signal is performed, followed by the selection of a voxel of interest, and lastly by the acquisition of the spectrum. For the spectra acquisition there are two types of sequences available: (a) Point-RESolved Spectroscopy (PRESS) and (b) STimulated Echo Acquisition Mode (STEAM). It is worth mentioning that the analyzed volume is selected by three selective radiofrequency pulses (accompanied by gradients) in the three directions in space (either 90°–90°–90° in STEAM, or 90°–180°–180° in PRESS). These pulses determine three orthogonal planes, whose intersection corresponds to the studied volume. Only the signal within this voxel will be recorded, by selecting the echo resulting from a series of the three studied radiofrequency pulses.

Chemical Shift Imaging (CSI)

Chemical shift imaging (CSI) consists of spectroscopic data of a group of voxels, in slice(s) (2D) or in a specific volume (3D). It is based on a repetition of STEAM or PRESS type sequences to which a spatial phase encoding is added. The number and direction of phase encodings depend on the number of dimensions explored, having as a consequence though, a longer acquisition time. The results appear in the form of a matrix of the obtained spectra from the studied regions, or as parametric images (metabolic maps).

However, it has to be emphasized that CSI has several disadvantages. In this technique, voxels of interest (VOIs) are much larger than those in SVS, so it is more difficult to achieve magnetic field homogeneity. Localization of multiple VOIs is not as accurate as localization via a single voxel in SVS, as phase encoding causes much more spin dephasing. In addition, adjacent voxels' interference can add up to 10% of their signal to the voxel of interest, thus degrading the obtained spectra. As a result, there is a signal loss of approximately 13% per direction of phase encoding, which has to be appropriately multiplied in the case of 3D CSI. Another disadvantage of 3D CSI is the increased acquisition time, which can last up to 15 min.

Limitations of MR Spectroscopy

Though a promising advance, several technical limitations potentially compromise the efficacy of MRS as a diagnostic modality. Intraparenchymal calcification, contamination from adjacent bone and fat (from the skull), cerebrospinal fluid (CSF) or the presence of intratumoral hemorrhage may alter the MRS signal and, if inadvertently included in an assessed voxel, may confound the obtained results. In order to obtain a good and accurate H^{1}MRS analysis the following guidelines should be scholastically followed: good magnetic homogeneity, good water suppression, proper localization in respect to the lesion, well optimized pulse sequences, and finally a cooperative patient.

To obtain good homogeneity, excellent shimming is a prerequisite, and calibration of water suppression must be exceedingly efficient. This allows a good analysis of the metabolite intensities. Another important issue is to obtain adequate signal-to-noise ratio in order to permit reproducible peak area integration, avoiding artefacts. Finally, the appropriate voxel size should be selected, and has to be large enough to obtain a detectable metabolite signal, thus avoiding distortion from other peaks in the spectrum and should not be placed near the skull, to avoid contamination from bone and fat. However, when the voxel size has to be very small, the obtained spectrum requires a larger acquisition time, in order to obtain good shimming and water suppression.

Stronger magnetic fields, as 3 T, can spread out precession frequencies over a wider range and may double spatial and temporal resolution. Moreover, stronger magnetic fields may also allow the detection of compounds that are currently considered to be not clearly detectable with lower magnetic fields. Nevertheless, at

higher magnetic fields, water is much more difficult to be suppressed, due to the increased magnetic field inhomogeneity, poorer radiofrequency coil efficiency, poorer shimming, and different relaxation times. Kim et al. (2006) have concluded that although there is an increased signal to noise ratio at 3 T compared to 1.5 T, a better spectral resolution at a short TE (35 ms) but not at long TE (144 ms), there was no significant difference in the metabolite ratios at 3 T. Their findings are in agreement with our experience from using 3 T MRI and MRS. Another issue that needs to be taken into consideration is the usage of commercial MRS analysis packages, which may be user-friendly but should be used with extreme caution, since in these packages there are metabolites, which are not detected in a routine brain spectrum (Xu et al., 2008).

Proton Magnetic Resonance Spectroscopy Brain Metabolites

Choline (Cho)

At 3.2 ppm a prominent resonance arises from the methyl protons of choline (Cho) containing compounds. It constitutes a structural compound of the cell membrane and is routinely detected in a normal brain spectrum, but in small concentrations. Choline signals in brain tumor studies are considered as a surrogate marker of cellular membrane turnover. Ex vivo studies of perchloric acid extracts of intracranial tumor tissue indicate that Cho spectral signal represents mostly free Cho, phosphocholine (PC) and glycerophosocholine (GPC) molecules (Miller et al., 1996). Nevertheless, at routine clinical magnetic field strengths, these three compounds are seen as a single resonance, as they cannot be resolved, hence they are referred as the total Cho signal.

Possible causes for the elevated Cho signal seen in brain tumors can be separated into: (a) intracellular and (b) extracellular mechanisms. In the intracellular environment, Cho may be elevated as a result of enhanced transport, phosphocholine may be elevated as a result of accelerated phosphorylation and transport, and all three compounds (Cho, PC and GPC) may be elevated as a result of cellular membrane break down. In the extracellular environment and in the blood, Cho may be elevated as a result of hyperperfusion and/or systemic metabolic alterations. According to several in vitro MRS studies based on brain tumor biopsy material, increased intracellular PC is the predominant cause for the Cho signal elevation (Tzika et al., 2002). It has been demonstrated, that PC increases with cell proliferation rate, and that glioma cells have enhanced Cho transport and phosphorylation during their growing phase (Podo, 1999).

Recently, the technique of ^{1}H high-resolution magic angle spinning (HR-MAS) has been shown to produce high-quality data, allowing the accurate measurement of many metabolites present in unprocessed biopsy tissue, allowing better correlations between in vivo and in vitro studies (Wilson et al., 2009). It has to be emphasized however, that the exact interpretation of changes in total choline signal is complicated, due to multiple contributions to the observed total choline spectrum resonance. Therefore, more general terms as increased cellular membrane turnover or altered cellular membrane metabolism, are frequently used to explain elevated Cho in gliomas.

Creatine (Cr)

At 3.03 ppm a composite peak arises from the methyl and methylene protons of Cr and phosphorylated creatine (PCr), often called total Creatine (tCr). In the brain, Cr and PCr are present in both neuronal and glial cells, and together with ATP play a crucial role in the energy metabolism of neuronal tissues. Total Cr constitutes a metabolite routinely detected in normal brain spectrum, and is considered to be a measure of cellular density, while is especially high in glial cells. The concentration of total creatine is relatively constant, with no changes reported with brain aging. As such, its resonance is frequently used as an internal concentration reference and other metabolites are represented as ratios to Cr. While convenient, the use of any internal concentration reference should be used with extreme caution. There appears to be a substantial variation in Cr concentrations between grey and white matter, as well as within individual tumors of a certain type. Although under most conditions, the use of Cr as a constant is reliable, previous absolute quantification studies have demonstrated that in a number of brain tumours, Cr levels were found to be significantly less than those in normal brain (Howe et al., 2003), and are decreasing with increased grade of malignancy.

N-Acetyl Aspartate (NAA)

At 2.01 ppm a prominent resonance arises from the methyl group of NAA. In general, NAA is considered to be a highly specific neuronal marker, reflecting the number of intact neurons in the gray matter, and the density of intact axons in the white matter. NAA is exclusively localized in the central and peripheral nervous system. Its concentration varies in different parts of the brain, and undergoes significant changes following any developmental central and peripheral nervous system changes. It has been reported that NAA resonance is a marker of neuronal density, and its decreased concentration in tumors reflects neuronal loss (Majos et al., 2004). The reported NAA concentration reduction in brain tumor spectra is typically attributed to the displacement and destruction of neuronal tissue, which accompanies gliotic infiltration (Birken and Oldendorf, 1989). Indeed, the vast majority of in vivo H^{1}MRS studies have demonstrated that NAA signal is markedly decreased in brain tumor spectra, although it is not unusual to detect a small residual amount of NAA. When NAA is present in a brain tumor spectrum, it is difficult to exclude the possibility that a small amount of NAA-containing (normal) brain tissue has accidentally been included in the sampled volume. It needs to be pointed out however, that NAA also decreases in other pathological conditions such as in the chronic stages of stroke (Gideon et al., 1992), or in multiple sclerosis (Simone et al., 2001). Moreover, NAA levels may reflect neuronal dysfunction rather than actual neuronal loss. This is substantiated by recovery of NAA levels in cases of incomplete reversible ischemia (Brulatout et al., 1996) or reversible traumatic brain injury (Sinson et al., 2001).

Alanine (Ala)

At 1.47 ppm a prominent resonance arises from the three methyl protons coupled to a single methane in the alanine molecule. Alanine is known to be the substrate of several amino acid transporters. The signal from

Alanine is usually overlapped by lipids, therefore, the use of spectral editing or the application of longer echo times is necessary, in order to distinguish these two resonances. Alanine is a non essential amino acid, with its main function being in the metabolism of tryptophan and pyridoxine. It also assists in the metabolism of sugars and organic acids, providing energy for muscle tissues and brain, without any significant contribution however, to the actual energy metabolism, but mainly to the carbon recycling process (Broer et al., 2007). Yudkoff et al. (1986) found, in cultured astrocytes, an important flux of nitrogen from glutamate to alanine, corresponding to net alanine synthesis. They proposed that alanine released from astrocytes is utilized by neurons to synthesize glutamate, whereas we would suggest that in higher eukaryotes, alanine may actually be the substrate that feeds the neurons to sustain their energy needs.

The total concentration of Ala is very low and is almost not detectable in a normal brain spectrum. It is not usually detected in gliomas, but has been expressed in tumors of meningeal origin, and it may be a distinct metabolite for meningiomas. Manton et al. (1995) suggested that the presence of ala in meningiomas may indicate that their metabolism involves partial oxidation of glutamine rather than glycolysis. Nevertheless increased Ala has also been observed in cases of evolving ischemia.

Lipids (Lip)

Lipid signals arise at about 0.9 and 1.4 ppm. Lipids are normally absent from a normal MR brain spectrum. They have short transverse relaxation times thus, are relatively easier to be detected when using short TE SVS (35 ms or less). The appearance of lipid resonances in a tumor usually represents necrosis, thus Lip are present in high grade gliomas, which typically have a larger necrotic fraction than lower grade tumors. Lipid concentration increases with the increased cellularity of the tumor, however, Lip are not always specific and reproducible markers. Since free lipid signals appear to be associated with necrotic areas, they may indicate high degree of malignancy or a tumor of metastatic origin. Therefore, detection of lipids is indicative of a malignant tumor. Gotsis et al. (1996) have reported that lipids are detected in anaplastic gliomas and GBM, in metastatic lesions, but also in abscesses of bacterial origin. They are usually not detected in low grade tumors, but may be found in lipid containing meningiomas. It is widely known that lipids remain a perplexing finding in brain H[1]MRS.

Lactate (Lac)

At 1.33 ppm lactate arises as a doublet resonance from the three equivalent methyl protons, while the single methine proton resonates as a quartet at 4.10 ppm. Lac (or lactic acid) is the end-product, hence the reflection, of anaerobic glycolysis. In normal human brain, lactate is below or at the limit of detectability in most studies. Its absence may conversely correlate with increased neo-vascularization of a highly aggressive malignant tumor. Increased Lac concentrations have been observed in a wide variety of conditions that are associated with restricted blood flow, hence hypoxia, such as ischemic stroke (Barker et al., 1994), mitochondrial myopathy, encephalopathy, and lactacidosis. It is also present in aggressive tumors (Negendank et al., 1996), and abscesses.

The increased concentration of Lactate and lipids, are consistent with rapid tumor growth leading to hypoxia, hypoxic stress, and finally to central necrosis, as the tumor outgrows its blood supply. Although Lac concentration is considered to increase with astrocytoma grade (Auer et al., 2001), the statistical significance of this finding is questionable, due to its high variability within tumor groups. Moreover, lactate and lipid levels, as a marker of tumor grade, have shown varied results in long-TE studies (Negendank et al., 1996). Lipids and lactate may coincide since they appear in the same region of the spectrum. These resonances are better distinguished at higher magnetic fields and by using CSI, which produces inversion of the lactate peak but not of the lipid peak.

MyoInositol (mI)

MyoInositol is a rather complex sugar alcohol that gives rise to four groups of resonances. The main resonance peak can be seen at 3.56 ppm. MyoInositol is located in astrocytes and is considered to be a marker of glial cells, but its exact function is not known.

It has been found that, mI is elevated in low-grade astrocytomas and demyelinating lesions (as multiple sclerosis). Castillo et al. (2000) reported that elevated mI may be a marker of low-grade astrocytomas. Recent magic-angle spinning (MAS) studies of whole-tumor biopsies have demonstrated that mI is elevated in astrocytomas, and its concentration decreases as malignancy grade increases (Cheng et al., 1998). Moreover, in a recent study by Kallenberg et al. (2009) it was shown that in the contralateral normal-appearing white matter, mean myo-inositol levels were significantly increased in patients with GBM compared to the levels of control subjects. Similarly, mI levels were higher in patients with GBM, compared to those of patients with low grade gliomas. Hence, increased concentrations of mI in the contralateral normal-appearing white matter of GBM patients are consistent with mild astrocytosis, and may suggest an early widespread neoplastic infiltration.

A normal brain spectrum is characterized by a marked concentration of NAA and presence of Cho and Cr (Fig. 8.1). Other metabolites, as Ala, Lip or Lac, are not detectable in a normal brain spectrum. Pathological brain areas show variable amounts of decreased concentration of NAA. Depending on the histological profile of the lesion, there may be variable amounts of Cho, Cr, Lip, Lac, Ala, mI, or other metabolites. The absolute amount of these metabolites, but more importantly their ratios, may characterize a brain lesion. Benign and low grade lesions present NAA but in lower concentrations than the normal values (Table 8.1). Absolute metabolite values vary significantly in different normal individuals; therefore, evaluating their ratios is a more accurate marker in grading gliomas, than their absolute values. It is always helpful to compare metabolite values in both hemispheres. In establishing an H^{1}MRS diagnosis, the ratios of NAA/Cho, NAA/Cr and Cho/Cr are being calculated (Table 8.2). All other metabolites are being identified in pathological conditions.

The principal metabolites that are most commonly evaluated in Proton Magnetic Resonance Spectroscopy

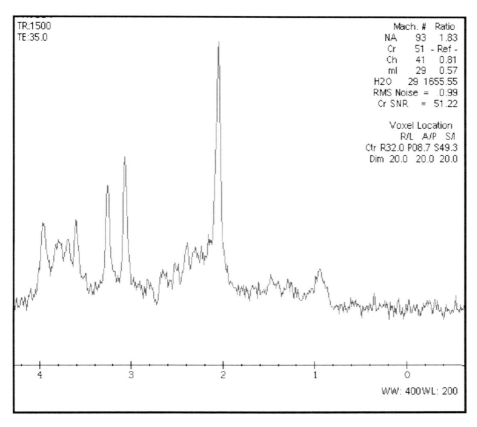

Fig. 8.1 MRS normal spectrum, demonstrating a dominant peak corresponding to NAA at 2 ppm, a peak at 3.03 ppm corresponding to Cr and a peak identified at 3.2 ppm corresponding to Cho

Table 8.1 The concentrations of the characteristic metabolites in gliomas

	Low grade (II)	Anaplastic (III)	GBM (IV)
NAA	Low	Very low	Very low or absent
Cho	High	Very high	Very very high
Cr	Low	Low	Very low
Cho/Cr	High	Very high	Very very high

Table 8.2 Approximate ratios of the normally detected metabolites in gliomas are shown, as reported by Fountas and Castillo

	Normal brain	Low grade (II)	Anaplastic (III)	GBM (IV)
NAA/Cr Fountas et al.	1.52	Increased	Increased	Very increased
NAA/Cr Castillo et al.	1.26	1.23	1.48	3.24
NAA/Cho	1.74	Decreased	Decreased	Very decreased
Cho/Cr Fountas et al.	1.51	2.15	2.78	5.40
Cho/Cr Castillo et al.	0.62	1.06	1.48	2.08
mI/Cr Castillo et al.	0.49	0.82	0.33	0.15

Table 8.3 Summary of the principal metabolites that are most commonly evaluated in proton magnetic resonance spectroscopy (H^{1}MRS)

Metabolite	Frequency/*Cerebral concentration*	Physiological role	TE	Variation impact
Cho	*3.2 ppm/0.9–2.5 mmol/kg*	Marker of cell membrane metabolism.	Long/short	↑ Tumors, inflammation, hypoxia, demyelization. *Caution:* *Higher in white matter than Grey matter.*
Cr *Creatine/Phosphocreatine*	*3.0 ppm/5.1–10.6 mmol/kg*	Compounds related to energy metabolism marker.	Long/short	Serves as reference peak as it is relatively constant. ↓ *Hypoxia, Stroke, Tumors*
NAA *N-Acetyl-Aspartate*	*2.02 ppm/7.9–16.6 mmol/kg*	Neuronal cell marker. Only seen in healthy nervous tissue.	Long/short	↓ Neuronal dysfunction. ↓ Ischaemia, trauma, inflammation, infection, tumors, dementia, gliosis.
Ala *Alanine*	*1.5 ppm/0.2–1.4 mmol/kg*	Is characteristic of mengingeal tumors	Long/short	Expressed in tumors of meningeal origin, may be discriminant metabolite.
Lipids *Free Lipids*	*0.9, 1.4 ppm/> 1.0 mmol/kg*	Membrane breakdown product.	Long/short	Indication of histological necrosis. *High grade tumors, metastatic lesions*
Lactate	*1.33 ppm/0.4 mmol/kg*	A product of anaerobic glycolysis.	Long	Nonspecific marker of tumor aggressiveness.
Myo-inositol (mI)	*3.6 ppm/3.8–8.1 mmol/kg*	Glial Marker	Long/short	A diagnostic modifier in diseases that affect Cho. ↓ *as glioma grade increases*

(H^{1}MRS) of the brain and a brief yet comprehensive explanation of their role in determining the obtained spectrum and potentially predicting their histopathological type and grade are summarised in Table 8.3.

Spectroscopic Tumor Profile

It is well known that gliomas are infiltrative tumors, which may extend and spread along the white matter tracts to the adjacent brain tissue, and frequently invade neighboring lobes, and even the contralateral hemisphere (Mikkelsen and Edvardsen, 1995). Gliomas are categorized into four grades: Pilocytic astrocytomas (WHO I), astrocytomas (WHO II), anaplastic astrocytomas, oligodendrogliomas and mixed glial tumors (WHO III) and Glioblastomas Multiforme (WHO IV). Anaplastic astrocytomas and GBM are more heterogeneous, may produce mass effect, and show variable degree of contrast enhancement. Gliomas frequently need to be differentiated from other tumors such as solitary metastases, lymphomas, but also non neoplastic lesions such as an abscess, or an evolving infarct.

There has been interest in using proton MR spectroscopic imaging (H[1]MRS) in the evaluation of the tumor borders and disease burden (Croteau et al., 2001). Moreover, several studies sought to determine a correlation between different proton H[1]MRS metabolic ratios and the degree of tumor infiltration, and examined the role of H[1]MRS in suggesting a preoperative histological diagnosis.

An important contribution of H[1]MRS is to identify the metabolic profile and the histological grade of a brain glioma. Negendank et al. (1996) and Fountas et al. (2004) concluded that glial tumors have significantly elevated Cho signals, and decreased Cr and NAA signal, compared to normal brain. Choline signal intensities were extremely high, while Cr signal intensities were very low, in anaplastic astrocytomas and GBMs in their series. They also described that anaplastic astrocytomas and GBMs demonstrated an increased Cho/Cr ratio (Table 8.2). Lipids may be detected in all grades of gliomas, however they usually present in higher concentrations in anaplastic astrocytomas and GBMs. Significant variability has been observed regarding the presence or absence of Lip peaks in low-grade gliomas. Likewise, the concentration of Lac varies significantly among patients with astrocytomas of the same histologic grade. Similarly, mI shows great variability in astrocytomas. The ratio of MI/Cr is a marker reported by Castillo et al. (2000) to be higher in low-grade astrocytomas, intermediate in control subjects, and lower in patients with anaplastic astrocytomas and GBMs.

Despite the accurate measurement of absolute metabolite concentrations, it seems that their ratios may be a more important marker in grading gliomas. Regarding the metabolite ratio findings, Fountas et al. (2004) reported NAA/Cr ratio to be decreased in all

gliomas however, they found no correlation between the degree of reduction and the tumor's histological grade. Likewise, the ratio of NAA/Cho is found to be inconsistent among tumors of the same histologic grade. Contrariwise, the Cho/Cr ratio is found to be a reproducible and consistent marker among astrocytomas of the same histologic grade. This metabolite ratio is lower in low-grade astrocytomas (grades II and III), but almost two-fold increased in GBMs. This finding suggests that the higher the Cho/Cr ratio is, the higher the tumor grade will be (Table 8.3). The ratios of Cho/Cr in grade II and III gliomas may not vary significantly, but in these cases, their conventional MRI characteristics may be helpful in their differentiation, since in grade III astrocytomas contrast enhancement is present in the vast majority of cases (Figs. 8.2 and 8.3). Moreover, the presence of lip in anaplastic astrocytomas may suggest a more aggressive histological type.

Nevertheless, gliomas need to be differentiated from other benign or malignant lesions. The most common differential diagnosis of glioma grade II and III is ischemia and infection, particularly when located in the temporal lobe. The concentration of lactate is increased in ischemia, and additionally the presence of lipids suggests necrosis in an infarcted brain area. Moreover, DWI may help differentiate acute/subacute ischemia from a low grade tumor, since ischemia shows markedly decreased diffusion. It cannot be overemphasized the importance of the patient's clinical history and symptomatology in the differential diagnosis process along with thorough interpretation of all available imaging studies.

In cases of *lymphomas*, H[1]MRS alone may not be able to distinguish them from gliomas, since both show increased Cho, reduced NAA and increased Cho/Cr and Cho/NAA ratios. In such cases, H[1]MRS combined with DWI may help in their differentiation, since lymphomas demonstrate characteristically decreased diffusivity. Furthermore, lymphomas have a more homogeneous contrast enhancement compared to gliomas, however this is certainly not a pathognomonic finding. The concordance of the above characteristics may help to establish a diagnosis in these cases.

GBM very often has conventional imaging characteristics indistinguishable from abscesses and metastases. Magnetic Resonance Spectroscopy may play an important role in the diagnosis and differentiation of these lesions. *Abscesses* uniquely contain

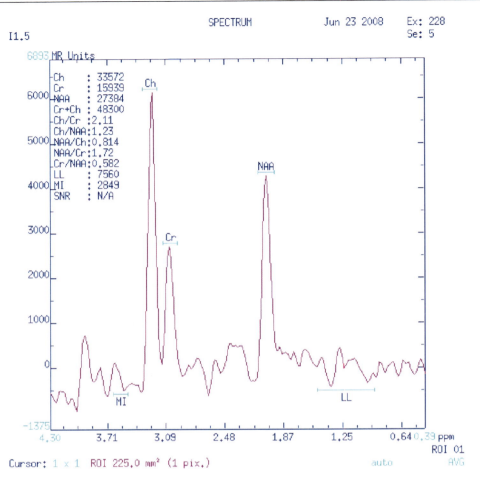

Fig. 8.2 A spectrum of a low grade astrocytoma (WHO II). Note the slightly decreased concentration of NAA and the relatively increased concentration of Cho. The concentration of Cr remains relatively unchanged. Lipids are almost undetectable

several aminoacids detectable on H[1]MRS. Moreover, abscesses have decreased diffusivity due to the decreased mobility of water protons, a finding that is not present in gliomas. Kapsalaki et al. (2008) reported the H[1]MRS characteristics of a wide variety of bacterial abscesses and also the usefulness of this methodology in distinguishing abscesses from gliomas and metastatic lesions. They outline in their study the role of H[1]MRS in identifying the causative agent of an abscess, and they point out its importance in following up the abscess's therapeutic response. The use of H[1]MRS in combination with DWI can significantly increase the diagnostic accuracy of conventional MR imaging and thus provide valuable preoperative information, regarding the nature of space occupying, ring-enhancing intracranial lesions.

Metastatic lesions, when solitary and ring enhancing, may also have indistinguishable imaging characteristics from necrotic GBMs. Both lesions show decreased, almost absent NAA, elevated Cho and decreased Cr. Lipids may also be present in both GBM and metastatic lesions, with metastatic lesions usually showing higher concentrations of lipids. On the other hand, the overall appearance of the spectrum between GBM and metastasis may occasionally be indistinguishable. In this case, H[1]MRS can differentiate between the two tumor types by evaluating the spectra at the lesion's periphery, as seen in Fig. 8.4. An infiltrating tumor, as a GBM, would yield elevated Cho and Lipids signals at the periphery of the lesion, whereas a metastasis would yield a relatively normal spectrum.

a)   b)

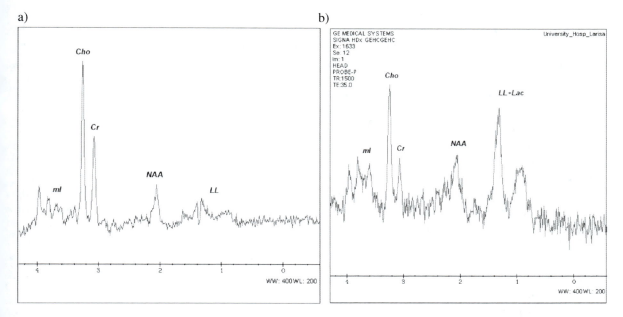

Fig. 8.3 A spectrum of an anaplastic astrocytoma (WHO III) (**a**) and (**b**): Note the decreased concentration of NAA and the markedly increased concentration of Cho in both spectra. In (**a**), the concentration of Cr remains relatively stable and lipids are almost undetectable. In (**b**), the concentration of Cr is slightly diminished and the lipids are increased, findings that possibly indicate a more aggressive type of glioma

a)   b)

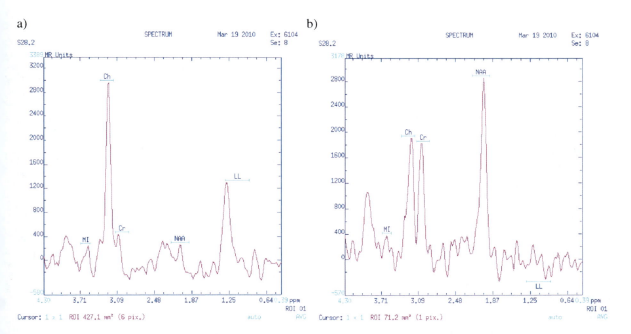

Fig. 8.4 (**a**) Spectrum obtained from the center of a tumor. Note the absence of NAA and Cr, and the markedly increased concentration of Cho. Also, there is a large amount of lipids in the tumor. These findings are characteristic of a necrotic GBM or a metastatic lesion. The presence of a normal spectrum identified in the periphery of the lesion (**b**) is more suggestive of a metastatic lesion

The major difficulty presents when we need to differentiate *radiation necrosis* from progressing or recurring glioma. Despite aggressive surgical resection along with chemotherapy and radiation, gliomas have the tendency to locally recur. An important question that is frequently raised is to differentiate in these cases between tumor recurrence versus radiation necrosis. In radiation necrosis spectrum, lipids are detected but Cho is usually not increased. However, increased levels of Cho may be seen in radiation necrosis due to the presence of inflammation. In such cases, differentiation with H[1]MRS alone is almost impossible. Other imaging modalities need to be combined, as DWI and perfusion MRI. A low Cerebral Blood Volume (CBV) through the area of contrast enhancement usually suggests radiation necrosis. On the contrary, high CBV along with increased levels of Cho and markedly increased Cho/Cr, Cho/NAA ratios is more suggestive of tumor recurrence. Despite all the recent MR advances, it is not unusual the differentiation between tumor recurrence and radiation necrosis to be still impossible. In these cases, thorough comparison with preoperative studies and close clinical and imaging follow up is of paramount importance.

Future of MRS Aided Diagnosis

It seems that we may have reached the limit of visual interpretation of spectra and as a result the field of neurospectroscopy should extend beyond qualitative analysis. Xu et al. (2008), propose at least two methods, which will take clinical MRS beyond the purely visual interpretation of a few metabolite peaks, to a richer, more automated neurochemical diagnostic concept. One is the wavelet analysis which extracts more information after data acquisition, than can currently be included in Fourier transform (FT). Another, is the widely disseminated LC Model (Provencher, 1993) which breaks the visible spectrum up into its presumed constituents, on the basis that any chemical already known to exist in the FT spectrum (so-called prior knowledge) can be outlined and quantified separately from the overlapping series of peaks we see on the screen of the MR scanner. This should only include patients in which the clinical/radiological diagnosis is uncertain.

Proton MRS is a promising diagnostic modality, which may be used to offer a better preoperative evaluation of intracranial gliomas. It may provide non invasive information regarding the histological grade of the examined tumor. It needs to be emphasized that H[1]MRS is not aiming to replace surgical biopsy in establishing a histological diagnosis. It is a complimentary method to the existent imaging modalities, which may attribute to a better preoperative evaluation of gliomas, and may also help differentiate between post-surgical radiation necrosis and tumor recurrence. H[1]MRS should be combined with conventional MR imaging and possibly all other available advanced MR imaging techniques, in order to suggest an accurate preoperative diagnosis, including tumor's histopathological type and grade.

References

Auer DP, Gossl C, Schirmer T, Czisch M (2001) Improved lipid analysis of [1]H-MR spectra in the presence of mobile lipids. Magn Reson Med 46:615–618

Barker PB, Gillard JH, van Zijl PCM, Soher BJ, Hanley DF, Agildere AM, Oppenheimer SM, Bryan RN (1994) Acute stroke: evaluation with serial proton MR spectroscopic imaging. Radiology 192:723–732

Birken DL, Oldendorf WH (1989) N-acetyl-L-aspartic acid: a literature review of a compound prominent in 1H-NMR spectroscopic studies of brain. Neurosci Biobehav Rev 13:23–31

Broer S, Broer A, Hansen J, Bubb WA, Balcar VJ, Nasrallah FA, Garner B, Rae C (2007) Alanine metabolism, transport, and cycling in the brain. J Neurochem 102:1758–1770

Brulatout S, Meric P, Loubinoux I, Borredon J, Correze JL, Roucher P, Gillet B, Berenger G, Beloeil JC, Tiffon B, Mispelter J, Seylaz J (1996) A one-dimensional (proton and phosphorus) and two-dimensional (proton) in vivo NMR spectroscopic study of reversible global cerebral ischemia. J Neurochem 66:2491–2499

Castillo M, Smith JK, Kwock L (2000) Correlation of myo-inositol levels and grading of cerebral astrocytomas. Am J Neuroradiol 21:1645–1649

Cheng LL, Chang IW, Louis DN, Gonzalez RG (1998) Correlation of high resolution magic angle spinning proton magnetic resonance spectroscopy with histopathology of intact human brain tumor specimens. Cancer Res 58: 1825–1832

Croteau D, Scarpace L, Hearshen D, Gutiérrez J, Rock J, Rosenblum M, Fisher J, Mikkelsen T (2001) Correlation between magnetic resonance spectroscopy imaging and image-guided biopsies: semi-quantitative and qualitative histo-pathologic analysis of patients with untreated glioma. Neurosurgery 49:823–829

Fountas KN, Kapsalaki E, Vogel R, Fezoulidis I, Robinson JS, Gotsis ED (2004) Noninvasive histologic grading of solid astrocytomas using proton magnetic resonance spectroscopy. Stereotact Funct Neurosurg 82:90–97

Gideon P, Henriksen O, Sperling B, Christiansen P, Olsen TS, Jorgensen HS, Arlien-Soborg P (1992) Early time course of N-acetylaspartate, creatine and phosphocreatine, and compounds containing choline in the brain after acute stroke. A proton magnetic resonance spectroscopy study. Stroke 23:1566–1572

Gotsis ED, Fountas K, Kapsalaki E, Toulas P, Peristeris G, Papadakis N (1996) In vivo proton MR spectroscopy: the diagnostic possibilities of lipid resonances in brain tumors. Anticancer Res 16:1565–1567

Howe FA, Barton SJ, Cudlip SA, Stubbs M, Saunders DE, Murphy M, Wilkins P, Opstad KS, Doyle VL, McLean MA, Bell BA, Griffiths JR (2003) Metabolic profiles of human brain tumors using quantitative in vivo 1H magnetic resonance spectroscopy. Magn Reson Med 49: 223–232

Jansen JF, Backes WH, Nicolay K, Kooi ME (2006) 1H MR spectroscopy of the brain: absolute quantification of metabolites. Radiology 240:318–332

Kallenberg K, Bock HC, Helms G, Jung K, Wrede A, Buhk JH, Giese A, Frahm J, Strik H, Dechent P, Knauth M (2009) Untreated glioblastoma multiforme: increased myo-inositol and glutamine levels in the contralateral cerebral hemisphere at proton MR spectroscopy. Radiology 253:805–812

Kapsalaki E, Gotsis ED, Fountas KN (2008) The role of proton magnetic resonance spectroscopy in the diagnosis and categorization of cerebral abscesses. Neurosurg Focus 24:E7

Kim JH, Chang KH, Na DG, Song IC, Kim SJ, Kwon BJ, Han MH (2006) Comparison of 1.5T and 3T 1H MR spectroscopy for human brain tumors. Korean J Radiol 7:156–161

Majos C, Julia-Sape M, Alonso J, Serrallonga M, Aguilera C, Acebes JJ, Arus C, Gili J (2004) Brain tumor classification by proton MR spectroscopy: comparison of diagnostic accuracy at short and long TE. Am J Neuroradiol 25:1696–1704

Manton DJ, Lowry M, Blackband SJ, Horsman A (1995) Determination of proton metabolite concentrations and relaxation parameters in normal human brain and intracranial tumours. NMR Biomed 8:104–112

Mikkelsen T, Edvardsen K (1995) Invasiveness in nervous system tumors. In Black P, Loeffler JS (eds) Cancer of the nervous system. Blackwell, Cambridge, MA

Miller BL, Chang L, Booth R, Ernst T, Cornford M, Nikas D, McBride D, Jenden DJ (1996) In vivo 1H MRS choline: correlation with in vitro chemistry/histology. Life Sci 58: 1929–1935

Negendank WG, Sauter R, Brown TR, Evelhoch JL, Falini A, Gotsis ED, Heerschap A, Kamada K, Lee BC, Mengeot MM, Moser E, Padavic-Shaller KA, Sanders JA, Spraggins TA, Stillman AE, Terwey B, Vogl TJ, Wicklow K, Zimmerman RA (1996) Proton magnetic resonance spectroscopy in patients with glial tumors: a multicenter study. J Neurosurg 84:449–458

Podo F (1999) Tumour phospholipid metabolism. NMR Biomed 7:413–439

Provencher SW (1993) Estimation of metabolite concentrations from localized in vivo proton NMR spectra. Magn Reson Med 30:672–679

Simone IL, Tortorella C, Federico F, Liguori M, Lucivero V, Giannini P, Carrara D, Bellacosa A, Livrea P (2001) Axonal damage in multiple sclerosis plaques: a combined magnetic resonance imaging and 1H-magnetic resonance spectroscopy study. J Neurol Sci 182:143–150

Sinson G, Bagley LJ, Cecil KM, Torchia M, McGowan JC, Lenkinski RE, McIntosh TK, Grossman RI (2001) Magnetization transfer imaging and proton MR spectroscopy in the evaluation of axonal injury: correlation with clinical outcome after traumatic brain injury. Am J Neuroradiol 22:143–151

Tzika AA, Cheng LL, Goumnerova L, Madsen JR, Zurakowski D, Astrakas LG, Zarifi MK, Scott RM, Anthony DC, Gonzalez RG, Black PM (2002) Biochemical characterization of pediatric brain tumors by using in vivo and ex vivo magnetic resonance spectroscopy. J Neurosurg 96: 1023–1031

Wilson M, Davies NP, Grundy RG, Peet AC (2009) A quantitative comparison of metabolite signals as detected by in vivo MRS with ex vivo 1H HR-MAS for childhood brain tumours. NMR Biomed 22:213–219

Xu V, Chan H, Lin AP, Sailasuta N, Valencerina S, Tran T, Hovener J, Ross BD (2008) MR spectroscopy in diagnosis and neurological decision-making. Semin Neurol 28: 407–422

Yudkoff M, Nissim I, Hummeler K, Medow M, Pleasure D (1986) Utilization of [15 N]glutamate by cultured astrocytes. Biochem J 234:185–192

Chapter 9

Infiltration Zone in Glioma: Proton Magnetic Resonance Spectroscopic Imaging

Oliver Ganslandt and A. Stadlbauer

Abstract In conventional magnetic resonance imaging (MRI) it is often difficult to delineate the border zone of gliomas. Proton magnetic resonance spectroscopic imaging (^{1}H-MRSI) is a noninvasive tool for investigating the spatial distribution of metabolic changes in brain lesions. In this chapter we describe the improvements in delineation of gliomas based on segmentation of metabolic changes measured with ^{1}H-MRSI. Metabolic maps for choline (Cho), N-acetyl-aspartate (NAA) and Cho/NAA ratios were calculated and segmented based on the assumption of Gaussian distribution of the Cho/NAA values for normal brain. Areas of hyperintensity on T2-weighted MR images were compared with the areas of the segmented tumour on Cho/NAA maps. Stereotactic biopsies were obtained from the MRSI/T2w difference areas. We found that the segmented MRSI tumour areas were greater than the T2w hyperintense areas on average by 20% (range 6–34%). In nearly half of the patients biopsy sampling from the MRSI/T2w difference areas showed tumour infiltration ranging from 4 to 17% (mean 9%) tumour cells in the areas detected only by MRSI. This method for automated segmentation of the lesions related metabolic changes achieves significantly improved delineation for gliomas compared clinical routine. In this chapter we demonstrate that this method can improve delineation of tumour borders compared to imaging strategies in clinical routine. Metabolic images of the segmented tumour may thus be helpful for therapeutic planning.

Keywords Infiltration · Tumor cells · MRI · MRSI · Choline · Histogram

Introduction

Gliomas are a group of brain tumors that account for ~40–67% of primary brain tumors. The incidence rate is calculated with ~4.0/100,000. Unfortunately, for the past 30 years no significant improvement in the survival rate of gliomas has been achieved in spite of significant progress both in neurosurgical techniques and molecular and cytogenetic science. Imaging and treatment of gliomas still pose one of the greatest challenges in cancer medicine and require a multidisciplinary cooperation of neuroradiologists, neurosurgeons, radiation oncologists and neurologists. A fundamental problem in imaging of glioma, is the fact that the true extent of tumor cell infiltration into the brain tissue is not depicted sufficiently by conventional magnetic resonance imaging (MRI). This problem is caused by the diffuse and infiltrative growth pattern of gliomas leading to an ill defined tumor border which, in consequence, makes every therapeutic approach difficult. Magnetic Resonance imaging techniques like T2-weighted and contrast enhanced MRI usually represents the methods of choice in clinical routine imaging. These imaging protocols, however, are not specific for gliomas and can result in ambiguous and misleading results. For this reason, innovative imaging modalities are needed to provide additional information on the extent of these lesions.

Magnetic Resonance spectroscopic imaging (MRSI) is a non-invasive tool for investigating the

O. Ganslandt (✉)
Department of Neurosurgery, University of
Erlangen-Nuremberg, 91054 Erlangen, Germany
e-mail: ganslandt@nch.imed.uni-erlangen.de

M.A. Hayat (ed.), *Tumors of the Central Nervous System, Volume 1*,
DOI 10.1007/978-94-007-0344-5_9, © Springer Science+Business Media B.V. 2011

spatial distribution of biochemical changes in brain lesions. Although in vivo MR spectroscopy is not able to detect metabolites which provide information about the infiltration of tumor cells per se, it is possible to detect specific patterns in the changes of metabolite concentrations compared to normal brain. Several studies have reported increased levels of choline-containing compounds (Cho) and a reduction in signal intensity of N-acetyl-aspartate (NAA) and creatine (Cr) in brain tumors. Choline-containing compounds are composed of choline, phosphocholine, and glycerophosphocholine and are thought to be markers for increased membrane turnover or higher cellular density. N-acetyl-aspartate is regarded as a neuronal marker mainly contained within neurons. The Cr peak is a signal from both creatine and phosphocreatine, and plays a role in tissue energy metabolism. The range of Cho increase and NAA decrease is compatible with the range of tumor infiltration (Stadlbauer et al., 2006). For pathologies that appear similar to brain tumors in conventional MR, imaging variations in changes of the above mentioned, as well as in other metabolites (inositol, lactate, lipids, glutamine/glutamate, alanine) can be used for differential diagnosis. This chapter outlines the strategies of visualization and intraoperative detection of biochemical changes in the infiltration zone of gliomas using MRSI.

Principle of Magnetic Resonance Spectroscopic Imaging

The basic principle of MR spectroscopy as in MR imaging, is the phenomenon of nuclear magnetic resonance. While MRI employs protons in water molecules to create images, MR spectroscopy offers the possibility to detect the chemical environment of protons in biologically significant molecules. Protons in different molecules are electromagnetically shielded according to the specific structure of the chemical bindings forced by the electrons. This results in a shift of the resonance frequency relative to the resonance frequency of water, thus leading to a profile of different resonance frequencies, a so-called spectrum. Two common approaches in MR spectroscopy are single voxel spectroscopy and chemical shift imaging.

Magnetic Resonance Imaging and Proton Magnetic Resonance Spectroscopic Imaging

Magnetic Resonance imaging and proton MR spectroscopic imaging (^{1}H-MRSI) were performed on a 1.5 T clinical whole body scanner (MAGNETOM Sonata, Siemens, Erlangen, Germany) equipped with the standard head coil. For evaluation of metabolic changes caused by tumor infiltration in the tumor border of 20 glioma patients (WHO grade II and III gliomas) we used the following MR protocol. Conventional MR imaging for diagnosis of glioma grade II or III consisted of (1) an axial turbo spin echo (TSE) sequence (T2-weighted, 5 mm section thickness, TR/TE 5600-6490/98 ms), (2) an axial fluid-attenuated inversion recovery (FLAIR) sequence (5 mm section thickness, TR/TE 10000/103 ms), and (3) pre- and post-gadolinium contrast enhanced coronal gradient echo (GE) sequences (T1-weighted, 5 mm section thickness, TR/TE 430/12 ms and 525/17 ms, respectively).

In each ^{1}H-MRSI session, a localization scan and an axial spin echo (SE) sequence (T1-weighted, TR/TE 500/15 ms, 256×256 matrix size, 16×16 cm FOV, 20 slices with no gap and a slice thickness of 2 mm) were acquired and used for both planning the MRSI experiment and integration of spectroscopic data into a stereotactic system. The volume of interest (VOI) of the MRSI experiment with PRESS (Point-RESolved Spectroscopy) volume preselection was aligned parallel to the axial T1w SE slices, and positioned to exclude lipids of the skull and subcutaneous fat. Water suppression was achieved using three CHESS (CHEmical Shift Selective) pulses prior to the PRESS excitation. The MR spectroscopic imaging parameters were TR/TE 1600/135 ms, 24×24 circular phase encoding scheme across a 16×16 cm FOV, slice thickness 10 mm, 50% Hamming filter and 2 NEX, spectral width 1000 Hz and 1024 complex points acquisition size. The total spectroscopic data acquisition time was < 13 min. The nominal voxel size was $0.67 \times 0.67 \times 1.0$ cm^3 (~0.45 cm^3 resolution). After zero-filling to 32×32 matrix size, the volume of a voxel relevant for post-processing with LCModel (Linear Combination of Model spectra) was 0.25 cm^3.

For registration to the frameless stereotactic system, six adhesive skin fiducials were placed in a scattered pattern on the head surface. To obtain a neuronavigation MR data set a three-dimensional (3D) anatomic magnetization prepared rapid acquisition gradient echo (MPRAGE) sequence was performed before surgery with the following parameters: TR/TE 2020/4.38 ms, 25 × 25 cm FOV, 1 mm isotropic and 160 slices.

Magnetic Resonance Spectroscopic Imaging Data Analysis

MRSI data sets were processed with the freely available reconstruction program csx (for Linux), obtained from PB Barker (Baltimore, USA). Spectroscopic imaging data were exponentially filtered with a line broadening factor of 3 Hz, zero filled to 2048 data points and Fourier transformed with respect to the spectral dimension. To remove the residual water peak we used a high-pass convolution filter (50 Hz stop band). Magnitude spectra were calculated, the position of NAA was set to 2.02 ppm and a susceptibility correction was applied. The peak areas for Cho, Cr and NAA were calculated by integration over the frequency range of 3.34—3.14 ppm, 3.14–2.94 ppm, and 2.22–1.82 ppm, respectively. Smooth linear interpolation to a 256 × 256 matrix resulted in the metabolic maps. Cho and NAA images were used to calculate a map of Cho/NAA ratios.

The procedure for segmentation of the tumor border due to the biochemical changes was based on the following assumptions: (1) the values for Cho/NAA in normal brain follow a Gaussian distribution, and (2) those for the tumor, including the border zone, are significantly increased (Stadlbauer et al., 2004a). A "healthy region" of predominantly white matter on the contralateral side and sufficient distance from the lesion according to the Cho/NAA ratio map was selected. The size of this region should be sufficient for statistical evaluation, i.e., to proof Gaussian distribution, and should have no relation, to the size of the tumor. The characteristics of Gaussian distribution are: unimodal, symmetric, and mean = median = modal value (mode). The first and the second properties were checked by inspection of the histogram, the latter by calculation and comparison of the three characteristic parameters for the Cho/NAA values of the selected region. The test for Gaussian distribution

given by David et al., (1954) was additionally performed. As it pertains to the Gaussian distribution, there is a relationship between the proportion of cases in between + or − each standard deviation (SD) from the mean. The relationships are: mean ± 1SD is related to 68.3% proportion of cases, mean ± 2SD is related to 95.4% proportion of cases and mean ± 3SD is related to 99.7% proportion of cases. The mean and the standard deviation of the Cho/NAA ratios were calculated for the selected region and all Cho/NAA values in the whole map less than the mean + 3SD were set to zero. This enabled the elimination of all but 0.3% normal brain areas in the Cho/NAA map and hence the segmentation of the tumor (Stadlbauer et al., 2004a).

The user-independent spectral fit program LCModel (version 6.0) was used for quantification of MRSI data (Provencher, 1993). The spectra were analyzed as a linear combination of a set of reference basis spectra for PRESS and TE 135 ms. Metabolite values in arbitrary units (a.u.) for Cho, Cr and NAA for the voxel positions of the MRSI data at biopsy sampling points were calculated on a workstation (SGI, Mountain View, CA, USA), using the LCModel program. Additionally 20 – 30 voxels of predominantly white matter in contralateral brain tissue were selected to obtain metabolite values from normal appearing white matter (NAWM). Spectral fits were performed in an analysis window from 1.0 to 3.85 ppm. Spectra with a signal-to-noise ratio (SNR) < 2 and a full width at half maximum (FWHM) > 0.075 ppm were not included. The metabolite values of Cho, Cr and NAA of the individual voxels were used for calculation of metabolite ratios Cho/Cr, NAA/Cr, and Cho/NAA.

Magnetic Resonance Imaging Evaluation

The T2w TSE data set of the routine tumor MRI of the patients was contoured automatically by the medical imaging software OSIRIS (version 4.17) obtained from the University Hospital of Geneva, Switzerland. The T2w area was contoured as the area of hyperintensity on the TSE images. The maximum of the calculated T2w hyperintensity areas covered by the PRESS-box delineated on the TSE images, corresponding to the MRSI slab, was used for comparison with the area of the segmented tumor in the Cho/NAA map.

Magnetic Resonance Spectroscopic Image – Guided Stereotactic Bopsy and Histopathologic Evaluation

Integration of MR spectroscopic data, as segmented Cho/NAA ratio map, were obtained using a combined data set consisting of MR imaging and MR spectroscopic imaging data, a

So-called MRI/MRSI hybrid data set (Fig. 9.1a) (Stadlbauer et al., 2004b). The hybrid data set was transferred to the planning workstation of the navigation system (VectorVision Sky, Brain LAB, Heimstetten, Germany) and a semi-automated coregistration (VV2 Planning 1.3, BrainLAB, Heimstetten, Germany) to the 3D MPRAGE data set was applied using a rigid registration algorithm. This fused 3D MR data set was used for frameless stereotaxy and MR spectroscopy guided biopsy sampling.

Prior to the tumor resection, biopsies were sampled in several regions according to the segmented metabolic map representing the pathological metabolite change of tumor tissue by using a stereotactic needle which was tracked by the navigation system. This procedure, performed before the tumor resection, ensured a minimal interference of brain shift which otherwise, would render the neuronavigation inaccurate. The coordinates of each biopsy locus were labeled and documented in the fused 3D MR data set by neurosurgeons. The histopathological findings of each specimen were traced back to the exact voxel positions in the fused MR data set containing the spectroscopic information. All glioma specimens were histologically examined according to the WHO classification of tumors of the nervous system. Tumor cells were identified using formalin-fixed and paraffin-embedded sections, either stained with hematoxylin-eosin (HE) or monoclonal antibodies against p53 (Dako, Glostrup,

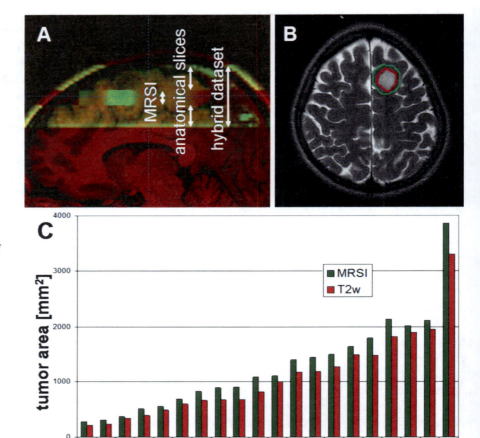

Fig. 9.1 (**a**) Image fusion of the MRI/MRSI hybrid data and a 3D MRI dataset (3D-MPRAGE). (**b**) Comparison of MRI/MRSI-defined tumor areas. Anatomical images (T2w) overlaid with tumor border contours of the MRSI experiment (*green*) and T2w hyperintensity (*red*). (**c**) Quantitative comparison of MRI/MRSI-defined tumor areas of 20 patients. Tumor areas in the segmented Cho/NAA maps are shown in *green* and T2w hyperintense areas in *red*

Denmark), MAP2c (clone), or Ki67 (Dako). MAP2c is a microtubule associated protein which is solely expressed in neuronal cells and glial tumor cells (48). Semiquantitative assessment of tumor cells versus pre-existing brain parenchyma was obtained microscopically using analysis software (Soft Imaging System, Leinenfeld-Echterdingen, Germany) at 200 times magnification in five different subfields of 348×261 µm in size. Only cells with a distinct nucleus were considered. All data were calculated as mean tumor cell number as a percentage of the number of whole cells (% tumor infiltration, %TI).

Results

Metabolic Maps and Segmentation

The values of the selected contralateral regions in the Cho/NAA ratio maps were checked for Gaussian distribution. All histograms showed an almost unimodal and symmetric distribution. Also the test of David (David et al., 1954) confirmed our assumption. The mean, median and modal value for the ratios in the selected normal brain region differed by less than 3%. These results also confirmed our assumption of Gaussian distribution of the Cho/NAA ratios in normal brain.

MRI/MRSI Tumor Area Comparison and Biopsy Sampling

Our method for coregistration of MRI and MRSI data using a MRI/MRSI hybrid data set (Fig. 9.1a) allows the direct comparison of T2w hyperintense areas (red line in Fig. 9.1b) and the areas of the segmented tumor in the Cho/NAA ratio map (green line in Fig. 9.1b). Also, the fact that the PRESS selected region (PRESS-box) did not always include the entire T2w hyperintense area, was thus unproblematic. All patients had segmented MRSI tumor areas that were greater than the T2w hyperintense areas covered by PRESS-box (Fig. 9.1c). The tumor areas according to the T2w hyperintensity ranged from 220–3301 mm^2, and those according to MRSI ranged from 277 to 3864 mm^2. The

amount of larger MRSI tumor areas compared to T2w areas was 20% on average (range 6–34%).

The frameless stereotactic software allowed tracking back the biopsy locations to the exact voxel position in the MR data set. For verification of the higher sensitivity in detection of pathologic changes of the MRSI experiment combined with the segmentation algorithm, we used biopsies obtained from the difference area (Fig. 9.2a, b). In nine patients, biopsy sampling from a predefined area was successful, and histological findings showed tumor infiltration ranging from ~4 to 17% (mean 9%) p53 or Map2c positive cells (e.g., 5% Map2c positive cells in Fig. 9.2c).

Figure 9.2 depicts an illustrative case of a 20 year old female patient with an astrocytoma WHO grade II. A screenshot from a view through the eyepieces of the navigation microscope and from the neuronavigation system is shown in Fig. 9.2a, b, respectively. The biopsy sampling point at the tumor border (orange cross), and the voxel positions #1 (contralateral normal brain) and #2 (biopsy sampling point) are superimposed on an axial T1-weighted MR image (red squares in Fig. 9.2B). Histopathologic evaluation of the biopsy reveals a %TI of 5% (Fig. 9.2c). Spectra fitted by LCModel for the voxel position #1 and #2, are given in Figures 2D (contralateral NAWM) and E (tumor border), respectively. Overlaid onto these images are the metabolite values for Cho, Cr, and NAA in arbitrary units (a.u.) which calculated for these individual voxels.

For the nine patients with biopsies from the tumor border, the metabolite values and metabolite ratios for the voxels at the biopsy locus were: Cho = 443 ± 82 a.u. (303–534 a.u.), NAA = 1897 ± 376 a.u. (1376–2419 a.u.), and Cr = 1028 ± 264 a.u. (682–1432 a.u.); and Cho/Cr = 0.45 ± 0.11 (0.32–0.69), NAA/Cr = 1.93 ± 0.49 (0.96–2.68), and Cho/NAA = 0.24 ± 0.07 (0.18–0.39), respectively. The metabolite values and metabolite ratios for contralateral normal brain were found with the following values: Cho = 451 ± 68 a.u. (343–562 a.u.), NAA = 2522 ± 340 a.u. (2056–3140 a.u.), and Cr = 1235 ± 172 a.u. (1020–1543 a.u.); and Cho/Cr = 0.37 ± 0.06 (0.29–0.46), NAA/Cr = 2.07 ± 0.34 (1.33–2.45), and Cho/NAA = 0.18 ± 0.03 (0.14–0.22), respectively.

Two-sided paired t tests only revealed significant differences between spectroscopic finding at biopsy site and contralateral normal brain for NAA

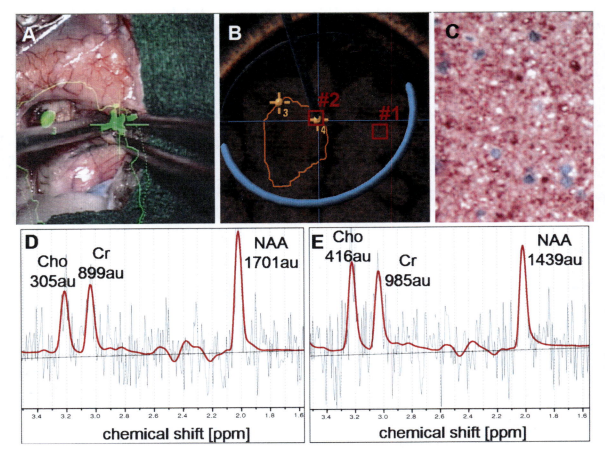

Fig. 9.2 (**a**) Intraoperative view through navigation microscope with tumor segmentation *(green line)* and biopsy site *(green marker)*. (**b**) Screenshot from navigation system with tumor segmentation *(orange line)*, biopsy site *(orange markers)*, and voxel positions #1 (contralateral normal brain) and #2 (tumor border) of the spectra shown in 2D and 2E, respectively. '2C: histologic result with 5% tumor cells

$(P = 0.001)$, Cr $(P = 0.013)$, Cho/Cr $(P = 0.028)$, and Cho/NAA $(P = 0.026)$, but not for Cho and NAA/Cr.

Discussion

Magnetic Resonance Spectroscopic Imaging is a promising tool to detect changes in the spatial distribution of metabolites in the brain. So far this technique has been used in a number of studies for mainly four clinical purposes: differential diagnosis (e.g., radionecrosis vs. viable tumor, grading of gliomas) (Pirzkall et al., 2002), delineation of treatment planning in radiation therapy, planning of stereotactic brain biopsy and response to treatment (Dowling et al., 2001).

However, due to the lack of standardized methods for evaluation of multidimensional spectroscopic data, MRSI has not yet become a routine, clinical tool. Therefore T2-weighted MRI, and pre- and post-gadolinium contrast enhanced T1-weighted MRI are usually the basis for surgical or radiation therapy treatment planning for brain tumors. In an attempt to overcome these limitations, we developed an automated method for delineation and segmentation of the lesion's metabolic changes. We achieved significantly improved delineation for gliomas, compared to the imaging strategies performed during a routine clinical. Biopsy samples from the area detected as tumor only by MRSI were obtained to proove our findings. However, it is possible that p53 and Map 2c could be found beyond our calculation of tumor pathology based on metabolic changes determined by ^{1}H-MRSI.

Visualization of metabolic changes in brain tumors has been achieved via different approaches. Images of different metabolite ratios (Cho/NAA, Cho/Cr and Cr/NAA) were utilized by Li et al. (2002) for evaluating and characterizing gliomas. De Edelenyi et al. (2000) showed six major metabolite peaks (Cho, Cr, NAA, alanine, lactate and/or lipids, and lipids) and information contained in T2-weighted MR images in a profile, so-called nosologic images, and used them for characterization of brain tumors.

In a recent publication McKnight et al. (2001) showed that the use of Cho/NAA ratios is suitable for delineation of the tumor border . They assumed that the relation between Cho and NAA in normal brain could be modeled as a linear function and used this to select voxels as internal controls for quantifying the probability of abnormality at each voxel location in patients with gliomas. In further studies of this group they achieved segmentation of brain tumors using this method and the definition of abnormality index contours (Pirzkall et al., 2001, 2002). These contours and contours for T1w region of contrast enhancement and T2w region of hyperintensity were overlaid onto anatomical images, or on maps of Cho/NAA, and used for target delineation in radiation therapy treatment planning (Nelson et al., 2002). For low grade glioma they found that in 55% of their patients the MRSI contour was contained totally within the T2w contour. Furthermore, MRSI defined pathologic changes extending beyond the hyperintense T2w region were quite small, and not distributed uniformly. For high grade glioma they found that a metabolically active tumor extended outside the hyperintense T2w region in 88% of their patients. However, their findings were not validated by histology and, in contrast to their methods, our approach is to segment the tumor in the metabolic image. This method reflects the pathology of the tumor in a more realistic way because tissue containing different levels of tumor infiltration is displayed according to its spatial distribution.

In this chapter, we present a technique for the integration of high-resolution MRSI information into the neurosurgical operating room. We used a combined imaging data set consisting of conventional MRI slices and segmented metabolic maps of the MRSI slice, a so-called MRI/MRSI hybrid data set, for merging biochemical information in a global 3D MRI. Drawing ROIs based on metabolic images allows intraoperative visualization of these ROIs to be displayed through the eyepieces of the microscope, leading to a MRSI guided tumor resection.

Furthermore, we used MRSI for determining changes in metabolite values of Cho, Cr, and NAA and metabolite ratios (Cho/Cr, Cho/tNAA and Cho/tNAA) at the tumor border with low tumor cell infiltration. The findings were compared to values on contralateral NAWM. We demonstrated that NAA, Cr, Cho/Cr, and Cho/NAA showed significant differences in comparison to a normal brain, but interestingly, not Cho and NAA/Cr. These results demonstrated that the assumption of a stable Cr concentration, which is required for quantification of metabolite values using ratios with Cr as denominator, is not supportable for the border zone of gliomas. Hence the calculation of NAA/Cr and Cho/Cr for determination of metabolic changes led to delusive results suggesting significant changes for Cho but not for NAA. 1H MRSI seems to be a promising method to characterize the non visible extent of glioma invasion into the brain. Progress will be expected from measurements at higher field strengths as 3T MR scanners emerge into wider use. However, it will be necessary to implement 3D chemical shift imaging and achieve a higher spatial resolution.

References

David HA, Hartley HO, Pearson ES (1954) The distribution of the ratio, in a single normal sample, of range to standard deviation. Biometrika 41:482–493

De Edelenyi FS, Rubin C, Esteve F, Grand S, Decorps M, Lefournier V, Le Bas JF, Remy C (2000) A new approach for analyzing proton magnetic resonance spectroscopic images of brain tumors: nosologic images. Nat Med 6: 1287–1289

Dowling C, Bollen AW, Noworolski SM, McDermott MW, Barbaro NM, Day MR, Henry RG, Chang SM, Dillon WP, Nelson SJ, Vigneron DB (2001) Preoperative proton MR spectroscopic imaging of brain tumors: correlation with histopathologic analysis of resection specimens. AJNR Am J Neuroradiol 22:604–612

Li X, Lu Y, Pirzkall A, McKnight T, Nelson SJ (2002) Analysis of the spatial characteristics of metabolic abnormalities in newly diagnosed glioma patients. J Magn Reson Imaging 16:229–237

McKnight TR, Noworolski SM, Vigneron DB, Nelson SJ (2001) An automated technique for the quantitative assessment of 3d-MRSI data from patients with glioma. J Magn Reson Imaging 13:167–177

Nelson SJ, Graves E, Pirzkall A, Li X, Chan AA, Vigneron DB, McKnight TR (2002) In vivo molecular imaging for planning radiation therapy of gliomas: an application of 1h MRSI. J Magn Reson Imaging 16:464–476

Pirzkall A, McKnight TR, Graves EE, Carol MP, Sneed PK, Wara WW, Nelson SJ, Verhey LJ, Larson DA (2001) MR-spectroscopy guided target delineation for high-grade gliomas. Int J Radiat Oncol Biol Phys 50: 915–928

Pirzkall A, Nelson SJ, McKnight TR, Takahashi MM, Li X, Graves EE, Verhey LJ, Wara WW, Larson DA, Sneed PK (2002) Metabolic imaging of low-grade gliomas with three-dimensional magnetic resonance spectroscopy. Int J Radiat Oncol Biol Phys 53:1254–1264

Provencher SW (1993) Estimation of metabolite concentrations from localized in vivo proton NMR spectra. Magn Reson Med 30:672–679

Stadlbauer A, Gruber S, Nimsky C, Fahlbusch R, Hammen T, Buslei R, Tomandl B, Moser E, Ganslandt O (2006) Preoperative grading of gliomas by using metabolite quantification with high-spatial-resolution proton MR spectroscopic imaging. Radiology 238:958–969

Stadlbauer A, Moser E, Gruber S, Buslei R, Nimsky C, Fahlbusch R, Ganslandt O (2004a) Improved delineation of brain tumors: an automated method for segmentation based on pathologic changes of 1 h-MRSI metabolites in gliomas. Neuroimage 23:454–461

Stadlbauer A, Moser E, Gruber S, Nimsky C, Fahlbusch R, Ganslandt O (2004b) Integration of biochemical images of a tumor into frameless stereotaxy achieved using a magnetic resonance imaging/magnetic resonance spectroscopy hybrid data set. J Neurosurg 101:287–294

Chapter 10

Malignant Gliomas: Role of E2F1 Transcription Factor

Marta M. Alonso, Juan Fueyo, and Candelaria Gomez-Manzano

Abstract E2F1 is a transcription factor regulated by the Rb pathway. Its role in the G1/S transition and S-phase entry in the cell cycle has been extensively reported. E2F1 regulates the biosynthetic activity of nucleotides, the activation of replication, the progression through M-phase of the cell cycle, and the regulation of genes related with chromosomal stability. In addition to the E2F1 crucial involvement in the cell cycle progression, E2F1 participates in both p53-dependent and independent apoptotic pathways. Our group has previously published the presence of high expression of E2F1 in malignant gliomas and the correlation of levels of expression with prognostic factor. Moreover, we reported the direct implication of E2F1 in tumorigenicity using transgenic animal models. Recent results from The Cancer Genome Atlas Research Network confirms the presence in human glioblastomas of the genetic alterations in the Rb tumor suppressor pathway, supporting previous reports describing high E2F1 activity in gliomas. In this chapter, we describe methodology to examine the presence of high expression and activity of E2F1, and a practical approach to examine the targeting of this major transcription factor.

Keywords E2F · Glioma · Expression · Transcription · Methodology

Introduction

E2F1 was first identified in 1986, when it was described as a cellular transcription factor that was bound to the adenoviral E2 gene promoter (Kovesdi et al., 1986a, b; Kovesdi et al., 1987). It was not until 1991 that its regulation by the tumor suppressor retinoblastoma (Rb) protein was described (Bandara and La Thangue, 1991; Chellappan et al., 1991). Rb was initially identified as a genetic locus associated with the development of an inherited eye tumor (Friend et al., 1986; Knudson, 1971). The realization that the loss of Rb function was associated with disease established the tumor suppressor paradigm (Cavenee et al., 1983). Rb was found to be an important target of oncoproteins that are expressed by DNA tumor viruses, such as adenovirus E1A, simian virus 40 T antigen, and the E7 proteins of human papillomaviruses (Classon and Harlow, 2002). Evaluation of this hypothesis led to the identification of the E2F1 transcription factor, the first identified cellular target of Rb (Helin et al., 1992; Kaelin et al., 1992; Nevins, 1992). E2F1 was later found to be a member of a family of closely related proteins, several of which were found to also directly interact with Rb (Trimarchi and Lees, 2002).

According to most current models, Rb controls cell cycle progression through its repressive effects on gene expression, which are mediated by the E2F family of transcription factors (Classon and Harlow, 2002; Dyson, 1998). The number of identified E2F family members has been steadily increasing: so far, eight human E2F genes have been described (E2F1-E2F8) (Christensen et al., 2005; Dyson, 1998; Harbour and Dean, 2000; Trimarchi and Lees, 2002), which can be divided into three categories on the basis of their

C. Gomez-Manzano (✉)
Department of Neuro-Oncology, University of Texas M.D. Anderson Cancer Center, Houston, TX 77030, USA
e-mail: cmanzano@mdanderson.org

M.A. Hayat (ed.), *Tumors of the Central Nervous System, Volume 1*,
DOI 10.1007/978-94-007-0344-5_10, © Springer Science+Business Media B.V. 2011

transcriptional properties and interaction potential with pocket proteins (Rb, p107, p130). E2F1, 2, and 3 are potent transcriptional activators that interact directly with Rb protein. E2F4 and 5 are classified as weak activators and appear to be able to interact with all three pocket proteins (Trimarchi and Lees, 2002). E2F6, 7, and 8 do not associate with pocket proteins and are believed to repress transcription (Trimarchi et al., 2001). E2F members interact with a DP protein (either DP1 or DP2) to form a heterodimer that is functionally capable of binding a consensus E2F site with high affinity. However, the function of the E2F-DP heterodimer is determined by the E2F subunit. E2F consensus binding sites are found in the promoter region of many, if not all, genes required for cellular proliferation, but how repressor and activator E2F complexes regulate E2F targets remains largely unknown. Evidence suggests that additional levels of transcriptional binding regulation exist within the cell and that different E2F complexes accumulate in different phases of the cell cycle (Sardet et al., 1995; Won et al., 2004).

The most intensively studied and best-understood function of E2F is its regulation of the G1/S transition and S-phase entry in the cell cycle (Dyson, 1998; Nevins, 1998), by regulating the expression of proteins responsible for DNA replication and cell cycle progression, such as DNA polymerase and proliferating cell nuclear antigen. E2F also regulates the biosynthetic activity of nucleotides by regulating expression levels of thymidine kinase, thymidylate synthase, and ribonucleotide reductase. In addition, initiation factors that assemble into a pre-replication complex at the origin of replication are under the transcriptional control of E2F (Leone et al., 1998). In cell cycle progression, E2F directs the synthesis of both cyclin E and cdk2, creating the kinase activity responsible for the activation of replication. In a feedback mechanism, cyclin E/cdk2 enhances the inactivation of Rb, thus inhibiting the release of E2F1 that was initiated by cyclin D/cdk4 (Harbour et al., 1999; Lundberg and Weinberg, 1998). The Rb/E2F pathway controls virtually the entire activation process of DNA replication and G1/S transition regulation.

Recent evidence demonstrates that E2F regulates the expression of several genes involved in the progression through M-phase of the cell cycle, such as cyclin B1 and B2, Bub1, and cdc2 (Muller et al., 2001). In addition, E2F has been found to directly regulate the transcription of genes involved in chromatin condensation (smc2 and smc4), the spindle checkpoint (Bub3 and mad2), and chromosome segregation (centromere protein and securin) (Ren et al., 2002). Some of these genes are known to induce aberrant spindle behavior when overexpressed, and deregulated expression of these targets may contribute to chromosomal instability. It is not clear how E2F contributes to the regulation of these promoters in vivo. One model suggests that in normal cells, these targets are initially repressed by E2F in G0 or G1 phase and then strongly activated at later stages of the cell cycle (Stevaux and Dyson, 2002). Functional studies also suggest that the role of E2F and the effects of deregulated activity extend beyond the G1/S transition (Hernando et al., 2004).

In addition to cell cycle progression, E2F1 participates in a protective apoptotic pathway that eliminates cells that have lost normal cell cycle control. Early studies indicated that increased E2F1 levels resulted in increased stability of the p53 protein and thus, induction of apoptosis. Ectopic expression of E2F1 led to apoptosis, and this phenomenon was observed in quiescent cultured cells subsequent to S-phase entry and also in transgenic mice (La Thangue, 2003). E2F1 can transcriptionally activate several other pro-apoptotic genes, such as Apaf-1 and other members of the caspase gene family that may contribute to p53-independent apoptosis. However, recent evidence suggests that p53-independent, E2F1-mediated apoptosis occurs mostly through direct transcriptional activation of the p53 homologue p73 (Irwin et al., 2000).

The mechanisms that determine proliferation and death in cells with deregulated E2F1 are unknown. Many researchers are using a model of E2F action that is based predominately on thresholds: activating E2Fs contribute to a pool of free E2F activity that induces inappropriate proliferation at a critical threshold level but apoptosis at another, higher threshold level (Ziebold et al., 2001). Furthermore, E2F1 acetylation has been shown to promote p73 induction, which leads to apoptosis (Irwin et al., 2000), suggesting that apoptotic regulation by E2F1 is post-transcriptionally mediated. An E2F transactivation-independent mechanistic model has also been proposed in which increased levels of the E2F1 protein complex and p53 or cyclin A result in apoptosis or survival, respectively (Kowalik et al., 1998).

Evaluation of E2F Expression in Gliomas and Prognostic Significance

Glioblastoma is the most common and malignant primary neoplasm of the central nervous system. Despite advances in surgery, radiotherapy, and chemotherapy, glioma patients have a poor prognosis, with a median survival duration of a little over 1 year (Wen and Kesari, 2008). Genetic alteration that affects the proteins that govern phosphorylation of Rb, inducing uncontrolled cell cycle progression, are commonly found in human brain tumors (Ueki et al., 1996). Indeed, there is evidence of mutations, deletions, or amplifications in several members of this pathway. The resultant inactivation of this pathway leads to an excess of free E2F. Interestingly, even though no gene amplification or mutation has been reported, E2F1 activity is high in these tumors. Parr and colleagues showed that E2F-responsive promoters were more active in gliomas than in normal cells because of free E2F and loss of phosphorylated Rb/E2F repressor complexes (Parr et al., 1997).

We reported elevated E2F1 expression at the protein or mRNA levels in 61 tumor samples (Alonso et al., 2005). We also showed that a transgenic mouse model engineered to express E2F1 specifically within glial cells (GFAP-tgE2F1), to the end of mimicking our findings in human samples, developed a highly penetrant tumorigenic phenotype: 20% of the animals developed brain tumors (Olson et al., 2007). Importantly, the distribution of tumors according to mouse age suggested the existence of a bimodal pattern of tumor development, similar to that in human disease. At an early age, mice with deregulated E2F1 show the formation of embryonal brain tumors such as medulloblastoma, choroid plexus carcinoma, and primary neuroectodermal tumor. Conversely, at an older age, mice that escaped embryonic tumor formation developed malignant gliomas, which are typically found in human adults. This study provided the first evidence of a global role for E2F1 in the formation and maintenance of multilineage brain tumors, thus establishing E2F1 as an oncogene in the brain.

Several research groups have reported an association between E2F1 overexpression and poor outcome in tumors such as oesophageal squamous cell carcinomas (Yamazaki et al., 2005); gastrointestinal stromal tumors (Haller et al., 2005); lymph node-positive breast cancers treated with fluorouracil, doxorubicin, and cyclophosphamide (Han et al., 2003); and breast neoplasias (Zhang et al., 2000). We found that E2F1 was overexpressed in two independent collections of patient samples consisting of 34 and 27 glioma specimens. Longer median survival was statistically significantly associated with lower E2F1 expression in tumors (103.6 weeks) rather than with higher expression (difference = 57.5 weeks; 95% confidence interval = 14.7 to 159.7; log-rank P = .002) (Alonso et al., 2005). At the present time, the value of E2F1 as a prognostic factor still remains under investigation, partly because of its paradoxical function in cancer (i.e., oncogene versus tumor suppressor) and the scarcity of studies on this topic.

In the following section, we describe the methodology used by our group for quantifying the expression of E2F1 in surgical tumor samples. Specifically, RNA levels were analyzed by quantitative PCR (Q-PCR) (Fig. 10.1).

Materials

1. Frozen tumor samples
2. Mortar and pestle
3. Blades
4. Dry ice
5. Liquid nitrogen
6. Trizol (Invitrogen, Eugene, OR)
7. DNAzap (ABI Systems, Foster City, CA)
8. 21-gauge needles
9. Isopropanol (Sigma, St. Louis, MO)
10. dNTPs (Invitrogen, Eugene, OR)
11. Oligo (dt) (Invitrogen, Eugene, OR)
12. Reverse transcriptase (Invitrogen, Eugene, OR)
13. E2F1 and GAPDH taqman probes (ABI Systems, Foster City, CA)
14. Polymerase chain reaction (PCR) master mix (ABI Systems, Foster City, CA)
15. Optical plates (ABI Systems, Foster City, CA)
16. Plate caps (ABI Systems, Foster City, CA)
17. QT-PCR machine

Methods

1. Immediately store tumor samples in liquid nitrogen after surgical resection.

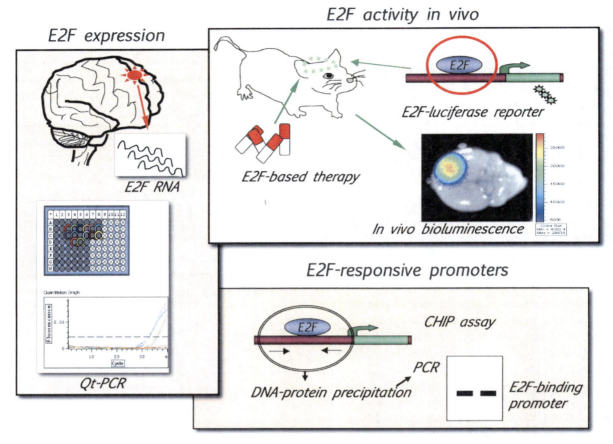

Fig. 10.1 Schematic illustration of three representative approaches used to examine the role of E2F in cancer. Prognostic value of E2F1 can be studied by quantifying E2F expression in surgical human samples by QT-PCR. Therapeutic modifications on the E2F1 transcriptional activity can be tested in preclinical studies using in vivo bioluminescence and chromatin immunoprecipitation assays

2. During RNA extraction, maintain tumor samples over dry ice covered with aluminum foil for RNA extraction.

3. Grind each sample (∼100 mg of tissue) into a fine powder with a mortar and pestle. Maintain the temperature by adding liquid nitrogen. The mortar and pestle should be cleaned with soap and water after each sample preparation and then sprayed with DNAzap.

4. Add Trizol to the tissue. Four mL of solution per 100 mg of tissue is necessary for adequate aqueous and organic phase separation.

5. Homogenize the mixture by passing it through a 21-gauge needle three or four times.

6. Incubate the homogenized samples for 5 min at 15–30°C to permit the complete dissociation of nucleoprotein complexes.

7. Add 0.2 mL of chloroform per 1 mL of Trizol.

8. Cap the sample tubes securely. Shake them vigorously by hand for 15 s and incubate them at 15–30°C for 2–3 min.

9. Centrifuge the samples at 12,000g for 15 min at 2–8°C. The mixture will separate into a red lower phenol-chloroform phase, an interphase, and a colorless upper aqueous phase. RNA will remain exclusively in the aqueous phase. The volume of the aqueous phase will be about 60% of the volume of Trizol used for homogenization.

10. Transfer the aqueous phase to a fresh tube and save the organic phase if isolation of the DNA or protein is desired.

11. Precipitate the RNA from the aqueous phase by mixing it with isopropyl alcohol. Use 0.5 mL of isopropyl alcohol per 1 mL of Trizol used for the initial homogenization.

12. Incubate the samples at 15–30°C for 10 min and centrifuge them at 12,000*g* for 10 min at 2–8°C. The RNA precipitate, often invisible before centrifugation, will form a gel-like pellet.

13. Remove the supernatant. Wash the RNA pellet once with 75% ethanol, adding at least 1 mL of 75% ethanol per 1 mL of Trizol used for the initial homogenization. Mix the sample by vortexing and centrifuge it at 7500*g* for 5 min at 2–8°C.

14. At the end of the procedure, briefly dry the RNA pellet (air-dry or vacuum-dry for 5–10 min). Do not dry the RNA by centrifugation under vacuum. It is important not to let the RNA pellet dry completely as this will greatly decrease its solubility.

15. Dissolve the RNA in RNase-free water or by passing the solution through a pipette tip a few times and incubate it for 10 min at 55–60°C.

16. Measure the RNA concentration (optimum ratio A260/280 < 1.6).

17. Copy 1 μg of RNA from each sample to cDNA.

18. Bring 1 μg of RNA to a final volume of 13 μL with RNAse-free water.

19. Add 1 μL of dNTPs (10 μM) and 1 μL of oligo (dT) and incubate the sample for 5 min at 55°C.

20. Place the samples on ice and add 4 μL of 10X buffer and 2 μL of dithiothreitol (1 M). Incubate them for 2 min at 42°C.

21. Briefly spin the samples and add 1 μL of reverse transcriptase. Incubate them for 45 min at 42°C.

22. Incubate the samples for 15 min at 70°C to ablate the enzyme activity.

23. Dilute the product to a ratio of 1:5.

24. Prepare two separate PCR master-mix reactions (one for each set of primers) using the PCR master mix and primers for glyceraldehyde 3-phosphate dehydrogenase (GAPDH) and E2F1 (for a 25 μL reaction: 2x PCR master mix, 12.5 μL; left, 0.5 μL; right, 0.5 μL; H$_2$O, 10 μL; sample: 1 μL).

25. Distribute 1 μL per sample (duplicates for each sample and each set of primers).

26. Perform the PCR. The cycling conditions are as follows: 10 min at 95°C for 1 cycle and 15 s at 95°C and 1 min at 60°C for 40 cycles.

27. Normalize input RNA with the amplification of GAPDH RNA. Use the comparative threshold cycle method to determine relative gene expression (Livak and Schmittgen, 2001).

E2f1 Activity and Therapeutic Interventions

As described above, the end result of an abnormal Rb pathway is E2F1 deregulation. Indeed, this excess E2F1 expression and activity can serve as a target for therapeutic interventions. Our research group has characterized a genetically engineered oncolytic adenovirus based on this concept. The adenovirus E1A protein is able to bind and abrogate the effect of Rb, thus releasing E2Fs and promoting S-phase entry. Apart from activating many E2F-responsive cellular genes, including E2F1 itself, E2Fs regulate the E2 region of the adenoviral genome; indeed, this is how E2F activity was first recognized. On the basis of this, our research at Alemany's laboratory generated ICOVIR-5, an adenovirus construct in which both the level and function of E1A are controlled at the transduction, transcription, and protein/protein interaction levels (Alonso et al., 2007; Majem et al., 2006). ICOVIR-5 expresses a mutant form of E1A that cannot bind to Rb, replicates selectively, and kills cells lacking functional Rb, as our group previously reported (Fueyo et al., 2000). In addition, the native E1A promoter is replaced by E2F-responsive elements. Thus, the construct is only functional in settings with high E2F activity and a mutant Rb pathway. We characterized ICOVIR-5 antiglioma effect and whether ICOVIR-5 infection enhanced E2F1 transcriptional activity in vivo (Alonso et al., 2007). To this end, we implanted U87 MG cells, previously transfected with a construct that contained the E2F promoter leading luciferase expression, into the brains of nude mice and measured E2F1 activity using bioluminescence imaging technology. The intratumoral injection of ICOVIR-5 resulted in strong luciferase expression, indicating an increase in the E2F activity. In experiments performed in parallel, we assessed whether there was prolonged interaction between free cellular E2F1 and recombinant E2F-responsive elements of ICOVIR-5 in vivo. To determine the E2F1 occupancy of the ectopic E2F1 promoter, we performed chromatin immunoprecipitation (ChIP) assays in U87 MG xenografts that had been treated with ICOVIR-5 intratumorally. Consistent with our previous findings, the E2F1 promoter contained in ICOVIR-5 genome was occupied by cellular E2F1 (Alonso et al., 2007).

In the following part, we detail the methodology used to determine in vivo both the E2F activity and the E2F occupancy of E2F-responsive elements in vivo (Fig. 10.1). Both aspects can be extrapolated to the study of other therapeutic interventions based on E2F1 high activity in malignant gliomas, as well as to the study of E2F transcriptional activity that will ultimately modify the expression of key molecules involved in the neoplastic phenotype of gliomas (Alonso et al., 2005).

Evaluation of E2F1 Activity In Vivo

Materials

1. Human glioblastoma U87 MG cell line (American Type Culture Collection, Manassas, VA) or other tumorigenic glioma cell line
2. Dulbecco's modified Eagle medium: F-12 (vol: 1:1) (GibcoBRL)
3. Fetal bovine serum (GibcoBRL Life Technologies, Rockville, MD)
4. Phosphate-buffered saline (PBS)
5. 100-mm tissue culture dishes (Corning-Costar, Corning, NY)
6. 0.05% trypsin and 0.5 mM EDTA in PBS (GibcoBRL)
7. 15 mL conical tube (BD Falcon, Franklin Lakes, NJ)
8. E2F1 reporter construct (kind gift from Dr. David Johnson, Department of Carcinogenesis, The University of Texas M. D. Anderson Cancer Center, Houston, TX)
9. FuGENE 6 transfection reagent (Roche Diagnostic Corp., Indianapolis, IN)
10. D-luciferin (Pierce, Rockford, IL)
11. IVIS imaging system (Caliper Lifesciences, Hopkinton, MA)

Methods

1. Seed cells (1×10^6 in 100-mm dishes) the day before transfection.
2. For transfection, mix E2F1 reporter construct (2 μg/dish) with 500 μL (dish) of serum-free media. Vortex briefly and incubate for 5 min.
3. Mix FuGENE 6 at a concentration of 3:1 v/w (μg of DNA to be transfected) in 500 μL of serum-free media. Vortex the mixture briefly and incubate for 5 min.
4. Mix the reagents from steps 1 and 2 and incubate them at RT for 45 min.
5. Dilute the adenovirus in serum-free media (100 μL/dish) to the appropriate concentration.
6. Wash the cells twice with PBS and add 1 mL of serum-free media.
7. When incubation has finished, add 1 mL of the DNA/FuGENE mixture to each dish.
8. Incubate the cells with the mixture for at least 4 h.
9. At the completion of the incubation time add 7 mL of 10% fetal bovine serum media and place the cells in the incubator at 37°C for up to 48 h.
10. Harvest the cells by trypsinization.
11. Spin the cells down for 5 min at 1500 rpm.
12. Resuspend the cells in PBS to a final 10 μL volume.
13. Implant the cells into the brains of athymic mice (Lal et al., 2000).
14. Forty-eight hours later, anesthetize the mice with isoflurane.
15. Inject the mice with D-luciferin (4 mg/g of body weight) intraperitoneally.
16. Image the mice for E2F-induced luciferase expression using an IVIS imaging system.

Acquisition parameters: Exposure time, 5 min; binning, 4; no filter; f/stop, 1; field of view, 10 cm.

Note: At the completion of step seven, E2F1-based therapeutic agents could be added to examine their effect in E2F activity.

Assessment of E2F1 Occupancy of E2F-Responsive Elements In Vivo

Materials

1. U87 MG cells (human glioblastoma cell lines) (American Type Culture Collection, Manassas, VA)
2. ICOVIR-5, or ultraviolet-inactivated ICOVIR-5
3. Dulbecco's modified Eagle medium: F-12 (vol: 1:1) with (GibcoBRL)
4. Fetal bovine serum (GibcoBRL)
5. PBS

6. 100-mm tissue culture dishes (Corning-Costar, Corning, NY)

7. 0.05% trypsin and 0.5 mM EDTA in PBS (GibcoBRL)

8. 15-mL conical tube (BD Falcon, Franklin Lakes, NJ)

9. Wild-type adenovirus and ICOVIR-5

10. Formaldehyde

11. ChIP assay kit (Upstate Biotechnology, Lake Placid, NJ)

12. Manual homogenizer

13. E2F1 (KH-95) or mouse immunoglobulin antibodies (Santa Cruz Biotechnology, Santa Cruz, CA) to immunoprecipitate cross-linked chromatin.

14. Primers to amplify a 272-bp fragment in the E2F1 promoter and the adjacent viral genome (5′-TGTCTGTCCCCACCTAGGAC-3′ and 5′-GCGGTTCCTATTGGCTTTAAC-3′) and E2 primers designed to amplify a 52-bp fragment in the E2 promoter that contains two binding sites for E2F1 (5′-TCGAACAAAAGCGCG AATTTAA-3′ and 5′-TTAAACTCTTTCCCGCG CTTTGATCAGT-3′)

15. Buffers/reagents: Salmon sperm DNA/protein A agarose (1.5 mL of packed beads with 600 μg of sonicated salmon sperm DNA [300 bp], 1.5 mg of bovine serum albumin, and 4.5 mg of recombinant protein A), sodium dodecyl sulfate (SDS) lysis buffer (1% SDS, 10 mM EDTA, and 50 mM Tris-HCl [pH 8.1 stored at ambient temperature]), ChIP dilution buffer (0.01% SDS, 1.1% Triton X-100, 1.2 mM EDTA, 16.7 mM Tris-HCl (pH 8.10), and 167 mM NaCl), low-salt immune complex wash buffer (0.1% SDS, 1% Triton X-100, 2 mM EDTA, 20 mM Tris-HCl [pH 8.1], and 150 mM NaCl), high-salt immune complex wash buffer (0.1% SDS, 1% Triton X-100, 2 mM EDTA, 20 mM Tris-HCl [pH 8.1], and 500 mM NaCl), LiCl immune complex wash buffer (0.25 M LiCl, 1% Nonidet P-40, 1% deoxycholate, 1 mM EDTA, and 10 mM Tris-HCl [pH 8.1]), and Tris-EDTA buffer (10 mM Tris-HCl and 1 mM EDTA [pH 8.0]).

Methods

1. Extract the brains from animals previously engrafted with the U87 MG glioma cell line (5 ×

10⁵) and treated with ICOVIR-5 or UV-inactivated ICOVIR.

2. Fix the brains by exposing them to 1% formaldehyde for 15 min at ambient temperature.

3. Wash the brains twice with PBS containing a mixture of protease inhibitors and 0.1 M glycine.

4. Resuspend the brains in 200 μL of lysis buffer (1% SDS, 10 mM EDTA, and 50 mM Tris-HCl [pH 8.1]) and protease inhibitors and homogenize the tissue with a manual homogenizer (pass through a 25-gauge syringe, if necessary), and incubate them for 10 min on ice.

5. Pellet the nuclei by centrifugation (5000 rpm for 5 min).

6. Resuspend the nuclei in nuclear lysis buffer (containing the same protease inhibitors as in the cell lysis buffer). Incubate them on ice for 10 min.

Note: The ChIP assay can be performed with the ChIP assay kit (Upstate Biotechnology, Lake Placid, NJ) by following the manufacturer's instructions. In brief, sonicate the lysate to shear DNA to lengths between 200 and 1000 bp, keeping the samples ice-cold. If longer genomic fragments are desired, use optimized conditions to produce the appropriate fragment size. Centrifuge the samples for 10 min at 13,000 rpm at 4°C and add 150 μL of the sonicated cell pellet suspension to a new 1.5-mL Eppendorf tube. Dilute the sonicated cell pellet suspension 10-fold in ChIP dilution buffer, adding protease inhibitors as described above, by adding 1350 μL of ChIP dilution buffer for a final volume of 1.5 mL in each immunoprecipitation condition.

To perform a PCR, use a portion of this suspension 1% [~15 μL] to quantitate the amount of DNA present in different samples. This sample is considered the 1% input/starting material, and the histone-DNA crosslinks must be reversed by heating it at 65°C for 4 hs and processing it with experimental samples. This sample can be stored at −80°C and processed with other samples the next day.

7. To reduce the non-specific background, pre-clear the 1.5-mL diluted cell pellet suspension with 60 μL of salmon sperm DNA/protein A agarose-50% slurry, 10 μL of pre-immune serum (Pierce: cat #31884), and 5 μg of sheared salmon sperm DNA for 2 h at 4°C with agitation.

8. Pellet the agarose by brief centrifugation (1 min @ 1000 rpm) and collect the supernatant fraction.

9. Add the immunoprecipitating antibody (E2F1 or immunoglobulin; 2 μg per sample) to the 1.5-mL supernatant fraction and incubate it overnight at 4°C with rotation.

10. Add 40 μL of salmon sperm DNA/protein A agarose slurry and 2 μg of sheared salmon sperm DNA for 2 hs at 4°C with rotation to collect the antibody and protein complex.

11. Pellet the agarose by gentle centrifugation (700–1000 rpm at 4°C for 1 min). Carefully remove the supernatant that contains unbound, non-specific DNA. Wash the protein A agarose/antibody/protein complex for 3 min on a rotating platform with the following buffers (listed in the order):

    (a) Low-salt immune complex wash buffer (1 × 1 mL)
    (b) High-salt immune complex wash buffer (1 × 1 mL)
    (c) LiCl immune complex wash buffer (1 × 1 mL)
    (d) 1 X Tris-EDTA buffer (2 × 1 mL)

    Washing conditions may differ slightly depending on the antibody's affinity for the antigen.

12. Prepare elution buffer (1% SDS, 0.1 M $NaHCO_3$)(84 mg $NaHCO_3$; 1 mL 10% SDS; 9 mL dH20, for 10 mL).

13. Elute the histone complex from the antibody by adding 1 × 100 μL and 2 × 75 μL elution buffer to the pelleted protein A agarose/antibody/protein complex. Place the tubes on a vortexer and mix at the medium setting for 15 min/elution. Spin down the agarose, carefully transfer the supernatant fraction (eluate) to another tube, and repeat the elution. Combine the eluates (total volume is ~200 μL).

14. Add 10 μL of 5 M NaCl to the combined eluates (250 μL) and reverse protein/histone-DNA cross-links by heating the sample at 65°C for at least 4 h. The sample can then be stored at −20°C, and the protocol can be continued the next day (Include the input/starting material and a transcriptionally inactivated DNA sample as the negative and background controls for the PCR reaction).

15. Add 10 μL of 0.5 M EDTA, 20 μL of 1 M Tris-HCl [pH 6.5], and 2 μL of 10 mg/mL proteinase K to the combined eluates and incubate for 1 h at 45°C.

16. Recover DNA using the Qiagen PCR purification kit. The final elution is in 25 μL in water.

17. Perform the PCR.

18. Run the products in a 2% agarose gel.

Acknowledgement We thank Ann Sutton (Department of Scientific Publication, The University of Texas M. D. Anderson Cancer Center, Houston, TX) for editorial assistance. This work was supported by an Institutional Research Grant from M. D. Anderson Cancer Center.

References

Alonso MM, Cascallo M, Gomez-Manzano C, Jiang H, Bekele BN, Perez-Gimenez A, Lang FF, Piao Y, Alemany R, Fueyo J (2007) ICOVIR-5 shows E2F1 addiction and potent antiglioma effect *in vivo*. Cancer Res 67:8255–8263

Alonso MM, Fueyo J, Shay JW, Aldape KD, Jiang H, Lee OH, Johnson DG, Xu J, Kondo Y, Kanzawa T, Kyo S, Bekele BN, Zhou X, Nigro J, McDonald JM, Yung WK, Gomez-Manzano C (2005) Expression of transcription factor E2F1 and telomerase in glioblastomas: mechanistic linkage and prognostic significance. J Natl Cancer Inst 97:1589–1600

Bandara LR, La Thangue NB (1991) Adenovirus E1a prevents the retinoblastoma gene product from complexing with a cellular transcription factor. Nature 351:494–497

Cavenee WK, Dryja TP, Phillips RA, Benedict WF, Godbout R, Gallie BL, Murphree AL, Strong LC, White RL (1983) Expression of recessive alleles by chromosomal mechanisms in retinoblastoma. Nature 305:779–784

Chellappan SP, Hiebert S, Mudryj M, Horowitz JM, Nevins JR (1991) The E2F transcription factor is a cellular target for the RB protein. Cell 65:1053–1061

Christensen J, Cloos P, Toftegaard U, Klinkenberg D, Bracken AP, Trinh E, Heeran M, Di Stefano L, Helin K (2005) Characterization of E2F8, a novel E2F-like cell-cycle regulated repressor of E2F-activated transcription. Nucleic Acids Res 33:5458–5470

Classon M, Harlow E (2002) The retinoblastoma tumour suppressor in development and cancer. Nat Rev Cancer 2:910–917

Dyson N (1998) The regulation of E2F by pRB-family proteins. Genes Dev 12:2245–2262

Friend SH, Bernards R, Rogelj S, Weinberg RA, Rapaport JM, Albert DM, Dryja TP (1986) A human DNA segment with properties of the gene that predisposes to retinoblastoma and osteosarcoma. Nature 323:643–646

Fueyo J, Gomez-Manzano C, Alemany R, Lee PS, McDonnell TJ, Mitlianga P, Shi YX, Levin VA, Yung WK, Kyritsis AP (2000) A mutant oncolytic adenovirus targeting the Rb pathway produces anti-glioma effect *in vivo*. Oncogene 19:2–12

Haller F, Gunawan B, von Heydebreck A, Schwager S, Schulten HJ, Wolf-Salgo J, Langer C, Ramadori G, Sultmann H,

Fuzesi L (2005) Prognostic role of E2F1 and members of the CDKN2A network in gastrointestinal stromal tumors. Clin Cancer Res 11:6589–6597

Han S, Park K, Bae BN, Kim KH, Kim HJ, Kim YD, Kim HY (2003) E2F1 expression is related with the poor survival of lymph node-positive breast cancer patients treated with fluorouracil, doxorubicin and cyclophosphamide. Breast Cancer Res Treat 82:11–16

Harbour JW, Dean DC (2000) The rb/E2F pathway: expanding roles and emerging paradigms. Genes Dev 14:2393–2409

Harbour JW, Luo RX, Dei Santi A, Postigo AA, Dean DC (1999) Cdk phosphorylation triggers sequential intramolecular interactions that progressively block Rb functions as cells move through G1. Cell 98:859–869

Helin K, Lees JA, Vidal M, Dyson N, Harlow E, Fattaey A (1992) A cDNA encoding a pRB-binding protein with properties of the transcription factor E2F. Cell 70: 337–350

Hernando E, Nahlâe Z, Juan G, Diaz-Rodriguez E, Alaminos M, Hemann M, Michel L, Mittal V, Gerald W, Benezra R, Lowe SW, Cordon-Cardo C (2004) Rb inactivation promotes genomic instability by uncoupling cell cycle progression from mitotic control. Nature 430:797–802

Irwin M, Marin MC, Phillips AC, Seelan RS, Smith DI, Liu W, Flores ER, Tsai KY, Jacks T, Vousden KH, Kaelin WG Jr (2000) Role for the p53 homologue p73 in E2F-1-induced apoptosis. Nature 407:645–648

Kaelin WG Jr, Krek W, Sellers WR, DeCaprio JA, Ajchenbaum F, Fuchs CS, Chittenden T, Li Y, Farnham PJ, Blanar MA (1992) Expression cloning of a cDNA encoding a retinoblastoma-binding protein with E2F-like properties. Cell 70:351–364

Knudson AG Jr (1971) Mutation and cancer: statistical study of retinoblastoma. Proc Natl Acad Sci USA 68:820–823

Kovesdi I, Reichel R, Nevins JR (1986a) E1A transcription induction: enhanced binding of a factor to upstream promoter sequences. Science 231:719–722

Kovesdi I, Reichel R, Nevins JR (1986b) Identification of a cellular transcription factor involved in E1A trans-activation. Cell 45:219–228

Kovesdi I, Reichel R, Nevins JR (1987) Role of an adenovirus E2 promoter binding factor in E1A-mediated coordinate gene control. Proc Natl Acad Sci USA 84:2180–2184

Kowalik TF, DeGregori J, Leone G, Jakoi L, Nevins JR (1998) E2F1-specific induction of apoptosis and p53 accumulation, which is blocked by mdm2. Cell Growth Diff 9:113–118

La Thangue NB (2003) The yin and yang of E2F-1: balancing life and death. Nat Cell Biol 5:587–589

Lal S, Lacroix M, Tofilon P, Fuller GN, Sawaya R, Lang FF (2000) An implantable guide-screw system for brain tumor studies in small animals. J Neurosurg 92:326–333

Leone G, DeGregori J, Yan Z, Jakoi L, Ishida S, Williams RS, Nevins JR (1998) E2F3 activity is regulated during the cell cycle and is required for the induction of S phase. Genes Dev 12:2120–2130

Livak KJ, Schmittgen TD (2001) Analysis of relative gene expression data using real-time quantitative PCR and the 2(-delta delta C(T)) method. Methods 25:402–408

Lundberg AS, Weinberg RA (1998) Functional inactivation of the retinoblastoma protein requires sequential modification by at least two distinct cyclin-cdk complexes. Mol Cell Biol 18:753–761

Majem M, Cascallo M, Bayo-Puxan N, Mesia R, Germa JR, Alemany R (2006) Control of E1A under an E2F-1 promoter insulated with the myotonic dystrophy locus insulator reduces the toxicity of oncolytic adenovirus ad-Delta24RGD. Cancer Gene Ther 13:696–705

Muller H, Bracken AP, Vernell R, Moroni MC, Christians F, Grassilli E, Prosperini E, Vigo E, Oliner JD, Helin K (2001) E2Fs regulate the expression of genes involved in differentiation, development, proliferation, and apoptosis. Genes Dev 15:267–285

Nevins JR (1992) E2F: a link between the Rb tumor suppressor protein and viral oncoproteins. Science 258:424–429

Nevins JR (1998) Toward an understanding of the functional complexity of the E2F and retinoblastoma families. Cell Growth Differ 9:585–593

Olson MV, Johnson DG, Jiang H, Xu J, Alonso MM, Aldape KD, Fuller GN, Bekele BN, Yung WK, Gomez-Manzano C, Fueyo J (2007) Transgenic E2F1 expression in the mouse brain induces a human-like bimodal pattern of tumors. Cancer Res 67:4005–4009

Parr MJ, Manome Y, Tanaka T, Wen P, Kufe DW, Kaelin WG Jr, Fine HA (1997) Tumor-selective transgene expression in vivo mediated by an E2F-responsive adenoviral vector. Nat Med 3:1145–1149

Ren B, Cam H, Takahashi Y, Volkert T, Terragni J, Young RA, Dynlacht BD (2002) E2F integrates cell cycle progression with DNA repair, replication, and G(2)/M checkpoints. Genes Dev 16:245–256

Sardet C, Vidal M, Cobrinik D, Geng Y, Onufryk C, Chen A, Weinberg RA (1995) E2F-4 and E2F-5, two members of the E2F family, are expressed in the early phases of the cell cycle. Proc Natl Acad Sci USA 92:2403–2407

Stevaux O, Dyson NJ (2002) A revised picture of the E2F transcriptional network and RB function. Curr Opin Cell Biol 14:684–691

Trimarchi JM, Fairchild B, Wen J, Lees JA (2001) The E2F6 transcription factor is a component of the mammalian bmi1-containing polycomb complex. Proc Natl Acad Sci USA 98:1519–1524

Trimarchi JM, Lees JA (2002) Sibling rivalry in the E2F family. Nat Rev Mol Cell Biol 3:11–20

Ueki K, Ono Y, Henson JW, Efird JT, von Deimling A, Louis DN (1996) CDKN2/p16 or RB alterations occur in the majority of glioblastomas and are inversely correlated. Cancer Res 56:150–153

Wen PY, Kesari S (2008) Malignant gliomas in adults. N Engl J Med 359:492–507

Won J, Chang S, Oh S, Kim TK (2004) Small-molecule-based identification of dynamic assembly of E2F-pocket protein-histone deacetylase complex for telomerase regulation in human cells. Proc Natl Acad Sci USA 101:11328–11333

Yamazaki K, Hasegawa M, Ohoka I, Hanami K, Asoh A, Nagao T, Sugano I, Ishida Y (2005) Increased E2F-1 expression via tumour cell proliferation and decreased apoptosis are correlated with adverse prognosis in patients with squamous cell carcinoma of the oesophagus. J Clin Pathol 58:904–910

Zhang SY, Liu SC, Al-Saleem LF, Holloran D, Babb J, Guo X, Klein-Szanto AJ (2000) E2F-1: a proliferative marker of breast neoplasia. Cancer Epidemiol Biomark Prev 9:395–401

Ziebold U, Reza T, Caron A, Lees JA (2001) E2F3 contributes both to the inappropriate proliferation and to the apoptosis arising in Rb mutant embryos. Genes Dev 15:386–391

Chapter 11

The Role of Glucose Transporter-1 (GLUT-1) in Malignant Gliomas

Randy L. Jensen and Rati Chkheidze

Abstract Glioblastoma multiforme (GBM) is the most aggressive and lethal primary brain tumor in adults. Despite significant advances in surgery, radiotherapy, and chemotherapy, prognosis for patients with GBM remains dismal, and clinical outcome varies markedly between patients. To formulate appropriate treatment strategy, accurate prognostic markers are needed to predict survival for individual patients. The glucose transporter GLUT-1 has emerged as a novel prognostic factor given its association with poorer response to therapy and poorer prognosis in patients with many different cancers. This chapter explores the role GLUT-1 may play in GBM angiogenesis, proliferation, and tumorigenesis. We review the molecular biology and physiologic function of the GLUT family of glucose transporters. We also explore the role these proteins have in the blood–brain barrier and how GLUT-1 is regulated at the transcriptional and post-transcriptional level. We place special emphasis on the role of hypoxia in glioma tumorigenesis, resistance to therapy, and GLUT-1 regulation. The role of GLUT-1 as a marker of tumor hypoxia is also discussed. Finally, the potential strategies of targeting GLUT-1 for the treatment of malignant glioma are explored. GLUT-1 appears to have a significant role in glioma tumor biology and deserves further study to determine the potential for exploiting this role in therapeutic measures for patients with malignant gliomas.

Keywords Glucose transporter-1 · Hypoxia · Metabolism · Brain tumor · Meningioma · Glioblastoma multiforme

Introduction

Glioblastoma multiforme (GBM) is the most aggressive and most lethal primary brain tumor in adults. It represents 19% of all primary brain tumors in United States. Despite significant advances in surgery, radiotherapy, and chemotherapy, prognosis for GBM remains dismal, as the median survival rate is only about 1 year. Even within this short survival time, the disease course is unpredictable. Although there are several variables that affect GBM progression, including age, complete surgical resection, histology, and performance score, every GBM case is unique and their prognostic significance varies from patient to patient. Even in patients with GBM that have similar histology and receive the same treatment, clinical outcome varies markedly. To formulate appropriate treatment strategy, prediction of survival is very important. Thus, more accurate prognostic markers are needed to predict survival for individual patients, and an extensive search is underway to identify special molecular prognosis markers that could more precisely predict GBM clinical outcome. The glucose transporter GLUT-1 has emerged as a novel prognostic factor for cancer. According to recent studies, GLUT-1 overexpression is associated with poorer response to therapy and poorer prognosis in patients with bone and soft tissue tumors, head and neck cancers, colorectal cancer, gallbladder carcinomas, breast cancer, and cervical cancer (Jensen, 2006, 2009). This

R.L. Jensen (✉)
Department of Neurosurgery, University of Utah, Salt Lake City, UT 84132, USA
e-mail: randy.jensen@hsc.utah.edu

M.A. Hayat (ed.), *Tumors of the Central Nervous System, Volume 1,*
DOI 10.1007/978-94-007-0344-5_11, © Springer Science+Business Media B.V. 2011

chapter explores the role GLUT-1 may play in GBM angiogenesis, proliferation, and tumorigenesis.

Glucose Transporter-1

GLUT-1 belongs to a family of highly homologous transmembrane glycoproteins that mediate Na$^+$-independent transport of glucose into cells (Behrooz and Ismail-Beigi, 1999). There are at least 12 GLUT subtypes, with all isoforms exhibiting highly homologous integral membrane proteins with 12 membrane-spanning domains, a single glycosylation site, and cytoplasmic NH$_2$ and COOH termini. At least three glucose transporter isoforms are thought to play a significant role in the brain. These include GLUT-1, which is present at high concentration at the blood-brain barrier (BBB) (55-kDa form) as well as in astrocytes (45-kDa form), GLUT3 expressed in neurons, and GLUT5 in microglia (Maher et al., 1994; Stockhammer et al., 2008). Structurally, GLUT-1 is related to other facilitated glucose transporters, but functionally, it is more related to glucose-regulated proteins (GRPs). In most cells, GLUT1 is induced by the same stimuli as GRPs, such as low glucose concentration, increased intracellular calcium, and inhibition of N-glycosylation. GLUT1 levels are not increased by heat shock (Behrooz and Ismail-Beigi, 1999).

Glut-1 Function

The major metabolic substrate of the brain is glucose, and the transport of glucose from blood to brain is tightly coupled with cerebral glucose utilization (Nishioka et al., 1992). It appears that glucose transport is the rate-limiting factor for overall glucose metabolism in rapidly growing cancer cells as well (Nagamatsu et al., 1996). Glucose is an extremely hydrophilic molecule unlikely to cross the BBB without assistance. The presence of glucose transport proteins is essential to supply glucose to the neurons and glia within the brain. The transport of glucose into the brain is facilitated by the GLUT family, with the GLUT-1 isoform being the most widely expressed form (Nishioka et al., 1992). GLUT-1 is ubiquitously expressed in normal tissue and expressed at higher concentrations in some tumors (Airley et al., 2001). Owing

to its ubiquitous expression, GLUT-1 is thought to mediate the basal transport of glucose as well as much of the non-insulin-dependent transport of glucose in mammals (Behrooz and Ismail-Beigi, 1999).

The GLUT-1 gene is active early in development, and its expression persists in virtually all tissues of the adult animal, albeit to varying degrees (Behrooz and Ismail-Beigi, 1999). GLUT-1 deficiency syndrome (De Vivo syndrome) is characterized by infantile seizures, developmental delay, acquired microencephaly, spasticity, ataxia, and hypoglycorrhachia. Clinically, patients with this syndrome show lower than normal levels of glucose and lactate in cerebrospinal fluid (Evans et al., 2008). Neuroectodermal stem cells show strong membrane immunoreactivity for GLUT-1 at early developmental stages in rodents. The expression of GLUT-1 decreases as these cells differentiate and is confined to endothelial cells as BBB function develops (Loda et al., 2000). As mentioned above, the two isoforms have different locations in the normal central nervous system. The 45-kDa form is detected mainly in neuronal and glial cells, whereas the 55-kDa form is mainly expressed in microvessels, choroid plexus, and ependymal cells and seems to be associated with endothelial cell BBB function (Harik et al., 1990; Maher et al., 1994).

Glut-1 and the BBB

GLUT-1 is asymmetrically distributed on the BBB plasma membrane, with an approximately fourfold greater abundance on the ablumenal membrane than on the lumenal membrane. Approximately 40% of the endothelial glucose transporter protein is contained within the cytoplasmic space, which provides a mechanism for rapid up-regulation of the transporter by altered distribution of transporter between cytoplasmic and plasma membrane compartments. This suggests that the mechanisms of regulation of glucose transport from blood to brain might involve differential distribution of the BBB glucose transporter in subcellular compartments of brain capillary endothelial cells (Farrell and Pardridge, 1991). This arrangement allows for management of changes in glucose demand.

The 55-kDa GLUT-1 is responsible for the passage of glucose across the endothelial cells of the BBB, the 45-kDa GLUT-1 is responsible for transport of glucose into glial cells, GLUT-3 mediates the uptake of glucose into neurons, and GLUT-5 is a microglial transporter (Maher et al., 1994). In normal brain, GLUT-1 expression is localized to the plasma membrane of endothelial cells in only those brain vessels that have intact BBB, but this does not seem to be true in experimental models of intracranial malignant glioma, where GLUT-1 expression is independent of vascular permeability (Harik et al., 1990).

Regulation of Glut-1 Expression

Regulation of GLUT-1 expression is complex and involves multiple signaling pathways. Stimuli that influence GLUT-1 expression include hypoxia, extracellular glucose concentration, inhibition of oxidative phosphorylation, thyroid hormone, calcium ionophores, insulin (Barthel et al., 1999), endothelin-1 (Ismail-Beigi, 1993; Mitani et al., 1996; Sanchez-Alvarez et al., 2004), and the same stimuli that affect GRPs, including low glucose concentration, increased intracellular calcium, and inhibition of N-glycosylation.

Endothelin-1 (ET-1) stimulates the translocation and up-regulation of both glucose transporter and hexokinase in astrocytes (Sanchez-Alvarez et al., 2004). ET-1 induces a rapid change in the localization of GLUT-1 and hexokinase to rapidly increase the entry and phosphorylation of glucose. This appears to require communication through gap junctions between astrocytes. ET-1 promotes a rapid translocation of GLUT-1 from an intracellular pool to the plasma membrane in astrocytes. This, in turn, increases glucose uptake, and these events seem to be closely related to the inhibition of gap junctional communication between astrocytes (Sanchez-Alvarez et al., 2004). There also appears to be a different ET-1 mechanism of GLUT-1-mediated long-term regulation of intracellular glucose (Sanchez-Alvarez et al., 2004).

Glutamate triggers a rapid increase in glucose uptake in astrocytes, but this mechanism is more likely due to activation of the glucose transporter rather than to translocation (Loaiza et al., 2003). Increased intracellular calcium concentration enhances GLUT-1 mRNA expression, but induction of GLUT-1 transcription by inhibition of oxidative phosphorylation does not require changes of intracellular calcium concentration (Mitani et al., 1996). GLUT-1 gene transcription

is increased after stimulation by calf serum, epidermal growth factor (EGF), fibroblast growth factor (FGF), platelet-derived growth factor (PDGF), and insulin-like growth factor-1 (IGF-1) in a number of fibroblast cell lines (Hiraki et al., 1988). This process does not require new protein synthesis and is mediated by protein kinase C-dependent and -independent pathways. A similar effect is seen after insulin stimulation through AKT kinase cascade pathways (Barthel et al., 1999).

Glucose is another important regulator of GLUT-1 expression. High glucose concentrations reduce GLUT-1 mRNA and protein while the reverse is true under low glucose conditions (Alpert et al., 2002). Specifically, this effect is dependent on extracellular glucose levels: The increase of glucose concentration up to 15 mM induces GLUT-1 (Knott et al., 1996), and additional increases result in down-regulation of GLUT-1 expression (Alpert et al., 2002, 2005; Knott et al., 1996). Insulin is one of the important regulators of GLUT-1 expression. It increases GLUT-1 levels via PI3 kinase and its downstream target serine/threonine kinase Akt1 (Barthel et al., 1999). This is not surprising given that a number of tumor suppressor genes, oncogenes, and growth factors have been reported to affect hypoxia-inducible factor-1 (HIF-1) function in many non-central nervous system tumors (Jensen, 2006, 2009). HIF-1, as will be seen below, is a major regulation of GLUT-1 expression.

Depending on the stimulus, GLUT-1 may be regulated acutely, chronically, or both. Acute stimulation of GLUT-1-mediated glucose transport in response to some stimuli is observed within minutes of exposure and is mediated through either translocation of the transporter to the plasma membrane or activation of GLUT-1 transporters preexisting at the cell surface. These mechanisms have been shown to increase glucose transport in the absence of an increase in total cell GLUT-1 transporter content (Behrooz and Ismail-Beigi, 1999). On the other hand, a more prolonged exposure to some stimuli and conditions is associated with increased levels of GLUT-1 mRNA. This mode of regulation is accomplished by both transcriptional and post-transcriptional mechanisms and leads to an overall increase in cell and plasma membrane GLUT-1 content. Hypoxia-mediated regulation of GLUT-1 is accomplished by both of these mechanisms depending on the need for either rapid or sustained glucose needs of cells (Behrooz and Ismail-Beigi, 1999).

Hypoxic Regulation of Glut-1

Hypoxia is one of the major stimuli that regulates GLUT-1 gene transcription and subsequent protein expression in a wide variety of cells and tissues in many organisms including humans (Behrooz and Ismail-Beigi, 1999). The enhanced expression and function of Glut-1 in response to hypoxia represents fundamental adaption that is critical to the maintenance of cellular homeostasis (Behrooz and Ismail-Beigi, 1999). Increased glucose transport/uptake is an essential step in the adaptive response to cellular stress and adaptive response to hypoxia. This was first observed in cardiac and skeletal muscle, where enhanced glucose uptake by cells and tissues resulted after hypoxic stimulation. Glucose transport is the rate-limiting step for glucose utilization and subsequently the overall effectiveness of the adaptive response to hypoxia in the majority of cells (Behrooz and Ismail-Beigi, 1999; Ismail-Beigi, 1993). Hypoxia-mediated regulation of GLUT-1 operates by two pathways: (1) direct inhibition of oxidative phosphorylation due to lack of the oxygen and (2) induction of the HIF-1α pathway.

Inhibitors of oxidative phosphorylation increase both GLUT1 mRNA expression and intracellular Ca^{2+} concentration. This is in line with observations that hypoxia-mediated glucose uptake can be mimicked by exposure to pharmacological inhibitors of oxidative phosphorylation (Ismail-Beigi, 1993). It has been proposed that the decrement in mitochondrial respiration and ATP synthesis triggers the stimulation of glucose transport. During aerobic metabolism, the availability of molecular oxygen as an electron acceptor allows the bulk of the cellular energy, in the form of ATP and reducing power, to be derived by oxidative level phosphorylation. Inhibition of this process, secondary to the decreased supply of oxygen, leads to an increase in the cellular demand for glucose metabolism through the glycolytic pathway to generate lactate (Behrooz and Ismail-Beigi, 1999). Increased intracellular calcium, by itself, increases GLUT-1 expression, but the effect of inhibitors of oxidative phosphorylation is not mediated only with increased calcium. There might be other intermediates that have not been discovered yet (Mitani et al., 1996). The switch from oxidative phosphorylation to anaerobic glycolysis in hypoxic tumor cells is accompanied by an increase in glucose requirements and transport. Glucose transporters are up-regulated in cells of many different tumors and mediate passive glucose uptake. They are induced by hypoxia and decreased oxidative phosphorylation via HIF-1 (Jonathan et al., 2006).

The original and best-characterized hypoxia-regulated molecule is the transcription factor HIF-1, which is composed of two subunits, HIF-1β and HIF-1α. Each of these proteins is constitutively expressed at the transcriptional level without any regulation by hypoxic conditions. HIF-1β is unchanged by hypoxic conditions whereas the HIF-1α protein is tightly controlled at a post-transcriptional level by two independent mechanisms. The first described and most understood regulator involves hydroxylation of proline residues, which leads to proteasomal degradation mediated by the Von Hippel-Lindau protein (pVHL) complex (Jensen, 2006, 2009). The second involves hydroxylation of an asparagine, which inhibits interaction between HIF-1 and the nuclear coactivator CBP/p300 (Jensen, 2006, 2009). Both of these regulatory mechanisms are inhibited under hypoxic (1–2% O_2) conditions. HIF-1 activates DNA promoter regions known as the hypoxia response elements (HREs). HREs induce transcription of more than 100 genes that help the cell "cope" with low O_2 conditions (Jensen, 2006, 2009). Glut-1, vascular endothelial growth factor (VEGF), erythropoietin, carbonic anhydrase IX (CA-IX), enolase, lactate dehydrogenase, tyrosine hydroxylase, aldolase A, phosphoglycerate kinase (PGK), transferrin and its receptor, and certain growth factors are all examples of proteins regulated by an HIF-1 though an HRE (Jensen, 2006, 2009).

GLUT-1 As an Intrinsic Measure of Hypoxia

As mentioned above, GLUT-1 and CA-IX are regulated by HIF-1 and are potential cellular markers of tumor hypoxia (Jensen, 2006). In fact, there is a high degree of correlation between an intravenously injected hypoxia marker pimonidazole and GLUT1/CAIX localization in bladder (Hoskin et al., 2003) and cervical cancer (Jensen, 2006). GLUT-1 expression has been demonstrated to correlate with tumor hypoxia, and low expression of GLUT-1 predicted metastasis-free survival in advanced carcinoma of the cervix (Airley et al., 2001). Some authors have predicted that GLUT-1 might be the most accurate marker of hypoxia since it signals dual control in hypoxic conditions by both reduced oxidative phosphorylation and the HIF-1 oxygen-sensing pathways (Airley et al., 2001).

GLUT-1 and GLUT-3 are up-regulated in a number of primary human brain tumors, and their expression in tumor cells is correlated with the distance of the cell from blood vessels (Nishioka et al., 1992). GLUT-1 but not CAIX was helpful in predicting distant metastasis and overall survival of patients with head and neck cancers (Jonathan et al., 2006). These authors were concerned that the expression of these proteins was altered by treatment regimen and cautioned that they might not be a very specific and robust marker of tumor hypoxia during or after a given therapeutic measure. Nevertheless, it is clearly important to facilitate the routine study of tumor hypoxia in clinical trials and ultimately to use this as "standard of care" in routine clinical practice. GLUT-1 might be a biomarker that allows measurement of tumor hypoxia before and after a given treatment.

Hypoxia and Cancer

Levels of hypoxia in many different human cancers predict the likelihood of metastases, tumor recurrence, resistance to chemotherapy and radiation, invasion, and decreased patient survival (Jensen, 2006, 2009). Some of the phenotypic changes fundamental to malignant tumor progression, such as oncogene activation, alteration of gene expression profiles, genomic instability, loss of apoptotic potential, and induction of angiogenesis, are suspected to be triggered by cellular hypoxia (Jensen, 2006, 2009).

In a similar manner to hypoxia, HIF-1α overexpression is described in many human cancers, including prostate, squamous cell carcinoma, lung, breast, bladder, and pancreatic (Jensen, 2006, 2009). Many studies have also demonstrated that increased HIF-1α activity predicts a more aggressive tumor grade, tumor invasion, resistance to radiation therapy, metastatic potential, and poorer prognosis (Jensen, 2006, 2009). HIF-1α is expressed even in normoxic conditions in human cancers like prostate, squamous cell, lung, breast, bladder, and pancreatic (Jensen, 2006, 2009).

Tumors derived from cells with HIF-1α knockout show decreased cell growth in vivo and in vitro (Jensen, 2006, 2009). Expression of molecules controlled by HIF-1 and their association with cancer is less studied, although CA-IX and Glut-1 expression reportedly correlates with poor response to adjuvant treatments (Jensen, 2006, 2009).

Hypoxia and Gliomas

As described above, some of the phenotypic changes fundamental to malignant tumor progression are suspected to be triggered by cellular hypoxia in many human cancers (Jensen, 2006, 2009). These same phenotypic changes have all been described in GBM, although the role of hypoxia in this process is less clear (Jensen, 2006, 2009). It is clear that tumor hypoxia increases GBM cell migration and invasion in both in vitro and in vivo glioma models (Jensen, 2006, 2009). In examining surgical specimens of human GBM, the cells found directly surrounding intratumoral necrotic areas have been implicated in hypoxia-regulated migration away from these presumed low oxygen regions (Jensen, 2006, 2009).

One suspected manifestation of hypoxia in GBM is intratumoral necrosis. The histological diagnosis of GBM depends on the presence of tumor necrosis and the cluster of cells that surround the necrotic areas known as pseudopalisading. The degree of necrosis within a GBM correlates inversely with patient outcome and survival (Jensen, 2006, 2009), although our own group was unable to demonstrate this relationship in our patient series (Flynn et al., 2008). All GBM tumors demonstrate necrosis regardless of tumor size, but the mechanism by which this happens is unknown at this time. Rodent glioma models demonstrate that even some tumors <1 mm in diameter are intensely hypoxic, poorly perfused, and possess sparse tumor vasculature, whereas larger tumors, 1–4 mm in diameter, were found to be better perfused with widespread vasculature and not significantly hypoxic (Jensen, 2006, 2009). This is partially explained by evidence that although GBM is a highly vascularized tumor, this microcirculation is functionally very inefficient and may contribute to relative hypoxia and necrosis within a given tumor (Jensen, 2006, 2009). Direct and indirect measurements of tumor hypoxia in human GBM and attempts at correlating this with tumor blood flow and necrosis have not resolved this controversy (Jensen, 2006, 2009). It is also entirely possible that intratumoral necrosis in GBM may not simply be due to inadequate vascular supply but instead may be a result of intrinsic molecular or genetic changes within the tumor. This is supported by microarray analysis of GBM necrosis identifying specific genes and patterns of gene expression that may help elucidate the molecular basis of necrogenesis in the future (Raza et al., 2004). Along these lines, hypoxia and loss of the gene phosphatase and tensin homolog (PTEN) up-regulate tissue factor expression, which seems to promote microvascular thrombosis and subsequent intratumoral necrosis (reviewed in Jensen, 2006, 2009). CD133+ brain tumor stem cells populations are increased by hypoxia, and there are reports of genetic instability within these populations after hypoxic exposure suggesting a potential mechanism for cancer stem cell development. The role of hypoxia-regulated molecules in brain tumor development, methods of imaging and measuring tumor hypoxia, and how hypoxia might be used as a target for treatment of these tumors is not in the scope of this chapter and is examined elsewhere (Jensen, 2009).

Glut-1 and Gliomas

Glioma cell lines in culture overexpress HIF-1α in both normoxia and hypoxic conditions (Jensen, 2006, 2009). Research in our laboratory has demonstrated that most malignant glioma cell lines have higher VEGF and HIF-1 expression at baseline. When these malignant glioma cell lines are transfected with a dominant-negative HIF-1α (DN-HIF-1α) expression vector or siRNA constructs directed against the HIF-1 gene, HIF-1α and GLUT-1 expression and VEGF secretion are decreased, with subsequent in vitro and in vivo growth inhibition (Gillespie et al., 2007; Jensen et al., 2006). Conditioned medium from rat C6 glioma cells grown under hypoxic conditions up-regulates GLUT-1 expression in rat brain endothelial cells while the same condition medium derived from normoxic cells has no significant effect on GLUT-1 protein levels (Yeh et al., 2008). This is accomplished via a mechanism requiring VEGF secretion, and the GLUT-1 up-regulation is mediated by the phophoinositide-3-kinase/AKT pathway. These results suggest that hypoxic brain tumors may secrete VEGF to increase glucose transport across the BBB by increased GLUT-1 production and activity (Yeh et al., 2008).

GLUT-1 and CA-IX are overexpressed in higher-grade astrocytomas and malignant glioma cell lines (Jensen, 2006, 2009). CA-IX expression within malignant gliomas predicts radiographic response and survival of patients treated with bevacizumab and irinotecan (Sathornsumetee et al., 2008). GLUT-1 as a predictor of response to chemotherapy is unknown.

Decreased expression of GLUT-1 is found in low-grade astrocytomas (Loda et al., 2000; Nagamatsu et al., 1993; Nishioka et al., 1992). Expression of GLUT-1 is significantly reduced in low-grade oligodendroglial tumors harboring loss of heterozygosity (LOH) of chromosome 1p (Stockhammer et al., 2008). This is an interesting finding for a couple of reasons. First and foremost is the well-known prognostic factor of combined LOH of the short arm of chromosome 1 and the long arm of chromosome 19 (LOH 1p/19q) seen in anaplastic and low-grade oligodendrogliomas (Stockhammer et al., 2008). The second reason is that the gene for GLUT-1 is encoded on 1p31.3-p35, suggesting that this gene function could be lost in patients with 1p LOH. Taken together, this would imply that one possible explanation of why patients with 1p LOH do significantly better than patients without this genetic change is that GLUT-1 plays an important role in the transformation to higher grade and more aggressive tumor behavior.

Our examination of approximately 250 human gliomas suggests that high-grade gliomas are more likely to be immunohistochemically positive for HIF-1α, VEGF, GLUT-1, and CA-IX (Table 11.1) than are low-grade tumors ($p = 0.0001$) (Flynn et al., 2008; Jensen et al., 2006). Although this does not seem to hold completely true when comparing only oligodendrogliomas and anaplastic oligodendrogliomas, even in that case GLUT-1 as a biomarker differentiates between these two grades ($p = 0.001$). Expression of GLUT-1 and related hypoxia-regulated proteins does not seem to be different between primary and recurrent GBM. Increased expression of these molecules in higher-grade gliomas was confirmed by Western blot and enzyme-linked immunosorbent assay of protein extracts from human brain tumors at the time of surgery compared with lower-grade tumors (Flynn et al., 2008; Gillespie et al., 2007). This has been confirmed by other studies in which a correlation has been suggested between brain tumor grade, vascularity, and HIF-1α and CA-IX expression

Table 11.1   Immunohistochemistry for hypoxia-regulated molecules

All tumors

Protein	All low-grade gliomas (low-grade astrocytoma, oligodendroglioma)	All malignant gliomas (GBM, anaplastic astrocytoma, anaplastic oligodendroglioma)	χ^2
GLUT-1	37/81 (46%)	115/145 (79%)	26.69, $p < 0.0001$
HIF-1	44/81 (54%)	131/163 (80%)	18.10, $p < 0.0001$
VEGF	47/87 (54%)	149/179 (83%)	25.77, $p < 0.0001$
CA-IX	30/82 (37%)	123/147 (84%)	52.64, $p < 0.0001$

Astrocytomas only

Protein	Low-grade astrocytoma	Glioblastoma and anaplastic astrocytoma	χ^2
GLUT-1	6/46 (13%)	104/132 (79%)	62.45, $p < 0.0001$
HIF-1	19/47 (40%)	117/147 (79%)	26.07, $p < 0.0001$
VEGF	24/50 (48%)	131/161 (81%)	21.78, $p < 0.0001$
CA-IX	14/48 (29%)	110/134 (82%)	45.59, $p < 0.0001$

Oligodendrogliomas only

Protein	Oligodendroglioma	Anaplastic oligodendrogliomas	χ^2
GLUT-1	8/35 (23%)	11/13 (85%)	15.11, $p = 0.0001$
HIF-1	18/34 (53%)	14/16 (88%)	5.64, $p = 0.018$
VEGF	23/37 (62%)	16/18 (89%)	4.19, $p = 0.041$
CA-IX	29/39 (85%)	13/13 (100%)	2.14, $p = 0.14$

Recurrent GBM vs. primary GBM

Protein	All GBM	De novo GBM	Recurrent GBM	χ^2
Glut-1	92/117 (79%)	73/93 (78%)	19/24 (79%)	0.0051, $p = 0.94$
HIF-1	104/132 (79%)	84/106 (79%)	20/26 (77%)	0.067, $p = 0.79$
VEGF	118/144 (82%)	92/113 (81%)	26/31 (84%)	0.099, $p = 0.75$
CAIX	93/119 (80%)	74/92 (80%)	21/27 (78%)	0.091, $p = 0.76$

Data from Jensen et al. 2006

(Sathornsumetee et al., 2008). GLUT-1 is a downstream target of HIF-1α. Treatment of mouse C6 glioma model with YC-1, an inhibitor of HIF-1α, resulted in a significantly lower GLUT-1 expression and [$_{18}$F]fluorodeoxyglucose ($_{18}$F-FDG) uptake (Assadian et al., 2008). HIF-1α up-regulates VEGF, and VEGF induces GLUT-1 expression via PI3K/Akt pathway (Yeh et al., 2008). $_{18}$F-FDG uptake as measured by preoperative positron emission tomography (PET) has been show to correlate with GLUT-1 expression and increased cellular proliferation in malignant human gliomas (Chung et al., 2004).

Hypoxia and Resistance to Therapy

Radiation therapy has been standard of care in the treatment of human GBMs for many years. The fact that hypoxia is involved in cellular radioresistance is well documented by radiobiologists and likely plays a role in GBM treatment failures (Jensen, 2006, 2009). The volume and intensity of hypoxia in GBM before radiotherapy is strongly associated with decreased time to tumor progression or overall patient survival. CD133+ brain tumor stem cells numbers are increased after hypoxic stimulation in experimental models, with subsequent increased radioresistance. Transfection of human brain tumor cells with a construct that increases BAX expression driven by a hypoxia-regulated promoter increases radiosensitivity of these cells, suggesting a role of hypoxia-regulated therapies for GBM (reviewed in Jensen, 2006, 2009).

Chemotherapy has become a mainstay in the treatment of patients with GBM. Unfortunately, conventional chemotherapeutic treatments for malignant brain tumors still have many limitations, including an almost universal eventual development of resistance to a given chemotherapy by GBM. There are a number of studies that suggest that GBM chemoresistance is mediated through hypoxia-related mechanisms. In fact, inhibiting hypoxia-regulated survival mechanisms, such as HIF-1α, by transfecting glioma cells with HIF-1α siRNA, renders these cells more sensitive to chemotherapeutic treatment, probably through a multidrug resistance pathway. Noscapine, a small molecule inhibitor of HIF, induces apoptosis of human glioma cell lines. Hypoxia-mediated activation of the Bcl-2 family protein Bad inhibits chemotherapeutic-induced apoptosis in glioblastoma cells. Bcl-2 19-kDa interacting protein 3 (BNIP3) is a hypoxia-inducible proapoptotic member of the Bcl-2 family that induces cell death by associating with the mitochondria. BNIP3 expression is increased in the hypoxic regions of GBM and is localized to the nucleus in most of these tumors. Under hypoxic conditions in normal cells, BNIP3 becomes primarily cytoplasmic, promoting cell death. In gliomas, even under hypoxic conditions, BNIP3 remains in the nucleus and is unable to induce apoptosis. Malignant glioma cell lines secrete proteins that suppress hypoxia-induced endothelial cell apoptosis with subsequent promotion of angiogenesis (reviewed in Jensen, 2006, 2009).

GBM is one of the most highly vascularized of human tumors, with significant vascular proliferation and angiogenesis (Jensen, 2006, 2009). Antiangiogenic therapy, usually in the form of the anti-VEGF antibody therapeutic drug bevacizumab, is commonly used for patients with GBM. Clinical trial data suggest that the presence of tumor hypoxia markers predicts radiographic response and survival of patients treated with bevacizumab and irinotecan (Sathornsumetee et al., 2008). It has been proposed that GBM hypoxia caused by vessel regression during the course of antiangiogenic therapy leads to up-regulation of proangiogenic factors such as FGF, ephrin A1, and angiopoietin 1. This is turn promotes the recruitment of bone marrow-derived cells (BMDCs) that have the capacity to increase tumor growth through new blood vessel growth. This is supported by evidence to suggest that BMDCs are recruited by hypoxia- and HIF-1-mediated pathways (Jensen, 2006, 2009). Once within the tumor, the BMDCs express a variety of cytokines, growth factors, and proteases, which assist in the development of new blood vessels to "fuel" tumor growth. HIF-1 promotes angiogenesis and tumor growth by inducing recruitment of various proangiogenic bone marrow-derived CD45+

myeloid cells, F4/80+ tumor-associated macrophages, and endothelial and pericyte progenitor cells in human GBM. Furthermore, hypoxia and radiation therapy promote the recruitment of hematopoietic progenitor cells to xenograft intracranial gliomas though a mechanism involving HIF-1-mediated induction of stromal cell-derived factor-1/CXC chemokine ligand 12 (reviewed in Jensen, 2006, 2009). It is clear from the discussion above that hypoxia in general and possibly HIF-1 more specifically plays a role in treatment-resistant mechanisms of GBM survival. Although less studied, it would not be surprising to find that inhibition of GLUT-1 would have similar effects.

GLUT-1 As a Therapeutic Target

Transcriptional control of HIF-1 and its downstream regulated proteins such as GLUT-1 is tightly linked with the hypoxic conditions found within solid tumors. Thus, hypoxia-regulated genes offer promise as novel therapeutic targets (Evans et al., 2008). This concept is supported by evidence that inhibition of glucose transporters induces apoptosis in lung and breast cancer (Rastogi et al., 2007). Inhibition of GLUT-1 in hypoxic breast and colon cancer cell lines leads to chemosensitivity for daunorubicin (Cao et al., 2007) and vincristine for an erythroblastoma cell line (Martell et al., 1997). The mechanism by which this happens is unclear, but there is evidence to suggest that over-expression of GLUT-1 without a coordinate increase in either HIF-1 or other HIF-1-regulated glycolytic enzymes increases glucose uptake but not the rate of glycolysis. This appears to be associated with higher levels of phosphodiester activity and increased cell membrane turnover as markers of increased cellular proliferation (Evans et al., 2008). This suggests that GLUT-1 expression many have an effect on cellular proliferation that is independent of those requiring HIF-1 mediated pathways. This might be exploited as a potential therapy driving cells. Conversely, an inhibition of GLUT-1 could lead to decreased intracellular glucose uptake, which would be especially detrimental in the case of a highly metabolically active malignant glioma. High levels of GLUT-1 expression in the BBB help maintain basal glucose levels in the brain, which would be a major therapeutic problem to overcome if GLUT-1 were to be targeted (Evans et al., 2008).

References

Airley R, Loncaster J, Davidson S, Bromley M, Roberts S, Patterson A, Hunter R, Stratford I, West C (2001) Glucose transporter Glut-1 expression correlates with tumor hypoxia and predicts metastasis-free survival in advanced carcinoma of the cervix. Clin Cancer Res 7:928–934

Alpert E, Gruzman A, Riahi Y, Blejter R, Aharoni P, Weisinger G, Eckel J, Kaiser N, Sasson S (2005) Delayed autoregulation of glucose transport in vascular endothelial cells. Diabetologia 48:752–755

Alpert E, Gruzman A, Totary H, Kaiser N, Reich R, Sasson S (2002) A natural protective mechanism against hyperglycaemia in vascular endothelial and smooth-muscle cells: role of glucose and 12-hydroxyeicosatetraenoic acid. Biochem J 362:413–422

Assadian S, Aliaga A, Del Maestro RF, Evans AC, Bedell BJ (2008) FDG-PET imaging for the evaluation of antiglioma agents in a rat model. Neurooncology 10:292–299

Barthel A, Okino ST, Liao J, Nakatani K, Li J, Whitlock JP Jr., Roth RA (1999) Regulation of GLUT1 gene transcription by the serine/threonine kinase akt1. J Biol Chem 274:20281–20286

Behrooz A, Ismail-Beigi F (1999) Stimulation of glucose transport by hypoxia: signals and mechanisms. News Physiol Sci 14:105–110

Cao X, Fang L, Gibbs S, Huang Y, Dai Z, Wen P, Zheng X, Sadee W, Sun D (2007) Glucose uptake inhibitor sensitizes cancer cells to daunorubicin and overcomes drug resistance in hypoxia. Cancer Chemother Pharmacol 59:495–505

Chung JK, Lee YJ, Kim SK, Jeong JM, Lee DS, Lee MC (2004) Comparison of [18f]fluorodeoxyglucose uptake with glucose transporter-1 expression and proliferation rate in human glioma and non-small-cell lung cancer. Nucl Med Commun 25:11–17

Evans A, Bates V, Troy H, Hewitt S, Holbeck S, Chung YL, Phillips R, Stubbs M, Griffiths J, Airley R (2008) Glut-1 as a therapeutic target: increased chemoresistance and HIF-1-independent link with cell turnover is revealed through COMPARE analysis and metabolomic studies. Cancer Chemother Pharmacol 61:377–393

Farrell CL, Pardridge WM (1991) Blood-brain barrier glucose transporter is asymmetrically distributed on brain capillary endothelial lumenal and ablumenal membranes: an electron microscopic immunogold study. Proc Natl Acad Sci USA 88:5779–5783

Flynn JR, Wang L, Gillespie DL, Stoddard GJ, Reid JK, Owens J, Ellsworth GB, Salzman KL, Kinney AY, Jensen RL (2008) Hypoxia-regulated protein expression, patient characteristics, and preoperative imaging as predictors of survival in adults with glioblastoma multiforme. Cancer 113:1032–1042

Gillespie DL, Whang K, Ragel BT, Flynn JR, Kelly DA, Jensen RL (2007) Silencing of hypoxia inducible factor-1α by RNA interference attenuates human glioma cell growth in vivo. Clin Cancer Res 13:2441–2448

Harik SI, Kalaria RN, Andersson L, Lundahl P, Perry G (1990) Immunocytochemical localization of the erythroid glucose transporter: abundance in tissues with barrier functions. J Neurosci 10:3862–3872

Hiraki Y, Rosen OM, Birnbaum MJ (1988) Growth factors rapidly induce expression of the glucose transporter gene. J Biol Chem 263:13655–13662

Hoskin PJ, Sibtain A, Daley FM, Wilson GD (2003) GLUT1 and CAIX as intrinsic markers of hypoxia in bladder cancer: relationship with vascularity and proliferation as predictors of outcome of ARCON. Br J Cancer 89:1290–1297

Ismail-Beigi F (1993) Metabolic regulation of glucose transport. J Membr Biol 135:1–10

Jensen RL (2006) Hypoxia in the tumorigenesis of gliomas and as a potential target for therapeutic measures. Neurosurg Focus 20(4):E24

Jensen RL (2009) Brain tumor hypoxia: tumorigenesis, angiogenesis, imaging, pseudoprogression, and as a therapeutic target. J Neurooncol 92:317–335

Jensen RL, Ragel BT, Whang K, Gillespie D (2006) Inhibition of hypoxia inducible factor-1α (HIF-1α) decreases vascular endothelial growth factor (VEGF) secretion and tumor growth in malignant gliomas. J Neurooncol 78:233–247

Jonathan RA, Wijffels KI, Peeters W, de Wilde PC, Marres HA, Merkx MA, Oosterwijk E, van der Kogel AJ, Kaanders JH (2006) The prognostic value of endogenous hypoxia-related markers for head and neck squamous cell carcinomas treated with ARCON. Radiother Oncol 79:288–297

Knott RM, Robertson M, Muckersie E, Forrester JV (1996) Regulation of glucose transporters (GLUT-1 and GLUT-3) in human retinal endothelial cells. Biochem J 318(Pt 1):313–317

Loaiza A, Porras OH, Barros LF (2003) Glutamate triggers rapid glucose transport stimulation in astrocytes as evidenced by real-time confocal microscopy. J Neurosci 23:7337–7342

Loda M, Xu X, Pession A, Vortmeyer A, Giangaspero F (2000) Membranous expression of glucose transporter-1 protein (GLUT-1) in embryonal neoplasms of the central nervous system. Neuropathol Appl Neurobiol 26:91–97

Maher F, Vannucci SJ, Simpson IA (1994) Glucose transporter proteins in brain. FASEB J 8:1003–1011

Martell RL, Slapak CA, Levy SB (1997) Effect of glucose transport inhibitors on vincristine efflux in multidrug-resistant murine erythroleukaemia cells overexpressing the multidrug resistance-associated protein (MRP) and two glucose transport proteins, GLUT1 and GLUT3. Br J Cancer 75:161–168

Mitani Y, Dubyak GR, Ismail-Beigi F (1996) Induction of GLUT-1 mRNA in response to inhibition of oxidative phosphorylation: role of increased [Ca2+]i. Am J Physiol 270:C235–C242

Nagamatsu S, Nakamichi Y, Inoue N, Inoue M, Nishino H, Sawa H (1996) Rat C6 glioma cell growth is related to glucose transport and metabolism. Biochem J 319(Pt 2):477–482

Nagamatsu S, Sawa H, Wakizaka A, Hoshino T (1993) Expression of facilitative glucose transporter isoforms in human brain tumors. J Neurochem 61:2048–2053

Nishioka T, Oda Y, Seino Y, Yamamoto T, Inagaki N, Yano H, Imura H, Shigemoto R, Kikuchi H (1992) Distribution of the glucose transporters in human brain tumors. Cancer Res 52:3972–3979

Rastogi S, Banerjee S, Chellappan S, Simon GR (2007) Glut-1 antibodies induce growth arrest and apoptosis in human cancer cell lines. Cancer Lett 257:244–251

Raza SM, Fuller GN, Rhee CH, Huang S, Hess K, Zhang W, Sawaya R (2004) Identification of necrosis-associated genes in glioblastoma by cDNA microarray analysis. Clin Cancer Res 10:212–221

Sanchez-Alvarez R, Tabernero A, Medina JM (2004) Endothelin-1 stimulates the translocation and upregulation of both glucose transporter and hexokinase in astrocytes: relationship with gap junctional communication. J Neurochem 89:703–714

Sathornsumetee S, Cao Y, Marcello JE, Herndon JE 2nd, McLendon RE, Desjardins A, Friedman HS, Dewhirst MW, Vredenburgh JJ, Rich JN (2008) Tumor angiogenic and hypoxic profiles predict radiographic response and survival in malignant astrocytoma patients treated with bevacizumab and irinotecan. J Clin Oncol 26:271–278

Stockhammer F, von Deimling A, Synowitz M, Blechschmidt C, van Landeghem FK (2008) Expression of glucose transporter 1 is associated with loss of heterozygosity of chromosome 1p in oligodendroglial tumors WHO grade II. J Mol Histol 39:553–560

Yeh WL, Lin CJ, Fu WM (2008) Enhancement of glucose transporter expression of brain endothelial cells by vascular endothelial growth factor derived from glioma exposed to hypoxia. Mol Pharmacol 73:170–177

Chapter 12

Malignant Gliomas: Role of Platelet-Derived Growth Factor Receptor A (PDGFRA)

Olga Martinho and Rui Manuel Reis

Abstract Platelet-derived growth factor receptor A (PDGFRA), a type III receptor tyrosine kinase, is frequently up-regulated in cancer, constituting therefore an attractive pharmacological target. Several lines of evidence indicate that PDGFRA plays an important role in gliomagenesis. In the present chapter we will discuss the frequency and type of PDGFRA molecular alterations present in malignant gliomas. Furthermore, we will address the implication of such PDGFRA alterations in malignant glioma patients' therapy response to PDGFRA targeted therapies.

Keywords PDGFRA · Molecular alterations · Gliomas

Introduction

Brain tumors represent the leading cause of cancer related-death in children and the fourth in middle-aged men (Louis et al., 2007). Malignant gliomas, accounting for approximately 70% of all primary brain tumors, are classified into several entities, being astrocytic tumors the most prevalent histological type, followed by oligodendroglial and mixed oligoastrocytic tumors (Louis et al., 2007). According to the World Health Organization (WHO), gliomas can be divided in 4 grades of malignancy. Despite advances in the treatment of glioma patients, the prognosis is dismal, mainly for glioblastomas (WHO grade IV) (Louis et al., 2007). Therefore, it is urgent to better understand glioma tumor biology in order to identify new therapeutic targets and more effective treatment strategies for these patients.

Platelet-derived growth factor receptor A (PDGFRA) is a transmembrane protein with five immunoglobulin-like repeats in the extracellular domain and with a split intracellular tyrosine kinase domain (Andrae et al., 2008). It belongs to class III family of receptor tyrosine kinases (RTKs), which also includes the receptors PDGFRB, KIT, the macrophage colony-stimulating-factor receptor (CSF1) and Fl cytokine receptor (Flt3) (Andrae et al., 2008; Blume-Jensen and Hunter, 2001). Ligand-activated receptors activate downstream signal cascades, including the MAP kinase, PI3-kinase/AKT and JAK/STAT pathways, regulating cellular proliferation, differentiation, invasion, and survival (Blume-Jensen and Hunter, 2001). In the central nervous system (CNS) PDGF signaling plays an important role in normal development, controlling glial cells proliferation of glial cells, mainly oligodendrocytes (Andrae et al., 2008; Richardson et al., 1988).

In malignant gliomas, PDGF receptors and its ligands are commonly co-expressed, suggesting that an autocrine PDGF receptor stimulation may contribute to glioma growth (Shih and Holland, 2006). In animal models, it has been shown that glioma-like tumors can be induced after PDGF overproduction (Uhrbom et al., 1998). Furthermore, it has been suggested that the activation of PDGFRA signaling, through the creation of a favorable microenvironment niche, can contribute to the transformation of neural stem/progenitor cells into glioma (Fomchenko and Holland, 2007). These

R.M. Reis (✉)
School of Health Sciences, Life and Health Sciences Research Institute, University of Minho, 4710-056 Braga, Portugal; Molecular Oncology Research Center, Barretos Cancer Hospital, CEP 14784 400, Barretos, S. Paulo, Brazil
e-mail: rreis@ecsaude.uminho.pt

M.A. Hayat (ed.), *Tumors of the Central Nervous System, Volume 1*,
DOI 10.1007/978-94-007-0344-5_12, © Springer Science+Business Media B.V. 2011

findings imply that PDGFRA signaling may be a driver of gliomagenesis. Consequently, it seems reasonable to hypothesize that PDGFRA constitutes a potential target for anticancer therapy in gliomas.

The interest in PDGFR as a cancer drug target has increased with the availability of small molecule RTK inhibitors, such as imatinib mesylate (Glivec®) and sunitinib (Sutent®), which bind to the target kinase ATP-binding-pocket, competing with ATP, thus blocking its kinase activity (Pietras et al., 2003). Imatinib was one of the first clinically available RTK inhibitor, with demonstrated efficacy in chronic myeloid leukemia (CML) and in gastrointestinal stromal tumors (GISTs), driven by activated forms of *BCR-ABL* and mutated *KIT/PDGFRA* genes, respectively (Capdeville et al., 2002). In malignant gliomas, clinical trials using imatinib are ongoing, however, with limited efficacy (De Witt Hamer, 2010). Nevertheless, the low number of studies and patients, involved so far, hampered the identification of molecular alterations predictive of PDGFR antagonists' response. Thus, we performed a comprehensive analysis of a large series of malignant gliomas (Martinho et al., 2009; Reis et al., 2005), aiming to define the frequency of PDGFRA overexpression and to determine whether PDGFRA overexpression is driven by PDGFA autocrine/paracrine stimulation loops, *PDGFRA* gene mutations, and/ or amplification mechanisms.

PDGFRA Alterations in Malignant Gliomas

Methodology

PDGFRA and PDGFA Immunohistochemistry

In order to determine the frequency and distribution of PDGFRA expression in malignant glioma patients, we analyzed a series of 157 glioma tumors. Additionally, to explore the presence of autocrine and/or paracrine stimulation loops, we also assessed in the same series of tumors, the expression levels of PDGFA, the main PDGFRA ligand. Representative 3 μm thick sections were cut from formalin-fixed and paraffin-embedded samples and subjected to immunohistochemical analysis using the streptavidin-biotin-peroxidase complex technique, with rabbit polyclonal antibodies raised

against human PDGFA (clone N-30, dilution 1:80; Santa Cruz Biotechnology, Santa Cruz, USA), and PDGFRA (dilution 1:175; LabVision Corporation, USA). In brief, deparaffinized and rehydrated sections used to study PDGFA expression were pretreated with microwaving in 10 mM citrate buffer (pH 6.0) three times for 5 min at 600 W. The sections used for PDGFRA expression were submitted to heat-induced antigen retrieval with 10 mM citrate buffer (pH 6.0) for 20 min in a water bath. After incubation of PDGFA and PDGFRA primary antibody at room temperature for 30 min, the secondary biotinylated goat anti-polyvalent antibody was applied for 10 min followed by incubation with streptavidin-peroxidase complex. The immune reaction was visualized with DAB as a chromogen (Ultravision Detection System Anti-polyvalent, HRP/DAB; LabVision Corporation, USA). Appropriated positive and negative controls were included in each run: for PDGFA and PDGFRA, coetaneous-mucosa transition of the anal region, namely medium caliber vessels with a muscular layer were used as positive controls. For negative controls, primary antibodies were omitted. All sections were counterstained with Gill-2 hematoxylin. The distribution and intensity immunoreactivity were semi-quantitatively scored as follows: (−) (negative), (+) (≤5%), (++) (5–50%), and (+++) (>50%). Samples with scores (−) and (+) were considered negative, and those with scores (++) and (+++) were considered positive.

PDGFRA Gene Mutations

To evaluate the presence of *PDGFRA* mutations in malignant gliomas, we screened a series of 92 cases for mutations in the known hotspot *PDGFRA* regions (exons 12, 18 and 23). The exons 12 and 18 are the most frequent mutated in GISTs (Gomes et al., 2008) and somatic mutations at exon 23 have been described in glioblastomas (Parsons et al., 2008; Rand et al., 2005). Mutations screening was done by PCR-single-strand conformational polymorphism (PCR-SSCP) followed by direct DNA sequencing of samples that showed a mobility shift in the PCR-SSCP analysis. Genomic DNA from tumors was isolated form serial 10 μm unstained sections of paraffin blocks. One adjacent hematoxylin and eosin-stained (H&E) section was taken for identification and selection of the tumor tissue. Selected areas containing at least 85% of tumor were marked and macroscopically dissected using a sterile needle (Neolus, 25 G-0.5 mm). Tissue was placed into a microfuge tube and DNA isolation was performed using QIAamp® DNA Micro Kit (Qiagen, Germany), following manufacture procedure.

PCR was carried out in a total volume of 25 μl, consisting of 1–2 μl of DNA solution, 0.5 μM of both sense and anti-sense primers, 200 μM of dNTPs (Fermentas INC., USA), 1.5–2 mM of MgCl2 (Bioron GmbH, Germany), 1× Taq Buffer Incomplete (Bioron GmbH, Germany) and 1U of Taq Superhot DNA Polymerase (Bioron GmbH, Germany). The reaction consisted of an initial denaturation at 96°C for 10 min, followed by 40 cycles with denaturation at 96°C for 45 s, annealing at 56–60°C for 45 s and extension at 72°C for 45 s, followed by a final extension for 10 min at 72°C, in a Thermocycler (BioRad, USA). Primer sequences for exons 12 were 5′-TCCAGTCACTGTGCTGCTTC-3′ (sense) and 5′-GCAAGGGAAAAGGGAGTCTT-3′ (antisense), for exon 18 were 5′-ACCATGGATCAGCCAGTCTT-3′(sense) and 5′-TGAAGAGGATGAGCCTGACC-3′ (anti-sense), and for exon 23 were 5′-GCTCTT CTCTCCCTCCTCCA-3′ (sense) and 5′-TTTCTGAA CGGGATCCAGAG-3′ (antisense). PCR products were mixed with an equivalent volume of the dena-turing loading buffer (98% formamide, 0.05% xylene cyanol and bromophenol blue). After denaturation at 98°C for 10 min and quenching on ice, 20 μl of the mixture were loaded onto a gel containing 0.8× MDE (Cambrex Corporation, USA) for exons 12 and 18 and 1× MDE for exon 23, and 0–3% glycerol (0% for exon 12 and 3% for exons 18 and 23). The gels were run for 20 h at 4°C for exons 12 and 18 and 20°C for exon 23. After the run, the gel was stained with Sybr Gold (Invitrogen Ltd, UK) and visualized under ultraviolet light in a UV transilluminator. Samples showing a mobility shift in the PCR-SSCP analy-sis different from the normal pattern were directly sequenced (Stabvida, Investigation and Services in Biological Sciences Lda, Portugal). All positive cases were confirmed twice with a new and independent PCR amplification, followed by direct sequencing.

PDGFRA Gene Amplification

To assess the presence of PDGFRA gene amplifica-tion in gliomas, we performed quantitative real-time PCR in 56 cases and further validate the results in 6 cases by chromogenic in situ hybridization and in 2 cases by microarray-based comparative genomic hybridization.

Quantitative Real-Time PCR

Quantitative real-time PCR (QPCR) was performed with LightCycler (Roche Molecular Biochemicals, Germany), using fluorescent hybridization probes and fluorescence resonance energy transfer for the detection of PCR amplification product, following the manufacturer's instructions. Briefly, primers and probes were designed to amplify a 124 bp (exon 18 from PDGFRA gene), and a 147 bp (18S gene) specific PCR product, where 18S was used as reference gene. PCR amplification was performed in a 10 μl reaction volume, under the following conditions: 1× reaction master mix (Lightcycler FastStart DNA Master hybridization Probes kit, Roche Molecular Biochemicals, Germany); 0.2 μM Probes (Roche Molecular Biochemicals, Germany); 0.5 μM primers; 4 mM MgCl2 (Roche Molecular Biochemicals, Germany) and 1 μl (20 ng/μl) of DNA. The reaction was initiated by a denaturation step for 10 min at 95°C, followed by 45 cycles with the following profile of amplification: incubation for 10 s at 94°C, specific annealing temperature (57°C for both genes) for 10 s and extension at 72°C for an amplicon dependent time (7 s for 18S and 5 s for PDGFRA), immediately followed by a cooling step for 2 min at 40°C. Primers and probes for 18S gene were previously described by our group (Gomes et al., 2007), for PDGFRA were as follow: 5′-TCAGCTACAGATGGCTTGATCC-3′ (forward primer), 5′-GCCAAAGTCACAGATCTTCACAAT-3′ (reverse primer), 5′-TGTGTCCACCGTGATCTG GCTGC-FL (donator probe), LC640-CGCAACGTC CTCCTGGCACAAGG-3′ (acceptor probe). The PCR was performed in duplicate for each studied sample. A series of 10 normal DNA from healthy individuals was investigated to determine the confidence interval and the standard deviations of the calculated ratios for reference and target gene. Evaluation of data was performed using the $\Delta\Delta Ct$ method: $\Delta\Delta Ct = \Delta Ct$ Tumor DNA $- \Delta Ct$ Normal blood DNA. ΔCt (threshold cycles) is the Ct of the reference gene minus the Ct of the target gene. Fold increase of the target gene PDGFRA was calculated by $2^{(\Delta\Delta Ct)}$ and values

>2 and <5 were defined as aneuploidy and values ≥5 were considered as gene amplification.

Chromogenic In Situ Hybridization

The presence of *PDGFRA* gene amplification was also assessed by means of chromogenic in situ hybridization (CISH) with an in-house generated probe made up with three contiguous, FISH-mapped and end-sequence verified bacterial artificial chromosomes (BACs) (RP11-626H04, RP11-231C18 and RP11-545H22), which map to the *PDGFRA* locus on 4q12 according to Ensembl V39 – June 2006 build of the genome (http://www.ensembl.org/Homo_sapiens/index.html). The in-house probe was generated, biotin-labeled and used in hybridizations as previously described (Gomes et al., 2007). Briefly, for heat pretreatment of deparaffinized sections, they were incubated for 15 min at 98°C in CISH pretreatment buffer (SPOT-light tissue pre-treatment kit, Zymed laboratories, USA) and digested with pepsin for 6 min at room temperature according to the manufacturer's instructions. CISH experiments were analyzed by 3 persons on a multi-headed microscope. Only unequivocal signals were counted. Signals were evaluated at 400×, and 630×, and 60 morphologically unequivocal neoplastic cells were counted for the presence of the gene probe signals. Amplification was defined as >5 signals per nucleus in >50% of tumor cells, or when large gene copy clusters were seen. CISH hybridizations were evaluated with observers blinded to the results of immunohistochemical and QPCR analysis.

Microarray-Based Comparative Genomic Hybridization

The microarray-based comparative genomic hybridization (aCGH) platform used for this study was constructed at the Breakthrough Breast Cancer Research Centre and comprises >16000 BAC clones tiled across the genome. This type of BAC array platform has been shown to be as robust as high density oligonucleotide arrays and its actual resolution is approximately 100 kb for >98% of the genome. Polymorphic BACs identified in an analysis of 50 male:female and female:female hybridizations were filtered out. This left a final dataset of 13711 clones with unambiguous mapping

information according to the March 2006 build (hg18) of the human genome (http://www.ensembl.org). Data were smoothed using the adaptive weight smoothing (aws) algorithm. A categorical analysis was applied to the BACs after classifying them as representing gain, loss, or no-change according to their smoothed Log2 ratio values Threshold values were chosen to correspond to three standard deviations of the normal ratios obtained from the filtered clones mapping to chromosomes 1–22, assessed in multiple hybridizations between DNA extracted from a pool of male and female blood donors (Log2 ratio of ± 0.08). Low level gain was defined as a smoothed Log2 ratio of between 0.12 and 0.40, corresponding to approximately 3–5 copies of the locus, whilst gene amplification was defined as having a Log2 ratio > 0.40, corresponding to more than 5 copies. Data processing and analysis were carried out in R 2.0.1 (http://www.r-project.org/) and BioConductor 1.5 (http://www.bioconductor.org/), making extensive use of modified versions of the packages aCGH, marray and aws in particular.

Statistical Analysis

Correlations between categorical variables were performed using the chi-square test (χ^2-test). Cumulative survival probabilities were calculated using the Kaplan-Meier method. Differences between survival rates were tested with the log-rank test. Two-tailed p values < 0.05 were considered significant. All statistical analysis was performed using SPSS software for Windows, version 16.0.

PDGFRA Expression

We observed that both PDGFRA and PDGFA are found to be overexpressed in glial tumors (Martinho et al., 2009; Reis et al., 2005). PDGFRA expression was detected in 31.8% (50/157) of gliomas, being more frequently expressed in astrocytic tumors (Fig. 12.1a and Table 12.1) (Martinho et al., 2009; Reis et al., 2005). Our data are in agreement with previous studies, where ~50% of malignant astrocytomas were reported to express this receptor (Liang et al., 2008; Ribom et al., 2002; Shih and Holland, 2006; Thorarinsdottir et al., 2008; Varela et al., 2004). PDGFA overexpression was found in 81% (127/157) of cases (Fig. 12.1b

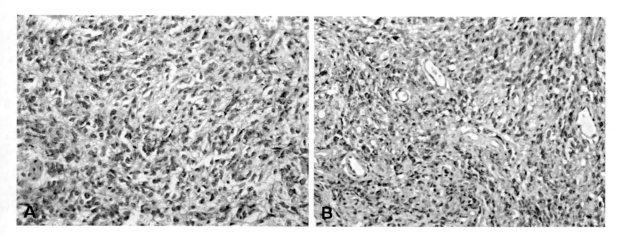

Fig. 12.1 Immunohistochemistry analysis of PDGFRA and PDGFA proteins in a glioblastoma with positive expression of: (**a**) PDGFRA (×200); and (**b**) PDGFA (×200). (Modified from Martinho et al., 2009)

and Table 12.1). PDGFA expression was also observed in tumor-associated endothelial cells and in basal membrane of blood vessels (Martinho et al., 2009; Reis et al., 2005). Previous studies on PDGFA mRNA expression reported high levels of PDGFA in gliomas (Andrae et al., 2008; Shih and Holland, 2006). It should be noted, however, that there is a paucity of data on prevalence of PDGFA protein expression in primary glioma specimens. Twenty seven percent (42/157) of gliomas coexpressed PDGFRA and its, ligand PDGFA, however, no statistically significant association was observed (Martinho et al., 2009; Reis et al., 2005). Particularly in gliosarcomas, positive co-expression of PDGFA and PDGFRA was observed in the glial component of 50% (3/6) of the cases, being negative in the mesenchymal portion (Reis et al., 2005).

A previous study demonstrated PDGFRA overexpression associated with poor prognosis in low-grade gliomas (Varela et al., 2004). In contrast, in a report of 40 patients with grade II astrocytomas and oligoastrocytomas, there was an association between high PDGFRA expression and favorable patient outcome (Ribom et al., 2002). Recently, Liang et al. (2008). in a pediatric high grade glioma series failed to find any significant impact of PDGFRA expression on survival. In our series, PDGFRA expression was not correlated with patients' survival. Interestingly, we found a trend for an association between the absence of PDGFA expression and a poor prognosis in patients with malignant glioma (Martinho et al., 2009).

PDGFRA Genetic Alterations

Overexpression of RTKs in cancer has been shown to be driven by underlying genetic events in a substantial proportion of cases. For instance, KIT overexpression in GISTs is driven by activating *KIT* mutations (Gomes et al., 2008), whereas HER2 overexpression in breast cancer is driven by *HER2* gene amplification (Arriola et al., 2008). In our studies no *PDGFRA* activating mutations were found (Martinho et al., 2009; Reis et al., 2005), which is in agreement with previous reports (Hartmann et al., 2004; Raymond et al., 2008; Sihto et al., 2005; Wen et al., 2006). Instead, four silent mutations and an intronic insertion were identified. In exon 12 there were three different silent transitions: a T to C change at base pair 1686 (I562I), a substitution of a G to A at position 1701 (P567P) and a transition of a C to T located at base pair 1777 (L593L). In exon 18 it was found at position 2472 a substitution of a C to T (V824V). At 50 bp downstream the 5′-end of exon 18 (between 2449 and 2450 bp), it was observed an insertion of an adenine nucleotide (IVS18-50insA) (Martinho et al., 2009; Reis et al., 2005). Apart from the two silent mutations in *PDGFRA* exon 12, the other mutations have been previously described and considered to be genetic polymorphisms.

Recent comprehensive genomic studies in gliomas have reported the presence of somatic mutations on *PDGFRA* coding region (Fig. 12.2) (Rand et al., 2005; McLendon et al., 2008; Greenman et al., 2007; Parsons

Table 12.1 PDGFA/PDGFRA expression and *PDGFRA* amplification in malignant gliomas

Parameter		PDGFA expression (N = 157)		PDGFRA expression (N = 157)		PDGFRA amplification[a] (N = 56)		
	N	Positive (%)	P value	Positive (%)	P value	N	Amplified (%)	P value
Histological type (WHO grade)								
Diffuse astrocytoma (II)	33	32 (97.0)	0.006*	15 (45.5)	<0.001*	10	5 (50.0)	0.227
Anaplastic astrocytoma (III)	5	5 (100)		3 (60.0)		2	0 (0)	
Glioblastoma (IV)	36	23 (63.9)		19 (52.5)		19	3 (15.8)	
Gliosarcoma (IV)	6	6 (100)		3 (50.0)			nd	
Oligodendroglioma (II)	32	23 (71.9)		4 (12.5)		10	1 (10)	
Anaplastic oligodendroglioma (III)	36	32 (88.9)		3 (8.3)		13	2 (15.4)	
Oligoastrocytoma (II)	2	1 (50.0)		0 (0)			nd	
Anaplastic oligoastrocytoma (III)	7	5 (71.4)		3 (42.9)		2	1 (50)	
Cellular lineage								
Astrocytic	80	66 (82.5)	0.519	40 (50.0)	<0.001*	32	8 (25.0)	0.334
Oligodendroglial	68	55 (80.9)		7 (10.3)		23	3 (13.0)	
Oligoastrocytic	9	6 (66.7)		3 (33.3)		2	1 (50.0)	
Malignancy grade (WHO)								
Low-grade (II)	67	56 (83.6)	0.298	19 (28.4)	0.263	21	6 (28.6)	0.232
High-grade (III and IV)	90	71 (78.9)		31 (34.4)		36	6 (16.7)	

[a] Assessed by QPCR

N: number of cases; nd: not done; (*) Statistically significant values ($p < 0.05$)

Table modified from Reis et al. (2005) and Martinho et al. (2009)

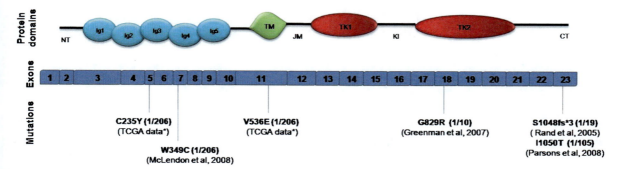

Fig. 12.2 Schematic representation of PDGFRA protein domains (*upper panel*) and coding exons (*middle panel*) with the indication of the *PDGFRA* gene mutations (*lower panel*) described in the literature. PDGFRA have five extracellular Ig domains (Ig-like domains), a transmembrane domain (TM), a juxtamembrane domain (JM), and a bipartite tyrosine kinase catalytic domain (TK1 and TK2) separated by a kinase insert region (KI) and a C-terminal tail (CT). The N-terminal is labeled N. (*) Data collected from the "The Cancer Genome Atlas" (TCGA) database: http://cancergenome.nih.gov/

et al., 2008; http://cancergenome.nih.gov). However, it is unclear the frequency and oncogenic role of these mutations in gliomas, since confirmatory studies are still missing. In fact, our studies did not show any of the described mutations at *PDGFRA* exons 18 and 23 (Reis et al., 2005; Martinho et al., 2009).

Our analysis of *PDGFRA* gene copy number status, as defined by QPCR, revealed *PDGFRA* copy number changes in 53.6% (30/56) of gliomas: 18 displayed aneuploidy/aneusomy and 12 (21.4%) were considered amplified (Table 12.1) (Martinho et al., 2009). The same frequency of *PDGFRA* amplification was described in previous studies (Holtkamp et al., 2007; Joensuu et al., 2005; Puputti et al., 2006; McLendon et al., 2008). In 12 cases, data on *PDGFRA* amplification status in the both primary and recurrent tumors were available. In all but one case primary and recurrent tumors displayed identical *PDGFRA* copy number status, suggesting that *PDGFRA* amplification is an early event (Martinho et al., 2009). To validate QPCR results we performed CISH in 6 cases and observed that the 3 cases harboring *PDGFRA* gene amplification by QPCR revealed clusters of *PDGFRA* signals in the nuclei of neoplastic cells (Fig. 12.3a), confirming gene amplification. In the 3 cases without *PDGFRA* gene amplification, only one-to-two *PDGFRA* gene signals per nucleus were found in neoplastic cells (Fig. 12.3b) (Martinho et al., 2009).

A significant association between *PDGFRA* amplification and overexpression was only found in diffuse astrocytomas (Martinho et al., 2009). Given that PDGFRA overexpression appears to be an early event in gliomagenesis (Hermanson et al., 1996), our results provide support to the contention that gene amplification may be one of the underlying mechanisms at this stage. In a way akin to other oncogenes, such as EGFR, overexpression of PDGFRA was more pervasive than gene amplification. It should be noted, however, that in our series there were ~42% of cases with *PDGFRA* amplification that lacked PDGFRA protein expression, suggesting that in some cases the target of 4q12 amplification may be a gene other than *PDGFRA* (Martinho et al., 2009). In fact, we and other authors have further demonstrated by techniques like aCGH (Fig. 12.3c) that the amplicon encompasses a region of 3.6 Mb, which, in addition to *PDGFRA*, also includes *KIT* and *KDR* oncogenes (Holtkamp et al., 2007; Joensuu et al., 2005; Puputti et al., 2006; McLendon et al., 2008; Martinho et al., 2009).

Clinical Implications of PDGFRA in Gliomas

Due to the high frequency of PDGFRA alterations in malignant gliomas, strategies aiming to inhibit PDGFRA signaling are under intensive clinical studies. The most frequently studied drug is imatinib, a small-molecule inhibitor of PDGFRA, PDGFRB and the BCR-ABL fusion protein (Capdeville et al., 2002). Despite the positive response, imatinib targeted therapy has not shown significant clinical activity as a single agent in adult and pediatric phase II studies (Baruchel et al., 2009; De Witt Hamer, 2010; Geoerger

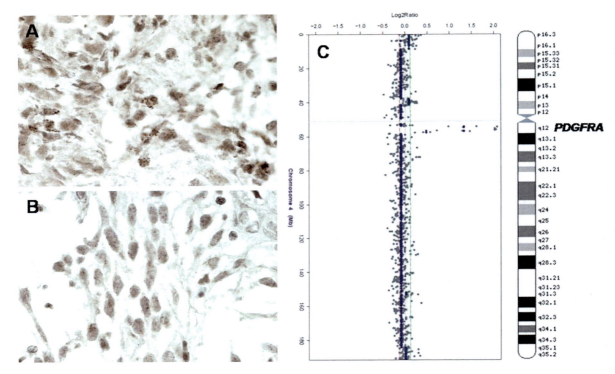

Fig. 12.3 CISH analysis of *PDGFRA* in glioblastomas: (**a**) case with *PDGFRA* amplification (×600, no H.E. counterstaining); and (**b**) case without *PDGFRA* amplification (×600, no H.E. counterstaining). (**c**) Ideogram and microarray CGH chromosome plots of chromosome 4 for a case exhibiting amplification of *PDGFRA* gene location. Log2 ratios are plotted on the X axis against each clone according to genomic location on the Y axis. The centromere is represented by a *horizontal dotted line. Vertical dashed lines* correspond to log2 ratios of 0.12 (*green*) and –0.12 (*red*). *Gray dots*: Log2 ratios; *Blue dots*: aws-smoothed Log2 ratios. (Modified from Martinho et al., 2009)

et al., 2009). Further studies are warranted to evaluate its efficacy in combination with gold-standard chemotherapy agents, such as temozolomide in CNS tumors.

Several reasons for these disappointing results can be raised. One fact can be the lack of biomarkers for PDGFRA antagonists' response, not allowing the selection of patients that truly could benefit from such therapies. Currently, some studies analyzed the prevalence of *PDGFRA* alterations in brain tumor patients enrolled in phase I/II studies of imatinib mesylate, yet, no associations were observed (Baruchel et al., 2009; Geoerger et al., 2009; Raymond et al., 2008; Wen et al., 2006). Other potential explanation is the development of resistance, through the constitutive activation of downstream intracellular effectors and coactivation of alternative RTKs in the neoplastic cells. To overcome this problem, combinations of targeted agents have been proposed and are currently being tested (Idbaih et al., 2008). In this line, cediranib, a multi-target RTK inhibitor which blocks PDGFRA, KIT, VEGFR1,

VEGFR2 and VEGFR3, is showing promising results in malignant glioma patients (Batchelor et al., 2007).

In conclusion, PDGFRA signaling is a major player in gliomagenesis. Despite the less encourage results of the initial clinical trials with anti-PDGFRA drugs, new, more effective and multi-target inhibitors are being designed and tested, supporting the potential therapeutic value of PDGFRA in patients with malignant glioma.

References

Andrae J, Gallini R, Betsholtz C (2008) Role of platelet-derived growth factors in physiology and medicine. Genes Dev 22(10):1276–1312

Arriola E, Marchiò C, Tan DS, Drury SC, Lambros MB, Natrajan R, Rodriguez-Pinilla SM, Mackay A, Tamber N, Fenwick K, Jones C, Dowsett M, Ashworth A, Reis-Filho JS (2008) Genomic analysis of the HER2/TOP2A amplicon in breast cancer and breast cancer cell lines. Lab Invest 88:491–503

Baruchel S, Sharp JR, Bartels U, Hukin J, Odame I, Portwine C, Strother D, Fryer C, Halton J, Egorin MJ, Reis RM, Martinho O, Stempak D, Hawkins C, Gammon J, Bouffet E (2009) A Canadian paediatric brain tumour consortium (CPBTC) phase II molecularly targeted study of imatinib in recurrent and refractory paediatric central nervous system tumours. Eur J Cancer 45(13):2352–2359

Batchelor TT, Sorensen AG, di Tomaso E, Zhang WT, Duda DG, Cohen KS, Kozak KR, Cahill DP, Chen PJ, Zhu M, Ancukiewicz M, Mrugala MM, Plotkin S, Drappatz J, Louis DN, Ivy P, Scadden DT, Benner T, Loeffler JS, Wen PY, Jain RK (2007) AZD2171, a pan-VEGF receptor tyrosine kinase inhibitor, normalizes tumor vasculature and alleviates edema in glioblastoma patients. Cancer Cell 11(1):83–95

Blume-Jensen P, Hunter T (2001) Oncogenic kinase signalling. Nature 411:355–365

Capdeville R, Buchdunger E, Zimmermann J, Matter A (2002) Glivec (STI571, imatinib), a rationally developed, targeted anticancer drug. Nat Rev Drug Discov 1:493–502

De Witt Hamer PC (2010) Small molecule kinase inhibitors in glioblastoma: a systematic review of clinical studies. Neurooncology 12(3):304–316

Fomchenko EI, Holland EC (2007) Platelet-derived growth factor-mediated gliomagenesis and brain tumor recruitment. Neurosurg Clin N Am 18:39–58

Geoerger B, Morland B, Ndiaye A, Doz F, Kalifa G, Geoffray A, Pichon F, Frappaz D, Chatelut E, Opolon P, Hain S, Boderet F, Bosq J, Emile JF, Le Deley MC, Capdeville R, Vassal G Innovative Therapies for Children with Cancer European Consortium (2009) Target-driven exploratory study of imatinib mesylate in children with solid malignancies by the Innovative Therapies for Children with Cancer (ITCC) European Consortium. Eur J Cancer 45(13): 2342–2351

Gomes AL, Gouveia A, Capelinha AF, de la Cruz D, Silva P, Reis RM, Pimenta A, Lopes JM (2008) Molecular alterations of KIT and PDGFRA in GISTs: evaluation of a Portuguese series. J Clinical Pathol 61(2):203–208

Gomes AL, Reis-Filho JS, Lopes JM, Martinho O, Lambros MB, Martins A, Schmitt F, Pardal F, Reis RM (2007) Molecular alterations of KIT oncogene in gliomas. Cell Oncol 29:399–408

Greenman C, Stephens P, Smith R, Dalgliesh GL, Hunter C, Bignell G, Davies H, Teague J, Butler A, Stevens C, Edkins S, O'Meara S, Vastrik I, Schmidt EE, Avis T, Barthorpe S, Bhamra G, Buck G, Choudhury B, Clements J, Cole J, Dicks E, Forbes S, Gray K, Halliday K, Harrison R, Hills K, Hinton J, Jenkinson A, Jones D, Menzies A, Mironenko T, Perry J, Raine K, Richardson D, Shepherd R, Small A, Tofts C, Varian J, Webb T, West S, Widaa S, Yates A, Cahill DP, Louis DN, Goldstraw P, Nicholson AG, Brasseur F, Looijenga L, Weber BL, Chiew YE, DeFazio A, Greaves MF, Green AR, Campbell P, Birney E, Easton DF, Chenevix-Trench G, Tan MH, Khoo SK, The BT, Yuen ST, Leung SY, Wooster R, Futreal PA, Stratton MR (2007) Patterns of somatic mutation in human cancer genomes. Nature 446(7132):153–158

Hartmann C, Xu X, Bartels G, Holtkamp N, Gonzales IA, Tallen G, von Deimling A (2004) Pdgfr-alpha in 1p/19q LOH oligodendrogliomas. Int J Cancer 112:1081–1082

Hermanson M, Funa K, Koopmann J, Maintz D, Waha A, Westermark B, Heldin CH, Wiestler OD, Louis DN, von Deimling A, Nister M (1996) Association of loss of heterozygosity on chromosome 17p with high platelet-derived growth factor alpha receptor expression in human malignant gliomas. Cancer Res 56:164–171

Holtkamp N, Ziegenhagen N, Malzer E, Hartmann C, Giese A, von Deimling A (2007) Characterization of the amplicon on chromosomal segment 4q12 in glioblastoma multiforme. Neurooncology 9:291–297

Idbaih A, Ducray F, Del Rio MS, Hoang-Xuan K, Delattre JY (2008) Therapeutic application of noncytotoxic molecular targeted therapy in gliomas: growth factor receptors and angiogenesis inhibitors. Oncologist 13(9):978–992

Joensuu H, Puputti M, Sihto H, Tynninen O, Nupponen NN (2005) Amplification of genes encoding KIT, PDGFRalpha and VEGFR2 receptor tyrosine kinases is frequent in glioblastoma multiforme. J Pathol 207:224–231

Liang ML, Ma J, Ho M, Solomon L, Bouffet E, Rutka JT, Hawkins C (2008) Tyrosine kinase expression in pediatric high grade astrocytoma. J Neurooncol 87:247–253

Louis DN, Ohgaki H, Wiestler OD, Cavenee WK, Burger PC, Jouvet A, Scheithauer BW, Kleihues P (2007) The 2007 WHO classification of tumours of the central nervous system. Acta Neuropathol 114:97–109

Martinho O, Longatto-Filho A, Lambros MB, Martins A, Pinheiro C, Silva A, Pardal F, Amorim J, Mackay A, Milanezi F, Tamber N, Fenwick K, Ashworth A, Reis-Filho JS, Lopes JM, Reis RM (2009) Expression, mutation and copy number analysis of platelet-derived growth factor receptor A (PDGFRA) and its ligand PDGFA in gliomas. Br J Cancer 15 101(6):973–982

McLendon R, Friedman A, Bigner D, Van Meir EG, Brat DJ, Mastrogianakis GM, Olson JJ, Mikkelsen T, Lehman N, Aldape K, Yung WK, Bogler O, Weinstein JN, VandenBerg S, Berger M, Prados M, Muzny D, Morgan M, Scherer S, Sabo A, Nazareth L, Lewis L, Hall O, Zhu Y, Ren Y, Alvi O, Yao J, Hawes A, Jhangiani S, Fowler G, San Lucas A, Kovar C, Cree A, Dinh H, Santibanez J, Joshi V, Gonzalez-Garay ML, Miller CA, Milosavljevic A, Donehower L, Wheeler DA, Gibbs RA, Cibulskis K, Sougnez C, Fennell T, Mahan S, Wilkinson J, Ziaugra L, Onofrio R, Bloom T, Nicol R, Ardlie K, Baldwin J, Gabriel S, Lander ES, Ding L, Fulton RS, McLellan MD, Wallis J, Larson DE, Shi X, Abbott R, Fulton L, Chen K, Koboldt DC, Wendl MC, Meyer R, Tang Y, Lin L, Osborne JR, Dunford-Shore BH, Miner TL, Delehaunty K, Markovic C, Swift G, Courtney W, Pohl C, Abbott S, Hawkins A, Leong S, Haipek C, Schmidt H, Wiechert M, Vickery T, Scott S, Dooling DJ, Chinwalla A, Weinstock GM, Mardis ER, Wilson RK, Getz G, Winckler W, Verhaak RG, Lawrence MS, O'Kelly M, Robinson J, Alexe G, Beroukhim R, Carter S, Chiang D, Gould J, Gupta S, Korn J, Mermel C, Mesirov J, Monti S, Nguyen H, Parkin M, Reich M, Stransky N, Weir BA, Garraway L, Golub T, Meyerson M, Chin L, Protopopov A, Zhang J, Perna I, Aronson S, Sathiamoorthy N, Ren G, Yao J, Wiedemeyer WR, Kim H, Kong SW, Xiao Y, Kohane IS, Seidman J, Park P, Kucherlapati R, Laird PW, Cope L, Herman JG, Weisenberger DJ, Pan F, Van den Berg D, Van Neste L,

Yi JM, Schuebel KE, Baylin SB, Absher DM, Li JZ, Southwick A, Brady S, Aggarwal A, Chung T, Sherlock G, Brooks JD, Myers RM, Spellman PT, Purdom E, Jakkula LR, Lapuk AV, Marr H, Dorton S, Choi YG, Han J, Ray A, Wang V, Durinck S, Robinson M, Wang NJ, Vranizan K, Peng V, Van Name E, Fontenay GV, Ngai J, Conboy JG, Parvin B, Feiler HS, Speed TP, Gray JW, Brennan C, Socci ND, Olshen A, Taylor BS, Lash A, Schultz N, Reva B, Antipin Y, Stukalov A, Gross B, Cerami E, Wang WQ, Qin LX, Seshan VE, Villafania L, Cavatore M, Borsu L, Viale A, Gerald W, Sander C, Ladanyi M, Perou CM, Hayes DN, Topal MD, Hoadley KA, Qi Y, Balu S, Shi Y, Wu J, Penny R, Bittner M, Shelton T, Lenkiewicz E, Morris S, Beasley D, Sanders S, Kahn A, Sfeir R, Chen J, Nassau D, Feng L, Hickey E, Barker A, Gerhard DS, Vockley J, Compton C, Vaught J, Fielding P, Ferguson ML, Schaefer C, Zhang J, Madhavan S, Buetow KH, Collins F, Good P, Guyer M, Ozenberger B, Peterson J, Thomson E (2008) Comprehensive genomic characterization defines human glioblastoma genes and core pathways. Nature 455(7216):1061–1068

Parsons DW, Jones S, Zhang X, Lin JC, Leary RJ, Angenendt P, Mankoo P, Carter H, Siu IM, Gallia GL, Olivi A, McLendon R, Rasheed BA, Keir S, Nikolskaya T, Nikolsky Y, Busam DA, Tekleab H, Diaz LA Jr, Hartigan J, Smith DR, Strausberg RL, Marie SK, Shinjo SM, Yan H, Riggins GJ, Bigner DD, Karchin R, Papadopoulos N, Parmigiani G, Vogelstein B, Velculescu VE, Kinzler KW (2008) An integrated genomic analysis of human glioblastoma multiforme. Science 321(5897):1807–1812

Pietras K, Sjoblom T, Rubin K, Heldin CH, Ostman A (2003) PDGF receptors as cancer drug targets. Cancer Cell 3:439–443

Puputti M, Tynninen O, Sihto H, Blom T, Maenpaa. H, Isola J, Paetau A, Joensuu H, Nupponen NN (2006) Amplification of KIT, PDGFRA, VEGFR2, and EGFR in gliomas. Mol Cancer Res 4:927–934

Rand V, Huang J, Stockwell T, Ferriera S, Buzko O, Levy S, Busam D, Li K, Edwards JB, Eberhart C, Murphy KM, Tsiamouri A, Beeson K, Simpson AJ, Venter JC, Riggins GJ, Strausberg RL (2005) Sequence survey of receptor tyrosine kinases reveals mutations in glioblastomas. Proc Nat Acad Sci 102:14344–14349

Raymond E, Brandes AA, Dittrich C, Fumoleau P, Coudert B, Clement PM, Frenay M, Rampling R, Stupp R, Kros JM, Heinrich MC, Gorlia T, Lacombe D,, van den Bent MJ European organisation for research and treatment of cancer brain tumor group study (2008) Phase II study of imatinib in patients with recurrent gliomas of various histologies: a European Organisation for Research and Treatment of Cancer Brain Tumor Group Study. J Clin Oncol 26: 4659–4665

Reis RM, Martins A, Ribeiro SA, Basto D, Longatto-Filho A, Schmitt FC, Lopes JM (2005) Molecular characterization of PDGFR-alpha/PDGF-A and c-KIT/SCF in gliosarcomas. Cell Oncol 27:319–326

Ribom D, Andrae J, Frielingsdorf M, Hartman M, Nister M, Smits A (2002) Prognostic value of platelet derived growth factor alpha receptor expression in grade 2 astrocytomas and oligoastrocytomas. J Neurol Neurosurg Psychiatry 72:782–787

Richardson WD, Pringle N, Mosley MJ, Westermark B, Dubois Dalcq M (1988) A role for platelet-derived growth factor in normal gliogenesis in the central nervous system. Cell 53:309–319

Shih AH, Holland EC (2006) Platelet-derived growth factor (PDGF) and glial tumorigenesis. Cancer Lett 232:139–147

Sihto H, Sarlomo-Rikala M, Tynninen O, Tanner M, Andersson LC, Franssila K, Nupponen NN, Joensuu H (2005) KIT and platelet-derived growth factor receptor alpha tyrosine kinase gene mutations and KIT amplifications in human solid tumors. J Clin Oncol 23:49–57

Thorarinsdottir HK, Santi M, McCarter R, Rushing EJ, Cornelison R, Jales A, MacDonald TJ (2008) Protein expression of platelet-derived growth factor receptor correlates with malignant histology and PTEN with survival in childhood gliomas. Clin Cancer Res 14:3386–3394

Uhrbom L, Hesselager G, Nister M, Westermark B (1998) Induction of brain tumors in mice using a recombinant platelet-derived growth factor B-chain retrovirus. Cancer Res 58:5275–5279

Varela M, Ranuncolo SM, Morand A, Lastiri J, De Kier Joffe EB, Puricelli LI, Pallotta MG (2004) EGF-R and PDGF-R, but not bcl-2, overexpression predict overall survival in patients with low-grade astrocytomas. J Surg Oncol 86:34–40

Wen PY, Yung WKA, Lamborn KR, Dahia PL, Wang YF, Peng B, Abrey LE, Raizer J, Cloughesy TF, Fink K, Gilbert M, Chang S, Junck L, Schiff D, Lieberman F, Fine HA, Mehta M, Robins HI, DeAngelis LM, Groves MD, Puduvalli VK, Levin V, Conrad C, Maher EA, Aldape K, Hayes M, Letvak L, Egorin MJ, Capdeville R, Kaplan R, Murgo AJ, Stiles C, Prados MD (2006) Phase I/II study of imatinib mesylate for recurrent malignant gliomas: North American Brain Tumor Consortium Study 99-08. Clin Cancer Res 12:4899–4907

Chapter 13

Molecular Methods for Detection of Tumor Markers in Glioblastomas

Marie E. Beckner and Mary L. Nordberg

Abstract Glioblastoma (grade IV/IV astrocytoma), the most malignant type of brain tumor, occurs in all age groups with the highest incidence in older patients. Novel therapeutic strategies and molecular assays to follow treatments of suppressible targets are urgently needed. Surveys of large numbers of genes in the initial phase of tumor marker identification are currently being performed in multi-center studies. Queries of the results in national databases, such as the Respository of Molecular Brain Neoplasia Database (REMBRANDT) can yield candidate tumor markers, such as those involved with upregulated glycolysis. We found that *ENO1*, encoding enolase 1, emerged as a tumor marker in glioblastomas. Although treatments directed at glycolytic enzymes, such as enolase, are not technically feasible, *ENO1* can be used to identify associated genes that are feasible targets. Real-time quantitative polymerase chain reaction (RQ-PCR) provides the sensitivity required to detect *ENO1*-associated tumor markers that can serve as suppressible treatment targets. The sensitivity of RQ-PCR is also ideal for monitoring treatment response to successful cancer drugs that are developed for molecular targets. This approach to tumor marker discovery in glioblastomas is described.

Keywords Tumor markers · Glioblastomas · Real-time quantitative PCR · REMBRANDT · Enolase

Introduction

Glioblastoma (grade IV/IV astrocytoma), the most malignant type of brain tumor, occurs in all age groups with the highest incidence in older patients (median age at diagnosis is 64 years). This is the major type of glioma in adults. Glioblastomas are characterized by invasive behavior within the central nervous system (CNS), resistance to therapy, and a poor prognosis. The five year patient survival rate is <4% CBTRUS, (2005). However, this type of tumor usually does not metastasize. Thus, glioblastomas can be considered as a model for the study of malignant, invasive behavior without considering the biology of metastasis. Novel therapeutic strategies and molecular assays to follow treatments of glioblastomas are urgently needed in view of the poor quality of life and survival in these patients. The genome of gliomas is highly unstable, leading to a myriad of genetic abnormalities whose full extent has only recently been appreciated. The Glioma Molecular Diagnostic Initiative discovered "a wealth of new genomic abnormalities in gliomas" (Kotliarov et al., 2006). A study of a large number of pediatric gliomas, utilizing single nucleotide polymorphism arrays, has detected areas of allelic imbalance in the glioblastomas (Wong et al., 2006). Array-based comparative genomic hybridization and microarray expression profiling have demonstrated deletion of 35 loci (median size of 1.86 Mb, median number of 16 genes) in primary glioblastomas (no previous history of a low grade glioma) and deletion of 54 loci (median size of 3.02 Mb, median number of 27 genes) in secondary glioblastomas (previous history of a low grade glioma present) (Maher et al., 2006).

M.E. Beckner (✉)
Department of Neurology, Louisiana State University Health Sciences Center School of Medicine in Shreveport, Shreveport, LA, USA
e-mail: mbeckner@sprynet.com

M.A. Hayat (ed.), *Tumors of the Central Nervous System, Volume 1*,
DOI 10.1007/978-94-007-0344-5_13, © Springer Science+Business Media B.V. 2011

In view of the genetic instability in glioblastomas it is not surprising that tumor suppressor genes, such as *PTEN*, are often lost. Although the effects of losing negative regulators includes increased downstream effects that aid neoplastic transformation, restoration of tumor suppressors is not feasible with the current limitations of gene therapy. However, suppressible treatment targets are found by identifying unique structural genetic defects or increased expression of key wild type genes and their products. Constitutively activated oncogenes resulting from missing or altered exons, novel fusion products of translocations, etc., constitute promising candidates for tumor specific therapies. Examples in glioblastomas include certain sequence alterations in the gene encoding epidermal growth factor receptor (*EGFR*). One mutation is a deletion of exons 2–7, known as the *EGFRvIII* variant. The protein encoded by *EGFRvIII* has activity that is independent of ligand binding. There are several other mutated *EGFR* products which also are ligand independent. Amplification of *EGFR* is also commonly found. Accordingly, identification of *EGFR* and its variants as tumor markers in glioblastomas has led to clinical trials of new therapeutic regimens directed against EGFR, but in unselected patients their success has not been clearly established (de Groot et al., 2008; Preusser et al., 2008). Although patients with brain tumors have been unselected for most clinical trials, patients with lung and colorectal carcinomas treated with the EGFR inhibitors are commonly selected according to their *EGFR* status. To aid in the selection of cancer patients for directed therapy, fluorescent in situ hybridization (FISH) analysis for *EGFR* amplification in clinical specimens is commonly performed. Requests for *EGFR* studies are increasing. During the last few months of 2008, amplification of *EGFR* was documented in several cases of primary or metastatic lung and colorectal carcinomas by FISH in our laboratory.

Molecular Methods for Tumor Markers

It is logical that tumor markers of therapeutic importance are associated either directly or indirectly with increased expression of basic functional genes required for malignant adaptations. The success of cells in genetically unstable tumors to emerge as a dominant proliferating or invasive clone is thus determined by mutations that lead to altered expression levels of genes encoding functional proteins. The proteins that participate in unchecked mitotic divisions, glycolysis, adaptation to hypoxia, proteolysis, migration, etc. contribute to the success of cancer cells. The intact genes in malignant cells are in complex biological networks under the influence of genes that harbor key transforming mutations. Various types of gene arrays are used for surveys of large numbers of genes in the initial phase of tumor marker identification. Once these genes are confirmed as tumor markers with other methods, such as real-time quantitative PCR (RQ-PCR), they can be evaluated for their clinical use as therapeutic targets and prognostic indicators in glioblastomas. For some of the structurally altered or amplified genes used as tumor markers, FISH and allele specific PCR are DNA based methods of detection that are appropriate for clinical assays of individual tumors. However, real-time quantitative RNA expression analysis by RQ-PCR exceeds the capabilities of all other methods in sensitivity of detection, both during the discovery phase and the clinical application of tumor markers. Due to its high level of sensitivity, RQ-PCR is preferred when subtle amplifications of genes and their products in a biological network are suspected to be "bad actors" responsible for tumors. Part of the difficulty in identifying tumor markers is attributed to the relatively low level of amplification for some key genes and their products in complex biological networks that can result in large functional effects, such as increased enzyme activity in glycolysis. Also, when targeted clinical therapies with small molecules are available (for example, in hematologic malignancies) RQ-PCR is needed to detect minimal residual disease. Detection of molecular relapses with RQ-PCR permits vital, timely treatment decisions prior to the emergence of morphologic and clinical relapses that are much more difficult to treat. It also provides guidance to avoid over-treatment. Therefore, RQ-PCR is anticipated to play a similar role in the future treatment of brain tumors when small molecule drugs for specific targets become available. Although achieving the level of sensitivity required for detection of tumor markers circulating in the peripheral blood from brain tumors may be an unrealistic goal, RQ-PCR has a good chance of detecting brain tumor markers in the cerebrospinal fluid that could be used to predict molecular relapses.

In comparison to proteomics for the study of biological networks, identifying RNA transcripts by sequence-related information can be more reliable. Protein identification that utilizes molecular weight determinations, such as mass spectrometry and immunoblotting, is less reliable if the genes of interest have been altered in genetically unstable tumors. In a small survey of proteins in frozen tissue samples of glioblastomas performed in our laboratory, one-third of the proteins identified with antibodies on immunoblots had aberrant molecular weights. In addition to genetic instability, the conspicuous activation of proteases in tumors resulting in partial degradation of proteins in vivo may also help to explain variation in the size of suspected tumor markers on immunoblots. However, studies based on RNA expression overcome the limitation of utilizing molecular weight as a parameter in identifying proteins as tumor markers. Primers for PCR can be designed to target a relatively small but crucial portion of a tumor marker's gene that is known to be selectively retained due to the functional relevance of the encoded protein fragment. Thus, genetic instability and degradation that are commonly found in highly malignant brain tumors can be minimized as confounding variables in RNA based searches for tumor markers.

Real-Time Quantitative Polymerase Chain Reaction

Among the PCR methods that rely on reverse transcriptase (RT) to generate complementary DNA (cDNA) from RNA for amplification, RQ-PCR offers the widest dynamic range of detection for expression of a marker. Rather than using the plateau region of a PCR reaction for quantification, RQ-PCR relies on the crossing threshold (C_t) of reactions during the exponential phase of PCR for quantifying results. The C_t is determined when the amplification product reaches a threshold above the background of initial cycling (such as at least ten times (or more) than the background noise of early cycles). In the presence of a fluorescent dye, such as SYBR Green that binds DNA, the signal for accumulating product is read in a closed tube system during RQ-PCR. The dynamic range of measurement is much wider than when the plateau of the PCR reaction is used as an endpoint. The amount of

amplified target is directly proportional to the original amount of the target marker's RNA only during the exponential phase of PCR amplification, which is reliably present at the C_t. Thus the C_t reflects accumulation of target amplicon at a stage of thermal cycling when substrates are not limiting and there is no product degradation. The dynamic range of RQ-PCR in recent translational oncology studies has been ten-fold to greater than eight orders of magnitude (Skrzypski, 2008; Vaananen et al., 2008).

Quantification can be accomplished in absolute amounts via standard curves or alternatively in relative amounts based on the expression levels of one or more housekeeping genes. A mathematical model termed the "*delta delta C_t*" equation is applied to reliably measure relative quantification (Livak and Schmittgen, 2001; VanGuilder et al., 2008). The expression of a tumor marker in a tumor sample can be compared with a reference sample (non-malignant tissue sample) using this equation. The dC_t for each gene in an assay equals C_t (tumor marker gene) – average C_t (house keeping genes). The ddC_t for each gene equals dC_t (tumor sample) – dC_t (reference non-malignant tissue sample). The fold-change for each gene from the normal reference sample to the tumor sample is calculated as 2^{-ddC_t} (the negative ddC_t exponential function of 2) assuming that the amount of product doubles during each cycle of amplification. The "*delta delta C_t*" equation converts the non-linear C_t results to linear results that are appropriate for analysis by standard statistical tests (VanGuilder et al., 2008). The efficiencies of RNA extraction, reverse transcription, and primer amplification during PCR should be equivalent for the tumor marker and housekeeping genes. Alternatively, variances in efficiencies, if present, can be detected and corrected with software programs that are available online from manufacturers of commercial kits and real-time PCR equipment.

Relative versus absolute quantification with RQ-PCR offers advantages in that standard curves are not needed. For unique tumor markers, such as those produced by fusions of broken genes, it is difficult for manufacturers of commercial kits to provide their standards consistently. The other major disadvantage is that extra tubes for dilutions are required during PCR reactions to establish standard curves. Also, if candidate tumor markers are under investigation for identification, relative quantification has the advantage of simultaneously providing results for multiple genes of interest, such as those constituting an entire pathway, without the requirement of multiple standard curves.

During studies to identify tumor markers, the *delta-delta C_t* method requires a reference sample. A reference sample can be provided by pooling purified RNA from nearby normal tissues in studies of tumors. Alternatively, a pooled sample of nonmalignant or "normal" RNA for a specific organ site can be obtained commercially. It is important to use the same reference sample for an entire study to establish a tumor marker. However, once a tumor marker is established and is being applied clinically to monitor treatment responses, the reference sample used is often entirely different. For each patient being followed for disease progression or response to therapy, the baseline tumor burden prior to any treatment is the preferred reference sample. When the patient's baseline tumor sample is not available, then the averaged results of baseline values in the laboratory for twenty or more patients with the same type of malignancy can be used as the reference sample. At the present time, the lack of effective, specific therapies for glioblastomas prevents the clinical use of tumor markers to follow patients for minimal residual disease.

Queries of the Rembrandt Brain Tumor Database

Although the wide dynamic range of RQ-PCR has clear advantages over other RT-PCR assays, global microarray surveys are still very useful. Semiquantitative RNA results from microarrays of RT-PCR products play an important role in the initial phase of establishing tumor markers. The National Cancer Institute and the National Institute of Neurological Diseases and Strokes at the National Institutes of Health (NIH) provide the Repository of Molecular Brain Neoplasia Database (REMBRANDT) that includes clinically relevant data from multiple institutions for free on-line retrieval on their website (http://rembrandt.nci.nih.gov). Queries of the REMBRANDT database can be used to perform surveys of potential tumor markers in brain tumors based on levels of gene expression and copy number. Information on genes of interest is obtained by searches using the names of genes from the Online

Mendelian Inheritance in Man (OMIM) database, an NIH resource. Expression analysis via Affymetrix microarrays, patient survival data, and gene copy number information can be correlated. For analysis of each gene in REMBRANDT either of two types of probe sets or "locators", Affymetrix or Unified Gene, can be used. For most genes, the expression of each one has been analyzed with multiple locators, each one identified with an unique alpha-numeric name on a pull down menu placed on the Kaplan Meier survival plot. The default locator is the Affymetrix probe set that produced the highest mean intensity of signal. Unified Gene locators are based on algorithms recently developed by the NIH to select the best performing Affymetrix probes. Prior to mid January, 2009, the default values were the average of all the Affymetrix locators (communication with NIH personnel). However, individual multiple locators are now available. Genes can be queried for each to obtain a range of expression results with survival data (REMBRANDT, 2009). Similar tumor databases for other organ systems are currently being developed by the NIH.

In our studies, the REMBRANDT database allowed selection of tumor marker candidates based on decreased patient survival. Expression levels in the database are quantified in a discontinuous manner for both increases and decreases at 2-fold, 3-fold, and up to 10-fold breakpoints to define groups of patients for ranking survival results. Primary brain tumors are grouped collectively as gliomas and also in subgroups, such as astrocytomas, glioblastomas (grade IV/IV astrocytomas, the most malignant brain tumors), oligodendrogliomas and mixed oligoastrocytomas. Because "gliomas" includes high and low grade glial (mostly astrocytic) tumors, queries of this broad group can be performed to detect tumor markers associated with poor survival. Up regulated pathways in tumors are encoded by multiple genes that can be surveyed in their entirety to select candidates for tumor markers.

Tumor Markers in the Glycolytic Pathway

Glycolysis is the favored energy production pathway in glioblastomas. Whereas the activities of mitochondrial enzymes are decreased in gliomas compared to normal cortical brain tissue, the activities of glycolytic enzymes are increased, most notably in glioblastomas (Meixensberger et al., 1995; Oudard et al., 1996, 1997, Oude Weernink, 1991; Weernik, 1990; Graham et al., 1985; Tanizaki et al., 2006). A high rate of glycolysis has been found in correlation with the loss of chromosome 10 in gliomas (Oudard et al., 1996). Our queries of the REMBRANDT database determined expression levels of genes encoding glycolytic pathway constituents to see (1) if a sizable number of the gliomas in REMBRANDT expressed the gene of interest at increased levels compared to "normal", and (2) if there was a correlation with decreased survival using Kaplan Meier plots. In a survey performed in February, 2009, the following glycolytic genes, listed in order of the metabolic pathway steps, were queried in gliomas: *hexokinases and glucokinase (HK1, HK2, HK3, GCK), glucophosphoisomerase (GPI), phosphofructokinases (PFKL, PFKM, PFKP), aldolases (ALDOA, ALDOC), triose phosphate isomerase (TPI1), glyceraldehyde-3-phosphate dehydrogenase (GAPDH), phosphoglycerate kinases (PGK1, PGK2), phosphoglycerate mutases (PGAM1, PGAM2, PGAM3), enolases (ENO1, ENO2, ENO3), and pyruvate kinases (PKLR, PKM2)*. The following genes: *HK3, HK2, PFKL, ALDOA, GAPDH, PGK1, PGAM2 and ENO1*, had upregulated expression levels with p values indicative of significantly poorer survival or a trend as shown in Table 13.1.

Note that the genes with significantly ($p < 0.05$) poorer survival included *HK*s that encode enzymes responsible for initiating glycolysis and genes encoding four of the five enzymes that mediate the "energy generation phase" of the glycolytic pathway. The Kaplan Meier survival plots consistently indicated decreased survival of the patients with upregulation of *ENO1* ($p < 0.01$) for all locators (left to right), Affymetrix type (201231_s_st, 217294_s_st, and 240258_at) and Unified Gene type (2023 and 240258_at), as shown in Table 13.1 and in Fig. 13.1. The survival data included other highly significant p values (< 0.001) for *HK2, HK3, and PGK1*. However, for *HK2* and HK3 there were only one and two locators, respectively, available in REMBRANDT to evaluate at the time of inquiry and one of six locators for *PGK1* yielded a much smaller group with an insignificant p value.

The consistently increased expression of *ENO1* in medium to relatively large groups of gliomas, that were associated with significantly decreased survival, indicates that it is an example of a glycolytic tumor marker. However, further investigation to detect related tumor markers is necessary due to the longstanding view that glycolytic enzymes, such as enolase, are not promising targets for new drug development. Evolution has provided barrel-shaped secondary structures around the active sites in glycolytic

Table 13.1 Glycolytic pathway genes with increased expression associated with decreased survival on Kaplan Meier plots in REMBRANDT, February, 2009, for multiple locators (probe sets). Numbers of tumors with at least 2-fold upregulated gene expression in 201 gliomas are listed with the corresponding p values for decreased survival listed in parentheses below the numbers. For multiple locators, the results are listed left to right according to the mean level of signal intensity for each

Genes	Affymetrix locators (listed left to right: highest to lowest mean intensity)							Unified gene locators	
HK2			127 (1.0E–4)						
HK3			20 (0.0351)					29 (5.0E–4)	
PFKL			1 (0.0361)					1 (0.0361)	
ALDOA		2 (0.0546)	2 (0.0546)	5 (0.0683)				2 (0.0521)	
GAPDH	0 (N/A)	1 (0.0692)	0 (N/A)	2 (0.02)	0 (N/A)	2 (0.02)	1 (0.0692)	3 (0.6385)	3 (0.6385)
PGK1	10 (0.0059)	34 (3.0E–4)	36 (0.0513)	30 (0.0353)	4 (0.998)			11 (0.0029)	
PGAM2			107 (0.0152)					107 (0.0152)	
ENO1		17 (0.0057)	29 (0.0013)	88 (6.0E–4)				34 (0.0014)	44 (0.0010)

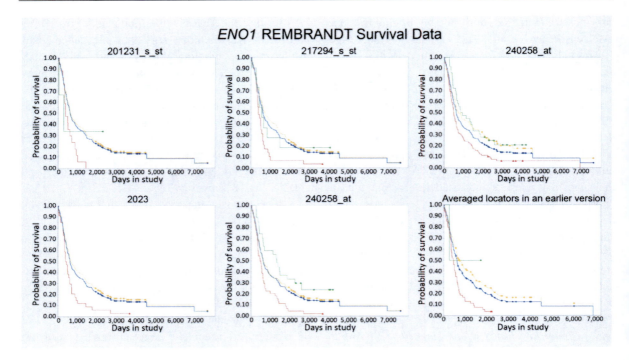

Fig. 13.1 Kaplan Meier survival plots for gene expression levels in gliomas for *ENO1* that encodes enolase, an enzyme in the "energy generation phase" of the glycolytic pathway. Unlike some of the other glycolytic enzymes, enolase is known to be variable in tumors. *ENO1*, chromosomal locus 12p13, was consistently up regulated for all of the locators (probe sets) with significant *p* values (<0.01) in gliomas included in REMBRANDT. The results listed for *ENO1* in Table 13.1 (201 gliomas, February, 2009) correspond to five plots, left to right, starting in the *top row*. The plot on the *bottom row* at the far right side represents the average of all the locators previously available in REMBRANDT (193 gliomas) in December, 2008. The average of all locators is no longer available in the latest version of REMBRANDT. *Red* = up regulated. *Green* = down regulated. *Yellow* = intermediate regulation

enzymes to exclude all molecules except their appropriate substrates with an efficiency that has frustrated efforts to develop drugs targeting specific glycolytic enzymes. Alternatively, regulators of glycolysis that lack these protective barrel-shaped structures should serve as secondary targets to suppress aberrant glycolysis. Therefore, expression of *ENO1*, as a gene encoding an effector for aberrant energy metabolism in tumors, should be associated with altered expression of related upstream and/or downstream tumor markers or "bad actors" that allow aberrant levels of glycolysis via control of *ENO1* expression. Glycolysis is known to be controlled by acidosis and a role for regulation by growth factors expressed in brain tumors is also a possibility. The hypothesis is that mediators of acid balance or growth factors whose levels of gene expression change in parallel with that of *ENO1* are tumor markers in the same biological network, either upstream or as part of feedback loops

for regulation of glycolysis. Gene products that control glycolysis, detected by relationships of their gene expression with *ENO1*, should be considered as candidates for anti-cancer drug development to control glycolysis.

Investigations of the REMBRANDT database for expression levels of genes that encode mediators of acid balance in cells and several growth factors led to the identification of a group of genes whose expression levels were associated with decreased survival among glioma patients. This parameter indicated that these genes should be further investigated for an association with the expression of *ENO1*. As mentioned earlier, genes encoding EGF and its receptor, EGFR, are of interest in brain tumors. The genes encoding platelet derived growth factor (PDGF) and receptors are also of interest in brain tumors. Queries of survival data in REMBRANDT were performed to establish candidates for further investigation among the growth factors and their receptors based on significantly poorer survival in glioma patients.

Of the growth factors and their receptors queried in REMBRANDT, two-fold or more increased levels of gene expression for *EGF*, *PDGFA*, and *PDGFRB* showed significantly decreased patient survival for "all gliomas" with at least some of the locators (Affymetrix and Unified Gene). The results available for analysis ranged from one Affymetrix and one Unified Gene locator for *EGF* to eight Affymetrix and six Unified Gene locators for *EGFR*. Results for all locators available at this time are listed in Table 13.2. Most of the corresponding Kaplan Meier plots that demonstrated significantly decreased survival ($p < 0.05$) are shown in Fig. 13.2. Variability in the results according to the locator was demonstrated for *EGFR* and *PDGFA* in Table 13.2. Thus, although REMBRANDT's gene expression data based on Affymetrix assays is invaluable due to the availability of survival data from multiple institutions, caution is required in interpretation of results for the genes with variability present.

Although testing associations for expression of genes such as *EGFR* would be problematic due to the variability among the different locators in REMBRANDT, associations for genes that demonstrate fairly stable results with multiple locators is possible with *chi square* analysis. Identification numbers for each patient with up regulated or down regulated gene expression in their tumor are listed in REMBRANDT by clicking on the category for each gene so that the patients can be cross-referenced. Associations between increased expression levels of a gene such as *ENO1* and other genes of interest in REMBRANDT can be tested by cross-referencing results for multiple genes in the tumors of individual patients. However, the disadvantages of relying on REMBRANDT data for establishing co-expression of genes include derivation of the reference control from averaged global results in the microarrays, small dynamic ranges for expression levels, discontinuous categories of results (2-fold, 3-fold, etc.), and the ability to only look for associations in one direction (increased or decreased) at a time with simple statistical methods. For these reasons, relationships indicated by microarray data between genes of interest and *ENO1* need to be confirmed with RQ-PCR. This is especially true until REMBRANDT accumulates more data.

Housekeeping Genes for Normalization of RQ-PCR

Surveys of multiple candidates as tumor markers with RQ-PCR can be performed by applying the *delta delta* C_t method for relative quantification. Design of a RQ-PCR study with *delta delta* C_t analysis includes choosing housekeeping genes and a reference sample. Candidates for housekeeping genes in brain tumors can be tested in queries of the REMBRANDT

Table 13.2 Genes for growth factors and receptors with increased expression associated with decreased survival for at least some locators (probe sets) on Kaplan Meier plots in REMBRANDT, February, 2009. Numbers of tumors with at least two-fold up regulated expression in 201 gliomas are listed with the *p* values for decreased survival listed in parentheses below the numbers. When multiple locators were used, their results are listed left to right according to the mean level of intensity for each (highest to lowest for each type)

Genes	Affymetrix locators				Unified gene locators		
EGF	38				40		
	(0.0)*				(1.0E–4)		
EGFR	170	142	41	89	134	45	91
	(0.838)	N/A	(0.2249)	(0.0215)*	(0.1917)	(0.23)	(0.0203)
EGFR cont.	143	4	134	46	90	61	43
	(0.8034)	(0.125)	(0.123)	(0.0217)*	(0.1174)	(0.2946)	(0.0074)*
PDGFA	50	75	51		57		
	(0.0010)*	(0.0133)*	(0.7672)		(6.0E–4)*		
PDGFRB	43				48		
	(0.0025)*				(6.0E–4)*		

*Corresponding Kaplan Meier survival plots are shown as Fig. 13.2 to illustrate significant results ($p < 0.05$). Only the Unified Gene locator results that included different numbers of patients (at least three) than those for Affymetrix locators are shown in Fig. 13.2.

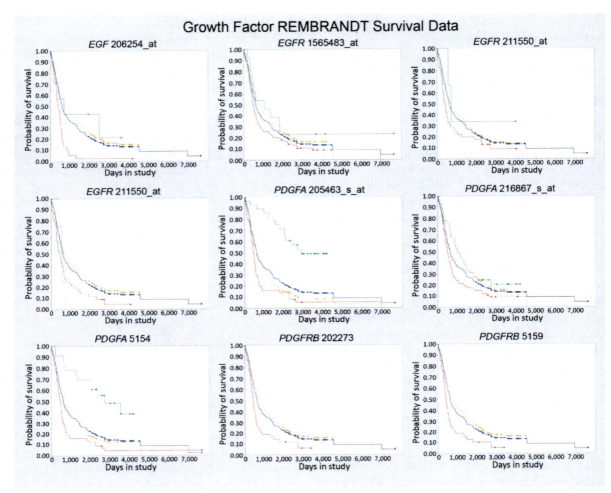

Fig. 13.2 Kaplan Meier survival plots for expression levels of genes encoding growth factors and receptors. *EGF, PDGFA, and PDGFRB* from chromosomal loci, 4q25, 7p22, and 5q31-q32, respectively, had results that included significant *p* values (<0.05) for decreased survival when their levels of expression were increased at least two-fold in 201 gliomas in the REMBRANDT database (February, 2009). For *EGF* with the locator 206254_at, there were 38 patients with increased expression. For *EGFR* with the locators 1565483_at, 211550_at, and 211550_at, there were 89, 46, and 43 patients with increased expression, respectively. For *PDGFA* with the locators 205463_s_at, 216867_s_at, and 5154 there were 50, 75, and 57 patients with increased expression, respectively. For *PDGFRB* with the locators 202273 and 5159 there were 43 and 48 patients with increased expression, respectively. These plots correspond with data, including *p* values, that are marked by asterisks in Table 13.2. *Red* = up regulation. *Green* = down regulation. *Yellow* = intermediate regulation

database to determine if their expression is altered in a high grade tumor, such as glioblastoma. Only genes whose expressions remain relatively stable in glioblastomas can function as housekeeping genes. Inclusion of multiple housekeeping genes is recommended for performing RQ-PCR in tumors, so that their averaged expression minimizes the likelihood that a genetic aberration in a single housekeeping gene in an occasional tumor would significantly affect the results. The stability of expression in glioblastomas for genes commonly considered as potential

housekeeping genes was determined in several queries of the REMBRANDT database over the past year. The latest results (February, 2009) are shown in Table 13.3.

As seen in Table 13.3, none of the commonly used housekeeping genes were ideal (no changes in expression levels) but the expression levels of *glyceraldehyde-3-phosphate dehydrogenase* (*GAPDH*) and *actin B* (*ACTB*) appeared to be the most stable among this group of genes in glioblastomas. Therefore the averaged expressions of *GAPDH* and *ACTB* can be used to normalize expression data

Table 13.3 Numbers of tumors with altered expression levels of candidate housekeeping genes in 109 glioblastomas in REMBRANDT, February, 2009. "Increased (↑)" and "decreased (↓)" categories represent 2-fold changes in gene expression from normal. None of the *p* values for the association of decreased survival and increased expression on Kaplan Meier plots were significant (*p* < 0.05) and * indicates the only two *p* values that were less than 0.1 in glioblastomas (note not gliomas). The expression levels of *GAPDH* and *ACTB* were the most stable in glioblastomas among this group of commonly used housekeeping genes

Gene	↑ or ↓	Affymetrix locators						Unified gene locators			
GAPDH	↑	1	2	0	0	2	0	1	3	3	
	↓	0	0	0	0	0	0	0	0	0	
ACTB	↑	4	3	2	4	6	13	4	9	7	20*
	↓	0	0	0	0	0	1	0	0	0	1
GUSB	↑			88	32				88		
	↓			0	8				0		
B2M	↑		35*	11	54				15		
	↓		0	0	3				0		
HPRT1	↑			0	20				0		
	↓			93	7				93		
RPL13A	↑		13	16	24	49			36		
	↓		0	0	0	0			0		

Abbreviations: GAPDH = glyceraldehyde-3-phosphate dehydrogenase, ACTB = actin B, GUSB = glucosidase B, B2M = beta 2 microglobulin, HPRT1 = hypoxanthine (guanine) phosphoribosyltransferase 1, RPL13A = ribosomal protein L13A. *p values < 0.1 but > 0.05.

in RQ-PCR assays of these tumors and the reference sample. Normalization corrects for small variations in pipeting, DNA extraction, reverse transcription, etc. The reference sample for investigational studies is easily obtained commercially as pooled human brain RNA in a quantity sufficient for large studies.

Investigations of Multiple Genes

For investigations of multiple genes of interest, the process of designing primers for all the genes and testing their efficiencies of amplification is daunting. Fortunately, commercial suppliers supply matched primers in a freeze-dried condition on customized 96 or 384 well plates for genes of interest in replicate wells along with controls for reverse transcription, amplification, genomic DNA contamination, etc. The appropriate master mix is also supplied commercially for loading samples.

Clinical Tumor Sample Preparation for RQ-PCR

Clinical tumor samples are obtained when glioblastomas are debulked by surgical dissection, ultrasonic aspiration, or a combination of both procedures. Tissue banks freeze solid tumor samples at –80°C or in liquid nitrogen. Tissue samples become available to investigators once Institutional Review Board approval is obtained. The tissue is processed to obtain intact RNA either with an automated or manual method. In our laboratory, pulverization of frozen tissue into a few drops of lysate buffer from a commercial RNA purification kit, followed by homogenization with a syringe and narrow (22–25) gauge needle, has worked well. Although traditionally, pulverization has been accomplished by mortal and pestle with tissue immersed in liquid nitrogen, our method of using dry ice is more convenient. In this method a few drops of lysate buffer are added to a tiny fragment (1–2 mm^3) of frozen tissue placed in the crease of a small, folded piece of aluminum foil lying in a metal pan sitting on dry ice (preferably a slab). The pan holding the tissue wrapped in foil is quickly removed from the dry ice to a concrete surface and the wrapped tissue is pounded with a cold hammer a few times in the pan. Except for the few seconds during pulverization, the pan with tissue wrapped in foil is kept on dry ice so that the tissue never thaws. Once the frozen tissue in lysate buffer is completely flattened into a smear, the pan is returned to the dry ice and the smear is immediately pipetted from the foil with the addition of more lysate buffer. The tissue is then homogenized with repeated needle aspirations into lysate buffer. Yields and quality of the RNA determined by the 260/280 method have been consistently good. Also, manufacturers of customized plates provide control plates to evaluate the quality of the samples in batches prior to using the customized plates. Second attempts at processing tissue often succeed on occasions when the first attempt at purification does not yield adequate amounts of good quality RNA. Commercial RT kits can be used to obtain cDNA from RNA. Once cDNAs of the tumor and reference samples are prepared, they are loaded with master mix into tubes or plates for RQ-PCR on a real-time PCR instrument. The same amount of total RNA is used for all samples in an experiment.

RQ-PCR Assays

Standard protocols for real-time PCR are followed with the option of including a melting curve analysis at the end of assays to ensure single amplicons. Analysis parameters, such as manual settings for the baseline and threshold for analysis, are recommended by the manufacturer. Tubes or plates in which PCR amplification has been performed are tightly sealed

at all times to prevent DNA contamination of future runs. An example of a RQ-PCR assay of multiple genes, including *EGF, PDGFA, ENO1*, etc. and controls is shown in Fig. 13.3. The threshold for analysis for all assays was set at twenty-fold greater than the baseline variation to ensure that analysis was performed during the exponential phase of amplification in every PCR run. Visually this was confirmed for each assay. The assay in Fig. 13.3 was performed using commercially prepared primers pre-loaded in triplicate wells of a 96-well plate (Custom R^2 PCR Array, SuperArray Biosciences Corp., Frederick, MD) on an ABI 7500 Prism Thermocycler System (Applied Biosystems, Foster City, CA). Only one-half of the plate was used to generate the results shown. Analysis using the *delta-delta* C_t method revealed increased expressions of *EGF* and *PDGFA* for 8 and 11 of 21 glioblastomas, respectively, relative to pooled non-malignant "normal" brain RNA (First Choice Human Brain Reference RNA, Ambion Applied Biosystems, Austin, TX) obtained from 23 adults. The anatomic sites for harvesting brain tissues for the tumor and reference samples could not be matched for specific

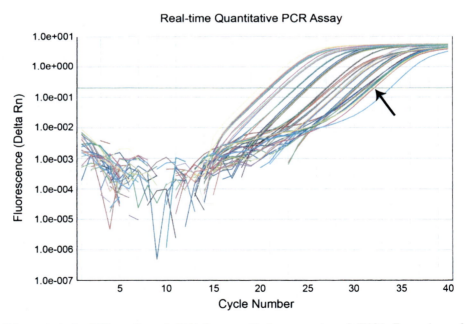

Fig. 13.3 Real-time quantitative PCR reactions of cDNA from RNA expressed by a group of genes in glioblastomas (frozen tissue samples). The expressions of these genes are under investigation for their relative levels in glioblastomas compared to a reference sample, non-malignant brain (unmatched for region), and to detect those genes whose levels of expression correlate with the expression of *ENO1*. Expressions of housekeeping genes, *GAPDH* and *ACTB*, were used for normalization. The *arrow* indicates the curves of PCR amplification for *EGF* in triplicate. In this tumor sample the expression of *EGF* was not increased relative to its expression in "normal" brain

lobe, etc. The patients with glioblastomas had an average age of 60.5 years, range of 19–81 years, which was comparable to the pooled "normal" brain RNA (average age of 68.3 years, range of 23–86 years). The sensitivity of RQ-PCR provided detection of changes in levels of gene expression in tumors compared to "normal" brain that were less than two-fold. Results of RQ-PCR are a continuous set of data points rather than being restricted to the intervals of 2-fold, 3-fold, etc. in the REMBRANDT database. Therefore the relationships of genes of interest with *ENO1* can be explored with greater sensitivity and reliability by using RQ-PCR to determine if there are tumor markers whose changes in expression parallel that of *ENO1*. Detection of genes whose regulation is related to *ENO1*, a known "bad actor", should include useful drug targets to control aberrant levels of glycolysis. In our RQ-PCR studies, no significant correlation of gene expression has been found yet for either *EGF* or *PDGFA* with *ENO1*. However, a significant correlation has been found for a gene encoding ATP citrate lyase a mediator of intracellular acid balance in our ongoing studies (Beckner et al., 2010).

In conclusion, important information can be gleaned from queries of the NIH's national tumor database, REMBRANDT, to use in planning focused studies of gene expression in tumors. In our ongoing RQ-PCR studies, expression of at least one gene encoding a mediator of acid balance has shown a significant correlation with the expression of a glycolytic enzyme, *ENO1*. It should be possible to dissect out regulatory mechanisms for aberrant levels of glycolysis that can be suppressed with drugs. In view of the difficulty in directly inhibiting glycolytic enzymes, suppressing regulators that control acidosis as "secondary" treatment targets represents a reasonable approach for suppressing glycolysis in glioblastomas. Also, the negative results for expression of genes encoding several growth factors and their receptors in reference to expression levels with *ENO1* may indicate that they do not stimulate glycolysis in glioblastomas. This information could help to define complex networks of tumor markers that predict which treatments are additive or cooperative versus those that are redundant, possibly with undesirable side effects. This approach will be increasingly important for designing new therapies when multiple small molecule inhibitors are combined as treatments in clinical trials. Although results of treatments targeted to

growth factors as single targets in glioblastomas are not encouraging, their combination with drugs directed toward unrelated targets resulting in additive effects may be more promising. Adding complementary drugs that suppress glycolysis to small molecule inhibitors of growth factors or their receptors should enhance the effects of small molecule inhibitors. The sensitivity of RQ-PCR for quantifying expression levels of genes selected by queries of REMBRANDT permits the efficient discovery of important relationships in tumor associated pathways. This is a novel approach for establishing new metabolic treatment targets in tumors.

Acknowledgements We acknowledge the Repository of Molecular for Brain Neoplasia Database (REMBRANDT) created and maintained by the NINDS, NCI, at the NIH for the availability of information on *ENO1* and other genes mentioned, including the Kaplan Meier survival plots shown. We thank Ronald L. Hamilton, MD and Colleen Lovell, Department of Pathology, University of Pittsburgh, with the University of Pittsburgh Brain Bank for provision of primary brain tumor tissue. We thank Jeffrey A. Kant, MD, PhD, Melissa Melan, PhD, and J.E. Dipaola, Department of Pathology, and Ian F. Pollack, MD and Naomi A. Agostino, Department of Neurological Surgery, University of Pittsburgh for advice and technical assistance. We thank The Walter L. Copeland Fund for Cranial Research of The Pittsburgh Foundation (D2006-0379) and the Louisiana State University-Shreveport School of Medicine 2008 Fall Grant for support.

References

Beckner ME, Fellows-Mayle W, Zhang Z, Agostino NR, Kant JA, Day BW, Pollack IF (2010) Identification of ATP citrate lyase as a positive regulator of glycolytic function in glioblastomas. Int J Cancer 126:2282–2295

CBTRUS (2005) Statistical report: primary brain tumors in the united states, 1998–2002. Central Brain Tumor Registry of the US, Hinsdale, IL, pp 12–48

De Groot JF, Gilbert MR, Aldape K, Hess KR, Hanna TA, Ictech S, Groves MD, Conrad C, Colman H, Puduvalli VK, Levin V, Yung WK (2008) Phase II study of carboplatin and erlotinib (tarceva, OSI-774) in patients with recurrent glioblastoma. J Neurooncol 90:89–97

Graham JF, Cummins CJ, Smith BH, Kornblith PL (1985) Regulation of hexokinase in cultured gliomas. Neurosurgery 17:537–542

Kotliarov Y, Steed ME, Christopher N, Walling J, Su Q, Center A, Heiss J, Rosenblum M, Mikkelsen T, Zenklusen JC, Fine HA (2006) High-resolution global genomic survey of 178 gliomas reveals novel regions of copy number alterations and allelic imbalances. Cancer Res 66:9428–9436

Livak KJ, Schmittgen TD (2001) Analysis of relative gene expression data using real-time quantitative PCR and the 2(-delta delta C(T)) method. Methods 25:2402–2408

Maher EA, Brennan C, Wen PY, Durso L, Ligon KL, Richardson A, Khatry D, Feng B, Sinha R, Louis DN, Quackenbush J, Black PM, Chin L, DePinho RA (2006) Marked genomic differences characterize primary and secondary glioblastoma subtypes and identify two distinct molecular and clinical secondary glioblastoma entities. Cancer Res 66: 11502–11513

Meixensberger J, Herting B, Roggendorf W, Reichmann H (1995) Metabolic patterns in malignant gliomas. J Neurooncol 24:153–161

Oudard S, Arvelo R, Miccoli L, Apiou F, Dutrillaux AM, Poisson M, Dutrillaux B, Poupon MF (1996) High glycolysis in gliomas despite low hexokinase transcription and activity correlated to chromosome 10 loss. Br J Cancer 74: 839–845

Oudard S, Boitier E, Miccoli L, Rousset S, Dutrillaux AM, Poupon MF (1997) Gliomas are driven by glycolysis: putative roles of hexokinase, oxidative phosphorylation and mitochondrial ultrastructure. Anticancer Res 17: 1903–1911

Oude Weernink PA, Rijksen G, Staal GE (1991) Phosphorylation of pyruvate kinase and glycolytic metabolism in three human glioma cell lines. Tumor Biol 12:339–352

Preusser M, Gelpi E, Rottenfusser A, Dieckmann K, Widhalm G, Dietrich W, Bertalanffy A, Prayer D, Hainfellner JA, Marosi C (2008) Epithelial growth factor receptor inhibitors for treatment of recurrent or progressive high grade glioma: an exploratory study. J Neurooncol 89:211–218

REMBRANDT (Repository of Molecular Brain Neoplasia Database) (2009) Generated and maintained by the NCI and NINDS at NIH http://rembrandt.nci.nih.gov. v1.5.2. Accessed Feb 2009

Skrzypski M (2008) Quantitative reverse transcriptase real-time polymerase chain reaction (qRT-PCR) in translational oncology: lung cancer perspective. Lung Cancer 59:147–154

Tanizaki Y, Sato Y, Oka H, Utsuki S, Kondo K, Miyajima Y, Nagashio R, Fujii K (2006) Expression of autocrine motility factor mRNA is a poor prognostic factor in high-grade astrocytoma. Pathol Int 56:510–515

Vaananen RM, Rissanen M, Kauko O, Junnila S, Vaisanen V, Nurmi J, Alanen K, Nurmi M, Pettersson K (2008) Quantitative real-time RT-PCR assay for PCA3. Clin Biochem 41:103–108

VanGuilder HD, Vrana KE, Freeman WM (2008) Twenty-five years of quantitative PCR for gene expression analysis. BioTechn 44:619–625

Weernik PA, Rijksen G, van der Heijden MC, Staal GE (1990) Phosphorylation of pyruvate kinase type K in human gliomas by a cyclic adenosine 5'-monophosphate-independent protein kinase. Cancer Res 50:4604–4610

Wong KK, Tsang YT, Chang YM, Su J, Di Francesco AM, Meco D, Riccardi R, Perlaky L, Dauser RC, Adesina A, Bhattacharjee M, Chintagumpala M,, Lau CC (2006) Genome-wide allelic imbalance analysis of pediatric gliomas by single nucleotide polymorphic allele array. Cancer Res 66:11172–11178

Chapter 14

Role of MGMT in Glioblastomas

Izabela Zawlik, Dorota Jesionek-Kupnicka, and Pawel P. Liberski

Abstract O^6-methylguanine DNA methyltransferase (MGMT) is a key DNA repair enzyme that specifically removes promutagenic methyl group from the O^6 position of guanine. Active MGMT protects cells against carcinogenesis induced by alkylating agents that makes it an important drug resistance factor and target for biochemical modulation of drug resistance. Loss of MGMT activity due to *MGMT* promoter methylation is a common occurrence in malignant gliomas. *MGMT* promoter methylation has been detected in approximately 50% of glioblastomas and is associated with the presence of G: C to A: T transition mutations in *TP53*. In many clinical studies, both methylation of *MGMT* and low MGMT level have been correlated with better clinical response of glioblastoma to chemotherapy with alkylating agents. This review will focus on the role of *MGMT* in glioblastoma and will show the results of several studies concerning association of *MGMT* status and survival among glioblastoma patients treated with alkylating agents.

Keywords MGMT · Methylation · Chemotherapy · Glioblastoma

Introduction

MGMT is a key DNA repair enzyme that specifically removes promutagenic methyl/alkyl group from the O^6 position of guanine by transferring it to cysteine

acceptor site on the protein itself and restores the guanine to its normal form without causing DNA strand breaks (Pegg, 2000). MGMT depleted cells are unable to repair O^6-methyloguanine (O^6MeG) and are more sensitive to the mutagenic and cytotoxic effect of ethylating agents (Yarosh et al., 1983). If O^6-methyloguanine (O^6MeG) is not repaired by MGMT it can cause chromosomal aberrations, point mutations, and malignant transformation. It has been shown that cells expressing MGMT (Mer$^+$ – methyl excision repair positive) are highly resistant to the killing effect of alkylating agents and display a lower frequency of apoptosis compared to MGMT-deficient (Mer$^-$) cells (Kaina et al., 1997; Meikrantz et al., 1998). Thus active MGMT protects cells against carcinogenesis induced by alkylating agents what makes it an important drug resistance factor and target for biochemical modulation of drug resistance. In gliomas, O^6MeG induces apoptosis by activating both the mitochondrial (in *P53* mutated tumors) and P53 controlled Fas dependent pathway (Roos et al., 2007).

It has been shown that O^6MeG is removed from rat brain DNA slower than from other tissues and MGMT activity is the lowest in human brain among several different tissues what suggests that brain may be more sensitive to alkylating agents than other tissues (Grafstrom et al., 1984; Margison and Kleihues, 1975). Possible involvement of diets containing *N*-nitroso alkylating compounds in glioma development has been reported (Lee et al., 1997). MGMT inactivation causes accumulation of G: C to A: T mutations resulting from preferential mispairing O^6MeG with thymine rather than cytosine during replication, which may initiate carcinogenesis if the mutations occur in the tumor-related genes (Toorchen and Topal, 1983). *MGMT* promoter methylation was associated with the presence

I. Zawlik (✉)
Department of Molecular Pathology and Neuropathology, Medical University of Lodz, Czechoslowacka 8/10 Str., 92-216 Lodz, Poland
e-mail: Izazawlik@yahoo.com

M.A. Hayat (ed.), *Tumors of the Central Nervous System, Volume 1*,
DOI 10.1007/978-94-007-0344-5_14, © Springer Science+Business Media B.V. 2011

of G:C to A:T transition mutations in *TP53* in many types of cancer, including glioblastoma (Esteller et al., 2001; Nakamura et al., 2001; Zawlik et al., 2009). The most frequent type of *TP53* mutations in glioblastomas is G: C to A: T transitions (Ohgaki et al., 2004). These data support the view that promutagenic O^6MeG adducts may be involved in glioblastoma development.

MGMT expression loss is rarely caused by deletion, mutation, rearrangement of the *MGMT* gene or mRNA instability (Day et al., 1980; Kroes and Erickson, 1995; Pieper et al., 1990; Yarosh et al., 1983), whereas is frequently caused by CpG islands hypermethylation within the *MGMT* promoter in a variety of primary tumors and gliomas cell lines (Costello et al., 1996; Esteller et al., 1999). Therefore, regulation of MGMT expression seems to be an epigenetic event directly dependent on *MGMT* promoter methylation. Method that is widely used for *MGMT* promoter methylation determination in glioblastomas is methylation-specific PCR (MSP) (Criniere et al., 2007; Hegi et al., 2005; Zawlik et al., 2009]. The MSP assay detects CpG islands methylation within the *MGMT* promoter with high sensitivity and specificity. *MGMT* promoter methylation has been studied extensively in glioblastomas, because it has significant clinical implications.

MGMT Expression/Methylation and Clinical Implications in Glioblastoma

MGMT promoter methylation was found in 45–57% of glioblastomas (Criniere et al., 2007; Hegi et al., 2005; Zawlik et al., 2009). At a population level *MGMT* promoter methylation was more frequent in secondary than in primary glioblastomas and was detected in a higher frequency in females than in males with glioblastoma (Zawlik et al., 2009). The tendency to the higher frequency of *MGMT* methylation in younger patients (<50 years) has been observed (Nakamura et al., 2001; Silber et al., 1999), however other studies did not confirmed these results (Jesien-Lewandowicz et al., 2009; Zawlik et al., 2009).

MGMT is the main single-acting factor responsible for resistance to alkylation agents chemotherapy in the first line treatment of glioblastoma such as nitrosoureas (chloroethylnitrosoureas, carmustine/BCNU, lomustine and fotemustine), temozolomide and procarbazine. The cytotoxicity of alkylating agents is reduced in the presence of MGMT by reversing the formation

of adducts at the O^6 position of guanine in CpG island, in consequence of that, MGMT prevents the formation of lethal cross-links of DNA and apoptosis (Pegg, 2000).

In many clinical studies, methylation of *MGMT*, low or lack of MGMT expression in glioblastoma have been correlated with better clinical response of glioblastoma to nitrosoureas and temozolomid improving progression of free survival (PFS) and overall survival (OS) (Criniere et al., 2007; Hegi et al., 2005; Jaeckle et al., 1998; Paz et al., 2004; Spiegl-Kreinecker et al., 2010; Stupp et al., 2009; Weller et al., 2009).

In the prospective trial (Southwest Oncology Group [SWOG] 8737), glioblastoma patients treated with radiotherapy and 1,3-bis-chloroethylnitrosourea (BCNU) that displayed low level of MGMT survived significantly longer than patients with high MGMT level (7 vs. 12 months). Furthermore, multivariate analysis showed that MGMT level was an independent of age, performance status and histology prognostic value (Jaeckle et al., 1998).

Positive association between *MGMT* methylation and clinical response for various alkylating drugs in glioma patients has been shown by Paz et al. (2004). The study showed that the most positive (partial or complete) response to the treatment of patients with *MGMT* promoter methylation has been achieved in first-line chemotherapy with temozolomide (68%) in comparison with procarbasine/CCNU (60%) and BCNU (55%) (Paz et al., 2004).

Other clinical trial, conducted by the European Organisation for Research and Treatment of Cancer and the National Cancer Institute of Canada (NCIC) (EORTC trial 26981/22981 and NCIC trial CE.3), reported that *MGMT* status had a prognostic value irrespective of treatment in a group of 206 glioblastoma patients. The median OS among patients with *MGMT* promoter methylation was 18.2 months vs. 12.2 months without *MGMT* promoter methylation ($P < 0.001$). Furthermore, a survival benefit was observed in patients with methylated *MGMT* promoter, treated with temozolomide and radiotherapy as compared with those who received only radiotherapy (median survival was 21.7 months vs. 15.3 months, two-year survival rate was 46.0% vs. 22.7% ($P = 0.007$). Among glioblastoma patients that did not show *MGMT* promoter methylation, the median survival was 12.7 months among those assigned to temozolomide and radiotherapy and 11.8 months among those assigned

Table 14.1 Median overall survival of a 5-year analysis in relation to radiotherapy and combined therapy with themozolomid in the whole group of patients ($N=573$) and in relation to MGMT status ($N=206$) (the randomized EORTC22981/26981–NCIC CE.3 [European Organisation for Research and Treatment of Cancer/National Cancer Institute of Canada] phase III trial). This study showed the benefits of adjuvant temozolomide with radiotherapy, most likely in patients with *MGMT* methylation status

	Radiotherapy			Radiotherapy+Temozolomide		
	MGMT+ (N=46)	MGMT– (N=54)	MGMT+/– (N=286)	MGMT+ (N=46)	MGMT– (N=60)	MGMT+/– (N=287)
Median survival (months)	15.3	11.8	12.1	23.4	12.6	14.6
2-ys (%)	23.9	1.8	10.9	48.9	14.8	27.2
3-ys (%)	7.8	0	4.4	27.6	11.1	16.0
4-ys (%)	7.8	0	3.0	22.1	11.1	12.1
5-ys (%)	5.2	0	1.9	13.8	8.3	9.8

Note: Data adopted from Stupp et al. (2009)

Abbreviations: MGMT, O^6-methylguanine methyltransferase; ys – years of survival; + methylated; – unmethylated; +/– irrespective of *MGMT* status

to radiotherapy, with 2-year survival rates of 13.8% and less than 2%, respectively (Hegi et al., 2005). This study surveyed the total group of 573 glioblastoma patients was finally finished with a 5-year analysis and confirmed that *MGMT* methylation status identifies patients who most likely benefit from the radiotherapy and chemotherapy with temozolomide (Table 14.1) (Stupp et al., 2009).

Recently, multivariate analysis in the study of German Glioma Network revealed younger age, higher performance score, *MGMT* promoter methylation, and temozolomide radiochemotherapy as independent factors associated with longer OS. *MGMT* promoter methylation was associated with longer PFS (relative risk of death; $RR = 0.5$) and OS ($RR = 0.39$; $P < 0.001$) in patients who received temozolomide (Weller et al., 2009).

Similarly, in a French series, *MGMT* promoter methylation assumed only predictive significance when patients received adjuvant nitrosoureas. *MGMT* promoter methylation had no impact on survival for the whole group, but showed a significant advantage (17.1 months vs. 13.1) for patients treated with radiochemotherapy (relative risk of death (RR) $= 0.53$; $P = 0.041$), particularly when patients received chemotherapy during the course of radiotherapy (median survival was 19.9 months vs. 12.5 months; $RR = 0.227$, $P = 0.001$) (Criniere et al., 2007).

Only in a single study, there was no relationship between the methylation status of the *MGMT* promoter and OS and response to alkylating agents (fotemustine or BCNU). Patient group with *MGMT* promoter methylation and treated only with radiotherapy exhibited similar medians of OS and PFS as patient group with *MGMT* promoter methylation and treated with a combination of radiotherapy and chemotherapy (Blanc et al., 2004).

The predictive value of *MGMT* gene promoter methylation was also validated in the outcome of glioblastoma therapy at recurrence (Metellus et al., 2009; Nagane et al., 2007; Sadones et al., 2009). Median PFS time reported by Nagane et al. (2007) was 2.2 months, and median OS time was 9.9 months from the initiation of therapy with temozolomid, in patients treated initially with chemotherapy or radiation 4 weeks or more before. Patients with low MGMT protein expression had a significantly improved PFS and OS compared to those with high expression (Nagane et al., 2007). Similar results were achieved in group of patients treated with carmustine (BCNU) wafer implantation. The median PFS and OS rates after recurrence were 3.6 months and 9.9 months, respectively, and the 6-month PFS rate after recurrence was 27.2%. On multivariate analysis, only age and *MGMT* promoter methylation at recurrence were correlated with better PFS and only *MGMT* promoter methylation at recurrence was associated with better OS (Metellus et al., 2009). However, other previous and more recent clinical studies failed to show the benefits from the radiochemotherapy with temozolomide in recurrent glioblastomas (Paz et al., 2004; Sadones et al., 2009).

Treatment of *MGMT*-deficient glioblastomas with alkylating therapy caused the loss of mismatch repair function. Initial methylation of *MGMT*, in conjunction with treatment, may lead to both a shift in

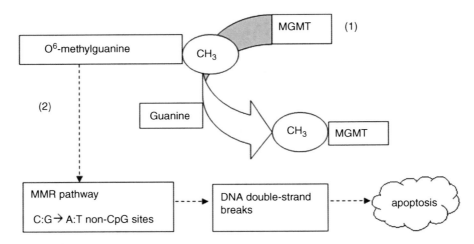

Fig. 14.1 The schematic role of MGMT in single-act DNA repair process (1) and in tumors treated with alkylating agents with *MGMT* promoter methylation (2)
(1) The MGMT enzyme removes the methyl group from the O^6-methylguanine DNA adduct to cysteine residue in the enzyme.
(2) In treated tumor samples with *MGMT* methylation unrepaired alkylated guanine residues shifted the mutation spectrum of *MMR* to a preponderance of G: C to A: T transition at non-CpG sites and may lead to the loss of mismatch repair function.

mutation spectrum affecting mutations at mismatch repair genes (MMR) and selective pressure to loss mismatch repair function. Patients with glioblastoma who initially respond to the frontline treatment, acquired an MMR-defective hypermutator phenotype and are mutated with characteristic C: G to A: T transitions at non-CpG sites resulting from unrepaired alkylated guanine residues (Fig. 14.1) (The Cancer Genome Atlas Research Network, 2008).

Focused on the predictive value of *MGMT* gene promoter methylation, the new alternative treatment strategies are required for patients, whose tumors do not have *MGMT* promoter methylation. The second aim seems to be the modulating chemoresistance to alkylating agents both in glioblastoma patients with methylated and unmethylated *MGMT* promoter. One of the ongoing randomised trials (EORTC 26082-22081) concerns study of radiation therapy and concurrent plus adjuvant temsirolimus (CCI-779) versus chemo-irradiation with temozolomide in newly diagnosed glioblastoma without methylation of the *MGMT* promoter (European Organisation for Research and Treatment of Cancer, 2010).

The other trials investigated the overcoming of the resistance to chemotherapy by a dose-dense continuous temozolomide administration or the combination treatment with MGMT inhibitors. The alternative dose-intensified schedules may also avoid this resistance in patients with unmethylated *MGMT* promoter (Wick et al., 2009).

The promising strategy to overcome chemoresistance to alkylating agents is inactivation of MGMT by potent MGMT-inhibiting agents, such as O^6-benzylguanine (O^6-BG) and other similar compounds (O^6-(4-bromothenyl) guanine (lomeguatrib), O^4-benzylfolates). O^6-benzylguanine lowers MGMT levels stichiometrically, but increasing toxicity from chemotherapy (reviewed by Hegi et al., 2008). The experimental studies and trial phase I and II, focused on the assignment of maximum-tolerated doses of O^6-BG, that would effectively suppress MGMT activity alone or in combination with chemotherapy. O^4-benzylfolates is considered a 30 time more effective than O^6-BG. This compound is also effective against the mutant P140K-MGMT that is resistant to O^6-BG and may have greater clinical potential (Hegi et al., 2008).

References

Blanc JL, Wager M, Guilhot J, Kusy S, Bataille B, Chantereau T, Lapierre F, Larsen CJ, Karayan-Tapon L (2004) Correlation of clinical features and methylation status of MGMT gene promoter in glioblastomas. J Neurooncol 68: 275–283

Cancer Genome Atlas Research Network. (2008) Comprehensive genomic characterization defines human glioblastoma genes and core pathways. Nature 455:1061–1068

Costello JF, Futscher BW, Tano K, Graunke DM, Pieper RO (1996) Graded methylation in the promoter and in the body of the O^6-methylguanine-DNA methyltransferase gene correlates with MGMT expression in human glioma cells. Cancer Res 56:13916–13924

Criniere E, Kaloshi G, Laigle-Donadey F, Lejeune J, Auger N, Benouaich-Amiel A, Everhard S, Mokhtari K, Polivka M, Delattre JY, Hoang-Xuan K, Thillet J, Sanson M (2007) MGMT prognostic impact on glioblastoma is dependent on therapeutic modalities. J Neurooncol 83:173–179

Day RS 3rd, Ziolkowski CH, Scudiero DA, Meyer SA, Lubiniecki AS, Girardi AJ, Galloway SM, Bynum GD (1980) Defective repair of alkylated DNA by human tumour and SV40-transformed human cell strains. Nature 288: 724–727

Esteller M, Hamilton SR, Burger PC, Baylin SB, Herman JG (1999) Inactivation of the DNA repair gene O6-methylguanine-DNA methyltransferase by promoter hypermethylation is a common event in primary human neoplasia. Cancer Res 59:793–797

Esteller M, Risques RA, Toyota M, Capella G, Moreno V, Peinado MA, Baylin SB, Herman JG (2001) Promoter hypermethylation of the DNA repair gene O (6) methylguanine-DNA methyltransferase is associated with the presence of G: C to A: T transition mutations in p53 in human colorectal tumorigenesis. Cancer Res 61:4689–4692

European Organisation for Research and Treatment of Cancer: Brain tumour group: Ongoing trials. (2010) http://groups.eortc.be/brain/html/trials.html. Accessed 22 Apr 2010

Grafstrom RC, Pegg AE, Trump BF, Harris CC (1984) O6-alkylguanine-DNA alkyltransferase activity in normal human tissues and cells. Cancer Res 44:2855–2857

Hegi ME, Diserens AC, Gorlia T, Hamou MF, de Tribolet N, Weller M, Kros JM, Hainfellner JA, Mason W, Mariani L, Bromberg JE, Hau P, Mirimanoff RO, Cairncross JG, Janzer RC, Stupp R (2005) MGMT gene silencing and benefit from temozolomide in glioblastoma. N Engl J Med 352: 997–1003

Hegi ME, Liu L, Herman JG, Stupp R, Wick W, Weller W, Mehta MP, Gilbert MR (2008) Correlation of O6-methylguanine methyltransferase (MGMT) promoter methylation with clinical outcomes in glioblastoma and clinical strategies to modulate MGMT activity. J Clin Oncol 26: 4189–4199

Jaeckle KA, Eyre HJ, Townsend JJ, Schulman S, Knudson HM, Belanich M, Yarosh DB, Bearman SI, Giroux DJ, Schold SC (1998) Correlation of tumor O6 methylguanine-DNA methyltransferase levels with survival of malignant astrocytoma patients treated with bis-chloroethylnitrosourea: a southwest oncology group study. J Clin Oncol 16: 3310–3315

Jesien-Lewandowicz E, Jesionek-Kupnicka D, Zawlik I, Szybka M, Kulczycka-Wojdala D, Rieske P, Sieruta M, Jaskolski D, Och W, Skowronski W, Sikorska B, Potemski P, Papierz W, Liberski PP, Kordek R (2009) High incidence of MGMT promoter methylation in primary glioblastomas without correlation with TP53 gene mutations. Cancer Genet Cytogenet 188:77–82

Kaina B, Ziouta A, Ochs K, Coquerelle T (1997) Chromosomal instability, reproductive cell death and apoptosis induced by O6-methylguanine in mex−, mex+ and methylation-tolerant mismatch repair compromised cells: facts and models. Mutat Res 381:227–241

Kroes RA, Erickson LC (1995) The role of mRNA stability and transcription in O6-methylguanine DNA methyltransferase (MGMT) expression in Mer+ human tumor cells. Carcinogenesis 16:2255–2257

Lee M, Wrensch M, Miike R (1997) Dietary and tobacco risk factors for adult onset glioma in the San Francisco bay area (California, USA). Cancer Causes Control 8:13–24

Margison GP, Kleihues P (1975) Chemical carcinogenesis in the nervous system. Preferential accumulation of O6-methylguanine in rat brain deoxyribonucleic acid during repetitive administration of N-methyl-N-nitrosourea. Biochem J 148:521–525

Meikrantz W, Bergom MA, Memisoglu A, Samson L (1998) O6-alkylguanine DNA lesions trigger apoptosis. Carcinogenesis 19:369–372

Metellus P, Coulibaly B, Nanni I, Fina F, Eudes N, Giorgi R, Barrie M, Chinot O, Fuentes S, Dufour H, Ouafik L, Figarella-Branger D (2009) Prognostic impact of O6-methylguanine-DNA methyltransferase silencing in patients with recurrent glioblastoma multiforme who undergo surgery and carmustine wafer implantation: a prospective patient cohort. Cancer 115:4783–4794

Nagane M, Kobayashi K, Ohnishi A, Shimizu S, Shiokawa Y (2007) Prognostic significance of O6-methylguanine-DNA methyltransferase protein expression in patients with recurrent glioblastoma treated with temozolomide. Jpn J Clin Oncol 12:897–906

Nakamura M, Watanabe T, Yonekawa Y, Kleihues P, Ohgaki H (2001) Promoter methylation of the DNA repair gene MGMT in astrocytomas is frequently associated with G: C >O A: T mutations of the TP53 tumor suppressor gene. Carcinogenesis 22:1715–1719

Ohgaki H, Dessen P, Jourde B, Horstmann S, Nishikawa T, Di Patre PL, Burkhard C, Schuler D, Probst-Hensch NM, Maiorka PC, Baeza N, Pisani P, Yonekawa Y, Yasargil MG, Lutolf UM, Kleihues P (2004) Genetic pathways to glioblastoma: a population-based study. Cancer Res 64: 6892–6899

Paz MF, Yaya-Tur R, Rojas-Marcos I, Reynes G, Pollan M, Aguirre-Cruz L, Garcia-Lopez JL, Piquer J, Safont MJ, Balana C, Sanchez-Cespedes M, Garcia-Villanueva M, Arribas L, Esteller M (2004) CpG island hypermethylation of the DNA repair enzyme methyltransferase predicts response to temozolomide in primary gliomas. Clin Cancer Res 10:4933–4938

Pegg AE (2000) Repair of O (6)-alkylguanine by alkyltransferases. Mutat Res 462:83–100

Pieper RO, Futscher BW, Dong Q, Ellis TM, Erickson LC (1990) Comparison of O-6-methylguanine DNA methyltransferase (MGMT) mRNA levels in Mer+ and Mer – human tumor cell lines containing the MGMT gene by the polymerase chain reaction technique. Cancer Commun 2:13–20

Roos WP, Batista LF, Naumann SC, Wick WM, Weller MCF, Kaina B (2007) Apoptosis in malignant glioma cells triggered by the temozolomide-induced DNA lesion. Oncogene 26:186–197

Sadones J, Michotte A, Veld P, Chaskis C, Sciot R, Menten J, Joossens EJ, Strauven T, D'Hondt LA, Sartenaer D, Califice SF, Bierau K, Svensson C, De Grève J, Neyns B (2009) MGMT promoter hypermethylation correlates with a survival benefit from temozolomide in patients with recurrent anaplastic astrocytoma but not glioblastoma. Eur J Cancer 45:146–153

Silber JR, Blank A, Bobola MS, Ghatan S, Kolstoe DD, Berger MS (1999) O6-methylguanine-DNA methyltransferase-deficient phenotype in human gliomas: frequency and time to tumor progression after alkylating agent-based chemotherapy. Clin Cancer Res 5:807–814

Spiegl-Kreinecker S, Pirker C, Filipits M, Lötsch D, Buchroithner J, Pichler J, Silye R, Weis S, Micksche M, Fischer J, Berger W (2010) O^6-methylguanine DNA methyltransferase protein expression in tumor cells predicts outcome of temozolomide therapy in glioblastoma patients. Neuro-Oncology 12:28–36

Stupp R, Hegi ME, Mason WP, van den Bent MJ, Taphoorn MJ, Janzer RC, Ludwin SK, Allgeier A, Fisher B, Belanger K, Hau P, Brandes AA, Gijtenbeek J, Marosi C, Vecht CJ, Mokhtari K, Wesseling P, Villa S, Eisenhauer E, Gorlia T, Weller M, Lacombe D, Cairncross JG, Mirimanoff RO (2009) European organisation for research and treatment of cancer brain tumour and radiation oncology groups; national cancer institute of Canada clinical trials group. Effects of radiotherapy with concomitant and adjuvant temozolomide versus radiotherapy alone on survival in glioblastoma in a randomised phase III study: 5-year analysis of the EORTC-NCIC trial. Lancet Oncol 10:459–466

Toorchen D, Topal MD (1983) Mechanisms of chemical mutagenesis and carcinogenesis: effects on DNA replication of methylation at the O^6-guanine position of dGTP. Carcinogenesis 4:1591–1597

Weller M, Felsberg J, Hartmann C, Berger H, Steinach JP, Schramm J, Westphal M, Schackert G, Simon M, Tonn JC, Heese O, Krex D, Nikkhah G, Pietach T, Wiestler O, Reinferberger G, von Deimling A, Loeffler M (2009) Molecular predictors of progression-free and overall survival in patients with newly diagnosed glioblastoma: a prospective translational study of the German glioma network. Clin Oncol 27(5743):5750

Wick W, Platten M, Weller M (2009) New (alternative) temozolomide regiment for the treatment of glioma. Neurooncol 11:67–69

Yarosh DB, Foote RS, Mitra S, Day III,RS (1983) Repair of O6-methylguanine in DNA by demethylation is lacking in mer- human tumor cell strains. Carcinogenesis 4:199–205

Zawlik I, Vaccarella S, Kita D, Mittelbronn M, Franceschi S, Ohgaki H (2009) Promoter methylation and polymorphisms of the MGMT gene in glioblastomas: a population-based study. Neuroepidemiology 32:21–29

Chapter 15

Glioblastomas: Role of CXCL12 Chemokine

Yasuo Sugita

Abstract Chemokines are small pro-inflammatory chemoattractant cytokines that bind to specific G-protein-coupled seven-span transmembrane receptors on the plasma membrane of target cells. They are also the major regulators of cell trafficking. Chemokines and their receptors were initially associated with the trafficking of leukocytes during physiological immune surveillance and with inflammatory cell recruitment in different diseases. CXCL 12, an alpha-chemokine that binds to G-protein-coupled CXCR4, plays an important and unique role in the regulation of stem/progenitor cell trafficking. Since CXCR4 is expressed on several tumor cells, these CXCR4-positive tumor cells may metastasize to organs that secrete/express CXCL12. In the specific case of gliomas, recent data show that CXCR4 and CXCL12 mRNAs colocalize to glioblastomas and that their expression increases with tumor grade and is associated with regions of necrosis and angiogenesis. This chapter summarises our current knowledge regarding the role of the CXCL12/CXCR4 axis in the central nervous system, focusing on the molecular mechanism by which the CXCL12/CXCR4 axis functions in the accelerated growth of glioblastomas, and further introduces the potential role of CXCL12/CXCR4-targeting compounds for the treatment of glioblastomas.

Keywords Chemokine · CXCL12 · CXCR4 · Glioblastoma

Introduction

Chemokines are small pro-inflammatory chemoattractant cytokines that bind to specific G-protein-coupled seven-span transmembrane receptors on the plasma membrane of target cells. They are also the major regulators of cell trafficking (Bajetto et al., 2001; Kucia et al., 2004). Chemokines and their receptors were initially associated with the trafficking of leukocytes during physiological immune surveillance and with inflammatory cell recruitment in different diseases. In addition, chemokines have been shown to play an important role in hematopoietic development by regulating migration, proliferation, differentiation, and survival of hematopoietic stem and progenitor cells (Kucia et al., 2004). Chemokines are classified into two main subfamilies, CXC (alpha) and CC (beta) chemokines based on the relative position of the four cysteine residues. Two other subfamilies of chemokines exist for which the prototypes are fractalkine: a membrane-bound glycoprotein in which the first two cysteines are separated by three amino acid residues (CXXXC), and lymphotactin, which has only two cysteines. The alpha-chemokines activate the CXC receptors (CXCR) 1–6, beta-chemokines signal to the CC receptors (CCR) 1–10, and fractalkine exerts its effects through the CX3CR1 receptor (Lazarini et al., 2003). Recently, compelling evidence has accumulated indicating that cancer cells employ several mechanisms to regulate their trafficking during metastasis. These mechanisms involve chemokine-chemokine receptor axes and regulate the trafficking of normal cells (Bajetto et al., 2001; Jiang et al., 2006; Singh et al., 2004; Smith et al., 2007; Stumm et al., 2002; Yasumoto et al., 2006).

Y. Sugita (✉)
Department of Pathology, Kurume University School of Medicine, Kurume, Fukuoka 830-0011, Japan
e-mail: sugita_yasuo@med.kurume-u.ac.jp

M.A. Hayat (ed.), *Tumors of the Central Nervous System, Volume 1*,
DOI 10.1007/978-94-007-0344-5_15, © Springer Science+Business Media B.V. 2011

CXCL 12, an alpha-chemokine that binds to G-protein-coupled CXCR4, plays an important and unique role in the regulation of stem/progenitor cell trafficking. Since CXCR4 is expressed on several tumor cells, these CXCR4-positive tumor cells may metastasize to organs that secrete/express CXCL12. In the specific case of gliomas, recent data show that CXCR4 and CXCL12 mRNAs colocalize to glioblastomas and that their expression increases with tumor grade and is associated with regions of necrosis and angiogenesis (Rempel et al., 2000).

This chapter focuses on the role of the CXCL12/CXCR4 axis in the central nervous system, particularly on the mechanism by which the CXCL12/CXCR4 axis functions in the accelerated growth of glioblastomas.

Role of CXCL12 in the Developing and Mature Central Nervous System

Chemokines have been traditionally defined as small (10–14 kDa) secreted leukocyte chemoattractants. However, chemokines and their cognate receptors are constitutively expressed in the central nervous system where immune activities are under stringent control. Why and how the central nervous system uses the chemokine system to carry out its complex physiological functions have intrigued investigators.

It was reported by Bajetto et al. (2001) that CXCL12 stimulates the proliferation of rat type-1 astrocytes in primary culture, and that activation of extracellular signal-regulated kinase (ERK1/2) is responsible for this effect. They suggested that the CXCR4/ CXCL12 axis likely plays an important role in physiological and pathological glial proliferation, such as during brain development and in reactive gliosis. Extensive evidence indicates that, under physiological conditions, CXCL12 is a key regulator of the early development of the central nervous system. Recently, it has been reported by Luo et al. (2008) that CXCL12 and its cognate receptor CXCR4 play an important role in neuronal development in the hippocampus. They have also shown that CXCL12/CXCR4/G protein/ERK signaling induces the expression of the GAD67 system via early growth response-1 (Egr1) activation, a mechanism that may promote the maturation of gamma-aminobutyric acid (GABA)ergic neurons during development. In addition, CXCL12/CXCR4 signaling is required for the migration of neuronal precursors, for axon guidance/pathfinding and for the maintenance of neural progenitor cells. In the mature central nervous system, CXCL12 modulates neurotransmission, neurotoxicity and neuroglial interactions. Thus, chemokines represent an endogenous system that helps to establish and maintain central nervous system homeostasis (Li and Ransohoff, 2008).

Extensive evidence indicates that CXCL12 is also a key regulator of the central nervous system under pathological conditions. Focal cerebral ischemia promotes subventricular zone-derived neuroblast differentiation and migration to the ischemic boundary region. It was reported by Liu et al. (2008) that the chemokine receptor CXCR4 and its ligand, CXCL12, regulate neuroblast migration towards the ischemic boundary after stroke. They also showed that CXCR4/CXCL12 primarily regulates adult neural progenitor cell motility but not differentiation, whereas overexpression of CXCR4 in the absence of CXCL12 decreases neural progenitor cell proliferation. Recently, CXCL12 has been shown to bind to, and signal through, the orphan receptor CXCR7. Interestingly, it was reported by Schönemeier et al. (2008) that CXCL12 may influence vascular, astroglial and neuronal functions via CXCR7 and may mediate cell recruitment to ischemic brain areas via CXCR4. In summary, the CXCR4/ CXCL12 axis is widely expressed in the central nervous system during development and after brain maturation and regulates the migration and proliferation of neuroprogenitor cells. In particular, CXCR4/ CXCL12 are present along deep white matter, which may be of relevance to the occurrence of glioblastomas.

Carcinoma, Sarcoma and Leukemia/ Lymphoma Cells Express CXCR4/CXCL12

Many studies of the CXCL12/CXCR4 signal system have been carried out, mostly in the fields of immunology and infection (Kucia et al., 2004). However, there is increasing evidence that altered expression of CXCL12 and CXCR4 plays an important role in carcinogenesis. For example, Jiang et al. (2006) have shown that CXCL12-CXCR4 interactions upregulate tumor necrosis factor and interglin beta 1 in ovarian tumor cell lines and promote angiogenesis, lymph node metastasis, and chemoattractant migration and invasion; such migration and invasion of tumor cells may result in tumor progression.

Smith et al. (2007) have also shown that the CXCL12/CXCR4 axis mediates primary central nervous system lymphoma cell migration and invasion. It was reported by Reddy et al. (2008) that CXCL12 stimulates vasculogenesis and enhances Ewing's sarcoma tumor growth in the absence of vascular endothelial growth factor in vitro. They speculated that the effects of CXCL12 on tumor neovascularization include augmentated chemotaxis of bone marrow cells, retainment of bone-marrow-derived pericytes in close association with the vessel endothelial lining, enhanced overall pericyte coverage of tumor neovessels and remodeling of the vascular endothelium into larger, functional structures. They propose that these processes act in combination to promote the growth of Ewing's sarcoma, even in the face of reduced vascular endothelial growth factor.

Metastasis is the major cause of mortality of malignant neoplasms. It is known that during metastasis tumor cells employ several mechanisms that also regulate the trafficking of normal cells. Therefore, the CXCL12/CXCR4 axis may regulate various mechanisms of tumor metastasis. If so, then how does the CXCL12/CXCR4 axis affect the mechanism of metastasis? Interestingly, it has been shown that CXCL12 induces a directional chemotaxis of several human tumor cell lines. This effect of CXCL12 on tumor cell motility corresponds to changes/rearrangement of cytoskeletal proteins, and tumor cells growing in the presence of CXCL12 display significant increases in the number and thickness of F-actin bundles (Kucia et al., 2004). The peritoneum carcinomatosis of stomach cancer is a good, concrete example of metastatic cancer. Peritoneal carcinomatosis is a frequent cause of death in patients with advanced gastric carcinoma. It was reported by Yasumoto et al. (2006) that the CXCL12/CXCR4 axis plays an important role in peritoneal carcinomatosis of gastric carcinoma. In their in vitro experiments, human gastric carcinoma cell lines, which were all highly efficient in generating malignant ascites in nude mice upon intraperitoneal inoculation, selectively express CXCR4 mRNA and protein. In particular, NUGC4 cells express CXCR4 mRNA at high levels and show vigorous migratory responses to its ligand CXCL12. CXCL12 enhances the proliferation

of, and induces rapid increases in the phosphorylation of protein kinase B/Akt and ERK1/2, in NUGC4 cells. They also showed that AMD3100 (a specific CXCR4 antagonist) effectively reduces tumor growth and ascitic fluid formation in nude mice inoculated with NUGC4 cells and found that CXCR4 positivity of primary gastric carcinomas significantly correlates with the development of peritoneal carcinomatosis in human clinical samples. Based on these results, they hypothesized that the CXCL12/CXCR4 axis is involved in the development of peritoneal carcinomatosis by gastric carcinoma. The collective evidence indicates the emergence of the CXCR4/ CXCL12 axis as an important regulator of the trafficking of various tumor cell types. Therefore, the CXCR4/ CXCL12 axis may be a potential therapeutic target for various neoplasms.

CXCR4/CXCL12 Promote Angiogenesis

Angiogenesis is a key event in the natural progression of malignant neoplasms. Vascular endothelial growth factor (VEGF), a major angiogenic factor, promotes the formation of leaky tumor vasculatures that are the hallmarks of tumor progression. A role for CXC-chemokine-modulation of VEGF signaling in tumorigenesis, especially with regard to interactions between the tumor and its microenvironment, has been recently elucidated in various cancers (Kryczek et al., 2005). For example, Matsuo et al. (2009) analyzed the potential co-operative role of CXCL8 and CXCL12 in tumor-stromal interactions in pancreatic cancer. They initially confirmed the expression of CXC-chemokine ligands and receptors respectively in pancreatic cancer and stromal cells. They then examined the co-operation between CXCL8 and CXCL12 in proliferation/invasion of pancreatic cancer and human umbilical vein endothelial cells. They showed that pancreatic cancer-derived CXCL8 and fibroblast-derived CXCL12 cooperatively induce angiogenesis in vitro by promoting human umbilical vein endothelial cell proliferation, invasion, and tube formation. It was reported by Liang et al. (2007) that CXCR4/CXCL12 induces Akt phosphorylation, which results in the upregulation of VEGF at both the mRNA and protein levels in breast carcinoma cell lines. Conversely, blocking the activation of Akt signaling leads to a decrease in VEGF protein levels. Furthermore, blocking CXCR4/CXCL12 interaction with a CXCR4 antagonist suppresses tumor angiogenesis and growth in vivo, while VEGF mRNA levels correlate well with those of CXCR4 in patient tumor samples. In summary, they demonstrated that the CXCR4/CXCL12 signaling axis can induce angiogenesis and cancer progression by increasing VEGF expression through activation of the PI3K/Akt pathway. Regarding malignant glial tumors, a role for these chemokines in tumorigenesis mediated by VEGF signaling has been recently elucidated. It was reported by Zagzag et al. (2006) that hypoxia and hypoxia-inducible factor-1 (HIF-1) play critical roles in glioblastomas. They hypothesized that CXCR4 would be upregulated by hypoxia and by HIF-1alpha in glioblastomas and suggested that hypoxia upregulates CXCR4 in glioblastomas by two different mechanisms: firstly, through the upregulation of HIF-1alpha in the pseudopalisading tumor cells themselves, and secondly, through the upregulation of the VEGF-stimulated angiogenic response in human brain microvascular endothelial cells. Yang et al. (2005) also investigated the role of CXCR4 in the production of the angiogenic factor, VEGF, in various human glioma cells of astrocytic origin. They detected mRNA and protein expression of CXCR4 in three glioma cell lines; U87-MG, SHG-44, and CHG-5. They also demonstrated that the mRNA and protein expression of functional CXCR4 in several human glioma cell lines correlates with the degree of differentiation of the tumor cells. It was reported by Maderna et al. (2007) that both nestin and CXCL12 are strongly expressed in glioblastomas, both by the tumor and by the endothelial cells. Nestin, a marker for multipotential neuroepithelial stem cells that is detected in neuroepithelial tumors and in proliferating endothelial cells, is involved in the early stages of lineage commitment, proliferation and differentiation. They therefore suggested that nestin-positive cells at least partly represent endothelial progenitors that are able to participate in angiogenesis via chemotactic CXCL12-mediated signals because of the colocalization of nestin and CXCL12. It was reported by Oh et al. (2009) that PAI-1 mRNA and protein expression are increased upon CXCL12 stimulation of CXCR4-positive glioma cells. In addition, they have shown that CXCL12 insults with TNF-alpha and TGF-beta 1 additive effects on the increase in PAI-1 expression. Glioma cells secrete a variety of soluble factors to promote their growth, including plasminogen activator inhibitor-1 (PAI-1). Based on these results, they suggested that the CXCL12/CXCR4 axis is linked to the PAI-1 system in glioma cells. Collectively, these studies suggest that expression of the CXCL12/CXCR4 axis facilitates angiogenesis and disease progression in various neoplasms.

CXCL12/CXCR4 Modulate Tumor Invasiveness Through Metalloproteinases

The invasive process of neoplastic cells involves the attachment of neoplastic cells to extracellular matrix components, degradation of the extracellular matrix, and subsequent tumor cell penetration into the adjacent interstitial stroma. Although many proteinases are capable of degrading the extracellular matrix, metalloproteinases (MMPs) appear to be particularly important for matrix degradation. Recent investigations have shown that malignant tumors use CXCL12-mediated mechanisms not only for tumor cell migration but also for invasion and MMP expression. It was reported by Singh et al. (2004) that CXCL12 and CXCR4 interaction modulates prostate cancer cell MMP expression and invasion as well as migration in vitro. Regarding gliomas, it was reported by Zhang et al. (2005) that CXCL12 increases the expression of membrane type-2 matrix metalloproteinase (MT2-MMP), but not that of the other MT-MMPs, MMP-2 or MMP-9. They therefore considered MT2-MMP as an effector of CXCR4 signaling in glioma cells and further revealed its novel role in modulating the invasive activity of glioma cells. These studies therefore suggest that expression of the CXCL12/CXCR4 axis facilitates the migration, invasion and MMP expression of various tumor cells.

CXCL12/CXCR4 Mediate Glioblastoma Progenitor Cell Proliferation

Although it has been accepted as a general principle that each glioma originates from a mature cell type based on the morphological similarity of the normal mature cells to neoplastic cells, this theory has not been verified, despite recent advances in cellular biology and molecular genetics. Growing evidence suggests that many neoplasms originate from aberrant proliferation of progenitor cells. With the discovery of neural stem cells/progenitor cells in the central nervous system, normal neural stem cells or progenitor cells have been speculated to be the principal targets of mutations that lead to glial tumors (Sugita et al., 2005). In addition, several recent reports suggest that tumor stem cells/progenitor cells exist in high-grade astrocytomas and can be isolated from these tumors (Ehtesham et al., 2009; Ma et al., 2008). Ma et al. (2008) have also shown in situ that astrocytomas contain a considerable number of cells with stem cell characteristics, and with increasing numbers of WHO grade of the astrocytoma. In addition, they reported a notable increase in the number of positively stained CXCR4 cells in astrocytomas Grade IV compared to other low grade tumors, which themselves had increased levels compared to normal brain tissue. It was also reported by Ehtesham et al. (2009) that CXCR4 is overexpressed in glioblastoma-derived sphere cultures compared to the corresponding differentiated tumor cells, and that co-expression of CXCR4 with progenitor cell markers was detected within cancerous cell populations in histopathological specimens of human glioblastoma. They also found that CXCL12 ligand-stimulated proliferation in glioblastoma-derived spheres, but not in differentiated glioblastoma cells. They therefore considered that CXCR4 is expressed at higher levels in neoplastic progenitor cells, and that the CXCL12 ligand specifically promotes glioma-derived spheres rather than differentiated tumor cell turn-over. They also speculated that CXCR4 plays an important role in the proliferation of glioma tumor stem cells. Thus, these studies suggest that the CXCL12/CXCR4 axis plays an important role as a regulator of glioma tumor stem cell biology.

Expression of CXCL12 on Pseudopalisading Cells and Proliferating Microvessels in Glioblastomas

The primary mechanism by which glioblastomas spread is different from that of other carcinomas. Notably, both CXCR4 and CXCL12 are overexpressed in glial tumor cells in vivo, suggesting a role for this chemokine in tumor growth (Barbero et al., 2003). Using immunohistochemical analysis of different glioblastomas, Rempel et al. (2000) reported that CXCR4 and CXCL12 do not colocalize to tumor regions that highly express the proliferation marker MIB-1, but localize to tumor regions characterized by necrosis and angiogenesis. They therefore speculated that CXCL12 promotes neoangiogenesis, which supplies nutrients to sustain tumor growth and/or modulation of the immune response.

In our previous study of astrocytomas, anaplastic astrocytomas, and glioblastomas, we showed that both tumor cells, and tumor cells associated with neighboring vessels, express CXCL12 (Komatani et al., 2009). We also detected CXCR4 expression in the cytoplasm of these tumors, suggesting that CXCR4/CXCL12 interactions play important roles in the growth, angiogenesis, and sustenance of the microenvironment of astrocytic tumors by both autocrine and paracrine mechanisms. However, there were obvious differences in the staining intensity and in the distribution of CXCL12 expression in subtypes of astrocytic tumors.

The pathologic features that distinguish glioblastomas from astrocyotmas in tissue sections include necrotic foci, usually with evidence of peripheral pseudopalisading cells and micovascular proliferation. It is also well known that numerous vascular changes occur at the transition of anaplastic astrocytomas to glioblastomas. Recent studies have shed light on the initial events of pseudopalisade formation in glioblastomas. A dramatic shift in biological behavior occurs following the transition from anaplastic astrocytomas to glioblastomas. The latter are characterized by pseudopalisading necrosis and increasing levels of angiogenesis, features that are pathophysiologically linked to, and mechanistically instrumental for, disease progression (Kleihues et al., 2006). Pseudopalisade formation results from the following sequence of events: (i) vascular occlusion, related to endothelial apoptosis and associated with intravascular thrombosis; (ii) hypoxia in regions surrounding vascular pathology; (iii) outward migration of glioma cells away from hypoxia, creating a peripherally directed wave of cell movement; (iv) death of nonmigrated cells leading to central necrosis; (v) an exuberant angiogenic response creating microvascular proliferation in regions peripheral to the central hypoxia; and (vi) enhanced outward expansion of infiltrating tumor cells toward a new vasculature (Brat and Van Meir, 2004). In this chapter, we show that tumor cells associated with pseudopalisades and neighboring vessels show intense and diffuse CXCL12 expression in glioblastomas (Fig. 15.1). Recently, investigators have demonstrated that CXCL12 regulates the cell growth and migration of hematopoietic stem cells but that it may also play a central role in brain development (Bajetto et al., 2001; Lazarini et al., 2003). More specifically, CXCL12 activates CXCR4 receptors that are expressed in a variety of neural cells, resulting in diverse biological effects. CXCL12-CXCR4 activation enhances the migration and proliferation of cerebellar granule cells, chemoattracts microglia, and stimulates cytokine production and glutamate release by astrocytes. It has also been shown that the tumorigenesis of neuroepithelial tumors reflects architectural changes in developing brain tissue (Sugita et al., 2005). Zagzag et al. (2006) demonstrated that CXCR4 expression is primarily under the control of HIF-1 in hypoxic pseudopalisading cells around areas of necrosis that overexpress HIF-1 alpha, whereas VEGF released by the psuedopalisading cells is, at least in part, responsible for CXCR4 upregulation in endothelial cells. Because hypoxia is known to be a potent stimulus for VEGF upregulation, they concluded that these molecular events are linked by hypoxia-induced upregulation of CXCR4 in glioblastomas. In summary, we propose the following model of hypoxic regulation of CXCR4/CXCL12 function in glioblastomas (Fig. 15.2). CXCR4/CXCL12 secretion by hypoxic pseudopalisading cells and by proliferating microvascular cells contributes to the outward migration of glioma cells away from hypoxia, thereby creating a peripherally moving wave of cells and subsequent microvascular proliferation.

In our previous study (Komatani et al., 2009), we also showed that the survival rate of glioblastoma patients with lower tumor expression of CXCL12 was significantly higher than that of patients with higher CXCL12 expression. By multivariate analysis, CXCL12 emerged as an independent prognostic factor for glioblastoma patients. In contrast, a comparison of patients with low and high CXCR4-expressing glioblastomas showed no significant difference in survival rates between these two groups. In addition, CXCR4 did not emerge as an independent prognostic factor for glioblastoma patients. These findings appear to be inconsistent with a previous report that CXCR4

staining of malignant neoplasms is associated with an unfavorable prognosis (Jiang et al., 2006). As our results indicated that CXCR4 plays an important role in tumor growth of both low- and high-grade astrocytic tumors, we consider that CXCR4/CXCL12 interaction is necessary for the growth of such astrocytic neoplasms and that additional high expression of CXCL12 in the glioblastoma cells themselves, and in the ensuing microvessels due to hypoxia, promotes tumorigenesis of primary glioblastomas de novo or promotes the transition from astrocytomas to glioblastomas. Indeed, pseudopalisades and the ensuing microvascular proliferation are considered to be associated with accelerated growth of glioblastomas (Kleihues et al., 2006). As such, expression of CXCL12 in glioblastomas could be a reliable and independent prognostic factor for patients with glioblastomas.

There remains the question of the role of CXCL12/CXCR4 expression at the invading edge of glioblastomas. The various patterns of local spread of glioblastomas are known as the secondary structures of Scherer. These patterns include perineuronal and perivascular satellitosis, subpial spread, and invasion along with white matter. These structures are referred to as "secondary" because their formation depends on underlying normal brain structures, as opposed to "primary" structures, such as pseudopalisading cells, necrosis, and microvascular proliferation. Zagzag et al. (2008) noted the relationship between the CXCL12/CXCR4 axis and the secondary structures of Scherer and proposed a biologically based mechanism for the nonrandom formation of Scherer's secondary structures applying the differential expression of CXCL12 and CXCR4 at the invading edge of glioblastomas. CXCL12 is highly expressed in neurons, blood vessels, subpial regions, and white matter tracts that form the basis of Scherer's secondary structures. In contrast, CXCR4 is highly expressed in invading glioma cells that are organized around neurons and blood vessels, in subpial regions, and along white matter tracts. Neuronal and endothelial cells exposed to vascular endothelial growth factor upregulate the expression of CXCL12. The CXCR4-positive tumor cells migrate toward a CXCL12 gradient in vitro, whereas inhibition of CXCR4 expression decreases their migration. Similarly, inhibition of CXCR4 decreases the levels of CXCL12-induced phosphorylation of FAK, AKT, and ERK1/2, suggesting CXCR4 involvement in the signaling of glioma invasion. This model was considered

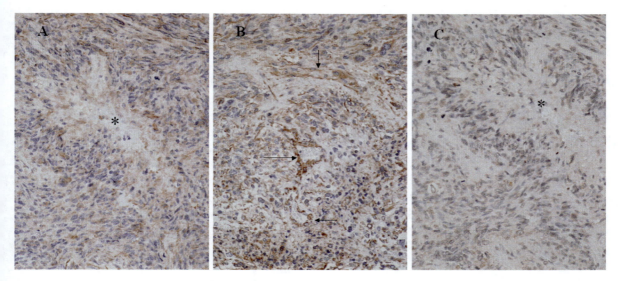

Fig. 15.1 Immunohistochemical distribution of CXCL 12 and CXCR4 in a glioblastoma. The distribution of CXCL12 and CXCR4 in a glioblastoma was analyzed by immunohistochemistry. Intense immunostaining of CXCL12 is observed in the psuedopalisading cells (asterions:necrosis) (**a**) and in proliferating microvessels (**b**, *arrows*). CXCR4-positive immunoreactivity is observed as diffuse staining of the cytoplasm of glioblastoma cells (asterions:necrosis) (**c**)

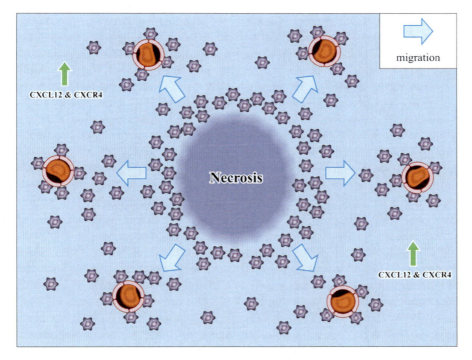

Fig. 15.2 Hypoxic regulation of CXCR4/CXCL12 function in glioblastomas. This scheme shows that the secretion of CXCR4/CXCL12 by hypoxic pseudopalisading cells and proliferating microvascular cells participates in the outward migration of glioma cells away from hypoxia, thereby creating a peripherally moving wave of cells and subsequent microvascular proliferation in the glioblastoma

to provide a plausible molecular basis for, and explanation of, the formation of Scherer's structures in glioma patients.

A Featured Therapeutic Trial of a Selective CXCR4/CXCL12 Inhibition for Glioblastoma Therapy

Inhibition of growth factor receptors may be useful as adjuvant therapy for the treatment of glioblastomas, following surgical resection, radiotherapy and chemotherapy. As outlined above, the CXCR4/CXCL12 axis plays a central role in tumorigenesis of glioblastomas. Thus, drugs that target CXCR4 or CXCL12 could disrupt the interactions between glioma cells and stromal cells. In addition, growing evidence implicates altered expression of CXCL12 and CXCR4 in the pathogenesis of CNS disorders such as HIV-associated encephalopathy, stroke and multiple sclerosis, making CXCL12 and CXCR4 plausible targets for future pharmacological intervention (Liu et al., 2008). It was reported by Rubin et al. (2003) that systemic administration of the CXCR4 antagonist AMD 3100 inhibits the growth of glioblastoma and medulloblastoma xenografts by increasing apoptosis and decreasing tumor proliferation. This result reflects the ability of AMD 3100 to reduce the activation of ERK1/2 and Akt, all of which are involved in signaling pathways downstream of CXCR4 that promote cell survival, proliferation, and migration. They also demonstrated that CXCR4 is critical for the progression of diverse brain malignances and they provided a scientific rationale for clinical evaluation of AMD 3100 in the treatment of both adults and children with malignant brain tumors. Redjal et al. (2006) also reported that CXCR4 signaling is implicated in tumor growth, survival, and migration in malignant brain tumors, and that pharmacologic inhibition of CXCR4 results in decreased tumor growth in preclinical models. To understand how CXCR4 inhibitors are incorporated into clinical therapy, they examined the determinants of tumor responsiveness to CXCR4 inhibition. Because optimal use of CXCR4 inhibition is likely to be one part of multimodality therapy, they also investigated the efficacy of CXCR4 inhibition combined with conventional cytotoxic chemotherapy. The effects of CXCR4 antagonists, AMD3100, alone or in combination with 1,3-bis(2-chloroethyl)-1-nitrosourea (BCNU), on cell growth were determined for several glioblastoma cell lines in vitro. In all cell lines tested, treatment of glioblastoma cells with BCNU followed by AMD3100 resulted in synergistic antitumor efficacy in vitro. Treatment with subtherapeutic doses of BCNU in combination with AMD3100 also results in tumor regression in vivo, and this result reflects both increased apoptosis and decreased proliferation following combination therapy. Their studies therefore support testing of CXCR4 inhibitors in patients with glioblastoma, and they established that inhibition of CXCR4 synergizes with conventional cytotoxic therapies in a clinically relevant combinatorial strategy.

Ping et al. (2007) reported that the lipoxygenase inhibitor Nordy can regulate CXCR4-mediated production of angiogenic factors by human glioblastoma cells. They found that Nordy potently inhibited CXCR4 ligand CXCL12-induced production of interleukin 8 and vascular endothelial cell growth factor, two important angiogenic factors implicated in the progression of malignant tumors. Their study further revealed that the effect of Nordy was attributable to its downregulation of the expression of functional CXCR4 in glioblastoma cells. They therefore considered that the anti-cancer activity of Nordy is due, at least in part, to its suppression of the chemokine receptor CXCR4 thus reducing the production of angiogenic factors by tumor cells.

To develop a therapeutic approach for inhibition of CXCL12 in tumors, Yang et al. (2007) investigated the signaling pathways that are critical for CXCL12 function in normal and malignant cells. They discovered that CXCL12-dependent tumor growth was dependent upon sustained inhibition of cyclic AMP (cAMP) production, and that the antitumor activity of the specific CXCR4 antagonist AMD 3465 was associated with the blocking of cAMP suppression. Consistent with these findings, they showed that pharmacologic elevation of cAMP with the phosphodiesterase inhibitor Rolipram suppresses tumor cell growth in vitro and, upon oral administration, inhibits intracranial growth in xenograft models of malignant brain tumors with comparable efficacy to AMD 3465. Thus, they considered that the clinical evaluation of phosphodiesterase inhibitors in the treatment of patients with brain tumors is warranted.

According to the review of Burger and Bürkle (2007), the CXCR4 antagonist AMD3100 is now being evaluated in phase III clinical trials for the mobilization of hematopoietic stem cells, and in preclinical studies for the treatment of leukemia. Therefore, the results of basic research could lead to a future therapeutic trial of a selective CXCR4/CXCL12 inhibitor therapy of glioblastomas.

References

Bajetto A, Barbero S, Bonavia R, Piccioli P, Pirani P, Florio T, Schettini G (2001) Stromal cell-derived factor-1 alpha induces astrocyte proliferation through the activation of extracellular signal-regulated kinases $\frac{1}{2}$ pathway. J Neurochem 77:1226–1236

Barbero S, Bonavia R, Bajetto A, Porcile C, Pirani P, Ravetti JL, Zona GL, Spaziante R, Florio T, Schettini G (2003) Stromal cell-derived factor 1 alpha stimulates human glioblastoma cell growth through the activation of both extracellular signal-regulated kinase $\frac{1}{2}$ and Akt[1]. Cancer Res 63:1969–1974

Brat DJ, Van Meir EG (2004) Vaso-occlusive and prothrombotic mechanisms associated with tumor hypoxia, necrosis, and accelerated growth in glioblastoma. Lab Invest 84:397–405

Burger JA, Bürkle A (2007) The CXCR4 chemokine receptor in acute and chronic leukaemia: a marrow homing receptor and potential therapeutic target. Br J Haematol 137:288–296

Ehtesham M, Mapara. KY, Stevenson CB, Thompson RC (2009) CXCR4 mediates the proliferation of glioblastoma progenitor cells. Cancer Lett 274:305–312

Jiang Y, Wu X-H, Shi B, Wu W-X, Yin G-R (2006) Expression of chemokine CXCL12 and its receptor CXCR4 in human epithelial ovarian cancer: an independent prognostic factor for tumor progression. Gynecol Oncol 103:226–233

Kleihues P, Burger PC, Aldape KD, Brat DJ, Biernat W, Bigner DD, Nakazato Y, Plate KH, Giangaspero F, von Deimling A, Ohgaki H, Cavenee WK (2006) Glioblastoma. In: Louis DN, Ohgaki H, Wiestler OD, Cavenee WK (eds) Pathology and genetics of tumours of the nervous system. International Agency for Research on Cancer, Lyon, pp 33–52

Komatani H, Sugita Y, Arakawa F, Ohshima K, Shigemori M (2009) Expression of CXCL12 on psuedopalisading cells and proliferating microvessels in glioblastomas: an accelerated growth factor in glioblastomas. Int J Oncol 34:665–672

Kryczek I, Lange A, Mottram P, Alvarez X, Cheng P, Hogan M, Moons L, Wei S, Zou L, Machelon V, Emilie D, Terrassa M, Lackner A, Curiel TJ, Carmeliet P, Zou W (2005) CXCL12 and vascular endothelial growth factor synergistically induce neoangiogenesis in human ovarian cancers. Cancer Res 65:465–472

Kucia M, Jankowski. K, Reca R, Wysoczynski M, Bandura L, Allendorf DJ, Zhang J, Ratajczak J, Ratajczak MZ (2004) CXCR4-SDF1 signalling, locomotion, chemotaxis and adhesion. J Mol Histol 35:233–245

Lazarini F, Than TN, Casanoa P, Arenzana-Seisdedos F, Dubois-Dalcq M (2003) Role of the alpha-chemokine stromal cell-derived factor (SDF1) in the developing and mature central nervous system. Glia 42:139–148

Li M, Ransohoff RM (2008) Multiple roles of chemokine CXCL12 in the central nervous system: a migration from immunology to neurobiology. Prog Neurobiol 84:116–131

Liang Z, Brooks J, Willard M, Liang K, Yoon Y, Kang S, Shim H (2007) CXCR4/CXCL12 axis promotes VEGF-mediated tumor angiogenesis through akt signaling pathway. Biochem Biophys Res Commun 359:716–722

Liu XS, Chopp M, Santra M, Hozeska-Solgot A, Zhang RL, Wang L, Teng H, Lu M, Zhang ZG (2008) Functional response to SDF1 alpha through over-expression of CXCR4 on adult subventricular zone progenitor cells. Brain Res 1226:18–26

Luo Y, Iathia J, Mughal M, Mattson MP (2008) SDF1alpha/CXCR4 signaling, via ERKs and the transcription factor egr1, induces expression of a 67-kDa form of glutamic acid decarboxylase in embryonic hippocampal neurons. J Biol Chem 283:24789–24800

Ma YH, Mentlein R, Knerlich F, Kruse ML, Mehdorn HM, Held-Feindt J (2008) Expression of stem cell markers in human astrocytomas of different WHO grades. J Nerooncol 86:31–45

Maderna E, Salmaggi A, Calatozzolo C, Limido L, Pollo B (2007) Nestin, PDGFRbeta, CXCL12, and VEGF in glioma patients: different profiles of (pro-angiogenic) molecule expression are related with tumor grade and May provide prognostic information. Cancer Biol Ther 6:1018–1024

Matsuo Y, Ochi N, Sawai M, Yasuda A, Takahashi H, Funahashi H, Takeyama H, Tong Z, Guha S (2009) CXCL8/IL-8 and CXCL12/SDF-1 alpha co-operatively promote invasiveness and angiogenesis in pancreatic cancer. Int J Cancer 124:853–861

Oh JW, Olman M, Benveniste EN (2009) CXCL12-mediated induction of plasminogen activator inhibitor-1 expression in human CXCR4 positive astroglioma cells. Biol Pharm Bull 32:573–577

Ping YF, Yao XH, Chen JH, Liu H, Chen DL, Zhou XD, Wang JM, Bian XW (2007) The anti-cancer compound nordy inhibits CXCR4-mediated production of IL-8 and VEGF by malignant human glioma cells. J Neurooncol 84:21–29

Reddy K, Zhou Z, Jia SF, Lee TH, Morales-Arias J, Cao Y, Kleinerman ES (2008) Stromal cell-derived factor-1 stimulates vasculogenesis and enhances Ewing's sarcoma tumor growth in the absence of vascular endothelial growth factor. Int J Cancer 123:831–837

Redjal N, Chan JA, Segal RA, Kung AL (2006) CXCR4 inhibition synergizes with cytotoxic chemotherapy in gliomas. Clin Cancer Res 12:6765–6771

Rempel SA, Dudas S, Ge S, Gutiérrez JA (2000) Identification and localization of cytokine SDF1 and its receptor, CXC chemokine receptor 4, to regions of necrosis and angiogenesis in human glioblastoma. Clin Cancer Res 6:102–111

Rubin JB, Kung AL, Klein R,S, Chan JA, Sun Y, Schmidt K, Kieran MW, Luster AD, Segal RA (2003) A small-molecule antagonist of CXCR4 inhibits intracranial growth of primary brain tumors. Proc Natl Acad Sci USA 100:13513–13518

Schönemeier B, Schulz S, Hoellt V, Stumm R (2008) Enhanced expression of the CXCL12/SDF-1 chemokine receptor CXCR7 after cerebral ischemia in the rat brain. J Neuroimmunol 198:39–45

Singh, S,, Singh, P,, Grizzle, WE,and, Lillard JW Jr. (2004) CXCL12-CXCR4 interactions modulate prostate cancer cell migration, metalloproteinase expression and invasion. Lab Invest 84:1666–1676

Smith JR, Faikenhagen KM, Coupland SE, Chipps TJ, Rosenblum JT (2007) Malignant B cells from patients with primary central nervous system lymphoma express stromal cell-derived factor-1. Am J Clin Pathol 127: 633–641

Stumm RK, Rummel J, Junker V, Culmsee C, Pfeiffer M, Krieglstein J, Höllt V, Schulz S (2002) A dual role for the SDF-1/CXCR4 chemokine receptor system in adult brain: isoform-selective regulation of SDF-1 expression modulates CXCR4-dependent neuronal plasticity and cerebral leukocyte recruitment after focal ischemia. J Neurosci 22:5865–5878

Sugita Y, Nakamura Y, Yamamoto M, Oda E, Tokunaga O, Shigemori M (2005) Expression of tubulin beta II in neuroepithelial tumors: reflection of architectural changes in the developing human brain. Acta Neuropathol 110:127–134

Yang SX, Chen JH, Jiang XF, Wang QL, Chen ZQ, Zhao W, Feng Y-H, Xin R, Shi J-Q, Bian X-W (2005) Activation of chemokine receptor CXCR4 in malignant glioma cells promotes the production of vascular endothelial growth factor. Biochem Biophys Res Commun 335:523–528

Yang L, Jackson E, Woerner BM, Perry A, Piwnica-Worms D, Rubin JB (2007) Blocking CXCR4-mediated cyclic AMP suppression inhibits brain tumor growth in vivo. Cancer Res 67:651–658

Yasumoto K, Koizumi K, Kawashima A, Saitoh Y, Arita Y, Shinohara K, Yamamoto A, Yamamoto H, Miyado K, Okano HJ, Fukagawa R, Higaki K, Minami T, Nakayama T, Sakurai H, Takahashi Y, Yoshie O, Saiki I (2006) Role of the CXCL12/CXCR4 axis in peritoneal carcinomatosis of gastric cancer. Cancer Res 66:2181–2187

Zagzag D, Esencay M, Mendez O, Yee H, Smirnova I, Huang Y, Chiriboga L, Lukyanov E, Liu M, Newcomb EW (2008) Hypoxia- and vascular endothelial growth factor-induced stromal cell-derived factor-1alpha/CXCR4 expression in glioblastomas: one plausible explanation of Schere's structures. Am J Pathol 173:545–560

Zagzag D, Lukyanov Y, Lan Li, Ali MA, Esencay M, Mendez O, Yee H, Voura EB, Newcomb EW (2006) Hypoxia-inducible factor 1 and VEGF upregulate CXCR4 in glioblastoma: implications for angiogenesis and glioma cell invasion. Lab Invest 86:1221–1232

Zhang J, Sarkar S, Yong VW (2005) The chemokine stromal cell derived factor-1 (CXCL12) promotes glioma invasiveness through MT2-matrix metalloproteinase. Carcinogenesis 26:2069–2077

Chapter 16

Cell Death Signaling in Glioblastoma Multiforme: Role of the Bcl2L12 Oncoprotein

Alexander H. Stegh

Abstract Malignant glioma (MG) represents the most prevalent and lethal primary central nervous system cancer. Despite aggressive surgical resection and treatment regimens, patients diagnosed with the highest grade MG, grade IV glioblastoma multiforme (GBM), survive for only 9–12 months after diagnosis. Multimodal approaches using radiation with conjunctive chemotherapy (temozolamide) resulted in only marginal increase in patients' survival up to 14.6 months. An incomplete understanding of how catalogued genetic aberrations dictate phenotypic hallmarks of the disease, particularly intense therapy (apoptosis) resistance, yet florid intratumoral necrogenesis, combined with a highly therapy-resistant cancer stem cell population (brain tumor stem cells, BTSC) as the putative cell-of-origin conspired to make GBM a highly enigmatic and incurable disease. Especially the continued lack of success in treating high-grade gliomas with targeted (receptor) tyrosine kinase inhibitors, which have been proven to be effective in other malignancies, has prompted a reevaluation of all aspects of glioma drug development and underlined the overarching need to identify and molecularly dissect genetic aberrations in cellular survival pathways that play pivotal roles in GBM's profound therapy resistance. This review focuses on apoptosis and necrosis pathways implicated in GBM development and evasion from therapy-induced cell death, and discusses the roles and potential therapeutical applications of the novel Bcl-2-like oncoprotein Bcl2L12 in driving cell death-related phenotypes in GBM.

A.H. Stegh (✉)
Department of Neurology, The Robert H. Lurie Comprehensive Cancer Center, The Brain Tumor Institute, Northwestern University, Chicago, IL, USA
e-mail: a-stegh@northwestern.edu

Keywords Apoptosis · Necrosis · Glioblastoma multiforme (GBM) · Bcl-2 family proteins · Bcl2L12 · αB-crystallin

Introduction

Malignant glioma is the most prevalent and lethal primary cancer of the central nervous system (CNS). Patients diagnosed with its most malignant manifestation Glioblastoma multiforme (GBM), survive for only 9–12 months (Furnari et al., 2007). Aggressive surgical resection combined with extant chemo- and radiotherapy improve life expectancy only marginally; recurrence is nearly universal and treatment options to combat such progression are limited and ineffective. Diffuse infiltration into normal brain parenchyma, intense therapy (apoptosis) resistance, combined with the seemingly paradoxical propensity for necrogenesis conspire to make GBM an incurable and debilitating disease. The past decade witnessed stunning progress in the systematic and genome-wide catalogization and functional validation of genetic aberrations driving GBM pathogenesis. Foremost the human cancer genome atlas project (TCGA) (The Cancer Genome Atlas Research Network, 2008) provided a comprehensive, large-scale analysis of the GBM genome and laid the foundation for further functional studies aiming to understand how genetic aberrations dictate phenotypic hallmarks of the disease, particularly therapy (apoptosis) resistance and florid intratumoral necrosis. Understanding the genetic, cell- and pathobiological underpinnings of apoptotic and necrotic death modalities, their complex interconnections and roles in gliomapathogenesis and therapy resistance is pivotal for the development of rational, molecularly targeted drugs. Such novel agents designed to modulate the activity of critical cell death modulators may overcome therapy resistance, alleviate neurologically debilitating symptoms caused by extensive necrogenesis and ultimately improve the dismal prognosis for GBM patients.

This chapter discusses cell death pathways important for GBM development and therapy resistance and focuses on *Bcl2-Like-12* (Bcl2L12) as a novel GBM oncoprotein and master regulator of the apoptosis/necrosis balance in GBM. Identified as an oncogene with frequent and robust amplification/over-expression in primary GBM (Stegh et al., 2007; 2008b), Bcl2L12 impacts a plethora of gliomagenic signaling circuits, including effector caspase activation, heat shock protein signaling and p53 tumor suppressive function and promotes tumorigenesis in orthotopic GBM mouse models. Here, we describe in detail Bcl2L12's *modus operandi* in glial cells and tumors and how Bcl2L12 biology complements our current understanding of apoptosis and necrosis signaling pathways. These detailed cell biological and in vivo gliomagenesis studies exemplify how genomic discoveries – when put into a cell biological and in vivo pathobiological context – will aid in decisively translating basic discoveries into drug development in the future.

Evasion from Apoptosis as a Tumorigenic and Resistance Mechanism in GBM

Genetic deregulation of apoptosis and necrosis, the two most prominent forms of mammalian cell death, is a decisive step in neoplastic transformation and is critical for the development of cell-intrinsic resistance mechanisms towards radio-, chemo- and targeted therapies (Hanahan and Weinberg, 2000). Apoptosis is an evolutionary highly conserved cellular process that plays fundamental roles in tissue homeostasis and consequently is frequently compromised in diverse pathological conditions, in particular in human cancers (Hotchkiss et al., 2009). As a genetically defined, hierarchically ordered cell death modality, apoptosis is triggered by the selective cleavage of foremost cytoskeletal and metabolic proteins by *cysteinyl aspartases* (caspases) (Stegh and Peter,

2001). Caspase activation induces a series of hallmark morphological changes in apoptosing cells that include cellular and nuclear shrinkage, chromatin condensation, DNA fragmentation and the formation of apoptotic, membrane encapsulated bodies (Hotchkiss et al., 2009).

The apoptosis signaling machinery relies on the complex interplay of extra- and intracellular sentinels and executioners. Death receptors (DRs), such as CD95/Fas, TNFR-1,-2 and the TRAIL-receptors DR4 and DR5, are important cell surface molecules that upon binding their cognate ligands relay environmental cues from the extracellular surroundings inwards. Instigated by ligand binding and subsequent receptor oligomerization, several intracellular signaling molecules, including caspases 8 and 10, are recruited to the cytoplasmic tail of a DR, culminating in the formation of a death-inducing signaling complex (DISC) (Stegh and Peter, 2001). DISC assembly results in proteolytic activation of caspases 8 and 10, which either directly cleave and activate downstream caspases, most importantly effector caspases 3 and 7, or induce mitochondrial disintegration to instigate the intrinsic apoptosis signaling pathway (Stegh and Peter, 2001). Here, caspase-8/10-mediated cleavage of the pro-apoptotic Bcl-2 family protein Bid generates a truncated product, tBid, which upon translocation to mitochondria induces mitochondrial outer membrane permeabilization (MOMP) (Stegh and Peter, 2001) – an irreversible process that can be inhibited by anti-apoptotic Bcl-2 proteins, such prototypic Bcl-2 or Bcl-x_L (Youle and Strasser, 2008).

In response to mitochondrial membrane damage, apoptogenic factors confined to the mitochondrial intermembrane or matrix space, most notably cytochrome c (cyt c), are released into the cytosol to modulate postmitochondrial caspase activation. Cyt c binds to the cytoplasmic scaffold protein Apaf-1 resulting in ATP-dependent recruitment and subsequent activation of caspase-9 (Stegh and Peter, 2001). As an initiator caspase, it promotes maturation of effector caspases, such as caspase-3 and -7, which in turn selectively cleave a limited number of cellular proteins with central functions in cell signaling, metabolism, cytoskeletal dynamics, DNA replication/transcription and protein translation to promote the ordered breakdown of cellular structures (Stegh and Peter, 2001).

The mitochondrial or intrinsic signaling pathway is not only an important signal amplification step in

DR-instigated apoptosis, but plays central roles in cellular responses to DNA damage, growth factor withdrawal and chemotherapy (Green and Kroemer, 2004). Here, the nuclear and cytoplasmic tumor suppressor p53 acts as a multifunctional stress sensor that in response to cellular damage can promote cell cycle arrest or induce apoptotic demise. Mechanistically, p53 acts as a transcription factor that induces expression of apoptosis activators or cell cycle inhibitors, such as caspase-9, Apaf-1 and p21, or triggers MOMP by modulating the activity of Bcl-2 family proteins (Green and Kroemer, 2009; Harris and Levine, 2005).

Many of these central apoptosis modulators are misappropriated in GBM on genomic, transcriptional and proteomic levels and their contribution to GBM pathogenesis and therapy evasion is indubitable. The definition of their precise *modi operandi* in driving tumor progression and dictating pathobiological phenotypes, however, remains an area of intensive research.

The Role of Death Receptors, Bcl-2 and IAP Protein Families in GBM Pathogenesis and Therapy Resistance

While CD95's pro-apoptosis functions in regulating the adaptive immune response is well documented and most notably involves the initiation of activation-induced cell death (AICD) of T cells, its role in cell death signaling in GBM is less well defined. Glioma cell lines are partially sensitive to CD95 ligation; receptor levels, however, do not correlate with sensitivity towards ligand-induced apoptosis and tumor grade, as CD95 expression increases during glioma progression from low-grade to anaplastic astrocytoma and are highest in GBM with most pronounced expression in perinecrotic areas (Ziegler et al., 2008). Interestingly, recent studies suggest unexpected, non-apoptotic roles for CD95 in GBM cell invasion and neural stem cell survival and specification. In GBM tumor cells, ligand-induced activation of CD95 does not lead to DISC formation, but instead promotes the recruitment of the Src family member Yes and the p85 subunit of phosphatidylinositol 3-kinase (PI3K) to the cytoplasmic portion of the receptor leading to upregulation of MMP-2 and MMP-9 via the Gsk3-β-catenin signaling pathway (Kleber et al., 2008). By triggering metalloproteinase activation and consequently breakdown

of the extracellular matrix, CD95 drives infiltration of GBM tumor cells into normal brain parenchyma and its neutralization reduces tumor cell invasion in vivo (Kleber et al., 2008). In addition, CD95 promotes neurogenesis by activating prosurvival pathways involving Src, PI3K, Akt and mTOR in neural stem cells (NSCs) leading to stem cell survival and neuronal differentiation (Corsini et al., 2009). Future studies will demonstrate, whether CD95-instigated neurogenic pathways in NSCs are also operative in brain tumor stem cells (BTSCs) as the putative GBM cell-of-origin, where they might play pivotal roles in promoting gliomagenesis by facilitating proliferation, migration and invasion.

The discovery of the death ligand (DL) TNF-related Apoptosis Inducing Ligand (TRAIL) as a selective inducer of apoptosis in tumor but not normal cells promised to be valuable for the selective induction of apoptosis in cancers in general and GBM in particular. Expressions analyses of two agonistic (TRAIL-R1 and -R2) and three antagonistic TRAIL-binding receptors (DcR1/TRAIL-R3; DcR2/TRAIL-R4; osteoprotegerin (OPG)) revealed preferential (over-) expression of agonistic, and decreased abundance of antagonistic receptors with some suggestion that such expression pattern correlate with favorable prognosis for patients with GBM (Ziegler et al., 2008). Interestingly, TRAIL is also expressed in GBM tumors, but is insufficient for prominent auto- or paracrine apoptosis induction and requires exogenous soluble TRAIL for profound tumoricidal activity (Ziegler et al., 2008). Besides insufficient endogenous TRAIL levels, aberrantly expressed apoptosis inhibitors downstream of the TRAIL-R DISCs, most notably Bcl-2 and IAP family proteins, might render GBM cells resistant towards TRAIL-mediated cell death.

Bcl-2 proteins belong to a family of evolutionary conserved, versatile apoptosis modulators that promote or inhibit apoptosis signaling by impacting intracellular organelle physiology, most importantly mitochondrial homeostasis (Youle and Strasser, 2008). While their contribution to the genesis and therapy resistance of several cancers, especially hematological malignancies, have been well studied, their impact on gliomagenesis is less well understood. Immunohistochemical studies in initial vs. recurrent GBM suggest a shift of the Bcl-2 rheostat towards anti-apoptotic adjustment: Protein abundance of anti-apoptotic members Bcl-2, Bcl-x_L and Mcl-1 increases, while pro-apoptotic factors, such as Bax, decrease (Ziegler et al., 2008). Quantification of canonical Bcl-2 family proteins during astrocytoma progression surprisingly and counterintuitively revealed predominant expression of anti-apoptotic members in low-grade tumors. As reported for other malignancy, e.g. mammary and gastric carcinomas, such expression profiles are linked to a more favorable prognosis (Ziegler et al., 2008).

While further experimental evidence is required to fully understand the molecular basis for downregulation of Bcl-2 cell death antagonists during astrocytoma progression, recent studies suggest that Bcl-2 family proteins have diverse functions beyond their dogmatic roles in apoptosis signaling. Anti-apoptotic Bcl-2 can induce apoptotic demise when bound to orphan nuclear receptor Nur77/TR3. Nur77 binding induces a Bcl-2 conformational change that exposes its BH3 domain, resulting in conversion of Bcl-2 from a protector to a killer (Cheng et al., 2006). Other studies reporting bimodal activity profiles of Bcl-2 family members identified Bax as a potent inhibitor of apoptosis in neurons of mice infected with Sindbis virus, Bak as a cell-type-specific anti- or pro-apoptotic protein in neurons depending on neuronal subtype and postnatal developmental stage and Bid that upon phosphorylation by ATM redirects the cellular program from apoptosis to S phase arrest to allow for DNA repair rather than cell death induction (Cheng et al., 2006). Finally, Bcl-2 has potent anti-growth activities, as it delays cell cycle progression through upregulation of the cyclin-dependent kinase (Cdk) inhibitor p27 and downregulation of phosphorylated retinoblastoma protein (Rb) and functional E2F (Cheng et al., 2006) Consequently, high-grade glioma may escape pro-apoptotic or cell cycle inhibitory functions of Bcl-2 by downregulating its expression.

While Bcl-2 family proteins impact organelle, foremost mitochondrial membrane integrity, Inhibitor of Apoptosis Proteins (IAPs) modulate postmitochondrial caspase signaling. Eight mammalian IAPs have been described: X-chromosome-linked IAP (XIAP, BIRC4, ILP1, MIHA), cellular IAP1 (cIAP1, BIRC2, HIAP2, MIHB) and cIAP2 (BIRC3, HIAP1, MIHC), neuronal apoptosis inhibitory protein (NAIP, BIRC1), survivin (BIRC5), Bruce (Apollon), melanoma IAP (ML-IAP, BIRC7, Livin, KIAP), and testis-specific IAP (Ts-IAP, ILP2, BIRC8). Based on sequence and domain conservation and broad anti-apoptotic activities, initial functional studies attributed caspase inhibitory activities to several members of the family, including cIAP-1 and cIAP-2. Structural studies that identified amino acid residues essential for effector caspase inhibition, however, revealed that XIAP and possibly the survivin:hepatitis B X-interacting protein (HBXIP) complex are likely the only true caspase inhibitors (Eckelman et al., 2006). Based on their frequent overexpression in many human malignancies and their central roles in diverse cancer-relevant signaling pathways, including caspase inhibition and NF-κB activation, members of this protein family emerged as promising targets for therapeutic intervention (Ziegler et al., 2008). While several members of this family, including Bruce, cIAP-1, cIAP-2 and XIAP are abundantly expressed in malignant glioma cell lines, survivin appears to be the only IAP protein that is overexpressed in GBM tumors, is linked to poor prognosis in patients (Ziegler et al., 2008) and plays pivotal roles in GBM cells' resistance towards radiotherapy likely by modulating DNA strand break repair, mitogenic and metabolic signaling (Ziegler et al., 2008).

Besides IAP and Bcl-2 family proteins as important mitochondrial and post-mitochondrial apoptosis modulators, Apaf-1 has also been implicated in GBM pathogenesis. Its precise role, however, is controversially discussed. *Apaf-1* localizes to chromosome 12q22-23, is frequently deleted by loss-of heterozygocity (LOH) and exhibits reduced mRNA and protein expression (Watanabe et al., 2003). Remarkably, Apaf-1 also shows frequent upregulation in GBM and medulloblastoma. Elevated protein levels of the caspase-9 activator account for increased sensitivity of tumor cells to cytochrome c-induced apoptosis (Johnson et al., 2007) pointing to heterogeneous and GBM tumor-specific Apaf-1 expression patterns and/or activity profiles.

Bcl2L12 Is Novel and Structurally Distinctive Member of the Bcl-2 Protein Family with IAP-Like Activities

The *Bcl2L12* gene localizes to chromosomal region 19q13 that together with other genomic 19q alterations is characteristic of GBM (Furnari et al., 2007). Detailed mRNA expression studies and in vitro oncogene cooperation assays of genes localizing to 19q13 including *Bcl2L12*, *IRF3*, *RRas*, *PPRG* and *FCTRG*, pointed distinctively to *Bcl2L12* as a gene with frequent and significant mRNA upregulation and potent transforming activity in vitro (Stegh et al., 2007). Subsequent expression analyses employing anti-Bcl2L12 immunohistochemistry on tissue microarrays (IHC-TMA) confirmed robust Bcl2L12 protein expression in 96% of primary GBM tumor specimens (Stegh et al., 2007).

Comprehensive homology analyses using different scoring matrices in pbalst searches (PAM30, PAM70, BLOSUM80), Pfam HMM database and Scansite queries identified a *C*-terminal Bcl-2 homology domain 2 (BH2) within the Bcl2L12 polypeptide with significant amino acid homology to the BH2 domains found in canonical Bcl-2 family proteins, most notably Bcl-2, Bcl-x_L or Mcl-1 (*e* values <0.05; Fig. 16.1). Strikingly, Bcl2L12 lacks additional BH domains and transmembrane motifs, and instead is characterized by six PxxP tetrapeptide and one proline-rich region with significant homology to corresponding motifs in well-described oncogenes, such as RRas (Scorilas et al., 2001; Stegh et al., 2007). The focally restricted homology to known Bcl-2 family proteins, the presence of a proline-rich region as a putative SH2/SH3 adapter and several phosphorylation sites for protein serine/threonine kinases (threonine117, serine121, threonine171, serine273) point to a mechanism of action at the intersection of cell death and mitogenic signaling.

Canonical anti-apoptotic Bcl-2 family proteins, such as Bcl-2 itself, rely on multiple BH and *C*-terminal hydrophobic membrane-spanning domains to exert their cytoprotective functions. In unstressed cells, Bcl-2 sequesters and inactivates the multi-BH domain containing, pro-apoptotic members Bax and Bak through heterodimer formation. Upon apoptosis induction and activation of BH3-only proteins (e.g. Bid, Bak or Bad) by transcriptional upregulation, limited proteolysis, or dephosphorylation, these apoptosis agonists translocate to mitochondria and displace Bax and Bak from an inhibitory Bax/Bak:Bcl-2 complex (Youle and Strasser, 2008). Here, a hydrophobic groove formed by the BH1, BH3 and BH4 domains of anti-apoptotic Bcl-2 binds the exposed BH3 domain of pro-death Bid, Bak or Bad. Such binding results in a conformational change in Bcl-2 provoking the release of Bax/Bak. Both proteins then oligomerize, insert into the outer mitochondrial membrane to induce MOMP, cytochrome c release and ultimately caspase activation (Youle and Strasser, 2008).

The lack of multiple BH domains and transmembrane motifs together with the presence of Bcl-2 atypical proline-rich motifs pointed to non-classical functions of Bcl2L12, which likely are independent of heterodimerization with Bcl-2-like death agonists and protection of mitochondrial membranes. Expectedly, subcellular fractionation and confocal immunohistochemistry studies of ectopic and endogenous Bcl2L12 proteins during apoptosis progression revealed predominant cytosolic and nucleoplasmic localization, without detectable constitutive or inducible association with intracellular membranes, including Golgi apparatus, endoplasmic reticulum, mitochondria and the nuclear envelope (Stegh et al., 2007).

Prompted by its distant, yet significant homology to Bcl-2 family proteins as master regulators of diverse cell death signaling pathways, cDNA complementation and RNAi-loss of-function studies revealed potent anti-apoptotic roles of Bcl2L12 in primary cortical astrocytes and transformed glioma cell lines. While ectopic expression of Bcl2L12 in murine cortical astrocytes null for the gliomagenic tumor suppressor *Ink4a/Arf* (Furnari et al., 2007) provoked profound resistance towards chemotherapy-, death receptor ligation- and DNA damage-induced apoptosis, RNAi-mediated knockdown of Bcl2L12 protein levels enhanced drug-induced apoptotic cell death (Stegh et al., 2007).

Bcl2L12 Is a Potent Inhibitor of Caspase-7 and Caspase-3 Downstream of Mitochondrial Membrane Disintegration

Reflecting its atypical domain structure and subcellular localization pattern, Bcl2L12 did not block cytochrome c release from the mitochondrial intermembrane space into the cytosol or the dissipation of the proton gradient across the inner mitochondrial membrane ($\Delta\Psi_M$) as two hallmark steps in mitochondrial membrane disintegration during apoptosis progression (Stegh et al., 2007). Forced Bcl2L12 expression also failed to inhibit cytochrome c-driven apoptosome assembly and subsequent caspase-9 activation, but potently inhibited the downstream maturation and activity of effector caspase 3 and 7 at the very distal end of the apoptosis signaling cascade (Stegh et al., 2007). A series of GST-pulldown,

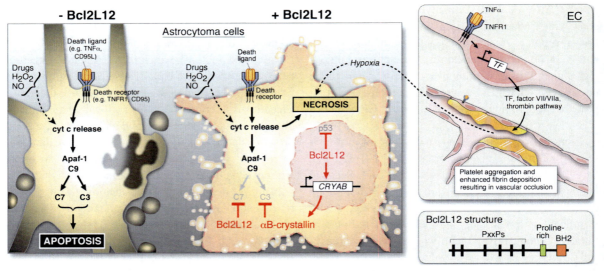

Fig. 16.1 Bcl2L12 is an anti-apoptoptic and pro-necrotic onco-protein in GBM. Upon apoptosis induction via death-receptors, chemotherapeutic drugs or as a consequence of an immune response executed by H_2O_2 or NO, astrocytoma cells undergo an apoptotic cell death ("-Bcl2L12", *left panel*): Cytochrome (cyt) c is released from the mitochondrial intermembrane space into the cytosol, where it acts in concert with Apaf-1 and dATP to activate caspase-9 (C9). C9 cleaves downstream effector caspases 3 and 7 (C3, C7) ultimately leading to chromatin condensation, DNA fragmentation, cellular shrinkage and formation of apoptotic bodies. In the presence of Bcl2L12 ("+Bcl2L12", *left panel*), effector caspase-3/7 activation is blocked. Mechanistically, Bcl2L12 can directly interact with and neutralize caspase-7 and up-regulates the small heat shock protein and caspase-3-specific inhibitor αB-crystallin to block caspase-3 activation/activity. Due to mitochondrial dysfunction provoking ATP depletion and a bioenergetic crisis, the cell death pathway deviates from apoptosis to necrosis. In parallel, other factors, such as TF-induced pro-coagulation initiated on endothelial cells (EC) and causing vaso-occlusion and hypoxia, contribute to necrogenesis of astrocytoma cells (upper *right panel*, "EC"). In addition, Bcl2L12 impacts the p53 tumor suppressor activity by preventing its binding to target gene promotes, thereby prominently inhibiting its transactivational activity. cyt c, cytochrome c; C9, caspase-9; C3, caspase-3; C7, caspase-7; TF, tissue factor; EC, endothelial cell; BH2, Bcl2 homology domain 2. Taken and modified from Stegh et al. (2008a)

co-immunoprecipitation and transcriptomic profiling studies provided detailed mechanistic insights into the IAP-like inhibitory activity of Bcl2L12: While direct and selective physical interaction with pro-caspase-7 matched well with Bcl2L12's ability to inhibit the proteolytic processing of the pro-enzyme into the catalytically active subunits (Stegh et al., 2007), transcriptional upregulation of the small heat shock protein and caspase-3-specific inhibitor αB-crystallin resulted in profound inhibition of caspase-3 (Stegh et al., 2008b). While caspase-3 plays essential and well documented roles in apoptosis propagation in various cells and tissues and is a crucial executioner of morphogenic cell death in the developing brain (Fig. 16.1; Stegh and Peter, 2001), caspase-7's role is less well defined, and involves prominent roles in signal propagation during IFN-β, cytotoxic drug- and Bcl-2/Bcl-x_L antisense-induced apoptosis in glioma cell lines (Furnari et al., 2007). In accord with these studies, RNAi-mediated knockdown of caspase-7 largely

phenocopied the effects of Bcl2L12 over-expression on cell death propagation in cortical astrocytes supporting the view that caspase-7 is a central apoptosis executioner in glial cells and that its inhibition represents an important aspect of Bcl2L12's gliomagenic activity profile (Stegh et al., 2007).

αB-Crystallin Is a Novel Gliomagenic Oncogene and Bcl2L12 Effector

Detailed analysis of the Bcl2L12 transcriptome in cortical astrocytes provided mechanistical insights into the caspase-3 inhibitory function of Bcl2L12. The small heat shock protein αB-crystallin exhibited robust, Bcl2L12-induced mRNA upregulation, while other heat shock proteins and postmitochondrial apoptosis signaling molecules, such as caspases, their activators (e.g. Apaf-1), or inhibitors (e.g.

IAPs, Bcl-2 family proteins) were not differentially expressed in control vs. Bcl2L12-transduced cultures (Stegh et al., 2008b). Correspondingly, human primary GBM tumors exhibited robust co-overexpression of Bcl2L12 and αB-crystallin and Bcl2L12-driven orthotopic glioma models displayed increased intratumoral αB-crystallin levels (Stegh et al., 2008b) further reinforcing a functional link between Bcl2L12 and αB-crystallin proteins. RNAi-loss of function and cDNA complementation studies revealed that αB-crystallin functions as a potent anti-apoptotic protein in glial through selective binding to and inhibition of caspase-3, but not caspase-7 (Stegh et al., 2008b). Finally, when ectopically expressed in glioma cells, αB-crystallin enhances the tumorigenic potential of intracranial glioma explants in vivo. These studies demonstrate the existence of a Bcl2L12-αB-crystallin signaling axis in glial cell in vitro and GBM tumors in vivo that connect the glioma oncogene and caspase-7 inhibitor Bcl2L12 with the small heat shock protein and caspase-3 inhibitor αB-crystallin (Stegh et al., 2008a; b).

αB-crystallin's functions as a molecular chaperone with potent cytoprotective effects against misfolded/denatured proteins. While its contribution to various pathological conditions, including myopathies, gliopathies and neurodegenerative conditions, has been well documented, its oncogenic functions, however, are only beginning to emerge. The study of the Bcl2L12-αB-crystallin interplay in GBM extends pervious cell and cancer biological studies that documented elevated expression of αB-crystallin in various cancer types (e.g. prostate cancer, oral squamous cell carcinomas, renal cell carcinomas and basal-like breast carcinomas) and attributed mitogenic, anti-apoptotic, invasive and angiogenic properties to the αB-crystallin oncoprotein (Arrigo et al., 2007). Consequently, αB-crystallin represents a novel and highly attractive target for pharmaceutical intervention in GBM, as it operates on key nodes of survival signaling important for tumor progression.

Bcl2L12 Inhibits the P53 Tumor Suppressor

While the above functional and biochemical studies of caspase-7 inhibition by Bcl2L12 provided insights into the activities of Bcl2L12 in the cytoplasm, the nuclear distribution pointed to a role of Bcl2L12 beyond cytoplasmic caspase inhibition, likely acting to modulate additional cancer-relevant pathways in the nucleus.

Deletion/mutation of the foremost nuclear tumor suppressor p53 is a common genetic event in primary GBM (The Cancer Genome Atlas Research Network, 2008; Zheng et al., 2008) and consequently, CNS-specific deletion of p53 in conjunction with genetic ablation of additional tumor suppressors, such as Pten and NF1, provoked an acute-onset, high grade glioma phenotype in mice (Alcantara Llaguno et al., 2009; Kwon et al., 2008; Zheng et al., 2008). The importance of p53 signaling for GBM development is further highlighted by the occurrence of astrocytoma in patients with Li-Fraunemi syndrome, a disorder characterized by p53 germline mutation. In addition, p53 pathway components are frequently altered in GBM tumors, most notably the Mdm family proteins and p53 antagonists Mdm2 and Mdm4 as well as $p14^{Arf}$ ($p19^{Arf}$ in mouse), which stabilizes p53 protein levels by blocking its proteosomal degradation (Harris and Levine 2005).

p53's prominent roles for GBM progression and the capacity of other Bcl-2 family proteins, such as Bcl-x_L, Bcl-2, Bax or Bak, to physically and functionally interact with the p53 tumor suppressor (Green and Kroemer 2009), prompted detailed oncogenomic and cell biological analyses of a potential Bcl2L12-p53 signaling axis. In silico analysis of the multidimensional TCGA dataset revealed higher levels of genomic amplification (non-focal 19q event) and consequently elevated mRNA levels of Bcl2L12 in tumors with an uncompromised p53 signalling pathway suggesting Bcl2L12 gain/overexpression represents an alternative genetic event to neutralize p53 (Stegh et al., 2010). In addition, Bcl2L12 prevents passage-induced senescence in mouse embryonic fibroblasts (Stegh et al., 2010) – a process that is attributed to a cellular stress-response mainly depending on a functional p53 pathway. In line with co-localization of Bcl2L12 and p53 in the nucleus of DNA-damaged cells, GST pull-down and immunoprecipitation assays with ectopic and endogenous proteins confirmed robust Bcl2L12-p53 complex formation that translates into potent inhibition of p53 transactivational potential by Bcl2L12 (Stegh et al., 2010; Fig. 16.1). Mechanistically, Bcl2L12 prevents p53 from binding to certain target gene promoters and consequently blocks p53's capacity to activate target genes governing cellular growth and apoptosis induction (Stegh et al., 2010). Thus, by virtue of its capacity to block caspase activation and p53's tumor suppressor activity, Bcl2L12 is a multi-functional modulator of key nodes of cytoplasmic and nuclear cell cycle and apoptosis signaling.

Necrosis Is a Trauma-Driven and Genetically Controlled Process in GBM

Sharply contrasting the ordered breakdown of the cellular scaffold during apoptosis, necrosis is characterized by early loss of plasma membrane integrity, subsequent cellular and organelle swelling and the release of intracellular content into the extracellular matrix provoking pronounced pro-inflammatory responses (Zong and Thompson, 2006). Recently, the concept of necrosis as a solely trauma-initiated process has been significantly expanded by the identification of genes that can actively regulate necrotic cell death. Consequently, "programmed necrosis" may represent yet another cell autonomous hallmark of cancer that by provoking an irreversible bioenergetic crisis triggers the release of oncogenic proteins into the extracellular matrix to stimulate proliferation, migration and invasion (Zong and Thompson, 2006). Necrotic cell death plays pivotal roles in GBM biology, as florid necrogenesis represents a pathobiological hallmark feature that distinguishes GBM from lower grade astrocytoma and negatively correlates with patient survival (Brat and Van Meir, 2004). Here, we will summarize our current understanding of necrosis signaling pathways, their modulation by Bcl2L12 and contributions to GBM pathogenesis.

Vascular Regression, Occlusion and Thrombosis Trigger Necrosis

Necrogenesis is a complex and multifactorial process that is instigated by vascular regression, as astrocytoma cells seeking access to surrounding blood vessels cause endothelial cells to undergo hypertrophy, discohesion and apoptosis. These processes are predominantly regulated by the Tie-2/angiopoietin-2 (Ang-2) receptor/ligand system that exhibits elevated expression in the vasculature of high, but not low-grade

astrocytomas (Brat and Van Meir 2004). Ang-2 is a Tie-2 antagonist that prevents receptor autophosphorylation and subsequent activation. Tie-2 inhibition causes endothelial cells to undergo apoptosis and/or structural changes and ultimately leads to vascular regression (Brat and Van Meir, 2004).

In addition, pro-thrombosis mechanisms are operative to further promote and sustain a hypoxic environment. Mechanistically, aberrant RTK activity in GBM tumors causes robust JunD/Ap-1-mediated upregulation of tissue factor (TF) (Brat and Van Meir, 2004). Upon binding to its activating ligand factor VII/VIIa in the plasma, TF promotes the conversion of pro-thrombin to thrombin causing platelet aggregation, fibrin deposition and ultimately occlusion of the blood vessel. Concomitant deregulation of the plasminogen activator or "fibrinolytic" system further amplifies TF-instigated thrombi formation and vascular occlusion: Reduced expression of the serine protease tissue-type plasminogen activator (tPA) with key functions in fibrin breakdown together with elevated levels of tPA inhibitor-1 (PAI-1) correlate with astrocytoma grade and patient survival (Brat and Van Meir, 2004). Caused by vessel regression and TF- and tPA/PAI-mediated vaso-occlusive processes, vascular dysfunction creates a hypoxic intratumoral microenvironment that provokes decline in nutrient and oxygen and consequently in intracellular ATP levels. In response, plasma membrane-bound ion pumps can no longer maintain cellular homeostasis resulting in disintegration, release of lysosomal enzyme and a local inflammatory response (Brat and Van Meir, 2004).

Compromised energy metabolism and the subsequent formation of intratumoral necrotic foci cause astrocytoma cells to move outwardly. These actively migrating cells form a hypercellular zone (pseudopallisades) around a central area of coagulative necrosis (Brat and Van Meir, 2004). On molecular levels, pseudopallisading cells are characterized by increased levels of hypoxia-inducible factor 1α (HIF-1α), a transcription factor that regulates cellular responses to low oxygen by regulation of a plethora of mitogenic, angiogenic, pro-migratory and invasive genes (referred to as hypoxia-responsive molecules, HRMs; for review see (Brat and Van Meir, 2004). HRMs, such as the receptor turosine kinases (RTKs) cMet and vascular endothelial growth factor receptor (VEGFR) together with elevated expression levels of metalloproteinases

MMP-2 and MMP-9 explain the soaring invasive and angiogenic potential of pseudopallisading cells that over time incorporate larger masses of tumor and non-tumor elements thereby expanding intratumoral necrotic areas (Brat and Van Meir, 2004).

Molecular Mechanisms of Programmed Necrosis

While degenerative processes in the tumor vasculature together with highly migratory and invasive pseudopallisades are instrumental for necrogenic processes in GBM tumors, this concept of trauma-driven necrosis has recently been expanded by the discovery of genetic events actively driving necrotic cell death. Similarly to unlimited proliferative capacity and resistance towards apoptosis, tumor cells acquire genetic aberrations that function to induce an irreversible bioenergetic crisis. In response, cells undergo necrosis and in the process release factors into the extracellular milieu, most notably high mobility group box 1 (HMGB1/amphoterin) and hepatoma-derived growth factor (HDGF) (Zong and Thompson, 2006) that trigger a plethora of pro-tumorigenic responses. HMGB1 binding to the Receptor for Advanced Glycation End products (RAGE) promotes proliferation, angiogenesis, invasion, metastasis and chemotherapy resistance. HDGF is overexpressed in many different cancer types and like HMGB1 exerts a plethora for tumorigenic functions, including invasion, metastasis and angiogenesis (Zong and Thompson, 2006).

While several signaling mechanisms have been shown to impact programmed necrosis, most importantly the inhibition of mitochondrial respiration through opening of the permeability transition (PT) pore, the cathepsin-mediated lysosomal pathway together with reactive oxygen species (ROS), Ca^{2+} and PARP signaling (Zong and Thompson, 2006), much attention focused on postmitochondrial cell death proteins as master regulators of the apoptosis/necrosis balance in tumor cells. Many laboratories established that post-mitochondrial caspase activation acts as a molecular switch between apoptotic and necrotic cell death. If caspase activation downstream of mitochondrial disintegration is blocked by genetically inactivating key components of the caspase signaling machinery, such as Apaf-1 or caspase-9, by

ATP depletion or pharmacological inhibition of caspase activity, apoptotic cell death execution is inhibited and cells undergo necrosis (Nicotera and Melino, 2004).

Mechanistically, mitochondrial membrane disintegration and extensive cytochrome c release in the absence of a functional caspase machinery result in decreased oxidative phosphorylation and intracellular ATP levels rendering cells unable to maintain ion homeostasis and provoking cellular edema, dissolution of organelles and plasma membranes (Nicotera and Melino, 2004). By blocking apoptosis signaling at the level of post-mitochondrial effector caspase activation and thereby redirecting the death program to necrosis, the molecular profile of caspase inhibitors, such as Bcl2L12 and IAPs, provides a rational explanation for a prime paradox in GBM – apoptosis resistance yet florid necrosis – and points to upregulation of postmitochondrial caspase inhibitors as a key progression event in malignant glioma (Fig. 16.1). Consequently, pharmacological inhibition of XIAP by the herbal anti-cancer compound embelin expectedly facilitated caspases activation and apoptosis execution and most importantly, reduced necrosis and inflammation in an experimental model of pancreatitis in vivo (Mareninova et al., 2006).

Similarly, upregulation of Bcl2L12 by grade IV astrocytoma cells may act in conjunction with necrosis-initiating vascular degeneration and local hypoxia-induced cell migration/invasion to promote intratumoral necrogenesis. While spontaneous apoptosis rates in GBM tumors are typically low, astrocytoma express high levels of death receptors, such CD95/Fas and DR5, that in conjunction with infiltrating immune-competent cells, such as microglia/macrophages and CD8-positive cytotoxic T cells create an apoptosis-prone environment that in the presence of caspase inhibitors propagate intratumoral necrotic cell death. In addition, Bcl2L12-driven necrotic cell death culminates in the release of HMBG1 (Stegh et al., 2007), which in turn may promote further tumor expansion via RAGE-mediated induction of proliferation, angiogenesis, metastasis and therapy-resistance. Thus, these studies support the interconnection of apoptosis and necrosis cell death paradigms downstream of mitochondrial membranes and open new avenues of therapeutic intervention at the level of Bcl2L12-driven, intertwined apoptosis/necrosis signaling pathways.

Conclusion and Future Perspectives: Roles of Bcl2L12 Beyond Caspase Inhibition

Advances in neurosurgery, radiation and conventional chemotherapy only marginally impacted GBM patients' survival; GBM as the most prevalent and malignant primary tumor of the CNS, remains a uniformly fatal disease. With a more detailed molecular and biological understanding of genetic abnormalities driving gliomagenesis, research has shifted towards the development of molecularly targeted therapies, especially those inhibiting the activity of RTKs, such as EGFR, the signature genetic aberration in GBM. Unfortunately, these and other single-targeted inhibitors have failed to demonstrate survival benefits as monotherapies, which is likely due to cytological, transcriptional and genotypic heterogeneity of GBM tumors, the existence of multiple parallel/compensatory (RTK) pathways and the deregulation of cell death signaling downstream of RTK activation. Key advances in the field of functional oncogenomics have begun to provide important clues underlying GBM's notorious therapy resistance. Among those was the identification and functional characterization of the novel GBM oncoprotein Bcl2L12 and its signaling surrogates that potently confer resistance to chemotherapy-induced apoptosis. Bcl2L12 is overexpressed in virtually all primary GBM samples, yet low or absent in low-grade disease and normal brain tissue. Extensive functional and biochemical studies have established that Bcl2L12 impacts various critical glioma signaling pathways as it potently inhibits effector caspase activation and p53 tumor suppressive function.

As one of several proof-of-principle studies, the characterization of this novel oncoprotein provided novel links between GBM tumor biology and phenotypes and will continue to mechanistically dissect additional gliomagenic signaling pathways impacted by Bcl2L12. In particular, future studies aim to explain Bcl2L12's role in mitogenic and possibly autophagic signaling and will assess the contribution of the proline-rich and phosphorylation motifs of the Bcl2L12 polypeptide to its overall pro-growth activities.

With the emergence of BTSCs as the putative GBM cell-of-origin, ongoing studies aim to assess Bcl2L12's role for BTSC biology, in particular its contribution to the therapy-resistant stem cell phenotype. BTSCs represent a small cell population embedded within GBM tissue that undergoes self-renewal in culture, forms diffusively invasive tumors in orthotopic transplants in vivo and can generate a diversified neuron and glia-like postmitotic progeny (Stiles and Rowitch, 2008). Importantly, the BTSC hypothesis may help explain why GBM are refractory towards extant chemo- and radiotherapies, as this cell population has a low mitotic index and may express a plethora of mitogenic and anti-apoptotic proteins, such as Bcl2L12, which render them resistant even towards targeted therapies, such as anti-RTK modalities (e.g. Tarceva, Iressa or Gleevec). Selective pressure and clonal expansion of those tumor-initiating cells with high levels of anti-apoptotic proteins may rationally explain the failures in treating GBM. Therefore, it will be important to unravel cell death mechanisms, in particular Bcl2L12-impacted signaling circuits, which will provide a mechanistic understanding of the therapy-refractory phenotype of GBM and may aid in therapeutically exploiting the biology of Bcl2L12 in cancer stem cells in the future.

References

Alcantara Llaguno S, Chen J, Kwon CH, Jackson EL, Li Y, Burns DK, Alvarez-Buylla A, Parada LF (2009) Malignant astrocytomas originate from neural stem/progenitor cells in a somatic tumor suppressor mouse model. Cancer Cell 15:45–56

Arrigo AP, Simon S, Gibert B, Kretz-Remy C, Nivon M, Czekalla A, Guillet D, Moulin M, Diaz-Latoud C, Vicart P (2007) Hsp27 (HspB1) and alphaB-crystallin (HspB5) as therapeutic targets. FEBS Lett 581:3665–3674

Brat DJ, Van Meir EG (2004) Vaso-occlusive and prothrombotic mechanisms associated with tumor hypoxia, necrosis, and accelerated growth in glioblastoma. Lab Invest 84:397–405

Cheng WC, Berman SB, Ivanovska I, Jonas EA, Lee SJ, Chen Y, Kaczmarek LK, Pineda F, Hardwick JM (2006) Mitochondrial factors with dual roles in death and survival. Oncogene 25:4697–4705

Corsini NS, Sancho-Martinez I, Laudenklos S, Glagow D, Kumar S, Letellier E, Koch P, Teodorczyk M, Kleber S, Klussmann S, Wiestler B, Brustle O, Mueller W, Gieffers C, Hill O, Thiemann M, Seedorf M, Gretz N, Sprengel R, Celikel T, Martin-Villalba A (2009) The death receptor CD95 activates adult neural stem cells for working memory formation and brain repair. Cell Stem Cell 5:178–190

Eckelman BP, Salvesen GS, Scott FL (2006) Human inhibitor of apoptosis proteins: why XIAP is the black sheep of the family. EMBO Rep 7:988–994

Furnari FB, Fenton T, Bachoo RM, Mukasa A, Stommel JM, Stegh A, Hahn WC, Ligon KL, Louis DN, Brennan C, Chin L, DePinho RA, Cavenee WK (2007) Malignant astrocytic glioma: genetics, biology, and paths to treatment. Genes Dev 21:2683–2710

Green DR, Kroemer G (2004) The pathophysiology of mitochondrial cell death. Science 305:626–629

Green DR, Kroemer G (2009) Cytoplasmic functions of the tumour suppressor p53. Nature 458:1127–1130

Hanahan D, Weinberg RA (2000) The hallmarks of cancer. Cell 100:57–70

Harris SL, Levine AJ (2005) The p53 pathway: positive and negative feedback loops. Oncogene 24:2899–2908

Hotchkiss RS, Strasser A, McDunn JE, Swanson PE (2009) Cell death. N Engl J Med 361:1570–1583

Johnson CE, Huang YY, Parrish AB, Smith MI, Vaughn AE, Zhang Q, Wright KM, Van Dyke T, Wechsler-Reya RJ, Kornbluth S, Deshmukh M (2007) Differential apaf-1 levels allow cytochrome c to induce apoptosis in brain tumors but not in normal neural tissues. Proc Natl Acad Sci USA 104:20820–20825

Kleber S, Sancho-Martinez I, Wiestler B, Beisel A, Gieffers C, Hill O, Thiemann M, Mueller W, Sykora J, Kuhn A, Schreglmann N, Letellier E, Zuliani C, Klussmann S, Teodorczyk M, Grone HJ, Ganten TM, Sultmann H, Tuttenberg J, von Deimling A, Regnier-Vigouroux A, Herold-Mende C, Martin-Villalba A (2008) Yes and PI3K bind CD95 to signal invasion of glioblastoma. Cancer Cell 13:235–248

Kwon CH, Zhao D, Chen J, Alcantara S, Li Y, Burns DK, Mason RP, Lee EY, Wu H, Parada LF (2008) Pten haploinsufficiency accelerates formation of high-grade astrocytomas. Cancer Res 68:3286–3294

Mareninova OA, Sung KF, Hong P, Lugea A, Pandol SJ, Gukovsky I, Gukovskaya AS (2006) Cell death in pancreatitis: caspases protect from necrotizing pancreatitis. J Biol Chem 281:3370–3381

Nicotera P, Melino G (2004) Regulation of the apoptosis-necrosis switch. Oncogene 23:2757–2765

Scorilas A, Kyriakopoulou L, Yousef GM, Ashworth LK, Kwamie A, Diamandis EP (2001) Molecular cloning, physical mapping, and expression analysis of a novel gene, BCL2L12, encoding a proline-rich protein with a highly conserved BH2 domain of the bcl-2 family. Genomics 72:217–221

Stegh AH, Brennan C, Mahoney JA, Folrloney KL, Jenq HT, Protopopov A, Chin L, DePinho RA (2010). Glioma Oncoprotein Bcl2L12 inhibits the p53 tumor suppressor. Genes Dev 24:2194–2204

Stegh AH, Chin L, Louis DN, DePinho RA (2008a) What drives intense apoptosis resistance and propensity for necrosis in glioblastoma? A role for Bcl2L12 as a multifunctional cell death regulator. Cell Cycle 7:2833–2839

Stegh AH, Kesari S, Mahoney JE, Jenq HT, Forloney KL, Protopopov A, Louis DN, Chin L, DePinho RA (2008b) Bcl2L12-mediated inhibition of effector caspase-3 and caspase-7 via distinct mechanisms in glioblastoma. Proc Natl Acad Sci USA 105:10703–10708

Stegh AH, Kim H, Bachoo RM, Forloney KL, Zhang J, Schulze H, Park K, Hannon GJ, Yuan J, Louis DN, DePinho RA, Chin L (2007) Bcl2L12 inhibits post-mitochondrial apoptosis signaling in glioblastoma. Genes Dev 21:98–111

Stegh AH, Peter ME (2001) Apoptosis and caspases. Cardiol Clin 19:13–29

Stiles CD, Rowitch DH (2008) Glioma stem cells: a midterm exam. Neuron 58:832–846

The Cancer Genome Atlas Research Network, (2008) Comprehensive genomic characterization defines human glioblastoma genes and core pathways. Nature 455:1061–1068

Watanabe T, Hirota Y, Arakawa Y, Fujisawa H, Tachibana O, Hasegawa M, Yamashita J, Hayashi Y (2003) Frequent LOH at chromosome 12q22-23 and apaf-1 inactivation in glioblastoma. Brain Pathol 13:431–439

Youle RJ, Strasser A (2008) The BCL-2 protein family: opposing activities that mediate cell death. Nat Rev Mol Cell Biol 9:47–59

Zheng H, Ying H, Yan H, Kimmelman AC, Hiller DJ, Chen AJ, Perry SR, Tonon G, Chu GC, Ding Z, Stommel JM, Dunn KL, Wiedemeyer R, You MJ, Brennan C, Wang YA, Ligon KL, Wong WH, Chin L, DePinho RA (2008) P53 and Pten control neural and glioma stem/progenitor cell renewal and differentiation. Nature 455:1129–1133

Ziegler DS, Kung AL, Kieran MW (2008) Anti-apoptosis mechanisms in malignant gliomas. J Clin Oncol 26:493–500

Zong WX, Thompson CB (2006) Necrotic death as a cell fate. Genes Dev 20:1–15

Chapter 17

Glioblastoma Multiforme: Role of Polycomb Group Proteins

Sabrina Facchino, Mohamed Abdouh, and Gilbert Bernier

Abstract Glioblastoma multiforme (GBM) is the most common and lethal primary brain tumor found in adult. Even with all the advances made in the field of cancer therapy for the last decade, the prognosis has not significantly changed, with a median survival of less than 1 year. Therefore, a better understanding of GBM biology is needed. Unraveling the basic mechanisms responsible for the initiation and progression of this tumor may open new fields for the development of efficient therapeutic strategies. Proteins of the polycomb (PcG) group family generally operate as transcription repressors and BMI1 is one of the best-characterized member. The implication of BMI1 in normal and cancerous stem cells survival, self-renewal and maintenance has been widely investigated. In most GBM, a relatively rare cell population, characterized as the tumor initiating cell population, expresses the stem cell marker CD133. In experimental systems, CD133-positive GBM cells are responsible for tumor initiation, maintenance, progression and resistance to chemo/radiotherapy. CD133-positive GBM "stem cells" thus possibly represent a valuable and specific cellular target to eradicate the tumor. Here, we report on the implication of BMI1 in GBM stem cell self-renewal and how BMI1 is indispensable for GBM tumor establishment and progression in a xenograft mouse model.

Keywords Glioblastoma multiforme · Glioma · Brain tumor · Cancer stem cell · Polycomb · BMI1 · Lentivirus · Small hairpin RNA · Mouse

Introduction

Glioblastoma multiforme (GBM) is the most common and lethal primary brain tumor occurring in adults. GBM can be classified into two families: primary and secondary. Primary GBM accounts for more than 90% of all GBM cases and is characterized by a rapid de novo development prior to symptomatic clinical features. In contrast, secondary GBM arises from the evolution of a recalcitrant low-grade astrocytoma (Louis et al., 2007; Maher et al., 2001). Despite significant progress in the treatment of cancers, the median survival of GBM-affected patients remains less than one year after diagnosis (Holland, 2001; Maher et al., 2001). The infiltrating nature of GBM tumors renders the surgical resection most difficult. Furthermore, the tumors are resistant to chemotherapies and radiotherapies. A better understanding of GBM biology will unravel the mechanisms underlying the initiation and progression of the cancer, and will open new gates for development of efficient therapeutic strategies.

The cancer stem cell hypothesis proposes the presence of a small population of cells within a tumor that shares common characteristics with normal stem cells, and the former is responsible for the origin and maintenance of the tumor. In experiment models, *cancer stem cells* should be sufficient for the formation of a secondary tumor when grafted into nude mice (Reya et al., 2001). In GBM, a subpopulation of cells expressing

G. Bernier (✉)
Department of Ophthalmology, Maisonneuve- Rosemont Hospital, University of Montreal, Montreal, QC H1T2M4, Canada
e-mail: gbernier.hmr@ssss.gouv.qc.ca

M.A. Hayat (ed.), *Tumors of the Central Nervous System, Volume 1*,
DOI 10.1007/978-94-007-0344-5_17, © Springer Science+Business Media B.V. 2011

the neural stem cell surface marker CD133 has been described and is considered as the tumor initiating cells (TICs) (Beier et al., 2007). Notably, Bao et al. (2006) demonstrated that the radioresistance of GBM tumor is procured by these cancer stem cells which express the CD133 marker through preferential activation of DNA damage response machinery. Therefore, an approach allowing to specially target these cancer stem cells is predicted to be an efficient treatment against GBM tumors.

Polycomb group (PcG) proteins are transcription regulators that act as repressors of gene expression through chromatin remodeling (Sparmann and van Lohuizen, 2006). PcG proteins form large multimeric complexes defined as *Polycomb Repressive Complex* (PRC) that are classically subdivided into two groups: PRC1 and PRC2 (Levine et al., 2002). PcG proteins of the PRC2 operate during early development and are essential regulators of embryonic stem cells maintenance. For example, EZH2, the core component of the PRC2, is required to prevent differentiation of embryonic stem cells by repressing the expression of transcription factors, such as Pax, Lhx, and Gata genes, implicated in organogenesis (Boyer et al., 2006; Sparmann and van Lohuizen, 2006). In contrast, PRC1 components appear to operate later during development and are important for the maintenance of the pool of adult stem cells. BMI1, a member of the PRC1 complex, is a key player in the self-renewal of hematopoietic and neuronal stem cells (Molofsky et al., 2003; Park et al., 2003). A large number of studies have also implicated PcG proteins in human cancers. *EZH2* is upregulated in lymphoma, prostate, and breast cancers (Kleer et al., 2003; Varambally et al., 2002; Visser et al., 2001), while *BMI1* is overexpressed in various human cancers, including medulloblastomas and neuroblastomas (Cui et al., 2006; Leung et al., 2004). In an experimental model, *Bmi1* was shown to be required for the self-renewal of leukemic stem cells (Lessard and Sauvageau, 2003; Park et al., 2003). We previously reported that BMI1 and EZH2 are both overexpressed in GBM tumors and enriched in tumor-initiating CD133+ stem cells. Inhibition of BMI1 or EZH2 expression in GBM cells cultured as neurospheres inhibited their growth and clonogenic potential. These observations correlated with depletion of the CD133+ cell population. Furthermore, BMI1 knockdown completely prevented brain tumor formation in mice. Thus, our work uncovered that PcG proteins are required in human GBM to sustain cancer-initiating stem cell renewal (Abdouh et al., 2009).

Methodology

Isolation and Culture of Primary GBM Cancer Stem Cells

Fresh GBM tumor samples were processed for cell culture within 1 h after reception. Tumors were washed and dissected into small pieces in DMEM/F12 medium. Necrotic tissues were extracted from the samples before mechanical dissociation. Obtained cell suspensions were passed trough a 40 μm filter mesh in order to remove any tissue debris. At this stage, we observe a bulk of red blood cell in our samples. To remove these cells, the samples were centrifuged using ficoll gradient (Ficoll-Paque™ PLUS, Amersham Biosciences). After centrifugation, cells were resuspended in neural stem cell medium. The medium is composed of DMEM/F12 medium (Invitrogen) containing 0.25% glucose, N2 and B27 supplements, Heparin (2 μg/ml; Sigma), Gentamycin (25 μg/ml; Invitrogen), human recombinant FGF2 (10 ng/ml; Peprotech), and human recombinant EGF (20 ng/ml; Sigma). The medium was changed once or twice a week to remove dead cells and the remaining red blood cells, if any. Subsequently, cultures were let to grow for several weeks until spherical colonies were observed (i.e., neurospheres). Formation of neurospheres is a main characteristic of neural stem cells. Obtained neurospheres can be maintained through several passages by incubating them in an enzyme free solution (Chemicon) at 37°C for 20 min, and mechanically dissociating them with a 20 G needle. After trituration, the single cell suspension was plated in the same culture medium as stated before. Finally, using an ultralow attachment plate (Corning) instead of a suspension plate will increase cancer stem cells (CD133+) proliferation and enrichment.

Polycomb Analysis

shRNA production: We have demonstrated by RNA and protein analyses that BMI1 and EZH2 are overexpressed in GBM and highly enriched in the cancer stem cell population (CD133+). To examine their function in GBM, we carried an efficient and stable knockdown of BMI1 and EZH2 by producing lentiviruses expressing different shRNA constructs. The basis of this technique relies on the defense mechanism of the cell against viral infection involving the RISK complex. At normal physiological level, the RISK complex can easily recognize viral double stranded RNA (dsRNA). Following the recognition phase, RISK will attach to the dsRNA, excise it, and then scan it for matches. When the RISK complex finds a match it will destroy it. shRNA sequence is made of two reverse complement oligonucleotides flanked by a loop sequence to produce the dsRNA. We designed different oligonucleotides that were complementary to regions in the ORF of BMI1 or EZH2. The PSICOLIGOMAKER program, from Jacks-lab, was used to predict the best target region in the ORF. The shRNA sequences were annealed to generate a double stranded shRNA and then were cloned downstream of the H1P promoter of the H1P-UbqC-HygroEGFP plasmid using Age1, Sma1, and Xba1 cloning sites (Ivanova et al., 2006).

Lentivirus production: The shRNA-expressing lentiviral plasmids were cotransfected with helper plasmids pCMVdR8.9 and pHCMV-G into 293FT packaging cells using Lipofectamin (Invitrogen) according to the manufacturer's instructions. Viral containing-media was collected at the second and the third day following post-transfection. The viral media was filtered and concentrated by ultracentrifugation. Viral titers were measured by serial dilution on 293T cells and followed by microscopic analysis for GFP fluorescence 48 h later. To improve viral transduction, lentiviruses were added to dissociated cells and incubated 1 h at 37°C in a final volume of 250 μl. Hygromycin selection (150 μg/ml) was added 48 h after infection.

Survival analysis: We analyzed the effect of BMI1 depletion on the self-renewal and survival of GBM cells. Self-renewal can be evaluated by different methods comprising cell expansion analysis through serial passages, colony formation (CFU), and differentiation. To measure cell expansion, we plated 1000 cells infected with control and experimental viruses. Thereafter, cells were counted and passaged every 2 weeks in order to follow cell expansion. We also investigated the ability of a single cell to form a colony using the colony formation assay (CFU). Preinfected

cells were dissociated to single cells in neural stem cell media and plated on a matrigel substrate, allowing them to adhere but not to differentiate. Cells were let to grow for 10 days and subsequently fixed and stained with cresyl violet. To examine spontaneous differentiation, preinfected cells were plated and cultured for 7 days on gelatin-coated chamber slides and analyzed for differentiation by immunofluorescence using antibodies against GFAP (astrocyte marker) and MAP2 (neuron marker). Cell survival was measured by comparing the percentage of apoptosis in control cells versus BMI1-depleted cells using Annexin-V staining and FACS analysis.

Stereotactic intracranial cell transplantation in NOD/SCID mice: Mice were handled in strict accordance with the Animal Care comity. GBM cells were dissociated and suspended in oxygenated HBSS. 3 μl of cell aliquots (15,000–100,000 cells per aliquot) were injected stereotactically into 60 days-old nonobese diabetic/severe combined immunodeficiency (NOD/SCID) mouse brain. Mice were anesthetized (Somnotol; 60 mg/kg), immobilized in a stereotactic frame, and the skull was drilled. The injection coordinates were 2 mm to the right of the midline, 2 mm posterior to the coronal suture and 3 mm deep. The scalp was closed using wound clips (Harvard). Animals were observed daily for development of neurological deficits.

Results

BMI1 and EZH2 Are Highly Expressed in GBM Tumors and Enriched in the CD133+ Cell Fraction

Immunohistological analysis of 5 archival paraffin-embedded and 4 newly surgically removed primary GBM tumors revealed high expression of BMI1 and EZH2 in tumor cells of all samples when compared to the surrounding normal brain tissue. We previously demonstrated that human astrocytes do not express BMI1 in vivo, in contrast with mouse astrocytes (Chatoo et al., 2009). Double-labeling analysis revealed that BMI1 is expressed in GFAP+ cells, thus showing BMI1 expression in transformed human astrocytes present in GBM tumors. BMI1 and EZH2 were also coexpressed with the stem cell markers CD133 and Nestin. Consistently, cultured GBM-derived neurospheres also expressed BMI1 and EZH2. Generated neurospheres could be maintained through serial passages; and while cultured in presence of serum, they could differentiate into neurons and astrocytes. Transcriptional analysis of GBM neurospheres by Real-time PCR revealed the expression of multiple neural stem cell markers such as CD133, SOX2, MUSASHI and LHX2. Thus, we can conclude that these cell culture conditions are optimal for the survival of cancer stem cells isolated from primary GBM samples. Most importantly, quantitative Real-time PCR analysis of CD133+ and CD133- cells isolated from GBM neurospheres using magnetic microbeads revealed that BMI1 and EZH2 are both highly enriched in the CD133+ fraction. Notably, high BMI1 expression could not be explained by gene amplification, since our analysis revealed that BMI1 is not amplified in these tumors. As control, gene amplification was observed for EGFr and PDGFr in most tumor samples.

BMI1 Knockdown Leads to the Depletion of CD133+ Cells

To address the function of BMI1 and EZH2 in GBM, we used lentiviruses to stably knockdown these proteins. A lentiviral construct encompassing an shRNA under the control of the U6 promoter and a fusion hygromycin/GFP protein under the control of the CMV promoter was used (Ivanova et al., 2006). BMI1 and EZH2 expression in GBM cells after infection and selection by hygromycin was evaluated by western blot and quantitative Real-time PCR analysis. In this study, two different lentiviruses were used to knockdown BMI1: shBMI1#1 and shBMI1#3, which deplete BMI1 to 95 and 50% respectively. A scramble construct (shScramble), which inefficiently targets BMI1, was used as a control.

Viruses were used to infect 3 independent GBM cell lines. To perform a colony-forming unit (CFU) assay, 1000 preinfected and selected cells were plated on matrigel in neural stem cell media and cultured for 2 weeks. GBM cells infected with the scramble virus produced large and dense adherent colonies, whereas BMI1 and EZH2 knockdown resulted in fewer, looser,

and smaller colonies. To evaluate self-renewal, we analyzed cells expansion through serial passages. We found that knockdown of BMI1 at 95% resulted in cells that were able to grow through serial passages, but at a slower pace than control cells (scramble). These results indicated a dose dependent response of GBM cells to BMI1 expression level.

Cells growth defect may results from increased apoptosis and/or cell differentiation. After knockdown of BMI1 in GBM cells, we found more apoptosis at different time points when compared to control cells. When plated on gelatin-coated slides, BMI1-depleted GBM neurospheres, in contrast to control neurospheres, displayed higher proportion of neurons and astrocytes, indicating an increased in cell differentiation. To better understand stem cell fate following BMI1 knockdown, we analyzed the expression of the stem cell genes CD133/PROMININ, MUSASHI, SOX2, and LHX2 by quantitative real-time PCR. BMI1 knockdown was accompanied by a drastic reduction in stem cell genes expression, suggesting depletion of the stem cell pool. Taking together, these results explained the cellular phenotypes we observed after BMI1 depletion in GBM cells.

BMI1 Is Required for Brain Tumor Formation

To delineate the role of BMI1 in tumor formation and growth in vivo, cells depleted of BMI1 or control cells were grafted by stereotactic injection in the brain of NOD/SCID mice. We previously demonstrated that in high cell density conditions, BMI1 knockdown had no effect on cell viability and CD133 expression, which allowed us to inject viable BMI1-depleted GBM cells in mice. Six to eight weeks after injection, control group animals started to develop neurological symptoms, and histological analysis of their brain showed the presence of typical hemorrhagic GBM tumors. Secondary neurosphere cultures could also be derived from these newly formed tumors. In contrast, mice grafted with BMI1-depleted GBM cells did not develop neurological symptoms and no evidence of tumor formation was found by histological analysis. Kaplan-Meyer survival curve demonstrated that control group mice died prematurely when compared to

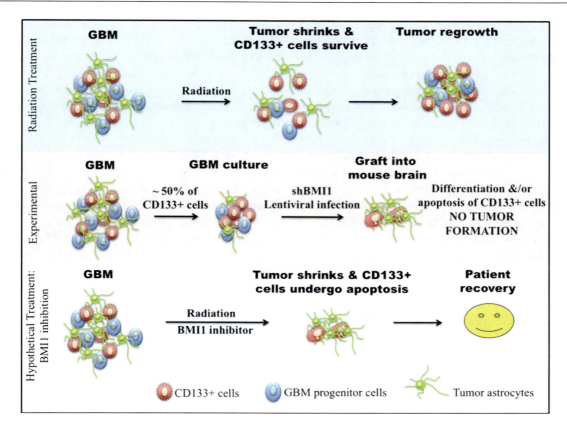

Fig. 17.1 Elimination of tumor initiating cells through inhibition of BMI1. In most GBM cases, tumor reappears after radiation therapy because resistant tumor initiating cells (CD133+) can survive the treatment. In an experimental model where BMI1 was depleted in vitro using the RNA interference technology, GBM cells cannot implant the brain of NOD/SCID mice owing to apoptosis induction and depletion of the CD133+ cell population. In a hypothetical therapeutic intervention where BMI1 activity could be inhibited using a pharmaceutical compound together with radiation therapy, it is predicted that specific destruction of the CD133+ cell population will lead to patient recovery and cure of the disease

naïve NOD/SCID, whereas mice injected with BMI1-depleted GBM cells exhibited a median survival comparable to that of normal NOD/SCID mice. These results demonstrated that BMI1 is required for GBM tumor formation in vivo (Fig. 17.1).

Discussion

BMI1 has been involved in several human malignancies (Lessard and Sauvageau, 2003; Bruggeman et al., 2007) and abnormal expression of BMI1 and EZH2 was found in multiple cancers. Our study demonstrated that BMI1 and EZH2 are robustly expressed in GBM tumors, enriched in CD133+ tumor-initiating cells, and essential for tumor cell growth. *BMI1* gene amplification has been identified in B-cell lymphoma;

however, no evidence of BMI1 amplification was found in GBM cell lines analyzed in this study (Abdouh et al., 2009; Bea et al., 2001). The mechanisms implicated in *BMI1* up-regulation in GBM may be attributed to the stemness state of GBM cells, since neuronal stem cells highly expressed BMI1 (Molofsky et al., 2003). Classical oncogenes overexpressed in GBM (such as *MYC* or *RAS*) and/or anti-oncogenes deleted or mutated in GBM (such as *P53*, *NF1* or *PTEN*) may also account for BMI1 upregulation. In this case, it is the transformed state of GBM cells that would influence BMI1 expression.

A gain-of-function activity of BMI1, attributed to its overexpression in GBM cells, may be required to confer new biological properties not usually found in normal cells. Indeed, we found that BMI1 knockdown enhanced the expression of a large group of HLA class

II molecules and to a lesser extent class I molecules. This is intriguing since GBM cells are known for their malignancy and invasion capacity, which implied their ability to evade from the immune system by down-regulating HLA molecules (Zagzag et al., 2005). This suggests that BMI1 may allow GBM tumor cells to bypass the host immune system through maintenance of a low immunogenic phenotype. Since it is known that neural stem cells exhibit a low immunogenic potential, in part because they do not express HLA molecules, BMI1 may thus confer GBM cells immune evasion either through direct repression of HLA genes expression or by preventing stem cell differentiation (Hori et al., 2003; Ubiali et al., 2007).

We have demonstrated that BMI1 knockdown induces an upregulation of genes involved in neurogenesis and gliogenesis, which is supported by our in vitro observations where BMI1 deple-tion increased neural and glial cell differentiation. BMI1 knockdown also leads to downregulation of *CD133/PROMININ* and *MUSASHI* expression. Collectively, our data suggested that BMI1 is required to maintain the undifferentiated state and self-renewal capacity of cancer initiating cells present in GBM tumors.

A meta-analysis performed with hundreds of independent GBM tumors recently showed that combined alterations of 3 major oncogenic path-ways is required for GBM tumor formation; ARF/MDM2/P53, P15^{INK4B}/P16^{INK4A}/P18^{INK4C}/RB, and RAS/PI(3)K/AKT pathways (CGAR, 2008). The main function of BMI1 is to repress the *INK4A/ARF* locus (which operates upstream of P53 and RB) and P53 activity (Chatoo et al., 2009; Jacobs et al., 1999). Moreover, it is important to note that the *INK4A/ARF* locus is deleted in $\geq$ 50% of GBM tumors and that *P53* is mutated in 35% of GBM tumors (CGAR, 2008). To identify possible new targets of BMI1 in GBM, we performed a gene expression profile analysis on two glioma cell lines having homozygous deletions of the *INK4A/ARF* locus. We found that *P21*^{Cip} transcripts were upregulated after BMI1 knockdown, and ChIP analysis confirmed direct binding of BMI1 to *P21*^{Cip} promoter regions. *P21*^{Cip} is also a direct positive target of P53, and P21^{Cip} inhibits cell growth and the RB pathway by blocking CDK4/CDK6 activity. BMI1 depletion also enhances *FOXOA3* and *P18*^{INK4C} expression, which are implicated in RAS/PI(3)K/AKT and P15^{INK4B}/P16^{INK4A}/P18^{INK4C}/RB pathways,

respectively. However, there is evidence that Bmi1 can also repress *p21*^{Cip1} expression in normal stem cells (Fasano et al., 2007), demonstrating that not all BMI1 activities ascribed here in GBM cells necessarily represent a gain-of-function. Our results provided a link between BMI1 and the 3 major pathways altered in GBM (Fig. 17.2).

Our data also revealed for the first time a direct involvement of EZH2 in human GBM. Because inhibitors of histone methyltransferase already exist and could represent a new therapeutic approach, more intensive investigations of EZH2 role in GBM tumors would be essential. Recently, a new cancer-specific polycomb complex (PRC4) containing EZH2, EED, SUZ12, and SIRT1 was identified in transformed cells lines. Notably, SIRT1 knockdown increases radio-sensitivity of CD133+ glioma cells (Chang et al., 2009). This raises the issue of whether EZH2 forms a complex with SIRT1 in GBM cells and/or whether increase PcG proteins expression levels in GBM leads to the formation of new molecular com-plexes having biochemical activities only found in cancer cells.

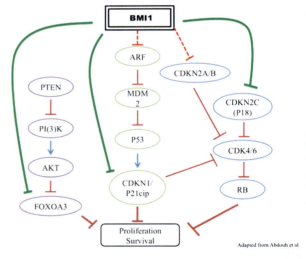

Fig. 17.2 BMI1 sustains tumor initiating cells renewal through inhibition of alternate tumor suppressor pathways. In most GBM cases (50%), the INK4A (CDKN2A/B)/ARF locus is deleted. Hence, BMI1 should not be required in these tumors since this locus is the main target of BMI1 activity. However, we found that BMI1 is still required for the survival of INK4A (CDKN2A/B)/ARF-null GBM cells. Experimental data from our laboratory suggest that BMI1 is also required in this context through inhibition of alternate tumor suppressor pathways that attempt to overcome P53 and RB inactivation and PI(3)K/AKT hyperactivity (adapted from Abdouh et al., 2009)

BMI1 or EZH2 depletion had a significant effect on GBM cell growth, but also on an astrocytoma grade III tumor sample. However, an oligodendroma tumor sample was resistant to BMI1 knockdown and was modestly affected by EZH2 depletion. Gliomas are histologically, immunohistochemically, and ultrastructurally classified as grade IV astrocytomas or oligodendromas (Maher et al., 2001). On the other hand, oligodendromas represent a distinct subtype of gliomas, probably due to a difference in the cell of origin when compared to astrocytoma and GBM. Polycomb dependency may be attributed to the astroglial nature of the cell of origin, which could explain the observed difference.

In conclusion, more evidences are pointing to the fact that brain malignancies may originate from NSC and contain cancer stem cells (Singh et al., 2003). Here we have demonstrated that BMI1 and EZH2, two PcG proteins, are highly expressed in CD133+ GBM stem cells and required to sustain their self-renewal. Polycomb proteins thus orchestrate important aspects of cancer stem cell biology and could represent prime molecular targets to cure GBM patients.

References

Abdouh M, Facchino S, Chatoo W, Balasingam V, Ferreira J, Bernier G (2009) BMI1 sustains human glioblastoma multiforme stem cell renewal. J Neurosci 29:8884–8896

Bao S, Wu Q, McLendon RE, Hao Y, Shi Q, Hjelmeland AB, Dewhirst MW, Bigner DD, Rich JN (2006) Glioma stem cells promote radioresistance by preferential activation of the DNA damage response. Nature 444:756–760

Bea S, Tort F, Pinyol M, Puig X, Hernandez L, Hernandez S, Fernandez PL, van Lohuizen M, Colomer D, Campo E (2001) BMI-1 gene amplification and overexpression in hematological malignancies occur mainly in mantle cell lymphomas. Cancer Res 61:2409–2412

Beier D, Hau P, Proescholdt M, Lohmeier A, Wischhusen J, Oefner PJ, Aigner L, Brawanski A, Bogdahn U, Beier CP (2007) CD133(+) and CD133(–) glioblastoma-derived cancer stem cells show differential growth characteristics and molecular profiles. Cancer Res 67:4010–4015

Boyer LA, Plath K, Zeitlinger J, Brambrink T, Medeiros LA, Lee TI, Levine SS, Wernig M, Tajonar A, Ray MK, Bell GW, Otte AP, Vidal M, Gifford DK, Young RA, Jaenisch R (2006) Polycomb complexes repress developmental regulators in murine embryonic stem cells. Nature 441:349–353

Bruggeman SW, Hulsman D, Tanger E, Buckle T, Blom M, Zevenhoven J, van Tellingen O, van Lohuizen M (2007) Bmi1 controls tumor development in an ink4a/arf-independent manner in a mouse model for glioma. Cancer Cell 12:328–341

CGAR. (2008) Comprehensive genomic characterization defines human glioblastoma genes and core pathways. Nature 455:1061–1068

Chang CJ, Hsu CC, Yung MC, Chen KY, Tzao C, Wu WF, Chou HY, Lee YY, Lu KH, Chiou SH, Ma HI (2009) Enhanced radiosensitivity and radiation-induced apoptosis in glioma CD133-positive cells by knockdown of SirT1 expression. Biochem Biophys Res Commun 380:236–242

Chatoo W, Abdouh M, David J, Champagne MP, Ferreira J, Rodier F, Bernier G (2009) The polycomb group gene bmi1 regulates antioxidant defenses in neurons by repressing p53 pro-oxidant activity. J Neurosci 29:529–542

Cui H, Ma J, Ding J, Li T, Alam G, Ding HF (2006) Bmi-1 regulates the differentiation and clonogenic self-renewal of I-type neuroblastoma cells in a concentration-dependent manner. J Biol Chem 281(45):34696–34704

Fasano CA, Dimos JT, Ivanova NB, Lowry N, Lemischka IR, Temple S (2007) ShRNA knockdown of bmi-1 reveals a critical role for p21-rb pathway in NSC self-renewal during development. Cell Stem Cell 1:87–99

Holland EC (2001) Gliomagenesis: genetic alterations and mouse models. Nat Rev Genet 2:120–129

Hori J, Ng TF, Shatos M, Klassen H, Streilein JW, Young MJ (2003) Neural progenitor cells lack immunogenicity and resist destruction as allografts. Stem Cells 21:405–416

Ivanova N, Dobrin R, Lu R, Kotenko I, Levorse J, DeCoste C, Schafer X, Lun Y, Lemischka IR (2006) Dissecting self-renewal in stem cells with RNA interference. Nature 442:533–538

Jacobs JJ, Kieboom K, Marino S, DePinho RA, van Lohuizen M (1999) The oncogene and polycomb-group gene bmi-1 regulates cell proliferation and senescence through the ink4a locus. Nature 397:164–168

Kleer CG, Cao Q, Varambally S, Shen R, Ota I, Tomlins SA, Ghosh D, Sewalt RG, Otte AP, Hayes DF, Sabel MS, Livant D, Weiss SJ, Rubin MA, Chinnaiyan AM (2003) EZH2 is a marker of aggressive breast cancer and promotes neoplastic transformation of breast epithelial cells. Proc Natl Acad Sci USA 100:11606–11611

Lessard J, Sauvageau G (2003) Bmi-1 determines the proliferative capacity of normal and leukaemic stem cells. Nature 423:255–260

Leung C, Lingbeek M, Shakhova O, Liu J, Tanger E, Saremaslani P, Van Lohuizen M, Marino S (2004) Bmi1 is essential for cerebellar development and is overexpressed in human medulloblastomas. Nature 428:337–341

Levine SS, Weiss A, Erdjument-Bromage H, Shao Z, Tempst P, Kingston RE (2002) The core of the polycomb repressive complex is compositionally and functionally conserved in flies and humans. Mol Cell Biol 22:6070–6078

Louis DN, Ohgaki H, Wiestler OD, Cavenee WK, Burger PC, Jouvet A, Scheithauer BW, Kleihues P (2007) The 2007 WHO classification of tumours of the central nervous system. Acta Neuropathol 114:97–109

Maher EA, Furnari FB, Bachoo RM, Rowitch DH, Louis DN, Cavenee WK, DePinho RA (2001) Malignant glioma: genetics and biology of a grave matter. Genes Dev 15:1311–1333

Molofsky AV, Pardal R, Iwashita T, Park IK, Clarke MF, Morrison SJ (2003) Bmi-1 dependence distinguishes neural stem cell self-renewal from progenitor proliferation. Nature 425:962–967

Park IK, Qian D, Kiel M, Becker MW, Pihalja M, Weissman IL, Morrison SJ, Clarke MF (2003) Bmi-1 is required for maintenance of adult self-renewing haematopoietic stem cells. Nature 423:302–305

Reya T, Morrison SJ, Clarke MF, Weissman IL (2001) Stem cells, cancer, and cancer stem cells. Nature 414:105–111

Singh SK, Clarke ID, Terasaki M, Bonn VE, Hawkins C, Squire J, Dirks PB (2003) Identification of a cancer stem cell in human brain tumors. Cancer Res 63:5821–5828

Sparmann A, van Lohuizen M (2006) Polycomb silencers control cell fate, development and cancer. Nat Rev Cancer 6:846–856

Ubiali F, Nava S, Nessi V, Frigerio S, Parati E, Bernasconi P, Mantegazza R, Baggi F (2007) Allorecognition of human neural stem cells by peripheral blood lymphocytes despite low expression of MHC molecules: role of TGF-beta in modulating proliferation. Int Immunol 19:1063–1074

Varambally S, Dhanasekaran SM, Zhou M, Barrette TR, Kumar-Sinha C, Sanda MG, Ghosh D, Pienta KJ, Sewalt RG, Otte AP, Rubin MA,, Chinnaiyan AM (2002) The polycomb group protein EZH2 is involved in progression of prostate cancer. Nature 419:624–629

Visser HP, Gunster MJ, Kluin-Nelemans HC, Manders EM, Raaphorst FM, Meijer CJ, Willemze R, Otte AP (2001) The polycomb group protein EZH2 is upregulated in proliferating, cultured human mantle cell lymphoma. Br J Haematol 112:950–958

Zagzag D, Salnikow K, Chiriboga L, Yee H, Lan L, Ali MA, Garcia R, Demaria S, Newcomb EW (2005) Downregulation of major histocompatibility complex antigens in invading glioma cells: stealth invasion of the brain. Lab Invest 85: 328–341

Chapter 18

Glioblastoma Multiforme: Role of Cell Cycle-Related Kinase Protein (Method)

Samuel S. Ng, Ying Li, William K.C. Cheung, Hsiang-Fu Kung, and Marie C. Lin

Abstract Glioblastoma multiforme (GBM), the most severe form of malignant brain tumor, is one of the deadliest cancers identified. Despite multimodal treatments with resection, chemotherapy, and radiotherapy, the prognosis of GBM remains poor over the past 30 years. Thus, the development of new and effective therapies is crucial. In this review, we discuss some alternative strategies for treating GBM by inhibiting the expression of cell cycle-related kinase (CCRK), a protein kinase which has recently been demonstrated to be a candidate oncogene in GBM.

Keywords Cell cycle-related kinase · Glioblastoma · siRNA

Introduction

Malignant gliomas are the most common and vicious type of primary brain tumor. In Europe and North America, the annual incidence is in the range of 2–3 cases per 100,000 individuals, accounting for ~30% of all intracranial neoplasms (Kanzawa 2003). They originate from poorly differentiated glia and are notorious for their high capacity of infiltrative growth. In its most severe manisfestation, glioblastoma multiforme (GBM; World Health Organization grade IV) (Louis et al., 2007), the median survival is just 12–15 months (Stupp et al., 2005). To date,

the standard treatment for GBM involves a combination of resection, chemotherapy and radiotherapy. Nevertheless, even with these multiple modalities, the prognosis has remained dismal for the past 30 years.

There are several reasons to explain why current therapies have limited benefit to GBM patients. First, GBM cells massively infiltrate the surrounding brain structures, making complete resection virtually impossible. Second, GBM is resistant to radiation. Third, penetration of chemotherapeutic agents into the tumor is limited by the blood – brain barrier in the brain. Therefore, the development of novel and effective therapeutic regimes is extremely important. In this review, we discuss some alternative methods for combating this devastating disease by the inhibition of cell cycle-related kinase (CCRK), a protein kinase which has recently been demonstrated to take part in GBM carcinogenesis (Ng et al., 2007).

Cell Cycle Regulation, Cell Cycle-Related Kinase, and Gliomagenesis

Most eukaryotic cell cycle transitions are controlled by various complexes formed between a CDK and a regulatory cyclin subunit. For full activation, CDK requires phosphorylation at a conserved threonine residue (e.g., Thr 160 in human CDK2) by another kinase known as a CDK-activating kinase (CAK) (Morgan, 1995). In mammals, CAK is a heterotrimeric complex consisting of CDK7, cyclin H, and a ring finger protein Mat 1 (Devault et al., 1995; Fisher and Morgan, 1994; Fisher et al., 1995). The CDK7/cyclin H/Mat 1 complex is also a subunit of the general transcription factor IIH (TFIIH), which phosphorylates the C-terminal

M.C. Lin (✉)
Brain Tumor Centre and Division of Neurosurgery, Department of Surgery, The Chinese University of Hong Kong, Shatin, Hong Kong, China
e-mail: mcllin@surgery.cuhk.edu.hk

M.A. Hayat (ed.), *Tumors of the Central Nervous System, Volume 1*,
DOI 10.1007/978-94-007-0344-5_18, © Springer Science+Business Media B.V. 2011

domain of the large subunit of RNA polymerase II (Akoulitchev and Reinberg, 1998; Roy et al., 1994; Shiekhattar et al., 1995).

Recently, CDKs, cyclins, and CDK-inhibitors have become major targets in GBM research. As such, hyperactivation of CDK4 (Burns et al., 1998), D-type cyclins (Buschges et al., 1999), as well as the loss of CDK-inhibitors such as p15 and p16 (Jen et al., 1994), have been implicated in gliomagenesis. Furthermore, it has been demonstrated that dysregulated CDKs and cyclins play an important role in the pathogenesis of GBM. For example, homologous deletion of the $p16^{INK4a}$ and $p14^{ARF}/p15^{INK4b}$ locus on chromosome 9p21.3 is a characteristic genetic abnormality that drives GBM carcinogenesis (Jen et al., 1994; Schmidt et al., 1994). This mutation simultaneously inactivates three tumor suppressor genes, namely the $p16^{INK4a}$ and $p15^{INK4b}$ CDK inhibitors and $p14^{ARF}$, which in turn regulates the activity of the p53 tumor suppressor (Lowe and Sherr, 2003; Ruas and Peters, 1998). Recently, two research groups have independently shown that deletion of $p18^{INK4c}$, another member of the INK4 family of CDK inhibitors, also leads to GBM (Solomon et al., 2008; Wiedemeyer et al., 2008). These data form the basis of developing various CDK or cell cycle inhibitors for GBM therapy.

Cell cycle-related kinase (CCRK) (also called p42 or PNQALRE) is a 42-kD protein kinase that shares 43% sequence identity with the CAK, CDK7 (Akoulitchev and Reinberg, 1998). CCRK has been reported to possess CAK activity by phosphorylating and activating CDK2, a major regulator of G1/S phase cell cycle transition (Liu et al., 2004). It is also a target for a specific chemical inhibitor of CDK protein family (RGB-286147) (Caligiuri et al., 2005). Cells lacking CCRK were incapable of growing and forming colonies in vitro, whereas cells with a reduced level of CCRK grew at significantly slower rates than control cells (Liu et al., 2004). Consistently, CCRK was identified as a suppressor of apoptosis in a large-scale siRNA screen (MacKeigan et al., 2005) and found to be essential for proliferation of cervical carcinoma HeLa cells, osteosarcoma U2OS cells, and colorectal carcinoma HCT116 cells (Liu et al., 2004; Wohlbold et al., 2006). Expression of CCRK protein has also been detected in different cancer cell lines, including cervical adenocarcinoma (HeLa cells), osteogenic sarcoma (U2OS cells), breast adenocarcinoma (MCF-7 cells), and prostate cancer (PC3 cells)

(Liu et al., 2004). These observations suggest that CCRK may possess oncogenic activity in various cancer types. Apart from its potential oncogenic functions, CCRK was found to be an activating kinase for male germ cell-associated protein kinase (MAK) and MAK-related kinase (MRK) (Fu et al., 2006). Moreover, a cardiac splice variant of CCRK was shown to promote cardiac cell growth and survival and was significantly downregulated in heart failure (Qiu et al., 2008), implying that CCRK is capable of performing multiple functions.

Recently, we have discovered that CCRK is a candidate oncogene in GBM. CCRK mRNA expression was elevated in 14 out of 19 (74%) of GBM patient samples as compared with normal brain tissue. Small interfering RNA (siRNA) suppression of CCRK inhibited the proliferation of two human GBM cell lines (U-373 and U-87), led to cell cycle arrest at the G1/S phase, and reduced phosphorylation of CDK2. In a subcutaneous nude mouse xenograft model, CCRK knockdown by short hairpin RNA (shRNA) suppressed the growth of GBM xenografts, whereas overexpression of CCRK conferred tumorigenicity to a non-tumorigenic U-138 GBM cell line (Ng et al., 2007). Collectively, these data have laid down the foundation for developing various anti-CCRK therapies for GBM.

Inhibition of Glioblastoma Growth Using siRNA or shRNA Targeting Cell Cycle-Related Kinase

In an attempt to suppress CCRK expression in GBM cells, we have designed two siRNA targeting human CCRK mRNA (siCCRK: 5'-GAAGGUGGCCCUAAGGCGG-3'; siCCRK2: 5'-GGCGGUUGGAGGACGGCUU-3'). We first transfected U-87 or U-373 human GBM cells with siCCRK (or siCCRK2; 200 nM) by Oligofectamine transfection reagent (Invitrogen) according to the manufacturer's instructions. In the control experiment, the cells were transfected with either an siRNA targeting firefly (*Photinus pyralis*) luciferase (siLuc; 5'-CGUACGCGGAAUACUUCGA-3') or Oligofectamine alone. To determine the effects of siCCRK and siCCRK2 on cell proliferation, cell number and viability were determined by trypan blue dye exclusion at 24, 48, and 72 hours after transfection. Both siCCRK and siCCRK2 were found to be effective in suppressing the growth of human GBM U-373 and U-87 cells in vitro. To examine the in vivo function of CCRK in GBM carcinogenesis, U-373 MG or U-87 MG cells (5×10^6 cells) were injected subcutaneously into the right flanks of nude mice that had been stably transfected an expression plasmid carrying shRNA targeting either CCRK (shCCRK; 5′-GAAGGTGGCCCTAAGGCGGTTGG AAGACG-3′) or luciferase (shLuc: 5′-GTGAA CATCACGTACGCGGAATACTTCGA-3′), and then the tumor volumes were measured weekly for 6 weeks. We found that stable transfection of shCCRK significantly reduced the volumes of both U-87 and U-373 xenografts, suggesting that CCRK knockdown is a potentially effective approach for GBM therapy (Ng et al., 2007).

To further examine the feasibility of treating GBM by CCRK suppression, we prepared

nanopolymer-DNA polyplexes consisting of high molecular weight 25kDa polyethylenimine (PEI) and a plasmid harboring shCCRK (PEI-25k-shCCRK). In nude mice subcutaneously xenografted with U-87 cells, repeated intratumoral injections of PEI-25k-shCCRK, but not the control PEI-shLuc or PEI alone, markedly reduced the tumor growth (Fig. 18.1), demonstrating the potential therapeutic value of suppressing CCRK in GBM gene therapy.

In conclusion, CCRK is a protein kinase which has recently been associated with human carcinogenesis. The observations showing that CCRK is expressed in different cancer cell lines and has tumorigenic activity in GBM suggest that it could be a bona fide oncogene. Although the molecular mechanism of CCRK-mediated oncogenesis has not been clarified, the recent discovery that CCRK can interact with cyclin H (Qiu et al., 2008) provides an important clue that it may, like CDK7, form a multimeric complex.

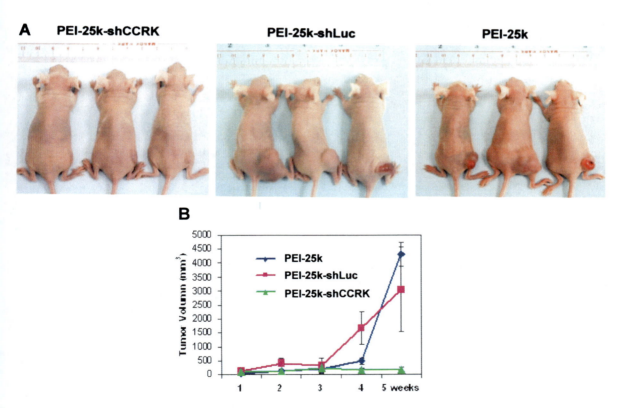

Fig. 18.1 Suppression of GBM tumor growth in vivo. (**a**) Nude mice were injected with U-87 cells at the right flanks subcutaneously. After the formation of tumor nodules, high molecular weight PEI (25kDa) mixed with shRNA targeting lucifierase (PEI-25k-Luc), PEI-25k alone, or PEI-25k-shCCRK was injected intratumorally twice a week. (**b**) Tumor volumes for PEI-25k, PEI-25k-shluc-, or PEI-25k-shCCRK-injected mice were calculated by the following formula: $V = 0.5 \times a \times b^2$, where a and b is the long and short diameters, respectively

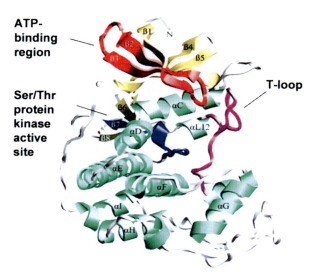

Fig. 18.2 The predicted 3D structure of human CCRK protein. The CCRK protein structure was constructed based on the crystal structure of human CDK2 protein (De Bondt et al., 1993). The amino acid sequence of CCRK was first aligned with CDK2 by T-coffee (Notredame et al., 2000) and then the pairwise alignment was manually refined and imported into SWISS-MODEL (http://swissmodel.expasy.org/). Using the program DeepView (Swiss-PdbViewer) (http://swissmodel.expasy.org/spdbv), the secondary structure of CCRK was obtained and it was further optimized by its built-in "Energy Minimisation" tool. The structure was stored in the SWISS-MODEL Repository (http://swissmodel.expasy.org/repository/smr.php?sptr_ac=Q8IZL9). According to this model, human CCRK protein consists of seven α-helices and eight β-strands. ProSite database analysis (http://www.expasy.org/prosite) indicated that it has a protein kinase domain (residues 4-288), with typical ATP-binding region and Ser/Thr protein kinase active site characteristic of CDKs. The ATP binding region (*red*), Ser/Thr protein kinase active site (*blue*), and T-loop (*pink*) are indicated

We hypothesize that this activated CCRK complex may in turn kick off the signalling cascade responsible for GBM carcinogenesis. With this in mind, discovery of small molecule CCRK inhibitors based on the predicted three-dimensional (3D) structure of CCRK protein (Fig. 18.2) as well as gene therapy regimes for delivering siRNA or shRNA targeting CCRK and/or its interacting partner(s) may serve as invaluable tools for blocking the carcinogenic pathway in GBM, and possibly, other cancers.

Acknowledgement The work was supported by the General Research Fund of the Research Grants Council of Hong Kong (773809 to S.S.N.).

References

Akoulitchev S, Reinberg D (1998) The molecular mechanism of mitotic inhibition of TFIIH is mediated by phosphorylation of CDK7. Genes Dev 12:3541–3550

Burns KL, Ueki K, Jhung SL, Koh J, Louis DN (1998) Molecular genetic correlates of p16, cdk4, and pRb immunohistochemistry in glioblastomas. J Neuropathol Exp Neurol 57:122–130

Buschges R, Weber RG, Actor B, Lichter P, Collins VP, Reifenberger G (1999) Amplification and expression of cyclin D genes (CCND1, CCND2 and CCND3) in human malignant gliomas. Brain Pathol 9:435–442

Caligiuri M, Becker F, Murthi K, Kaplan F, Dedier S, Kaufmann C, Machl A, Zybarth G, Richard J, Bockovich N, Kluge A, Kley N (2005) A proteome-wide CDK/CRK-specific kinase inhibitor promotes tumor cell death in the absence of cell cycle progression. Chem Biol 12: 1103–1115

De Bondt HL, Rosenblatt J, Jancarik J, Jones HD, Morgan DO, Kim SH (1993) Crystal structure of cyclin-dependent kinase 2. Nature 363:595–602

Devault A, Martinez AM, Fesquet D, Labbe JC, Morin N, Tassan JP, Nigg EA, Cavadore JC, Doree M (1995) MAT1 ('menage a trois') a new RING finger protein subunit stabilizing cyclin H-cdk7 complexes in starfish and xenopus CAK. EMBO J 14:5027–5036

Fisher RP, Morgan DO (1994) A novel cyclin associates with MO15/CDK7 to form the CDK-activating kinase. Cell 78:713–724

Fisher RP, Jin P, Chamberlin HM, Morgan DO (1995) Alternative mechanisms of CAK assembly require an assembly factor or an activating kinase. Cell 83:47–57

Fu Z, Larson KA, Chitta RK, Parker SA, Turk BE, Lawrence MW, Kaldis P, Galaktionov K, Cohn SM, Shabanowitz J, Hunt DF, Sturgill TW (2006) Identification of yin-yang regulators and a phosphorylation consensus for male germ cell-associated kinase (MAK)-related kinase. Mol Cell Biol 26:8639–8654

Jen J, Harper JW, Bigner SH, Bigner DD, Papadopoulos N, Markowitz S, Willson JK, Kinzler KW, Vogelstein B (1994) Deletion of p16 and p15 genes in brain tumors. Cancer Res 54:6353–6358

Kanzawa T, Ito H, Kondo Y, Kondo S (2003) Current and future gene therapy for malignant gliomas. J Biomed Biotechnol 2003:25–34

Liu Y, Wu C, Galaktionov K (2004) P42, a novel cyclin-dependent kinase-activating kinase in mammalian cells. J Biol Chem 279:4507–4514

Louis DN, Ohgaki H, Wiestler OD, Cavenee WK, Burger PC, Jouvet A, Scheithauer BW, Kleihues P (2007) The 2007 WHO classification of tumours of the central nervous system. Acta Neuropathol 114:97–109

Lowe SW, Sherr CJ (2003) Tumor suppression by ink4a-arf: progress and puzzles. Curr Opin Genet Dev 13: 77–83

MacKeigan JP, Murphy LO, Blenis J (2005) Sensitized RNAi screen of human kinases and phosphatases identifies new regulators of apoptosis and chemoresistance. Nat Cell Biol 7:591–600

Morgan DO (1995) Principles of CDK regulation. Nature 374:131–134

Ng SS, Cheung YT, An XM, Chen YC, Li M, Li GH, Cheung W, Sze J, Lai L, Peng Y, Xia HH, Wong BC, Leung SY, Xie D, He ML, Kung HF, Lin MC (2007) Cell cycle-related kinase: a novel candidate oncogene in human glioblastoma. J Natl Cancer Inst 99:936–948

Notredame C, Higgins D, Heringa J (2000) T-coffee: A novel method for multiple sequence alignments. J Mol Biol 302:205–217

Qiu H, Dai H, Jain K, Shah R, Hong C, Pain J, Tian B, Vatner DE, Vatner SF, Depre C (2008) Characterization of a novel cardiac isoform of the cell cycle-related kinase that is regulated during heart failure. J Biol Chem 283:22157–22165

Roy R, Adamczewski JP, Seroz T, Vermeulen W, Tassan JP, Schaeffer L, Nigg EA, Hoeijmakers JH, Egly JM (1994) The MO15 cell cycle kinase is associated with the TFIIH transcription-DNA repair factor. Cell 79:1093–1101

Ruas M, Peters G (1998) The p16INK4a/CDKN2A tumor suppressor and its relatives. Biochim Biophys Acta 1378:F115–F177

Schmidt EE, Ichimura K, Reifenberger G, Collins VP (1994) CDKN2 (p16/MTS1) gene deletion or cdk4 amplification occurs in the majority of glioblastomas. Cancer Res 54:6321–6324

Shiekhattar R, Mermelstein F, Fisher RP, Drapkin R, Dynlacht B, Wessling HC, Morgan DO, Reinberg D (1995) Cdk-activating kinase complex is a component of human transcription factor TFIIH. Nature 374:283–287

Solomon DA, Kim JS, Jenkins S, Ressom H, Huang M, Coppa N, Mabanta L, Bigner D, Yan H, Jean W, Waldman T (2008) Identification of p18^{INK4c} as a tumor suppressor gene in glioblastoma multiforme. Cancer Res 68:2564–2569

Stupp R, Mason WP, van den Bent MJ, Weller M, Fisher B, Taphoorn MJ, Belanger K, Brandes AA, Marosi C, Bogdahn U, Curschmann J, Janzer RC, Ludwin SK, Gorlia T, Allgeier A, Lacombe D, Cairncross JG, Eisenhauer E, Mirimanoff RO (2005) European organisation for research and treatment of cancer brain tumor and radiotherapy groups, and national cancer institute of Canada clinical trials group. Radiotherapy plus concomitant and adjuvant temozolomide for glioblastoma. N Engl J Med 352:987–996

Wiedemeyer R, Brennan C, Heffernan TP, Xiao Y, Mahoney J, Protopopov A, Zheng H, Bignell G, Furnari F, Cavenee WK, Hahn WC, Ichimura K, Collins VP, Chu GC, Stratton MR, Ligon KL, Futreal PA, Chin L (2008) Feedback circuit among INK4 tumor suppressors constrains human glioblastoma development. Cancer Cell 13:355–364

Wohlbold L, Larochelle S, Liao JC, Livshits G, Singer J, Shokat KM, Fisher RP (2006) The cyclin-dependent kinase (CDK) family member PNQALRE/CCRK supports cell proliferation but has no intrinsic CDK-activating kinase (CAK) activity. Cell Cycle 5:546–554

Chapter 19

Markers of Stem Cells in Gliomas

P. Dell'Albani, R. Pellitteri, E.M. Tricarichi, S. D'Antoni, A. Berretta, and M.V. Catania

Abstract Gliomas are the most common neoplasms of the Central Nervous System (CNS) and a frequent cause of mental impairment and death. Despite the improved responsiveness to primary therapy, survival of glioma patients is still very low. Therapies of malignant gliomas are often palliative because of their infiltrating nature and high recurrence. During the last decade, the concept that gliomas may arise from cancer stem cells (CSCs) has emerged. CSCs share with neural stem cells (NSCs) the capacity of cell renewal, multipotency and the expression of specific proteins, such as CD133 and nestin. This chapter describes similarities and differences between NSCs and CSCs, and summarizes the emerging knowledge on the possible role of stem cell markers as markers in gliomas, particularly in their tumoral grading. In addition, the importance of specific niches in maintaining pools of CSCs is considered. The involvement of signal transduction pathways, such as Notch, PDGF/PDGFR, Hedgehog-Gli1, and Bone morphogenetic protein and their implications in the control of CSCs function in gliomas are analyzed. Furthermore, certain proteins expressed in tumor migrating cells and possibly involved in recidive are evaluated.

Keywords Gliomas · Markers of cancer stem cells · Neural stem cells (NSCs) · Cancer stem cells (CSCs) · Side population cells (SP cells) · Signal transduction pathways

P. Dell'Albani (✉)
Department of Medicine, Italian National Research Council, Institute of Neurological Sciences, Section of Catania, Gaifami P., 18, 95126, Catania, Italy
e-mail: p.dellalbani@isn.cnr.it

Introduction

Gliomas represent the most frequent primary tumors of the Central Nervous System (CNS) and an important cause of mental impairment and death. Gliomas are histologically classified according to their hypothesized line of differentiation (e.g., astrocytes, oligodendrocytes, or ependymal cells), and are grouped into four clinical World Health Organization (WHO) grades according to their degree of malignancy. Gliomas of astrocytic origin (astrocytomas) are classified into pilocytic astrocytomas (Grade I), astrocytoma (Grade II), anaplastic astrocytoma (Grade III) and glioblastoma multiforme (GBM) (Grade IV). Tumors arising from oligodendrocytes include oligodendrogliomas (Grade II) and oligoastrocytomas (Grade III). Grade I tumors are biologically "benign", while grade II tumors are low-grade malignancies with long clinical courses. Grade III and IV are malignant gliomas and are lethal within a few years and 9–12 months, respectively. Furthermore, more than 50% of grade II gliomas transform into grade III and IV tumors within 5–10 years of diagnosis. Different therapeutic approaches are needed in each case. Even though, with the exception of grade I tumors, which are surgically curable if resectable at the time of diagnosis, all other grade gliomas are not curable with surgery because of their tendency to affect the cerebral hemispheres in a diffuse manner. Malignant gliomas are highly recurrent tumors even after surgery, chemotherapy, radiation, and immunotherapy. Ionizing radiation (IR) represents the most effective therapy for glioblastoma but radiotherapy remains only palliative because of radioresistance. The treatment strategies for gliomas have not changed appreciably for many years and most are based on a limited knowledge of the biology of the disease.

In the past most of the research on human brain tumors has been directed on the molecular and cellular analysis of the bulk tumor mass until during the last few years when it became clear that the tumor key cell is able to self-renew, proliferate, differentiate, and maintain the tumor mass. Essentially, in brain tumor two main cellular populations could be observed: the bulk of malignant cells, which are "cell death committed" cells, and a rare fraction of self renewing, multipotent and tumor initiating cells called cancer stem cells (CSCs). In 2003 Singh et al. published an article showing the identification of CSCs in human brain tumors, followed by another one relative to the identification of human brain tumor initiating cells (Singh et al., 2004). During the last 10 years numerous publications on CSCs appeared and this topic became the most fascinating subject of research in the tumor field. The majority of studies of brain CSCs have attempted to characterize and define the behaviour and the molecular mechanisms adopted by these cells to survive, proliferate, and repair any damage they can suffer escaping from apoptotic cell death. Brain tumor stem cells (BTSCs) resemble neural stem cells (NSCs) in terms of phenotype, signalling, and behaviour in vitro. Normal and CSCs share the expression of several markers, the ability for self-renewal and differentiation, and signalling pathways involved in the regulation of cellular survival and proliferation. Recently, a small population of stem cells, termed *Side Population* (SP), has been identified in several normal tissues and tumors. To develop anti-cancer and more specifically anti-CSCs therapies it will be important to analyze each piece of the puzzle "tumor". For this purpose the principal goal is the definition of specific protein markers that identify uniquely the CSCs versus NSCs to create a tumor targeted therapy. This chapter will discuss neural and cancer stem cell similarities and differences, the most accredited mechanisms of cancerogenesis and the emerging knowledge on markers of stem cells eligible as markers in gliomas, which in some instances could be correlated to the tumoral grading. The known strategies or methods to identify CSCs will be briefly mentioned. The importance of specific niches in maintaining pools of CSCs will also be discussed. The role of signalling pathways such as Notch, PDGF/PDGFR, Hedgehog-Gli1, and Bone morphogenetic protein and their implications in the control of CD133+ CSCs function in gliomas, will be discussed. Furthermore, certain proteins expressed in

tumor migrating cells and possibly involved in recidive will also be evaluated.

Neural and Cancer Stem Cells

Neural stem cells (NSCs) are the CNS tissue-specific stem cells. NSCs have self-renewal, proliferative capacities and multi-potentiality. In fact, NSCs are able to maintain the number of quiescent stem cells in a given brain region or to increase it in particular situations, and they are able to generate neurons, astrocytes, and oligodendrocytes (Gritti et al., 2002). During an early embryonic phase of development, NSCs divide symmetrically maintaining stemness and expanding the cellular population. In a second neurogenic phase, NSCs undergo asymmetric division, giving rise to new stem cells and to proliferating precursors belonging to the neuronal lineage. After this phase a glial progeny will develop with the progressive decline of stem cells, even though a small number of stem cells persists in specific regions of the adult brain, primarily in the subventricular zone (SVZ) of the forebrain lateral ventricles and in the dentate gyrus of the hippocampus.

In the past, tumor cells in the brain were hypothesized to derive mostly from the transformation of mature neural cells such as astrocytes, oligodendrocytes or neuronal precursors. Recently, this theory has changed because the concept of CSCs has been extended to brain tumors. To date, two models have been proposed to explain cellular cancer proliferation. In the classic *stocastic model* all the cells in a tumor have similar tumorigenic potential that is activated asynchronously and at a low frequency. In contrast, the *hierarchical model* proposes that only a rare subset of cells within the tumor have significant proliferation capacity and the ability to generate new tumors resembling the primary tumor, while the other tumor cells are terminally differentiated and committed to cell death. The hierarchical hypothesis correlates with the cancer-stem-cell theory now supported by accumulating experimental data showing that cancers, like normal organs, may be maintained by a hierarchical organization that includes stem cells, transient amplifying cells (precursor cells), and differentiated cells (Reya et al., 2001). Malignant gliomas contain both proliferating and differentiating cells, which express either neuronal or glial markers, and can be generated from both NSCs and glial lineage cells, such as oligodendrocyte precursor cells or astrocytes, which can behave as NSCs under appropriate conditions. These observations raise the possibility that they may contain multipotent neural-stem-cell (NSC)-like cells (Ignatova et al., 2002). Stem cells can be identified by the expression of specific markers, although they do not appear to be organ-specific. Normal stem cells and CSCs share the expression of several markers, the ability for self-renewal and differentiation, and signalling pathways involved in the regulation of cellular survival and proliferation. Furthermore, both show telomerase activity, resistance to apoptosis and increased membrane transporter activity.

Side Population Cells

Recently, a small population of stem cells, termed *Side Population* (SP), has been identified in several normal tissues and tumors on the basis of the ability to extrude fluorescent dyes, by the "flow cytometry-based side population technique" (Sing et al., 2003, 2004; Yuan et al., 2004). SP-stem cells have several fundamental properties: (1) they are generally very rare (~0.01–5% of total number of cells from tumors), (2) they rarely divide, even though they have an elevated proliferative potential, (3) they can self-renew. SP cells are capable of sustained expansion ex vivo and are able to generate, through asymmetric division, both SP and non-SP progeny (Hirschmann-Jax et al., 2004). SP cancer stem cells obtained from brain tumors form neurospheres, which have the capacity for self-renewal and are able to differentiate into phenotypically diverse populations including neuronal, astrocytic, and oligodendroglial cells when dissociated in single cell suspension. Recently, the presence of stem cell – enriched SP in long-term cultured human and rat glioma cell lines has been shown. SP stem cells demonstrate elevated chemoresistance. A recent report suggests that SP cells are heterogeneous with respect to the expression of drug transporter proteins belonging to adenosine triphosphate-binding cassette (ABC) superfamily, one of which is ABCG2 that is expressed in proliferating cells preferentially. SP cells also express high levels of the *ABCA3* transporter gene and have greater capacity to expel cytotoxic drugs,

such as mitoxantrone, resulting in better survival than non SP-cells. Thus, SP phenotype defines a class of CSCs with high resistance to chemotherapeutic agents that should be targeted during the treatment of malignant disease. These cells can undergo to asymmetrical division giving rise to ABCG2 positive (+) and negative (–) cancer cells. ABCG2+ cells have been identified as *tumor progenitor cells*, while among the ABCG2- cells both *primitive cancer stem cells*, which show high self-renewal, proliferative potential and high expression levels of "stemness" genes such as Notch-1, and *differentiated tumor cells*, which are partially or fully differentiated cells that constitute the bulk of tumor mass have been endowed.

Strategies for Cancer Stem Cells Identification

Since the identification and isolation of CSCs, the need to obtain a good number of these cells to study them both at cellular and molecular levels has becoming evident. Thus, it was important to find out specific methodologies to enrich and amplify CSCs from primary tumor tissue or even from tumor cell lines.

Four methods are available for the identification of CSC:

1. *Isolation of CSCs by Fluorescence Activated Cell Sorting (FACS) and Magnetic Cell Sorting (MACS) which use the presence of specific surface markers.*
   This method was used by Bonnet and Dick (1997) to isolate, from a patient affected by acute myeloid leukemia (AML), cells that were able to start leukaemia when transplanted in immuno-deficient mice. Now this method is adopted to isolate CSCs from various tumors such as breast cancer, malignant glioma, lung cancer, and others.
2. *Isolation of "Side Population" (SP cells) enriching CSCs.*
   This technique is based on the capability of some cells to extrude the fluorescent dye Hoechst 33342, which depends on the expression of an ATP – binding cassette (ABC) transporter on the surface of these cells. This technique is one of the most used method to select and identify CSCs from human cancers (such as glioma, neuroblastoma,

lung cancer). The SP method has a few disadvantages such as the high sensitivity to staining conditions (Hoechst concentration, cell concentration, staining time and staining temperature); furthermore, when the staining process is complete, the cells should be maintained at 4°C in order to inhibit further dye efflux. Another disadvantage is due to harvesting relatively small number of SP cells (0.01–0.05%). Moreover, Hoechst 33342 is cytotoxic because of its association with DNA, which determines the inhibition of DNA topoisomerase I causing DNA strand breaks; some researchers think that differences in clonogenicity and tumorogenicity between SP and non-SP cancer cells might depend on the Hoechst 33342 staining itself.

3. *Isolation of CSCs by using a serum-free medium that allows the formation of cellular aggregates called "tumorsferes"*

In 1992 Reynolds and Weiss published a method that allows the in vitro enrichment of NSCs in brain tissues. In this method, tissue is disrupted into single cells and cultured in the presence of epidermal growth factor (EGF) and basic fibroblast growth factor (bFGF) until the non-adherent cells form three-dimensional spheres that are enriched for NSCs. The same method has also been used for the isolation of CSCs from brain tumors and other malignancies.

4. *Isolation of CSCs by using their functional characteristics.*

Yu and Bian (2009) published an intriguing new method to isolate CSCs, which does not use any sorting based on stem cell markers, nor the Hoechst 33342 that could be toxic during SP-population selection. Four steps can be recognized, the first is based on the property that CSCs have to firmly adhere to extracellular matrix (ECM) while the bulk of committed tumor cells can be removed roughly; the second step is based on the higher chemotactic activity of CSCs versus tumor differentiated cells, the third step is based on the CSCs property of destructing and remodelling the ECM by which these cells can move earlier than committed cells; and the last step is to verify all the three important characteristics of CSCs: self-renewal, multipotency, and tumorigenicity. This method has recently appeared in the literature and needs to be further confirmed by other investigations. However, in addition to these methods, new protocols for the isolation and enrichment of CSCs based on their molecular functional characteristics are needed to study and understand their ability to escape pharmacological or ionizing radiation therapies, their infiltrating nature, and the possible role they have in angiogenesis and tumoral vascularisation.

Stem Cell Markers in Brain Tumors

As mentioned above in brain tumors two main cellular populations could be observed: (1) the bulk of malignant cells, which are "cell death committed" cells and (2) a rare fraction of self renewing multipotent and tumor initiating cells, the CSCs. The identification of protein markers that identify uniquely the CSCs versus NSCs is of paramount importance to create a tumor targeted therapy. Moreover, since from all published data the concept is emerging that a significant heterogeneity is evident within specific subtypes of solid tumors such as GBMs, it will be rational to develop specific molecular targeted drugs which could be personalized for individual tumors.

During this decade new important progress has been made in the recognition of possible markers of CSCs. Most important markers are: CD133, Nestin, Musashi, Sox-2 and CXCR4 as indicated in the summary presented in Fig. 19.1.

CD133

CD133 (prominin-1) was the first identified member of the prominin family of pentaspan membrane glycoproteins. It was identified in both human and mice and was originally classified as a marker of primitive haematopoietic stem cells and NSCs. CD133 is considered to be a marker for embryonic NSCs. In the early postnatal stage, CD133 is expressed in intermediate radial glial/ependymal cell types, while in the adult CNS it is present in a subset of NSCs (ependymal cells) and is down-regulated in normal differentiated cells (Kania et al., 2005). In spite of growing data present in literature, CD133 function is still not completely understood. Its restricted localization in membrane protrusions of epithelial and other cell types, in association with membrane cholesterol, suggests an involvement in the dynamic organization of membrane protrusions and in mechanisms such as migration

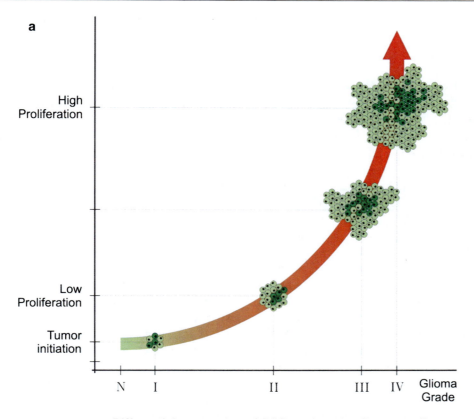

a

High Proliferation

Low Proliferation

Tumor initiation

N   I   II   III IV   Glioma Grade

b

Differential expression of CSC markers in glioma grading

	Grade I	Grade II	Grade III - IV
Cellular dedifferentiation Angiogenesis Brain infiltration	CD133- Nestin+ CXCR4+/-	CD133+/- Nestin+ CXCR4+	CD133+↑↑ Nestin+↑↑ CXCR4+↑
Proliferation	Musashi+ Ki67+/- Notch+ SOX-2+/-	Musashi+ Ki67+ Notch+ SOX-2+	Musashi+↑ Ki67+↑ Notch+↑ SOX-2+↑
Drug Transporters	ABCG2+/-	ABCG2+	ABCG2+↑ MDR-1+↑ MRP-1+↑
Apoptosis blockers			IAPs+↑ BCL-2↑ FLIP↑ BCL-XL↑
DNA repair	MGMT+/-	MGMT+	MGMT↑

Fig. 19.1 Scheme representing the differential expression of CSC markers in glioma grading. (**a**) Diagram showing glioma initiation and growth with a correlation among cell proliferation and tumor grading. (**b**) Summary of CSC markers expressed in the different gliomas grade related to prominent cellular functions altered in gliomas. The different proteins are grouped in cluster, which are related to specific cellular functions, but proteins position in a cluster is not stringent. (–) the negative sign is related to the absence or very low level expression of the protein; (+/–) is related to low levels of the protein; (+) the positive sign is related to the presence of the protein, while ↑ or ↑↑ is related to high or very high expression levels of the proteins

and interaction of stem cells with neighbouring cells and/or ECM.

CD133 also represents a marker of tumor – initiating cells. CD133 expression was investigated both at protein and mRNA levels in non-neoplastic brain tissue. No CD133 protein expression was observed in normal brain, while RT-PCR analysis displayed positivity in tumor samples. From these observations it was possible to hypothesize that there could be a potential post-translational down regulation of CD133 protein accompanying cell differentiation, while CD133 mRNA is constitutively transcribed even at very low levels in individual cells. CD133 expression pattern has been correlated with CSCs obtained from glioblastomas, but there are also experimental evidences of CD133+ cells in low grade tumors. Moreover, the number of CD133 cells quantitatively correlates with tumor grade indicating an involvement of these cells in glioma progression. CD133 cells have also the tendency to accumulate in dense clusters most of which have been found in highly vascularised regions of high grade gliomas; in parallel, NSCs have the tendency to accumulate in areas called "niches" within the SVZ during early cortical development. Because vascularisation is important to support tumor cell migration, it could be speculated that CD133 cells are present in strategic positions for tumor cell invasion, with single CD133 cells sporadically present within glioma tissue as the reminiscence of the invasive pathways.

In 2006, Liu et al. isolated two populations of CD133 positive (+) and negative (−) cells from primary culture of adult glioblastoma by FACS analysis. CD133+ cells exhibited stem cell properties in vitro and were able to initiate and drive tumor progression in vivo, strongly suggesting that CD133+ cells might be the brain tumor initiating cells. This notion has been challenged by studies demonstrating that glioblastoma CD133− cells have also properties of stem cells, even though, with lower proliferation index, and are tumorigenic when engrafted intra-cerebrally into nude mice (Beier et al., 2007). These data were confirmed by Wang et al. (2008), who observed that CD133− cells implanted in brain of nude mice gave rise to brain tumor demonstrating that CD133+ cells were not important for brain tumor initiation, but for tumor progression associated with increased angiogenesis and shorter survival. Thus, CD133 expression seems to be related to angiogenesis. CD133+ cells are strongly resistant to drugs and toxins because they express several ABC transporters and have active DNA repair capacity and resistance to apoptosis. Bao et al. (2006) demonstrated that CD133+ tumor cells isolated from both human glioma xenografts and primary patient glioblastoma specimens preferentially activate the DNA damage checkpoint in response to radiation, and repair radiation-induced DNA damage more effectively than CD133− tumor cells. Furthermore, these authors could reverse CD133+ glioma stem cells radioresistance by using a specific inhibitor of the Chk1 and Chk2 checkpoint kinases, and consequently hypothesized that CD133+ tumor cells represent the cellular population that confers glioma radioresistance and may be the source of tumor recurrence after radiation.

Other characteristics of CD133+ cells are derived from a gene expression analysis that revealed a higher expression of drug transporters BCRP1/ABCG2 and MGMT versus CD133− (Liu et al., 2006), but also higher levels of apoptosis suppressors such as Bcl-2, FLIP, BCL-XL and several inhibitor of apoptosis proteins (IAPs), such as (XIAP, cIAP1, cIAP2, NAIP and survivin) (Schimmer, 2004). IAPs bind and inhibit caspases 3, 7, and 9, preventing apoptosis, modulating cell division, cell cycle progression, and signal transduction pathways. Interestingly, CD133 expression is different in primary GBM and in recurrent GBM being significantly higher in recurrent GBM tissue obtained from patients as compared to their respective newly diagnosed tumors. In addition, it has been observed that CD133+ cells isolated from glioblastoma biopsies highly express the cell surface chemokine receptor CXCR4 (see below). From these data it appears that CD133+ CSCs may have importance not only in tumoral recurrence after chemo- and radio-therapies, but also in brain invasion. While this chapter was in preparation Lottaz et al. (2010) published an article that gives new insights into the possible sub-classification of GBM. These authors were able to distinguish two sub-groups of GBM by using a newly derived 24-gene signature: the type I CSC lines that display "proneural" signature genes and resemble fetal neural stem cell (fNSC) lines and type II CSC lines that show "mesenchymal" transcriptional profiles resembling adult NSC (aNSC) lines. The phenotype analysis of type I CSC lines evidenced that they express CD133 and grow as neurospheres, while type II CSC cells lack CD133 and display a (semi-) adherent growth. From these data and from an accurate molecular analysis of seventeen GBM CSC lines, authors hypothesize that GBM may derive from cells that have retained or acquired properties of either fNSC or aNSC, but that have lost the differentiation potential (Lottaz et al., 2010).

NESTIN

Nestin is a protein belonging to class VI of intermediate filaments (IFs), that is produced in stem/progenitor cells in the mammalian CNS during development (Zimmerman et al., 1994) and is a marker of proliferating and migrating cells. IFs are highly diverse intra-cytoplasmic proteins which show cell type specificity of expression. IFs are cytoskeleton constituents involved in various cellular functions such as the control of cell morphology, adhesion, proliferation, and cellular migration. Changes in the expression of IF proteins regulate remodelling of cell cytoskeleton during development. This is particularly evident in the CNS where IFs have sequential expression. Embryos in pre-implantation phase express cytokeratins (classes I and II). During embryogenesis, a developmental period characterized by tremendous cell migration, nestin (class VI) is coexpressed with vimentin (class III) in neuroephithelial and radial glial cells of the ventricular and the pial surfaces of the neural tube. When differentiation starts, cells leaving the cell cycle down-regulate nestin and subsequently up-regulate alternative IFs such as neurofilaments (NFs) (class IV) in committed neurons and glial fibrillary acid protein (GFAP) (class III) in glial precursors. In adult CNS, nestin expression persists in small populations of stem/progenitor cells of the SVZ and to a lesser extent in the choroid plexus even though several morphological types of nestin-positive cells (neuron-like, astrocyte-like, cells with smaller cell bodies and fewer processes) are detectable in different areas of forebrain of normal human adult brain. Moreover, nestin may be reexpressed in the adult organism under certain pathological conditions such as brain injury, ischemia, inflammation, and neoplastic transformation (Holmin et al., 1997). IF subtypes have been linked to enhanced motility and invasion in a number of different cancer subtypes. Nestin has been detected in brain tumors both of low grade, pilocytic astrocytomas, and of high grade, malignant gliomas including glioblastoma multiforme. Dahlstrand et al. (1992) showed high nestin expression in high malignant tumors, such as glioblastoma multiforme, when compared to less anaplastic glial tumors. Nestin expression in tumor cells may be related to their dedifferentiated status, enhanced cell motility, invasive potential, and increased malignancy. In addition, nestin has also been identified in the cell nucleus of tumor cell lines obtained from glioblastoma patients, suggesting that nuclear nestin may have a role in chromatin organization or may act as specific regulator of gene expression (Veselska et al., 2006). Further studies should be addressed regarding the relationship between nestin re-expression and tumor malignancy.

MUSASHI

Musashi is a conserved family of RNA-binding proteins. Its expression has been evolutionary conserved from nematodes to vertebrates. In mammals the MUSASHI family controls neural stem cell homeostasis, differentiation, and tumorigenesis by repressing translation of particular mRNAs. Musashi-1 is a member of the MUSASHI family in vertebrates, which is preferentially expressed in neural progenitor cells, including NSCs of the periventricular area and it is down-regulated during neurogenesis. Low levels of musashi are observed in periventricular neural stem/progenitor cells (ependymal cells and SVZ astrocytes) in the adult brain. Musashi-2 is a second gene belonging to the MUSASHI family, which was discovered by Sakakibara et al. (2001) through homology analysis. Musashi-1 and -2 cooperate to activate Notch signalling through repression of translation of the mRNA of the intracellular Notch signal repressor m-Numb, and to maintain the self-renewing ability of NSCs (Fig. 19.2). Elevated expression of musashi-1 (high mRNA and protein expression levels) has been reported in astrocytomas of different WHO grades and more specifically in grade IV, while in other tumors including melanomas and prostate cancer lower expression has been observed.

SOX-2

SOX (SRY-like HMG box) genes represent a family of transcriptional cofactors implicated in the control of diverse developmental processes. To date, more

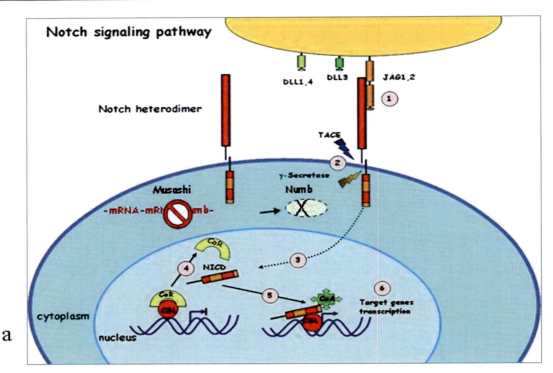

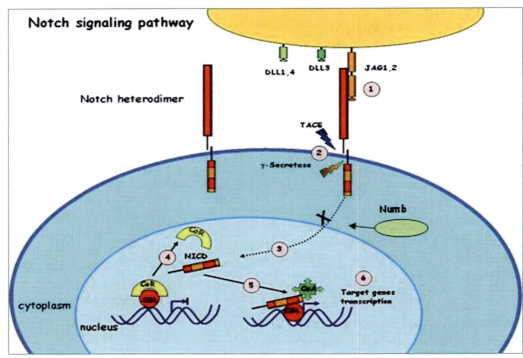

Fig. 19.2 Notch signalling is a ligand-receptor initiated pathway. The interaction between a ligand (DLL-1, -3,-4 and JAG-1, -2) (1) and Notch receptors triggers two successive cleavages (2), the first mediated by TACE (tumor necrosis factor-α-converting enzyme) and the second by γ-secretase, originating an intra-cytoplasmic fragment of Notch (NICD). NICD translocates to the nucleus (3) where it binds to the transcription factor CBF1/Su(H)/LAG1 (CSL). This interaction results in the displacement of the co-repressor (CoR) (4) and recruitment of the co-activator (CoA) (5) leading to transcriptional activation of target genes (6). Maintenance of activated signalling depends on positive or negative regulation through the action of Musashi (**a**) and Numb (**b**) respectively

than 20 SOX genes have been described in mammals and are divided into six distinct groups according to their HMG-box homology (Schepers et al., 2002). SOX genes exhibit highly dynamic expression patterns during embryogenesis. In early stages of mouse embryonic development SOX1-3 are highly expressed within the CNS and are down-regulated when neural cells are in the cell cycle and start to differentiate. SOX-2 has a role in growth and self-renewal of several stem cell types, both embryonic and adult. In fact, its activity is integrated in a complex network of transcription factors that influence both the pluripotency and differentiation of embryonic stem cell. In normal mouse brain SOX-2 is expressed in NSCs, early precursors and a few mature neurones. Recently, different research groups have shown the selective over-expression of SOX-2 in malignant gliomas both at mRNA and protein levels, whereas SOX-2 was not detectable in normal cortex (Gangemi et al., 2009).

CXCR4

Cancer cells obtained from glioblastoma biopsies highly express the cell surface chemokine receptor *CXCR4*. This chemokine in NSCs may have a significant role in directing NSC migration during CNS development. Interestingly, an over-expression of CXCR4 has been related to an highly invasive potential of gliomas (Ehtesham et al., 2006). Recent studies have analyzed the involvement of the CXCR4/CXCL12 signaling pathway to the proliferation, survival, and motility of a human GBM cell line (do Carmo et al., 2010). These authors demonstrated that CXCR4/CXCL12 axis determined an increase in cell proliferation and motility. Moreover, the blockage of CXCR4 induced a significant increase of apoptosis. These observations indicate that CXCR4/CXCL12 signalling pathway may contribute to the growth and invasive characteristic of GBM development. These data add new possible targets for improved glioma therapies.

Prognostic Roles of Cancer Stem Cell Markers in Glioma Grading

Numerous studies attempt to shed light on possible prognostic markers of CSCs in gliomas. *Nestin* could

be considered as a potential prognostic marker for GBM patients as highlighted by numerous experimental evidence. Immunohistochemical detection of nestin protein expression could be used as indicator of dedifferentiation and progression in astrocytomas. In this regard, it has been observed that low-grade astrocytomas contain low levels of nestin, while most high-grade gliomas express high levels of nestin with nestin-positive cells more abundant at the transition zone of the tumor. In addition to nestin, *musashi* expression was also investigated in low and high grade gliomas. Musashi-1 positive cells have been observed in a patch-like pattern in close proximity of tumor vessels; additionally, some musashi positive cells could be widely distributed within tumor parenchyma occasionally surrounding necrotic areas. Even though the expression pattern of *musashi* correlate with malignancy being high in glioblastoma, it is weaker than nestin in tumor cells of high grade gliomas, suggesting that these two proteins follow a differential pattern of expression. In fact, musashi expression, that is a marker of asymmetric cellular division may be stopped early, while nestin may be stopped late in the brain tumor stem cell dedifferentiation versus glioblastoma progression. Moreover, high level of nestin, but not musashi in brain cancer cells, indicates significantly shorter survival of glioma patients (Strojnik et al., 2007). Similar to nestin also CD133+ cells show a quantitative correlation with gliomas grade (low and high grade) and tissue distribution. In fact, CD133+ cells are present in cluster in surrounding tumor parenchyma and are frequently associated with tumor vessels. Nestin and CD133 expression may be considered an important feature of human gliomas. Low expression of these two markers significantly correlate with long survival of glioma patients. In addition to Nestin, CD133, musashi and SOX-2 have been shown to increase with increasing WHO grade. In conclusion, nestin and CD133 and other up-regulated markers may be potential indicators of biological aggressiveness of gliomas. Moreover, the presence of Ki67, a marker of cellular proliferation, together with CD133 could be considered independent prognostic factors of tumor recurrence and short survival. The ABCG2 drug transporter may also be used as a predictor for the outcome of glioma treatment. Enhanced expression of ABCG2 has been detected in human glioma tissue while low levels were found in normal brain. Furthermore, high-grade gliomas have the tendency to express higher levels of ABCG2 than low grade ones.

Cancer Stem Cell Markers Associated to Glioma Chemo- and Radio-Resistance

Despite the effort of biomedical research in the set-up of glioma therapies, the current treatments remain insufficient. From data present in literature it is known that the following two mechanisms are the main mechanisms by which cancer cells are able to survive and proliferate infiltrating surrounding tissue. The first mechanism is dependent on a *multidrug resistance* that is the result of over-expression of membrane proteins that pump-out from the tumoral cell anticancer agents decreasing the intracellular drug concentration; the second mechanism is the *resistance to apoptosis.*

Multidrug resistance (*MDR*) refers to the ability that cancer cells have to resist to a broad spectrum of structurally unrelated cytotoxic drugs that have different modes of action. MDR may be either intrinsic resistance (it could be established since the beginning of the chemotherapy) or acquired resistance (it could be acquired after the treatment period and could be determined by genetic mutations). MDR cancer phenotype could depend on the expression of drug transporters such as the over-expression of *adenosine triphosphate-binding cassette (ABC)* superfamily. This family consists of 48 human ABC genes that give rise to proteins known as ATP-dependent efflux pumps, which are able to translocate a range of substrate molecules, such as lipids and xenobiotic compounds across the cellular membranes using energy of ATP hydrolysis or forming membrane channels. ABC genes have been organized into seven subfamilies ranging from ABCA-ABCG, depending on their amino acid sequence and domain structure. ABCG2, also known as breast cancer resistance protein (BCRP), belongs to the ABC superfamily, and is a drug transporter that has been found to play an important role in conferring the MDR phenotype. ABCG2 is able to efflux > 20 different cytotoxic drugs such as mitoxantrone, daunorubicin, doxorubicin and topotecan (Doyle and Ross, 2003). ABCG2 has been detected in microvessel endothelial human brain and glioma cells, implicating an important role in both normal brain functions and glioma treatment. SP stem cells demonstrate elevated chemoresistance. Malignant SP cells export readily many cytotoxic drugs because of the high expression levels of drug-transporters such as MDR-1 (i.e., ABCB1 or P-glycoprotein), MRP-1 (ABCC1), ABCA2, ABCA3, and ABCG2. Moreover, the expression of the MRP-1 protein specifically has been verified in multiple human brain tumor types including astrocytomas, glioblastomas, meningiomas, neuroblastomas, and oligodendrogliomas. In addition to efflux pumps other defence mechanisms could be used by CSCs. Alkylating agents such as carmustine (BCNU) and temozolomide (TMZ) are drugs used for adjuvant glioma therapy. These and similar drugs act on cancer cells alkylating their DNA on specific bases and damaging surviving mechanisms.

CSCs appear to posses enhanced DNA repair capacity compared to other cells within the tumors. This capacity is dependent on the activity of the O^6-methylguanine-DNA-methyltransferase (*MGMT*) gene. MGMT gene encodes for an important DNA repair protein, which acts by removing alkylating products from the O6 position on guanine. The resulting alkylated MGMT, also called "suicide enzyme", is then marked for degradation by ubiquitinization. Physiological functioning of MGMT is important for maintaining cell integrity. Moreover, epigenetic silencing of the MGMT gene by methylation of the CpG islands of its promoter region has been demonstrated to determine loss of gene transcription and protein expression. Loss of MGMT expression will result in decreased DNA repair and retention of alkylated groups. The analysis of the MGMT expression level with immunohistochemistry, and the methylation status of its promoter could be used as valuable predictors for clinical response to alkylating agents. In fact, glioma patients lacking tumor MGMT expression have benefited from O^6-alkylating agent-based chemotherapy, meaning a prolonged survival compared to patients with MGMT-proficient tumors. Recently, Rivera et al. (2010) demonstrated that in GBM patients who received radiotherapy alone following resection, the methylation of MGMT promoter correlated with an improved response to radiotherapy, while unmethylated tumors demonstrated double progression during radiation treatment. Even the median time of interval between resection and tumor progression was approximately half that of methylated tumors. From these data authors suggest that MGMT promoter methylation could be a predictive biomarker of radiation response. Furthermore, because this biomarker has also been demonstrated to be predictive of response to alkylating agents, it could represent a general favourable prognostic factor in GBM.

Resistance to apoptosis is the main mechanism that is not mediated by efflux pumps, and it is known to depend on the activation of cellular anti-apoptotic defence. Recent data show that XIAP (X-linked inhibitor of apoptosis protein) is the most potent member of IAP gene family acting on caspase inhibition and apoptosis suppression. Moreover, XIAP is over-expressed in chemoresistant cancer cells (Zhang et al., 2008). It appears that chemo-and radio-resistance depends on diverse mechanisms that could act in concert or have a prominent role depending on the insult from which cancer cells would defend. New therapeutic approaches should target all sensitive proteins playing key roles in mechanisms of insults, repair and maintenance of CSCs survival and proliferation in order to obtain not only the reduction of tumor mass but the arrest of tumor growth and survival.

Brain Tumor Cell Niches

Recent data have provided evidence that stem cells of various tissues are present in protective niches. Stem cell niches are specialized microenvironments for normal stem cells. In adult mammalian brain, neurogenesis persists in two germinal areas, the subventricular zone (SVZ) of the forebrain lateral ventricles and the dentate gyrus of the hippocampus, where continuous postnatal neuronal production seems to be supported by NSCs. The central structural element of the neural stem cell niche is provided by capillaries within these areas. Stem cells reside in proximity of endothelial or other vascular cells facilitating communications among these cell types. Niches are not a simply repositories but also complex dynamic "places" that actively regulate the stem cell functions. Components and organization of the stem cell niches are different in various organisms and among tissues of the same organism and might include heterogeneous cell types, matrix glicoproteins, proteins secreted locally or distally that drive specific signals and specific-local metabolic conditions. Important functions of stem cell niches are the regulation of stem cell self-renewal and cell fate. Constitutive cells of niches provide a cell contact and secrete factors that essentially maintain stem cells in a quiescent status. The exact mix of secreted factors, that regulate NSCs, have not yet been determined, even though it is possible to indicate few possible factors or proteins such as the brain-derived neurotrophic factor (BDNF), the vascular endothelial growth factor C (VEGF-C) (Le Bras et al., 2006), the bone morphogenic proteins (BMPs) (Piccirillo and Vescovi, 2007) and the Pigment Epithelium-Derived Factor (PEDF) (Ramirez-Castillejo et al., 2006). It is important to note that in niches a bidirectional communication does exist among cells that constitute the niche and the stem cells. There is in fact in vitro evidence, showing the effects of NSCs on brain-derived endothelial cells which survive and form vascular tubes due to the secretion of VEGF and BDNF from NSCs. Thus, it is possible to hypothesize that diseased stem cell niches might contribute to tumorigenesis. In fact, recently published data have shown aberrant vascular niches in glioblastomas. A disorganized and excessive blood vessel formation is characteristic of glioblastoma. This feature could be explained by the fact that CSCs residing in diseased stem cell niches need a huge trophic support due to the rapid growth of tumoral cells. This observation is supported by reports that correlate the number of capillaries of glioblastoma with patient prognosis. Furthermore, there is evidence that CD133+ cells obtained from glioblastomas are able to form highly vascularized tumors in the brain of immuno-compromised mice. Like NSCs, glioblastoma stem cells appear to posses potent angiogenic activity and recruit vessels during tumorigenesis. Using multi-photon laser scanning microscopy it has been shown that CD133+/nestin+ cells within sections of human glioblastomas, oligo-dendrogliomas, medulloblastomas, and ependymomas are situated in close proximity of tumor capillaries. Moreover, a specific role has been assigned to endothelial cells present in neural niches; in fact, endothelial-derived factors have been shown to accelerate the initiation and growth of brain tumors. Despite the conspicuous number of studies in this field, numerous questions remain unanswered such as: Does the diseased stem cell niche drives the tumor development? Or do CSCs recruit other CSCs? How do cancer stem cells and their niches subvert the tight regulatory conditions that feature normal stem cell niches? Answering these questions will be of relevant interest, because with the disclosure of the pathologic strategies adopted by cancer stem cell niches, new therapeutic approaches could be adopted to stop aberrant tumoral growth.

Cancer Stem Cells and Invasiveness

In addition to the evaluation of niches, another important feature of tumor growth is the invasiveness. Despite the progress in early diagnosis of gliomas, surgery and radiation protocols, only 15% of gliomas patients who underwent radical surgery are still alive 2 years after diagnosis. This dismal prognosis is essentially due to the highly invasive nature of glioblastoma cells. Tumor cells that migrate into the surrounding brain parenchyma escape surgical resection and are the putative source of recurrent tumors. The invasion is triggered by several cell surface receptors including receptor tyrosine kinases (RTKs), G protein-coupled receptors (GPCRs), TGF- receptors, integrins, immunoglobulins, tumor necrosis factor (TNF) family, cytokine receptors, and protein tyrosine phosphatase receptors.

Local cell invasion involves the detachment from the original site, the attachment to extracellular matrix (ECM), the degradation of the ECM, and migration. In each step numerous proteins are involved. In detachment the down regulation of cell adhesion molecules is necessary, while the attachment to the extracellular matrix (ECM) is sustained by integrins. Furthermore, ECM should be remodelled through the action of several classes of proteases including matrix metalloproteinases (MMPs, e.g., MMP-2, MMP-9 and membrane-type MMP, MT-MMP), ADAMs (a disintegrin and metalloproteinase), plasmin, and cathepsins. Finally, last step of invasion is determined by cytoskeletal rearrangements and formation of lamellipodia and filopodia (Teodorczyk and Martin-Villaba, 2010). CSCs isolated from gliomas over-express a repertoire of molecules involved in infiltrating process such as CXC chemochine receptor 4 (CXCR4), CD44, vascular cell adhesion molecule-1 (VCAM-1) and integrins ($\alpha\nu\beta5$, $\alpha\nu\beta3$, $\alpha5\beta51$). Furthermore, there are experimental evidences that glioma stem cell over-express some proteins involved in destruction and remodelling of ECM such as matrix metalloproteinase -2 (MMP-2) and MMP-9. Analysis of spatial distribution of glioma cells under laser confocal microscopy performed by Yuan et al. (2004) showed an elevated proportion of CD133+ and nestin+ cells in the margin of the tumor. Moreover, numerous nestin+/Sox2+ glioma cells were observed to infiltrate into the surrounding normal brain tissue.

Notch, PDGF, Hedgehog-Gli1, and Bone Morphogenetic Protein Signalling Pathways Implications in Control of CD133+ CSC Function in Gliomas

Some of the signalling pathways that are involved in differentiation and proliferation of glial progenitors are altered in gliomas. The *Notch* family of transmembrane receptors comprise Notch-1, -2, -3 and -4. Mature Notch receptors are heterodimers derived from the cleavage of Notch pre-proteins into an extracellular and a trans-membrane subunits including the intracellular region. Mammalian Notch genes are widely expressed during embryonic development. Notch signalling is a ligand-receptor initiated pathway (Fig. 19.2). Maintenance of an activated Notch pathway is influenced by at least two factors, the negative regulator Numb, and the positive regulator Musashi-1. Numb negatively regulates Notch by promoting its ubiquitination and by interfering with nuclear translocation. The RNA-binding protein Musashi-1 increases Notch activity by inhibiting Numb translation by binding to its *cis*-acting repressor sequences in the 3'-untranslated region (Fig. 19.2).

Notch signalling activates a diverse repertoire of genes regulating different cellular functions, and it has been referred to as a *gatekeeper against differentiation*. In fact, Notch signalling blocks differentiation towards a primary differentiation fate in a cell, and instead directs the cell to a second alternative differentiation program or forces the cell to remain in an undifferentiated state. In the CNS, Notch is essential for the maintenance of the neural stem cell. Recently, Andreu-Agullò et al. (2009) have reported that treatment of NSCs with the *Pigment Epithelium-Derived Factor* (PEDF) enhances Notch-dependent transcription of the downstream effectors Hes1 and 5 of the HES family of basic helix-loop-helix transcription factors. Hes transcription factors negatively regulate the expression of pro-neurogenic genes, therefore Notch signalling enhances self-renewal by antagonizing differentiation, even though it can also regulate proliferation and survival. These authors suggest that PEDF maintains/induces the activity of CBF1 transcription factor in dividing NSCs, determining increased self-renewal and multi-differentiation potentials. In addition, the observation that *Egfr* promoter is a target of CBF1 has highlighted the involvement of Notch activation on proliferation. Moreover, because Hes1 and Hes5 block the execution of neurogenic programs, Notch signalling may act allowing the reversibility from the quiescent state of NSCs. Therefore, a coordinated expression of EGFR and Hes1 may determine stemness by promoting mitogenic response in a highly regulated quiescent population.

Studies performed in transgenic Notch activity-reporter (TNR) mice have demonstrated that high CBF1 activity discriminates stem cell from committed progenitors, while loss-of-function experiments have shown that down-regulation of Notch activity is necessary for the transition from radial glia/astroglia-like cells to committed progenitors (Mizutani et al., 2007). Furthermore, Notch promotes differentiation of various glial cell types (astrocytes, Müller glial cells, and radial glial cells). In addition to these functions, it has been shown that Notch activity prevents nestin degradation during stem cell differentiation (Mellodew et al., 2004). Recently, it has been observed that Notch-1 and its ligands are over-expressed in many glioma cell lines and primary human gliomas. In addition, the experimental knockdown of Notch-1 and its ligands determined apoptosis and inhibited proliferation of cultured glioma cell lines prolonging the survival in murine orthotopic brain tumor model (Purow et al., 2005). This evidence suggests that Notch-1 signalling might be critical for tumorigenesis and might represent an important target in the treatment of gliomas. Moreover, recent data suggest that Notch signalling promotes the formation of CSCs in gliomas.

Notch signalling can directly up-regulate nestin expression in gliomas and cooperate with KRAS to generate peri-ventricular lesions characterized by continued proliferation of stem cells in the SVZ. In addition, it has been observed that a constitutive activation of Notch signalling in glioma cell lines promotes growth and increases the formation of neurosphere-like colonies in the presence of growth factors. Moreover, it has been observed that in medulloblastoma cell cultures a blockade of Notch signalling through inhibition of γ-secretase drastically reduces the number of CD133+ cells, totally abolishes the SP cells, and inhibits the ability of forming tumors in vivo. These data suggest that the loss of tumor forming capacity could be due to the depletion of stem-like cells (Fan et al., 2006). Accordingly, Hes1 mRNA, a marker of Notch pathway activity, is substantially up-regulated in the CD133-enriched fraction of medulloblastoma cell line cultures. This confirms that Notch signalling is especially active in stem-like cancer cells and supports the possibility that Notch pathway inhibition may target this population.

PDGF was originally identified in platelets and in serum as a mitogen for fibroblasts, smooth muscle cells (SMC), and glial cells in culture. To date, four PDGF ligands PDGFA-D are known. The four PDGF polypeptide chains form five dimeric PDGF isoforms: PDGF-AA, -AB, -BB, -CC, and -DD. PDGF isoforms exert their cellular effects through tyrosine kinase α- (PDGFR-α) and β- (PDGFR-β) receptors. During embryogenesis, glial and neuronal progenitors express the PDGFR-α, whereas neurons and astrocytes express PDGF. The PDGFR-α is constantly expressed during differentiation of neural stem cells, but is phosphorylated only after PDGF-AA treatment, while the PDGFR-β is very low or not detectable in uncommitted cells, but its expression increases with differentiation. During the post-natal period, as glial progenitors differentiate into oligodendrocytes, PDGFR-α expression is down-regulated. In adult brain, PDGFR-α is present in the ventricular and sub-ventricular zone of the lateral ventricles possibly restricted to neural stem cells, whereas PDGF is widely expressed by neurons and astrocytes.

Ablation of the PDGFR-α in a subpopulation of post-natal neural stem cells shows that this receptor is required for oligodendrogenesis, but not for neurogenesis. Interestingly, the infusion of PDGF-AA alone into mice SVZ arrests neuroblast production and induces SVZ B cell proliferation contributing to the generation of large hyperplasias with some features of gliomas (Jackson et al., 2006). Thus, activation of PDGF signalling in SVZ B stem cells might represent an event contributing to initiate tumorigenesis. Numerous studies have demonstrated coexpression of the PDGF-A, PDGF-B, and of the PDGFRs in glioblastomas, suggesting that both autocrine and paracrine stimulation could play an important role in glial tumorigenesis. Lokker et al. (2002) observed a decrease in cellular survival and proliferation of glioma cell lines by blocking the PDGF autocrine signalling, providing evidence for a critical role of the autocrine loop in maintaining cell transformation. Furthermore, amplification of the PDGFR-α gene has been observed in low grade and in a subset of high-grade gliomas. In neural progenitors and in more mature astrocytes of newborn mice the overexpression of the PDGFR-β determines the formation of oligodendrogliomas and oligoastrogliomas, respectively. Data present in literature on PDGF/PDGFRs expression in gliomas show how important it is to understand the diverse molecular events that play a role in PDGF/PDGFRs expression, signalling activation, and cellular responses in gliomagenesis.

HedgeHog (HH)-GLI signaling also has a role in gliomas. SONIC HH (SHH) activates a signal transduction cascade with the involvement of membrane proteins such as PATCHED1 (PTCH1) and SMOOTHENED (SMOH), leading to the action of GLI transcription factors. Recently, Clement et al. (2007) demonstrated that human gliomas and their CSCs require HH-GLI pathway activity for proliferation, survival, self-renewal, and tumorigenicity. These authors showed that in human gliomas (grade III) HH-GLI signaling regulated the expression of stemness genes, such as *NANOG, OCT4, SOX,* and *BMI1* and the self-renewal of CD133+ glioma CSCs. The stemness signature observed in grade III could be extended to grade IV (GBM) and grade II tumors, even though with lower expression levels. The high stemness signature observed in grade III gliomas has been related to abundance of CSCs. The decreased levels in GBMs could be due to the increased number of more differentiated tumor-derived cells, to increased participation of non-tumor cells and to increased angiogenesis. Moreover, in GBMs with expressing SHH new vessels, angiogenesis provides not only the nutrients to the tumor, but also determines its growth and CSCs self-renewal. The involvement of HH-GLI signalling in the regulation of proliferation of normal brain and cancer stem cells has also been proved by the experimental use of cyclopamine, a specific SMOH inhibitor. Adherent primary cultures of gliomas treated with cyclopamine showed decreased cell proliferation. The cyclopamine treatment resulted in a decreased *GLI1* expression and complete cell death after 10 days of treatment. Interestingly, when the drug treatment was interrupted a culture recovery was observed, indicating temporally distinct cytostatic and cytotoxic effects. The authors have hypothesized that cyclopamine treatment could spare normal quiescent stem cells in their niches, and thus would allow the regeneration of normal adult tissues after cessation of treatment, offering new therapeutic prospectives.

Bone morphogenetic proteins (BMPs) are multifunctional growth factors that belong to the transforming growth factor beta (TGF-beta) superfamily. The roles of BMPs in embryonic development and cellular functions in postnatal and adult animals have been extensively studied in recent years. Signal transduction studies have revealed that the canonical proteins, Smad1, 5 and 8 are the immediate downstream molecules of the BMP receptors, playing a central role in BMP signal transduction (Chen and Panchision, 2007). Studies from transgenic and knockout mice for BMPs and related genes have shown that BMP signaling plays a critical role in heart, neural, and cartilage development. BMPs are well characterized inducers of CNS stem cell differentiation, astroglial fate, mitotic arrest, and apoptosis. In adult brain, BMPs play an instructive role in the stem cell niche, where the interaction of these proteins and their inhibitor Noggin regulates the acquisition of an astroglial phenotype in the stem cell progeny. BMP activities are regulated at different molecular levels. In addition to their physiologic roles, it has been observed that some BMPs are implicated in the development of several cancers. Recent data show that BMP4, a protein belonging to the BMPs family, strongly activates BMP receptors (BMPRs), triggering Smad signalling cascade in cells isolated from human GBMs. BMP4 treatment determined a decreased proliferation and an increased expression of differentiated neural markers, with no effect on cell viability. BMP4 treatment resulted in a reduced clonogenic ability (>70%), both in the size of the CD133+ side population (~50%) and in the growth kinetics of GBM cells, indicating that it is able to gain a reduction of the CSC pool. Moreover, human GBM cells transiently exposed to BMP4 were no more able to establish intracerebral GBMs when implanted in cerebral hemispheres of nude mice. Based on these data it has been hypotesized that the transient exposure to BMP4 depletes the brain tumor initiating cancer population and produces a significant decrease in the in vivo tumor-initiating ability of GBM cells (Piccirillo and Vescovi, 2007). These observations prompted the authors to hypothesize that BMP4, induces differentiation of the tumor-initiating cells rather than killing them; it could be used after surgery to block new GBM development. However, more experiments need to be done to better understand this mechanism and try to set a therapeutic approach.

Conclusion

In the past, most of the research on human brain tumors has been directed to the bulk of tumor mass, while only recently the attention of researchers is focused on tumor key cells, the CSCs. CSCs represent a small subset of cells within the tumor mass able to self-renew and proliferate, which are responsible of both the initiation of primary disease and of its recurrence. Considering that cancer initiation and progression is a multi-step process involving numerous cellular mechanisms, including altered gene expression, signal transduction pathway activation and/or inhibition and secretion of growth factors, new therapeutic protocols should take into account all these variables. The definition of a panel of CSC markers has a relevant interest for several reasons: CSC markers may serve as prognostic or predictive tools; they are fundamental both to select CSCs and attempt their depletion through specific therapeutic approaches. In fact, the definition of a specific GBM profile and the identification of markers predictive of survival will enable clinicians to use individualized therapies.

Because gliomas, as other tumors, are very heterogeneous in their cellular composition, molecular expression, and clinical outcomes, the design of individualized therapies will be one of the most ambitious goals for the biomedical research.

Acknowledgments We thank Mr. Francesco Marino for his helpful work for figure editing.

References

Andreu-Agulló C, Morante-Redolat JM, Delgado AC, Farinas I (2009) Vascular niche factor PEDF modulates notch-dependent stemness in the adult subependymal zone. Nat Neurosci 12:1514–1523

Bao S, Wu Q, McLendon RE, Hao Y, Shi Q, Hjelmeland AB, Dewhirst MW, Bigner DD, Rich JN (2006) Glioma stem cells promote radioresistance by preferential activation of the DNA damage response. Nature 444:756–760

Beier D, Hau P, Proescholdt M, Lohmeier A, Wischhusen J, Oefner PJ, Aigner L, Brawanski A, Bogdahn U, Beier CP (2007) CD133+ and CD133- glioblastoma-derived cancer stem cells show differential growth characteristics and molecular profiles. Cancer Res 67:4010–4015

Bonnet D, Dick JE (1997) Human acute myeloid leukemia is organized as a hierarchy that originates from a primitive hematopoietic cell. Nat Med 3:730–737

Chen HL, Panchision DM (2007) Concise review: bone morphogenetic protein pleiotropism in neural stem cells and their derivatives–alternative pathways, convergent signals. Stem Cells 25:63–68

Clement V, Sanchez P, de Tribolet N, Radovanovic I, Altaba RA (2007) HEDGEHOG-GLI1 signaling regulates human glioma growth, cancer stem cell self-renewal and tumorigenicity. Curr Biol 17:165–172

Dahlstrand J, Collins VP, Lendahl U (1992) Expression of the class VI intermediate filament nestin in human central nervous system tumors. Cancer Res 52:5334–5341

do Carmo A, Patricio I, Cruz MT, Carvalheiro H, Oliveira CR, Lopes MC (2010) CXCL12/CXCR4 promotes motility and proliferation of glioma cells. Cancer Biol Ther 9:56–65

Doyle LA, Ross DD (2003) Multidrug resistance mediated by the breast cancer resistance protein BCRP (ABCG2). Oncogene 22:7340–7358

Ehtesham M, Winston JA, Kabos P, Thompson RC (2006) CXCR4 expression mediates glioma cell invasiveness. Oncogene 25:2801–2806

Fan X, Matsui W, Khaki L, Stearns D, Chun J, Li YM, Eberhart CG (2006) Notch pathway inhibition depletes stem-like cells and blocks engraftment in embryonal brain tumors. Cancer Res 66:7445–7452

Gangemi RM, Griffero F, Marubbi D, Perera M, Capra MC, Malatesta P, Ravetti GL, Zona GL, Daga A, Corte G (2009) SOX2 silencing in glioblastoma tumor-initiating cells causes stop of proliferation and loss of tumorigenicity. Stem Cells 27:40–48

Gritti A, Vescovi AL, Galli R (2002) Adult neural stem cells: plasticity and developmental potential. J Physiol 96:81–90

Hirschmann-Jax C, Foster AE, Wulf GG, Nuchtern JG, Jax TW, Gobel U, Goodell MA, Brenner MK (2004) A distinct "side population" of cells with high drug efflux capacity in human tumor cells. Proc Natl Acad Sci USA 101:14228–14233

Holmin S, Almqvist P, Lendahl U, Mathiesen T (1997) Adult nestin-expressing subependymal cells differentiate to astrocytes in response to brain injury. Eur J Neurosci 9:65–75

Ignatova TN, Kukekov VG, Laywell ED, Suslov ON, Vrionis FD, Steindler DA (2002) Human cortical glial tumors contain neural stem-like cells expressing astroglial and neuronal markers in vitro. Glia 39:193–206

Jackson EL, Garcia-Verdugo JM, Gil-Perotin S, Roy M, Quinones-Hinojosa A, VandenBerg S, Alvarez-Buylla A (2006) PDGFRα-positive B cells are neural stem cells in the adult SVZ that form glioma-like growths in response to increased PDGF signalling. Neuron 51:187–199

Kania G, Corbeil D, Fuchs J, Tarasov KV, Blyszczuk P, Huttner WB, Boheler KR, Wobus AM (2005) Somatic stem cell marker prominin-1/CD133 is expressed in embryonic stem cell-derived progenitors. Stem Cells 23:791–804

Le Bras B, Barallobre MJ, Homman-Ludiye J, Ny A, Wyns S, Tammela T, Haiko P, Karkkainen MJ, Yuan L, Muriel MP, Chatzopoulou E, Bréant C, Zalc B, Carmeliet P, Alitalo K, Eichmann A, Thomas JL (2006) VEGF-C is a trophic factor for neural progenitors in the vertebrate embryonic brain. Nat Neurosci 9:340–348

Liu G, Yuan X, Zeng Z, Tunici P, Ng H, Abdulkadir IR, Lu L, Irvin D, Black KL, Yu JS (2006) Analysis of gene expression and chemoresistance of CD133+ cancer stem cells in glioblastoma. Mol Cancer 5:67–78

Lokker NA, Sullivan CM, Hollenbach SJ, Israel MA, Giese NA (2002) Platelet-derived growth factor (PDGF) autocrine signalling regulates survival and mitogenic pathways in glioblastoma cells: evidence that the novel PDGF-C and PDGF-D ligands May play a role in the development of brain tumors. Cancer Res 62:3729–3735

Lottaz C, Beier D, Meyer K, Kumar P, Hermann A, Schwarz J, Junker M, Oefner PJ, Bogdahn U, Wischhusen J, Spang R, Storch A, Beier CP (2010) Transcriptional profiles of CD133+ and CD133- glioblastoma-derived cancer stem cell lines suggest different cells of origin. Cancer Res 70: 2030–2040

Mellodew K, Suhr R, Uwanogho DA, Reuter I, Lendahl U, Hodges H, Price J (2004) Nestin expression is lost in a neural stem cell line through a mechanism involving the proteasome and notch signalling. Develop Brain Res 151:13–23

Mizutani K, Yoon K, Dang L, Tokunaga A, Gaiano N (2007) Differential notch signaling distinguishes neural stem cells from intermediate progenitors. Nature 449:351–355

Piccirillo SGM, Vescovi AL (2007) Bone morphogenetic proteins regulate tumorigenicity in human glioblastoma stem cells. Ernst Schering Found Symp Proc 5:59–81

Purow BW, Haque RM, Noel MW, Su Q, Burdick MJ, Lee J, Sundaresan T, Pastorino S, Park JK, Mikolaenko I, Maric D, Eberhart CG, Fine HA (2005) Expression of notch-1 and its ligands, delta-like-1 and jagged-1, is critical for glioma cell survival and proliferation. Cancer Res 65:2353–2363

Ramirez-Castillejo C, Sànchez-Sànchez F, Andreu-Agullò C, Ferròn SR, Aroca-Aguillar JD, Sànchez P, Mira E, Escribano J, Farinas I (2006) Pigment epithelium-derived factor is a niche signal for neural stem cell renewal. Nat Neurosci 9:331–339

Reya T, Morrison SJ, Clarke MF, Weissman IL (2001) Stem cells, cancer, and cancer stem cells. Nature 414:105–111

Reynolds BA, Weiss S (1992) Generation of neurons and astrocytes from isolated cells of the adult mammalian central nervous system. Science 255:1707–1710

Rivera AL, Pelloski CE, Gilbert MR, Colman H, De La Cruz C, Sulman EP, Bekele BN, Aldape KD (2010) MGMT promoter methylation is predictive of response to radiotherapy and prognostic in the absence of adjuvant alkylating chemotherapy for glioblastoma. Neurooncol 12:116–121

Sakakibara S, Nakamura Y, Satoh H, Okano H (2001) RNA-binding protein musashi2: developmentally regulated expression in neural precursor cells and subpopulation of neurons in mammalian CNS. J Neurosci 21:8097–8107

Schepers GE, Teasdale RD, Koopman P (2002) Twenty pairs of sox: extent, homology, and nomenclature of the mouse and human sox transcription factor gene families. Develop Cell 3:167–170

Schimmer AD (2004) Inhibitor of apoptosis proteins: translating basic knowledge into clinical practice. Cancer Res 64: 7183–7190

Singh SK, Clarke ID, Terasaki M, Bonn VE, Hawkins C, Squire J, Dirks PB (2003) Identification of a cancer stem cell in human brain tumors. Cancer Res 63:5821–5828

Singh SK, Hawkins C, Clarke ID, Squire JA, Bayani J, Hide T, Henkelman RM, Cusimano MD, Dirks PB (2004) Identification of human brain tumor initiating cells. Nature 432:396–401

Strojnik T, Røsland GV, Sakariassen PO, Kavalar R, Lah T (2007) Neural stem cell markers, nestin and musashi proteins, in the progression of human glioma: correlation of nestin with prognosis of patient survival. Surg Neurol 68:133–143

Teodorczyk M, Martin-Villalba A (2010) Sensing invasion: cell surface receptors driving spreading of glioblastoma. J Cell Physiol 222:1–10

Veselska R, Kuglik P, Cejpek P, Svachova H, Neradil J, Loja T, Relichova J (2006) Nestin expression in the cell lines derived from glioblastoma multiforme. BMC Cancer 6: 32–43

Wang J, Sakariassen PØ, Tsinkalovsky O, Immervoll H, Bøe SO, Svendsen A, Prestegarden L, Røsland G, Thorsen F, Stuhr L, Molven A, Bjerkvig R, Enger PØ (2008) CD133 negative glioma cells form tumors in nude rats and give rise to CD133+ cells. Int J Cancer 122:761–768

Yu SC, Bian XW (2009) Enrichment of cancer stem cells based on heterogeneity of invasiveness. Stem Cell Rev 5: 66–71

Yuan X, Curtin J, Xiong Y, Liu G, Waschsmann-Hogiu S, Farkas DL, Black KL, Yu JS (2004) Isolation of cancer stem cells from adult glioblastoma multiforme. Oncogene 23:9392–9400

Zhang Z, Wang X, Wang S (2008) Chemosensitization effects of simultaneous suppression of MDR1 and XIAP in multidrug resistant glioma cells. Med Oncol 25:367–373

Zimmerman L, Parr B, Lendahl U, Cunningham M, McKay R, Gavin B, Mann J, Vassileva G, McMahon A (1994) Independent regulatory elements in the nestin gene direct transgene expression to neural stem cells or muscle precursors. Neuron 12:11–24

Chapter 20

Efficient Derivation and Propagation of Glioblastoma Stem-Like Cells Under Serum-Free Conditions Using the Cambridge Protocol

T.M. Fael Al-Mayhani and Colin Watts

Abstract Traditionally, glioblastoma multiforme (GBM) can be grown in vitro as monolayer cultures under serum-enriched conditions. Recent data indicated that GBM can also be cultured as floating spheres under serum-free (SF) conditions in a manner similar to neural stem cells (NSC). Interestingly, GBM cultures under SF conditions can preserve many molecular and cellular characteristics of the original tumour making these cultures the best currently available model for GBM studies. However, cell line propagation using this standard approach is often difficult and cell lines can successfuly be obtained in <50% of cases. In this chapter we describe the Cambridge Protocol; a new, efficient, robust and reproducible method to derive and propagate GBM cell lines under SF conditions with a success rate of >90%. These GBM cell lines exhibit long-term expansion in vitro, form tumours in vivo and have a molecular and cytogenetic profile typical of their parent tumours.

Keywords Glioblastoma · Cancer stem cell · Cambridge protocol · Cell culture · Serum free

Introduction

Since its development in early 20th century, cell culture has contributed enormously to the development of biological studies of normal and neoplastic cells. Ideally, cell cultures should represent exactly the parent tissue at molecular, genetic, cytogenetic and subsequently functional levels. However, this ideal aim is confounded by the substantial difference between the in vitro and in vivo conditions. Nonetheless, it is worthwhile to develop culture techniques and conditions that can produce closer in vitro models to the tissue of origin in order to increase the chance of potential translational applications.

Traditionally, glioblastoma multiforme (GBM) can be grown in vitro as monolayer cultures under serum-enriched conditions. Recent data indicated that GBM can also be cultured as floating spheres under serum-free (SF) conditions in a manner similar to neural stem cells (NSC). Interestingly, GBM cultures under SF conditions can preserve many molecular and cellular characteristics of the original tumour making these cultures the best currently available model for GBM studies. However, cell line propagation using this standard approach is often difficult and cell lines can successfuly be obtained in <50% of cases.

In this chapter we describe the Cambridge Protocol; a new, efficient, robust and reproducible method to derive and propagate GBM cell lines under SF conditions with a success rate of >90%. These GBM cell lines exhibit long-term expansion in vitro, form tumours in vivo and have a molecular and cytogenetic profile typical of their parent tumours.

We are going first to discuss the effects of serum-enriched versus SF culture conditions and the growth as monolayer cultures versus spheroid cultures. This will be followed by a general overview on NSC culture and more specific description of GBM cell cultures.

As suggested by the American Tissue Culture Association (ATCA) terminology, normal and

C. Watts (✉)
Cambridge Centre for Brain Repair, Department of Clinical Neuroscience, E. D. Adrian Building, Forvie Site, Robinson Way, Cambridge, CB2 0PY
e-mail: cw209@cam.ac.uk

M.A. Hayat (ed.), *Tumors of the Central Nervous System, Volume 1*,
DOI 10.1007/978-94-007-0344-5_20, © Springer Science+Business Media B.V. 2011

neoplastic cells can be grown for short-term in vitro as *primary cultures* which may be passed as *cell lines*. Cell lines tend to stop dividing at some point (within days or weeks) and cannot be passaged indefinitely. However, in some cases, this limit can be passed and as a result *established cell lines* can be obtained. Establishing cell lines may occur spontaneously in neoplastic cell lines or, upon artificial immortalization, in normal cell lines. The point at which a cell line is described as established is discussed in more detail below. The ATCA terminology differs from the original suggestion made by Hayflick which used the term *cell strain* to describe cell cultures with limited lifespan and leave the term cell line to refer to established cell lines only (Hayflick and Moorhead, 1961; Ponten and Macintyre, 1968). In this work we will be using the ATCA terminology.

General Overview

Historical Background

Remak in 1856 and von Recklinghausen in 1868 published their observations regarding the viability of isolated amphibian hematopoetic cells in vitro. This was followed by the pioneer experiments of Sidney Ringer and Wilhelm Roux in late 19th century which can be considered as the earliest serious attempts to study animal cells after being separated from their original tissues. Perhaps, J. Jolly was the first to follow up the mitotic activity of isolated tissues in vitro for a longer period of 1 month. However, it was not until the first decade of 20th century when the principles of cell culture were established in 1907 by Ross Harrison when he conducted functional experiments showing the growth of neural fibers in vitro (Harrison et al., 1907).

A notable experimental work of that period was conducted by Earle in early 1940s to study the in vitro neoplastic transformation of normal murine cells. Earle's experiments led to the establishment of the first murine neoplastic cell lines in 1943. Similarly, in 1951 George Otto Gey of John Hopkins Hospital established the first human neoplastic cell line called HeLa after a female patient with an agressive glandular adenocarcinoma of the cervix (Gey et al., 1952).

With respect to GBM, short term cultures of GBM explants were known since the 1920s with the pioneer

work of Fischer, Cox and Pinkus. Occasional reports on establishing GBM cell lines appeared before 1965 (Manuelidis and Pond, 1959). However, in the late 1960s Jan Ponten published his detailed work on long-term propagation of established GBM cell lines including the famous U lines (Ponten and Macintyre, 1968). Since then, cell culture has been an essential tool in biological studies of gliomas.

Culture Shock Versus Cell Clock

In the first half of the 20th century, the cell culture field was dominated by the dogma of "culture shock" which states that all normal cells are capable of indefinite proliferation in vitro when the optimal conditions could be provided. This dogma was popularized by the Nobel laureate Alex Carrel who claimed the ability to culture chicken normal fibroblasts for more than 36 years. However, others challenged the "culture shock" concept insisting on the concept of "cellular clock" which states that all cells can undergo only definite number of divisions. These concepts of "culture shock" versus "cellular clock" were an issue of debate until the elegant series of experiments conducted by Leonard Hayflick and Paul Moorhead in the early 60s. Hayflick showed in 1961 that normal cells can only undergo certain number of cell divisions (50 $\pm$10 doublings) before undergoing a scenescence crisis in which cells stop dividing (Hayflick and Moorhead, 1961). Afterward, this phenomenon has been referred to as Hayflick limit. In addition, he linked the Hayflick limit to an intrinsic factor in the cell nucleus that counts and remembers the number of divisions the cell has undergone and called it the "replicometer". Further work has revealed that the "replicometer" is the telomeres at the ends of the chromosomes which undergo gradual shortening with each cell division. Later, it has been shown that preventing the telomeres shortening results in bypassing the Hayflick limit and gives the cell culture immortal properties.

In contrast to normal cells which respect the Hayflick limit, cancer cells are immortal and can proliferate beyond the limit to form established cell lines which are defined as cell lines that divided >60 doublings in culture. This is due to the ability to prevent the telomeres shortening by an enzyme called telomerase or by a process called alternative lengthening of telomeres (ALT). This immortality is considered, controversially, as one of the traditional hallmarks of cancer.

Serum-Enriched Versus Serum-Free Conditions

Traditionally, serum (usually fetal calf or bovine serum) is added to the culture media to support the growth of normal cells. Similarly, cancer cells can be cultured under serum-enriched conditions as primary cultures, cell strains or cell lines. Although it represents a rich source of nutrients, serum has significant disadvantages. First, the variable composition of serum batches means that cells cultured under serum-enriched conditions are exposed to different materials with different selective pressures. Second, the support of the growth of mature cells in serum cultures can interfere with stem cell growth resulting in non-pure and contaminated cultures. Furthermore, applying serum on GBM cultures may lead to the support of growth of cells that have abnormalities not representative of the parent tumours.

Cell culture under serum-free (SF) conditions provides several advantages. First of all, it facilitates the cell cultures under more defined environmental conditions (Bottenstein et al., 1979). Second, it supports the growth of immature stem-like phenotypes (Reynolds and Weiss, 1992; Richards et al., 1992). Based on these advantages, there have been attempts to grow cancer cells under SF conditions. Early and recent studies have shown the possibility of culturing cancer cells under SF conditions (Barnes et al., 1981).

Monolayer Versus Spheroid Cultures

Usually cells are grown in vitro as two-dimensional monolayer cultures. These cultures can be derived from normal and neoplastic tissues as primary cultures and sometimes propagated as cell lines or even established cell lines (in the case of cancer cells). Monolayer culture holds several advantages by ensuring that cells are homogeneously exposed to the culture environment. In addition, it helps in providing better quantitative evaluation and morphological and phenotypic cell characterization. However, cells in monolayer cultures undergo some changes. For example, although cell-cell contacts are formed but the two dimensional nature of the culture leads to profound dissimilarity to the in vivo situation. In addition, cells in monolayer cultures tend to secrete less extracellular matrix (ECM) and be more dependent on the artificial adhesive substrates in order to attach to the culture dish. Moreover, the fact that mature cells can grow as monolayers should be taken into account when intended to derive pure neoplastic or stem cell cultures.

Cells can also grow as floating spheroid bodies. The spheroid cultures have a long history beginning in developmental biology with the pioneering work of Holtfreter and Moscona in the 1940s and 1950s. Then, it was used to culture cancer cells isolated from melanoma and epithelioma patients before being applied to normal cells (Sutherland, 1988).

However, not all cells are able to form spheroids under these anchorage-independent conditions. Normal cells, for example, need to be grown in shaken cultures in order to form spheroid aggregates. Subsequent comparative studies revealed that primary spheroid cultures can efficiently and spontaneously be formed from embryonic and cancer cells but very rarely from normal cells (Carlsson et al., 1983). In fact, the spontaneous proliferation of cells as spheres in an anchorage-independent manner has later been considered as one of the classical features of transformed cells in culture (Macpherson and Montagnier, 1964). However, not all tumours can form spheroids, an observation that may probably be related to the location within the tumour mass. Cells in spheroid cultures are thought to represent the main features of the original normal tissues (Sutherland, 1988). This has been particularly useful for differentiation studies. This contradicts the inaccurate common notion claiming that spheres contain stem-like cells only. In fact, early and recent data have shown clearly that most viable cells within the spheres are differentiated cells. However, stem-like cells and other primitive phenotypes can be enriched in the spheroid bodies due to the fact that fully differentiated cells are more anchorage-dependent.

Regarding cancer, spheroids exhibit several similarities to tumours such as central necrosis, a rim of proliferating cells and the ability to synthesize and secrete ECM components (Sutherland, 1988). These features cannot be simulated by monolayer cultures. As a result, some investigators have proposed using spheroid cultures as intermediate model of complexity between the two dimensional monolayer cultures and the real situation in vivo (Sutherland, 1988).

But spheroid cultures have their own disadvantages. The 3D structure of spheroid bodies is highly artificial and does not guarantee better representation of the original tissues. Also, the feeding media cannot penetrate the central region of spheres leading to progressive central necrosis and loss of cell viability. Furthermore, the heterogeneous environment within the spheroids renders them difficult to interrogate and quantification of cells within the spheres is not possible without complete dissociation.

GBM and GBM Cell Cultures

GBM and the Cancer Stem Cell Hypothesis

There is an analogy between stem cells and cancer cells that was well recognized since the early 19th century in embryological terms (Recamier, 1829). This analogy has been based on observational data showing that both, stem cells and cancer cells, have proliferative activity, indefinite self-renewal ability and can produce progeny to maintain either the normal tissue (in the case of stem cells) or the cancer mass (in the case of cancer cells).

These observations led to the embryonal rest hypothesis by Cohenheim in 1868 and the stem cell-origin of cancers (Wylie et al., 1973). However, other experimental work has taken the relation between cancer and stemness further in a wider sense by introducing the concept of the stem-line (Makino, 1956; Richards, 1955) which becomes to be known later as the cancer stem cell (CSC) hypothesis (Reya et al., 2001). The CSC hypothesis does not address the possible stem cell origin of cancer. Rather it recognizes two cell populations within the cancer mass called CSC and non-CSC. According to the hypothesis, CSC populations exhibit stem-like characteristics with the ability to maintain the tumour growth, whereas non-CSC undergo terminal differentiation (Reya et al., 2001). If true, this hypothesis may explain different aspects of cancer biology such as cancer heterogeneity, growth, resistence to therapies, and recurrence.

There is good evidence to support the CSC hypothesis in heamatopoetic malignancies (Bonnet and Dick, 1997). However, although putative stem-like cells have been identified, the CSC hypothesis remains highly controversial in solid tumours of different types (Hill, 2006). These include breast cancer, lung cancer, colon cancer, prostate cancer, head and neck cancer, sarcomas and brain cancers (Sell, 2004). The identification of CSC in brain tumours (Galli et al., 2004; Hemmati et al., 2003; Ignatova et al., 2002) has been based on the expression of several NSC markers including CD133 (Singh et al., 2004), CD15 (Son et al., 2009) and nestin (Calabrese et al., 2007). However, none appears to be a universal or specific CSC marker in brain tumours, and it is possible that no such marker exists. The use of these markers is further complicated by our limited understanding of their function and the controversial data regarding their expression patterns in the nervous system under normal and pathological conditfions. In all cases, the available studies have not fully addressed the synonymous relation between cancer cells and stem cells and in particular the question of how CSC and non-CSC are organized within the tumour remains unanswered.

Leaving aside the CSC hypothesis, the analogy between cancer and stem cells has been exploited to refine and improve the culture of cancer cells. In fact, it is plausible to argue that this analogy can be extended to include the in vitro culture conditions and based on that, cancer cells and stem cells tend to grow under similar optimal conditions. As a result, NSC SF culture conditions could represent the optimal growth conditions for GBM cells in culture (Fael Al-Mayhani et al., 2009; Lee et al., 2006).

Culturing GBM Under NSC Culture Conditions

NSC can be cultured as free-floating spheres under defined SF conditions (Reynolds and Weiss, 1992; Richards et al., 1992), which include supplements such as B27 and N2 and growth factors EGF, and FGF (Caldwell et al., 2001; Carpenter et al., 1999). This spheroid approach has also been applied to embryonic and adult human NSC cultures (Moe et al., 2005; Nunes et al., 2003). Also, monolayer cultures have been successfully applied to murine NSC cultures. Similarly monolayer NSC cultures could be isolated from human fetal and adult nervous system (Conti et al., 2005). However, in all these cases long-term propagation of NSC is highly limited and cells cannot be kept expanding for more than a few passages in vitro (Moe et al., 2005).

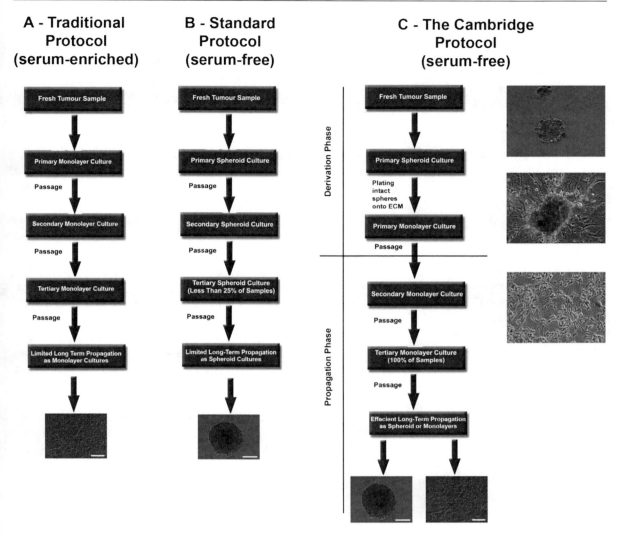

Fig. 20.1 shows the three culture protocols used for GBM cell lines derivation and propagation. (a) GBM can be cultured as monolayers under traditional protocol using serum-enriched conditions. It has been reported that cell lines can be established in less than 50% of cases (b) also, GBM can be cultured as spheres under serum-free conditions but the efficacy of obtaining long-term propagation is limited. In our experience, we could not propagate the spheres beyond passage 4. (c) the Cambridge Protocol combines both sphere and monolayer cultures under serum-free conditions with more than 90% success rate. Notably, cell lines can be propagated as either spheres in plain flasks or monolayers in ECM-coated flasks

It is well recognized that GBM cells can be cultured in vitro as either explants or monolayer cultures under traditional serum-enriched conditions (Traditional Protocol; Fig. 20.1a) (Carlsson et al., 1978). The serum provides substantial support for GBM growth that is thought to be linked to the high concentration of growth-promoting factors (Darling, 2004).

GBM cell cultures can also be derived according to the standard protocol under NSC SF culture conditions as spheroid bodies (Standard Protocol; Fig. 20.1b) (Hemmati et al., 2003; Ignatova et al., 2002; Singh et al., 2004). Several reports have showed that GBM cultures under these conditions are more representative of their parent tumours at the molecular and cytogenetic levels (De Witt Hamer et al., 2007; Lee et al., 2006). In fact, SF conditions can significantly change the behaviour of even well-established GBM cell lines in terms of tumour growth rate and similarity to the original tumour (Lee et al., 2006). All these observations indicate that SF conditions generate a better in vitro model of GBM.

Similar to NSC, GBM need to be cultured with growth factors such as EGF and FGF (Vescovi et al., 1993). However, due to the stressful nature of SF culture, obtaining GBM cell lines under these conditions can be difficult even after appropriate nutrient enrichment (Brewer and LeRoux, 2007). Spheroid cultures under SF conditions can be established successfully from <50% of the clinical samples (Table 20.1 and references therein). This figure has been reported by many investigators and supported by our own data (Galli et al., 2004; Gunther et al., 2007). The high rate of failure leads to a waste of effort and resources and can influence experimental design. It also results in the substantial loss of precious clinical samples which compromises the attempts to establish clinically annotated biobanks. All these factors highlight the importance of developing an improved method to improve the efficacy of derivation and long-term propagation of GBM cell lines under SF conditions.

Apart from the low efficacy, there is another disadvantage of the standard GBM SF cultures related to the nature of the spheroid bodies. As mentioned above, spheroids comprise aggregations of cells with a complex microenvironment that is difficult to interrogate, quantify or propagate. By contrast, monolayer cultures offer an excellent alternative to quantify the cells in vitro and investigate their characteristics. We therefore developed a technique that by combining primary spheroid cultures and monolayer cultures we could reliably and reproducibly derive human GBM cell lines. Here, we describe an efficient method to obtain and maintain GBM cell lines under SF conditions that preserves the clinical samples and produces material for subsequent applications including genetic studies, drug screening and patient-based studies.

Table 20.1 The efficiency of obtaining glioma cultures under SF conditions using the standard sphere protocol

Reference	GBM samples
Ignatova et al. (2002)	$n = 10$; Primary spheres
Hemmati et al. (2003)	$n = 2$; Secondary spheres
Galli et al. (2004)	$n = 12$; 50% efficiency
Singh et al. (2004)	$n = 1$; not determined
(Gunther et al. (2007)	$n = 19$; 47% efficiency

The Cambridge Protocol

GBM Cell Cultures Can Be Efficiently Derived from GBM Tumours Under Defined SF Conditions

The materials and practical step-by-step description of our protocol are provided in Appendix 1 and 2, respectively. The protocol comprises two phases; a derivation phase and a propagation phase as shown in Fig. 20.1c. To facilitate the selection of primitive cell phenotypes and remove debris and mature cells in the derivation phase, free floating primary spheroid bodies were allowed to form from dissociated surgical specimens under defined SF conditions. To generate long-term self-renewing cell lines, primary tumour spheres were collected after 1–3 weeks in culture and plated intact without dissociation onto ECM-coated flasks. Within 24 h, the spheroid bodies attached to the ECM and began to flatten as cells grew in a radial manner to form the primary monolayer culture (Fig. 20.1c). After a variable period of time (mean=10.7 weeks, range=3–26 weeks) this primary monolayer culture approached confluence (Fig. 20.1c). At this stage, it was passaged and viable cells were then reseeded at a standard density of $15,000/cm^2$ to generate a secondary monolayer culture.

GBM Cell Cultures Can Be Efficiently Propagated for Long-Term Under SF Conditions

In the propagation phase the secondary monolayer culture was allowed to approach confluence in a similar manner. The cells were then passaged and reseeded to generate a tertiary monolayer culture. This process could be then repeated to produce subsequent generations. From this stage cell lines can be propagated for long-term as monolayer on ECM-coated flasks (Fig. 20.1c). However, when plain uncoated flasks were used, most cell lines retain the ability to grow as spheroid aggregates. This was true for most cell lines, however, two cell lines failed to be propagated as long-term spheres, but did grow as adherent monolayer cultures. Using this protocol, we were able to derive self-renewing cultures from 19 patients with GBM under defined SF conditions with high efficiency and minimal loss of clinical material. One GBM cell line was lost due to infection. All other cell lines propagated successfully. Hence, our derivation was successful in 19/19 (100%), and successful long-term propagation was obtained in 18/19 (94%) (Fael Al-Mayhani et al., 2009).

Comparison with a Standard Protocol Shows the High Efficacy of the Cambridge Protocol

Early data generated in our lab showed the low efficacy of the standard protocol of sphere cultures (Fael Al-Mayhani et al., 2009). Secondary spheroids were observed in only 4/16 clinical samples and tertiary spheres were generated from 1/4 secondary spheroids; however, quaternary spheres could not be obtained and no GBM culture could be propagated.

We directly compared the derivation of GBM cell cultures according to our protocol with the standard sphere protocol. Three GBM samples from three different patients were resected, dissociated and seeded to generate the primary spheroid cultures. We then collected the primary spheres and seeded them into two cultures to generate secondary spheroid culture (standard protocol) or primary monolayer culture (according to our protocol). Notably, our culture approach efficiently generated long-term self-renewing cell lines from each sample when compared to the standard protocol (Fishers exact test $p < 0.001$). We observed that even after long-term growth as monolayer in ECM cultures, GBM lines retain the ability to grow as floating spheroid bodies if cultured under sphere-promoting conditions in the absence of adhesive substrate (ECM). In vitro cells propagation as sphere or monolayer cultures was directly compared over 8 consecutive passages in two GBM cell lines. When seeded at a constant density (15,000 cells per cm^2) the cells number from monolayer cultures was significantly higher compared to free floating spheroid cultures among all 8 passages ($F_{3,27} = 8.473$, $p < 0.001$).

GBM Cell Lines Conserve Characteristic Molecular Cytogenetic Abnormalities of Their Parent Tumours

To determine if the derived cells were cancer cells and representative of their parent tumors at the molecular cytogenetic level, we performed array comparative genomic hybridization (aCGH) analysis. We compared different GBM cell lines (at passage 5 and passage 20) with their tumour of origin. All tested tumors had Chromosome 7 gain and Chromosome 10 monosomy. These were conserved in all corresponding cell lines. Also, abnormalities in Chromosome 13, Chromosome 1, and Chromosome 9 were found in parent GBM tumours and their identical derived cell lines. However, EGFR amplification, which is a common finding in GBM tumours, was lost but one from the derived GBM cell lines tested. The aCGH data confirm that the parent tumours were typical GBM with a genomic profile that was highly conserved for long-term in their derived cell lines. In addition, we compared, using RT-PCR and Q-PCR, our GBM cell lines with the original GBM tumours in terms of the expression of genes associated with neural development. Our data showed a high level of conservation of the expression of a panel of developmental neural genes including Hes1, Mash1, Nkx2.2, Pax6, and Sox2 (Fael Al-Mayhani et al., 2009).

Our GBM Cell Lines Contain Cancer Cells of Neural Origin

The cytogenetic profile of the cell population was typical to GBM parent tumours. However, there is a possibility that our cultures may contain, in addition to neural cancer cells, contaminating non-neural cells such as microglia, pericytes, endothelial cells, muscular cells, and macrophages. We, therefore, explored the purity of our GBM cell cultures. CD90 (Thy1), a marker for mesenchymal and heamatopoetic cells, was used to stain our cell lines. We found that CD90 was not expressed by any of our cell lines. Similarly, we looked for contaminating endothelial cells and pericytes using anti CD31 and PDGFR-β antibodies, respectively. Both markers were not expressed in any tested cell line. It has been reported that macrophages can be maintained in vitro under SF conditions. We tested our cell lines for the positivity of CD68, a marker for macrophages and microglia. Again, our GBM cells in culture did not express CD68.

Characterization of GBM Cell Phenotypes Under SF and Differentiation Conditions

Next, we wanted to explore the phenotypes of the GBM cell lines under SF conditions. We observed the expression of markers associated with NSC in monolayer and spheroid cultures. These markers include the intermediate filament Nestin and the pentaspan transmembrane protein CD133. In addition, markers associated with glial progenitors were observed. These include the ganglioside A2B5, the proteoglycan NG2, and transcription factor Olig2. Except for CD133, the expression of all other markers was widely observed in our tested cell lines in early and late passages indicating a notably stable expression.

Regarding CD133, some cell lines were CD133$^-$, whereas others contained small numbers of CD133$^+$ cells. Interestingly, less than half of the parent tumour samples expressed CD133 and the pattern of CD133 expression in cell lines correlated with the original tumour. A small number of CD133+ cells in our cell lines could be observed at early passages, but using PCR no CD133 expression could be detected beyond passage 10.

Withdrawal of growth factors and enriching the culture media with 10% FCS is routinely used to induce NSC differentiation. When we tested the effect of differentiation conditions on our GBM cell lines we observed substantial change in cell morphology and phenotype. The cells began to flatten assuming more wide and irregular shape and the cell processes became more prominent. In parallel, the expression of the primitive neural markers (CD133, A2B5, NG2, and Olig2) was down-regulated. Instead, the expression of markers associated with mature neural cells was observed such as the astrocytic marker, GFAP. Interestingly, GFAP was often coexpressed with the early neuronal marker βIII-tubulin reflecting the abnormality of the cell phenotype. However, mature neuronal markers e.g., MAP2ab were not expressed. The expression of the early oligodendrocyte marker O4 was less common and only observed in a small number of cell lines after extended exposure to differentiation

conditions of >14 days. Again, these expression patterns under differentiation conditions were similar in monolayer and spheroid cultures. Quantitative analysis was performed for various cell lines regarding the expression of CD133, Nestin, NG2, A2B5, Olig2, GFAP and βIII-tubulin. The proportions were highly variable among different cell lines and the coexpression of GFAP and βIII-tubulin was common.

GBM Cell Lines Derived According to Cambridge Protocol Form Tumours In Vivo

In order to demonstrate that the GBM cell populations derived using the Cambridge Protocol were able to form tumours, we tested the tumourigeneity by subcutaneous and intra-cerebral implantation into immuno-compromised mice (SCID and nude mice). Suncutaneous (SC) implantation was performed by injecting 10^6 cells mixed with 100–200 µl of ECM under the dermal layer of the hind limbs of SCID mice. This produced obvious subcutaneous lumps within variable periods of 2–20 weeks. Next, we wanted to make sure that these grafts came from human cells and not formed by host reactive cells. Grafts were excised, fixed, sectioned and stained, with anti-human nuclei (HN) antibodies which recognize human cell nuclei. Results show that the grafts consisted of highly packed human cells.

To show orthotopic tumour formation we implanted 5×10^4 cells into the forebrain of SCID mice. Cells were allowed to grow for up to 18 weeks. Grafts at 6 and 18 weeks post-implantation were compared showing an increase in size. Grafts showed changes characteristic of high grade tumours including high cellularity with abnormal mitotic figures, increased vascularity, local invasion of the surrounding white matter, and extensive migration. However, pseudopalisading was not observed. The implanted HN+ GBM cells were also detected in the corpus callosum, cerebral cortex, ipsilateral hemisphere, contralateral hemisphere, subventricular zone (SVZ), rostral migratory stream, and olfactory bulb. These features are more characteristic of the clinical condition compared to traditional GBM cell lines such as U87 which form discreet tumour margin with minimal invasion of the host brain.

Implantations of primary, secondary, and tertiary spheroids, generated using the standard neurosphere protocol, were also observed to form grafts. These data support previous reports (Lee et al., 2006; Singh et al., 2004) and confirm that tumourigenic populations can be derived from GBM with high efficiency using the Cambridge Protocol.

Discussion

Several early reports have demonstrated the possibility of growing GBM as primary cultures. Also, GBM cell lines can be propagated as monolayers under serum-rich conditions according to the Traditional Protocol as shown in Fig. 20.1a (Carlsson et al., 1978; Manuelidis and Pond, 1959). Based on the potential similarity between cancer cells, and stem cells it has been proposed that both cell types grow optimally under similar culture conditions. In fact, recent reports have indicated that GBM cells can be more representative of their parent tumours if cultured under the NSC SF culture conditions (De Witt Hamer et al., 2007; Lee et al., 2006). The derivation of GBM cell lines under SF conditions has been reported from both adult and pediatric GBM samples as sphere culture using the standard protocol (Hemmati et al., 2003; Ignatova et al., 2002; Singh et al., 2004). However, this approach is successful in obtaining GBM cell cultures from less than half of the clinical samples (Table 20.1 and references therein). In addition to the low efficacy, sphere cultures have several weaknesses.

Monolayer cultures under SF conditions have been used to derive normal NSC cultures from embryonic cells and adult brain (Conti et al., 2005) but have not been applied on GBM cells.

We have combined spheroid and monolayer cultures to improve the efficiency of derivation of human GBM cell lines under SF conditions. The Cambridge Protocol comprises a derivation phase followed by a propagation phase. In the derivation phase spheres are allowed to form from dissociated clinical sample. This primary sphere culture may be important as enriching step for primitive phenotypes (Reynolds and Weiss, 1992). In addition, it helps in purifying our culture of mature phenotypes which are dependent on adhesive substrates and therefore cannot survive a non-adherent culture condition.

Another adherent approach has been introduced to culture the GBM-derived cells directly as a monolayer

under SF conditions without the sphere formation step (Pollard et al., 2009). In our experience, we previously compared GBM cell lines derivation with and without the initial step of sphere formation. Importantly, when the sphere step was ignored, the identification of the non-differentiated cell types was confounded by the presence of large quantities of debris and differentiated cells that also adhered to the substrate. Moreover, there is potential risk of supporting contaminating normal or non-neural cells particularly macrophages which can efficiently be cultured for long term under SF conditions. Based on our observations, we recommend using a spheroid formation step before starting the monolayer cultures.

In the propagation phase, we plate the intact primary spheres on ECM. We tried other adhesive materials such as PDL and laminin. However, most spheres do not attach to PDL and can only attach to laminin when it is used at a high concentration.

The improvement in the derivation and subsequent propagation of GBM cell lines in our cultures may be explained by the maintenance of appropriate environmental interactions which are lost upon the dissociation of spheres (Sutherland, 1988; Svendsen et al., 1998), showing the potential importance of cell-cell interaction.

Using our protocol, a stable cell line in terms of expansion rate is usually obtained by the 4th or 5th passage and established cell lines could be conferred by passage 20–36 depending on the doubling time which varies among different GBM samples. Our results compare favorably with reported cell lines derived from normal human NSC cultures (up to quaternary spheres) (Moe et al., 2005), established GBM cell lines under traditional serum-rich conditions (30–40%) (Ponten, 1975) and 48%, and GBM cell cultures and lines under standard SF conditions (Table 20.1 and references therein).

GBM cell line expansion begins as a phase of rapid growth followed by a stable expansion. This may reflect a period of selection of the expanding population during which the size of this compartment increases. This is then followed by a phase in which expansion of the proliferative population is balanced by loss of non-proliferative cells. Interestingly, we observed variation in the pattern of expansion between different GBM cell lines in vitro. This may reflect the heterogeneity among brain tumours with similar WHO grade, and it is not explained by the differences in the proportion of active colony-forming cells within the population.

We observed that after several passages as monolayers, our GBM cell lines were able to propagate as monolayers or spheres upon seeding onto ECM-coated or plain uncoated flasks, respectively. After each passage, we noted that the cell number from monolayer cultures was higher than the cell number from spheroid cultures. These observations may be explained by variation in the microenvironment in which the cells are proliferating. Cells within neurospheres may not receive the same level of exposure to mitogens and nutrients. This may result in variability in cell cycling, the emergence of areas of necrosis, and cell loss. Based on these observations we continue to use monolayer cultures for long-term propagation.

We have confirmed that our GBM cell lines contain no contaminating non-neural cells by showing no reactivity to anti CD90, CD31, and PDGFR-β antibodies. The negative expression of the glycophosphatydil CD90 (Thy1) excludes the contamination with heamatopoetic stem cells, mesenchymal stem cells, endothelial cells, fibroblasts, and mature neurons. CD31 is a surface glycoprotein expressed by different types of blood cells and used extensively to detect endothelial cells in normal and neoplastic tissues. The lack of its expression by our cell lines further supports the absence of endothelial cell in our cultures. The absence of PDGFR-β indicates no contamination with pericytes. In normal brain, PDGFR-β is expressed by pericytes around blood vessels. Similarly, in GBM, PDGFR-β is expressed by the pericytes of tumour blood vessels. Our GBM cell lines do not express CD68, a marker of macrophages and microglia. This observation is important as macrophages can survive and propagate under SF conditions. However, with respect to microglia, it is well known that it is very difficult to be cultured even under serum-enriched conditions as they cannot survive the initial steps of tissue digestion. In the best available studies, microglia may be cultured only for a short period of time (2–3 weeks) under the optimum conditions which are more supportive than our cell culture conditions.

Characterizing our cell lines under SF conditions reveals the expression of markers associated with neural precursors such as CD133, Nestin, NG2, A2B5,

and Olig2. CD133 is a pentaspan transmembrane protein that was first described in heamatopoetic system. However, some reports indicated its expression by NSC in developing brain. We should note, however, that CD133 is not expressed by germinal zones of adult brain (Pfenninger et al., 2007). In addition, a recent report demonstrates that CD133 is not a universal marker for NSC in the developing brain (Sun et al., 2009).

Nestin is an intermediate filament expressed by neural precursors. However, Nestin is not exclusive to the immature neuro-epithelial cells because it exists in endothelial cells, monocytes, pericytes, cardiac muscles and smooth muscles. Its expression is well documented in glioma of all grades especially GBM and it is thought to be correlated with WHO grade. However, again it is not exclusive to GBM neural cells as GBM proliferating endothelial cells can also express Nestin. Nestin expression by glioma cell lines is highly variable which may be related to the frequent use of serum-enriched conditions in traditional GBM cultures. NG2 is a surface proteoglycan expressed together with the ganglioside A2B5 and the transcription factor Olig2 by NG2+ glial progenitors.

Under serum-rich conditions each of our GBM cell lines expressed markers associated with astrocytes (GFAP), oligodendrocytes (O4), and neurons (βIII-Tubulin). We observed widespread co-expression of GFAP and βIII-tubulin in our cultures. This is consistent with previous reports and illustrates the phenotypic abnormality of these cells (Hemmati et al., 2003; Ignatova et al., 2002; Singh et al., 2004). Interestingly, Nestin, a marker expressed by neural precursors (see above), continues to be expressed even after prolonged exposure to serum. However, cancer cells are highly abnormal and applying observations of stem cell multipotentiality to this population may be of limited clinical and scientific importance particularly given the phenotypic variability within and between GBM cell lines and tumour samples.

Our data also indicate that GBM cell lines derived using our protocol conserve the genetic phenotype of the parent GBM tumour such as Chromosome 7 gain and Chromosome 10 monosomy (Ichimura et al., 2004). However, EGFR amplification, which is a common finding in GBM tumours (Libermann et al., 1984), was lost in the derived GBM cell lines. This is consistent with previous reports (Bigner et al., 1990), and may be explained by the in vitro effects on the derived cell lines. Also, this observation imposes a question concerning the importance of EGFR amplification for the survival of GBM cell lines. These results complement other work which has directly compared the effect of serum on GBM cells in vitro to suggest that culturing under defined SF conditions are more representative of GBM tumours at cellular (Lee et al., 2006) and molecular cytogenetic level (De Witt Hamer et al. (2007).

Our GBM cell lines are tumourigenic in vivo as shown by subcutaneous and intracerebral implantation in SCID mice. SC implantation is a quick and simple procedure. The graft growth and development can be followed and monitored easily and the animal remains in very good health even with large lumps. All these advantages render SC implantations as an ideal screening test of the tumurigenetic ability of our cell lines.

After orthotopic implantation, all our GBM cell lines tested formed tumour masses. It is obvious that the level of immunosupression of the in vivo model would affect the take rate of the tumour cells and as a result the evaluation of the tumourogenic competency. However, in our SCID mice model, we used 50,000 cells in order to obtain tumours after variable period of latency (2 months as an average). This is readily consistent with the results from experimental work on homologous and autologous implantation of cancer cells in mice and humans and represents, therefore, a more accurate model of human disease (Moore et al., 1957). In light of these data, the use of deeply immuno-compromised mice (e.g., IL2$^-$/SCID) may not be an ideal model for studying tumour-competency because of the obvious inconsistency with the results of homologous and autologous experiments which can be considered a more reliable reference point (Moore et al., 1957; Quintana et al., 2008).

Our GBM cell lines were able to form tumours with high vascularity, notable infiltration in the surrounding tissue, nests of tumour cells invading the normal stroma, and migration of tumour cells away from the injection site. Human cells could be observed in nearly every part of the host brain. These observations are consistent with GBM invasive behavior. However, graft growth and invasion of the host was highly variable between different lines from samples of the same histological grade. Such variability in

patterns of development closely reproduces clinical variability observed in patients but precise correlation with clinical data remains to be explored.

Our data show that using the Cambridge Protocol facilitates the derivation and propagation of GBM cell lines under SF conditions. The derived cell lines are a better model of GBM growth and invasion and are more representative of the parent tumours.

Appendix 1: Materials

Defined SF Culture Media

Cells were cultured in serum-free (SF) medium (phenol-free Neurobasal-A (NBA) with 20 mM L-glutamine (Sigma) and 1% v/v PSF solution with 20 ng/ml human epidermal growth factor (hEGF,), 20 ng/ml human fibroblast growth factor (hFGF) mixed with 20 ng/ml heparin, 2% v/v B27 supplement and 1% N2 supplement.

Differentiating Culture Media

For differentiating conditions, growth factors were withdrawn and fetal calf serum (FCS) (Gibco) was added to NBA with a final concentration of 10%.

Adhesive Substratum in Flasks and Coverslips

Extracellular matrix (ECM) from Engelbreth Holm-Swarm mouse sarcoma (Sigma) was diluted 1:10 in phenol-free Neurobasal-A (NBA) (Gibco) before coating the flasks and coverslips.

Red Blood Cells Buffer

In order to get rid of blood cells, single cell suspension was washed with filtered red cell lysis buffer (RCLB) which consists of 8.3 gr NH4Cl, 1 g KHCO3, 1.8 ml of 5% EDTA in 1 L dd water, pH 7.4.

Appendix 2: Practical Points

Derivation Protocol

Here we provide step-by-step description of the Cambridge protocol:

1. Tumour tissue collection: tumour tissues should be collected in chilled HBSS or PBS buffer and processed within < 6 h of collection.
2. Tumour tissue dissociation: the tissue should be micro-dissected to get rid of any clots, gross blood vessels or necrotic areas before being chopped into small pieces using sterile blades. The tissue pieces then are collected into 50 ml tube and spun for 5 min at 1000 g in HBSS or PBS buffer.
3. Next, 5 ml of PDD cocktail enzymes (Papain, Dispase, DNAse) mixture are added to the minced tissue and triturate continuously using 10 ml orange pipette for 5–10 min. This step is quite subjective as the user should proceed to the next step once the mixture becomes liquefied with no or very few observable fragments. Other types of digestive enzymes have been tried such as 1:5 diluted trypsin with EDTA and Accutase. All have produced satisfactory results. However, Accutase can take longer time and, depending on the sample, the cell dissociation may not be complete.
4. The dissociated contents are filtered through 40 μm filter, and 5 ml of red blood cell buffer is added before spinning for 5 min at 1000 g. This step can be repeated if required until there is no apparent blood band at the pellet.
5. The pellet is resuspended using 1 ml of fresh NBA and the number of viable cells is quantified using haemocytometer and trypan blue-exclusion. It should be noted that due to the dissociation process it is likely to end up with lots of debris and dead cells but this is highly variable between samples.
6. 1×10^6 cells are seeded into plain, uncoated T75 flask and then 8–10 ml of defined SF media are added. Making more than one flask is advisable but this depends on the final number of viable cells at the end of the process. The cells culture is kept in an appropriate incubator at 37°C, 5% CO_2. It is advisable to change the culture media every week.
7. Spheroid aggregates should be observed within few days and over the next 2–3 weeks these aggregates increase in number and size.
8. After variable period of time, spheroid aggregates are collected and spun once with HBSS or PBS in 1000 g centrifuge. Next, the aggregates are seeded without dissociation onto ECM-coated T75 flask. Ten millilitre of defined SF media are added and the cell culture is kept in an appropriate incubator at 37°C, 5% CO_2.

Propagation Protocol

Passage the cells once the culture is 90% confluent (on average every 7–10 days). For passaging follow the steps below:

1. The old media is discarded
2. The culture is rinsed once or twice with sterile HBSS or PBS (Ca/Mg free). This step will facilitate the action of the digestive enzymes in the next step
3. Accutase (3 ml to T225 flasks; 2 ml to T75 flasks) is added to the culture with incubation at room temperature for 5–10 min. Some cell lines may take up to 20 min to be fully detached. Diluted Trypsin (1:5) can be used but it may be harmful particularly to cultures at early passages.
4. A gentle smack can be given to the flask to make sure that nearly all cells are detached and floating (using light microscope).
5. The content of the flask is collected in a 15 ml tube.
6. The flask is rinsed with HBSS or PBS and any remaining cells are collected in the 15 ml tube
7. The cells are centrifuged once in 1000 g for 5 min
8. The supernatant is discarded and the pellet is resuspended in 1 ml HBSS or PBS
9. The viable cells are quantified using haemocytometer and trypan blue exclusion
10. Seeding 1×10^6 cells into new ECM-coated T225 with 15–20 ml feeding media or 0.5×10^6 cells into ECM-coated T75 with 8–10 ml feeding media. Note: in most cases, seeding the cells into plain un-coated flask will lead to spontaneous formation of spheroid aggregates.

References

Barnes D, van der Bosch J, Masui H, Miyazaki K, Sato G (1981) The culture of human tumor cells in serum-free medium. Methods Enzymol 79:368–391

Bigner SH, Humphrey PA, Wong AJ, Vogelstein B, Mark J, Friedman HS, Bigner DD (1990) Characterization of the epidermal growth factor receptor in human glioma cell lines and xenografts. Cancer Res 50:8017–8022

Bonnet D, Dick JE (1997) Human acute myeloid leukemia is organized as a hierarchy that originates from a primitive hematopoietic cell. Nat Med 3:730–737

Bottenstein J, Hayashi I, Hutchings S, Masui H, Mather J, McClure DB, Ohasa S, Rizzino A, Sato G, Serrero G (1979) The growth of cells in serum-free hormone-supplemented media. Methods Enzymol 58:94–109

Brewer GJ, LeRoux PD (2007) Human primary brain tumor cell growth inhibition in serum-free medium optimized for neuron survival. Brain Res 1157:156–166

Calabrese C, Poppleton H, Kocak M, Hogg TL, Fuller C, Hamner B, Oh EY, Gaber MW, Finklestein D, Allen M (2007) A perivascular niche for brain tumor stem cells. Cancer Cell 11:69–82

Caldwell MA, He X, Wilkie N, Pollack S, Marshall G, Wafford KA, Svendsen CN (2001) Growth factors regulate the survival and fate of cells derived from human neurospheres. Nat Biotechnol 19:475–479

Carlsson J, Collins P, Brunk U (1978) Plasma membrane motility and proliferation of human glioma cells in agarose and monolayer cultures. Acta pathologica et microbiologica Scandinavica 86:45–55

Carlsson J, Nilsson K, Westermark B, Ponten J, Sundstrom C, Larsson E, Bergh J, Pahlman S, Busch C, Collins VP (1983) Formation and growth of multicellular spheroids of human origin. Int J Cancer 31:523–533

Carpenter MK, Cui X, Hu ZY, Jackson J, Sherman S, Seiger A, Wahlberg LU (1999) In vitro expansion of a multipotent population of human neural progenitor cells. Exp Neurol 158:265–278

Conti L, Pollard SM, Gorba T, Reitano E, Toselli M, Biella G, Sun Y, Sanzone S, Ying QL, Cattaneo E, Smith A (2005) Niche-independent symmetrical self-renewal of a mammalian tissue stem cell. PLoS Biol 3:e283

Darling JL (2004) In: Vitro culture of malignant brain tumors. In: Pfranger R, Freshney RI (eds) Culture of human tumor cells. Wiley-Liss, New Jersey, p 355

De Witt Hamer PC, Van Tilborg AA, Eijk PP, Sminia P, Troost D, Van Noorden CJ, Ylstra B, Leenstra S (2007) The genomic profile of human malignant glioma is altered early in primary cell culture and preserved in spheroids. Oncogene 27:2091–2096

Fael Al-Mayhani TM, Ball SL, Zhao JW, Fawcett J, Ichimura K, Collins PV, Watts C (2009) An efficient method for derivation and propagation of glioblastoma cell lines that conserves the molecular profile of their original tumours. J Neurosci Methods 176:192–199

Galli R, Binda E, Orfanelli U, Cipelletti B, Gritti A, De Vitis S, Fiocco R, Foroni C, Dimeco F, Vescovi A (2004) Isolation and characterization of tumorigenic, stem-like neural precursors from human glioblastoma. Cancer Res 64:7011–7021

Gey GO, Coffman WD, Kubicek MT (1952) Tissue culture studies of the proliferative capacity of cervical carcinoma and normal epithelium. Cancer Res 12:264–265

Gunther HS, Schmidt NO, Phillips HS, Kemming D, Kharbanda S, Soriano R, Modrusan Z, Meissner H, Westphal M, Lamszus K (2007) Glioblastoma-derived stem cell-enriched cultures form distinct subgroups according to molecular and phenotypic criteria. Oncogene 27:2897–2909

Harrison RG, Greenman MJ, Mall FP, Jackson CM (1907) Observations of the living developing nerve fiber. Anat Rec 1:116–128

Hayflick L, Moorhead PS (1961) The serial cultivation of human diploid cell strains. Exp Cell Res 25:585–621

Hemmati HD, Nakano I, Lazareff JA, Masterman-Smith M, Geschwind DH, Bronner-Fraser M, Kornblum HI (2003) Cancerous stem cells can arise from pediatric brain tumors. Proc Nat Acad Sci USA 100:15178–15183

Hill RP (2006) Identifying cancer stem cells in solid tumors: case not proven. Cancer Res 66:1891–1895. discussion 1890

Ichimura K, Ohgaki H, Kleihues P, Collins VP (2004) Molecular pathogenesis of astrocytic tumours. J Neurooncol 70:137–160

Ignatova TN, Kukekov VG, Laywell ED, Suslov ON, Vrionis FD, Steindler DA (2002) Human cortical glial tumors contain neural stem-like cells expressing astroglial and neuronal markers in vitro. Glia 39:193–206

Lee J, Kotliarova S, Kotliarov Y, Li A, Su Q, Donin NM, Pastorino S, Purow BW, Christopher N, Zhang W (2006) Tumor stem cells derived from glioblastomas cultured in bFGF and EGF more closely mirror the phenotype and genotype of primary tumors than do serum-cultured cell lines. Cancer Cell 9:391–403

Libermann TA, Razon N, Bartal AD, Yarden Y, Schlessinger J, Soreq H (1984) Expression of epidermal growth factor receptors in human brain tumors. Cancer Res 44:753–760

Macpherson I, Montagnier L (1964) Agar suspension culture for the selective assay of cells transformed by polyoma virus. Virology 23:291–294

Makino S (1956) Further evidence favoring the concept of the stem cell in ascites tumors of rats. Ann N Y Acad Sci 63:818–830

Manuelidis EE, Pond AR (1959) Continuous cultivation of cells arising from human case of glioblastoma multiforme (glioma T.C.178). Proc Soc Exp Biol NY 102:693–695

Moe MC, Varghese M, Danilov AI, Westerlund U, Ramm-Pettersen J, Brundin L, Svensson M, Berg-Johnsen J, Langmoen IA (2005) Multipotent progenitor cells from the adult human brain: neurophysiological differentiation to mature neurons. Brain 128:2189–2199

Moore AE, Rhoads CP, Southam CM (1957) Homotransplantation of human cell lines. Science 125:158–160

Nunes MC, Roy NS, Keyoung HM, Goodman RR, McKhann G 2nd, Jiang L, Kang J, Nedergaard M, Goldman SA (2003) Identification and isolation of multipotential neural progenitor cells from the subcortical white matter of the adult human brain. Nat Med 9:439–447

Pfenninger CV, Roschupkina T, Hertwig F, Kottwitz D, Englund E, Bengzon J, Jacobsen SE, Nuber UA (2007) CD133 is not present on neurogenic astrocytes in the adult subventricular zone, but on embryonic neural stem cells, ependymal cells, and glioblastoma cells. Cancer Res 67:5727–5736

Pollard SM, Yoshikawa K, Clarke ID, Danovi D, Stricker S, Russell R, Bayani J, Head R, Lee M, Bernstein M, Squire JA, Smith A, Dirks P (2009) Glioma stem cell lines expanded in adherent culture have tumor-specific phenotypes and are suitable for chemical and genetic screens. Cell Stem Cell 4:568–580

Ponten J (1975) Neoplastic human glia cells in culture. In: Fogh J (ed) Human tumour cell in vitro. Plenum, New York, NY, p 557

Ponten J, Macintyre EH (1968) Long term culture of normal and neoplastic human glia. Acta Path Microbiol Scand 74:465–486

Quintana E, Shackleton M, Sabel MS, Fullen DR, Johnson TM, Morrison SJ (2008) Efficient tumour formation by single human melanoma cells. Nature 456:593–598

Recamier JCV (1829) Rechereches sur le traitment du cancer, par la compression methodique simple ou combinee, et sur l'histoire generale de la meme maladie. Gabon, Paris

Reya T, Morrison SJ, Clarke MF, Weissman IL (2001) Stem cells, cancer, and cancer stem cells. Nature 414: 105–111

Reynolds BA, Weiss S (1992) Generation of neurons and astrocytes from isolated cells of the adult mammalian central nervous system. Science 255:1707–1710

Richards BM (1955) Deoxyribose nucleic acid values in tumour cells with reference to the stem-cell theory of tumour growth. Nature 175:259–261

Richards LJ, Kilpatrick TJ, Bartlett PF (1992) De novo generation of neuronal cells from the adult mouse brain. Proc Natl Acad Sci USA 89:8591–8595

Sell S (2004) Stem cell origin of cancer and differentiation therapy. Crit Rev Oncol Hematol 51:1–28

Singh SK, Clarke ID, Hide T, Dirks PB (2004) Cancer stem cells in nervous system tumors. Oncogene 23:7267–7273

Son MJ, Woolard K, Nam DH, Lee J, Fine HA (2009) SSEA-1 is an enrichment marker for tumor-initiating cells in human glioblastoma. Cell Stem Cell 4:440–452

Sun Y, Kong W, Falk A, Hu J, Zhou L, Pollard S, Smith A (2009) CD133 (prominin) negative human neural stem cells are clonogenic and tripotent. PLoS One 4:e5498

Sutherland RM (1988) Cell and environment interactions in tumor microregions: the multicell spheroid model. Science 240:177–184

Svendsen CN, ter Borg MG, Armstrong RJ, Rosser AE, Chandran S, Ostenfeld T, Caldwell MA (1998) A new method for the rapid and long term growth of human neural precursor cells. J Neurosci Methods 85:141–152

Vescovi AL, Reynolds BA, Fraser DD, Weiss S (1993) BFGF regulates the proliferative fate of unipotent (neuronal) and bipotent (neuronal/astroglial) EGF-generated CNS progenitor cells. Neuron 11:951–966

Wylie CV, Nakane PK, Pierce GB (1973) Degree of differentiation of nonproliferating cells of mammary carcinoma. Differentiation 1:11–20

Chapter 21

Glioma Cell Lines: Role of Cancer Stem Cells

John R. Ohlfest and Stacy A. Decker

Abstract In this chapter, we review the cancer stem cell hypothesis and discuss implications for this paradigm in considering whether glioma cell lines contain bonafide cancer stem cells, the source material used for tissue culture, and experimental methods used in preclinical research. We identify three key modifications to standard tissue culture protocols that allow for enrichment of cancer stem cells that closely reflect the genetics, gene expression, and phenotype of the primary tumors. These modifications are the use of: (i) primary tumors exclusively cultured in serum-free media, (ii) cellular adherence to artificial extracellular matrix, (iii) physiologic oxygen in tissue culture. Widespread acceptance of this tissue culture protocol should lead to in vitro and in vivo preclinical models that more faithfully recapitulate the human disease and thereby increase the rate of successful therapeutic development.

Keywords Glioma · Brain tumor stem cell · Serum-free culture · Cancer stem cell · Oxygen

Introduction

The consensus definition for a cancer stem cell, as established by the American Association for Cancer Research (AACR), requires classification based on the "ability to recapitulate the generation of a continuously growing tumor" that resembles the heterogeneous phenotype and morphology of the primary tumor (Clarke et al., 2006). In practice, the identification of a cancer stem cell is accomplished through the use of transplantation systems. This requires injection of a limited number of tumor cells into immunocompromised mice at an orthotopic site (e.g.: brain tumor into brain, breast tumor into mammary pad) and assessment of tumor formation. This experimental platform provides a standard method for evaluating putative cancer stem cells for the capacity to engraft and differentiate into all neoplastic cell types present in the primary tumor. The ability of transplanted cells to propagate a tumor that can phenocopy the original tumor is a key operational criterion that must be met for any tumor cell to be labeled as a cancer stem cell. Additionally, self-renewal potential must be demonstrated by serial transplantation into secondary and tertiary recipients. These self-renewing, tumor initiating cells that phenocopy the primary tumor are hereafter referred to as cancer stem cells.

The existence of cancer stem cells was first established in leukemia through transplantation into severe combined immune-deficient (SCID) mice (Lapidot et al., 1994). These leukemia-initiating cells were not functionally homogenous, however. Two populations of leukemia initiating cells were able to engraft in NOD-SCID mice, but only the cells with self-renewal potential were capable of long-term repopulation as demonstrated by serial transplantation (Hope et al., 2004). Thus, an apparent hierarchy exists in leukemia in which a rare cancer stem cell divides asymmetrically to self-renew itself and generates a short-lived progenitor to propagate the disease. However, recent evidence suggests that cancer stem cells may not be "rare" across all tumor types and stages. Quintana et al.

J.R. Ohlfest (✉)
Department of Neurosurgery, University of Minnesota Medical School, Minneapolis, MN 55455, USA
e-mail: Ohlfe001@umn.edu

M.A. Hayat (ed.), *Tumors of the Central Nervous System, Volume 1*,
DOI 10.1007/978-94-007-0344-5_21, © Springer Science+Business Media B.V. 2011

(2008) demonstrated that as many as 27% of malignant melanoma cells could initiate tumors that phenocopy the human disease in severely immunocompromised SCID/γcR –/– mice. The tumor initiating frequency was an order of magnitude lower in SCID mice with functional γc receptor subunits, which are required for IL-2 signaling and murine natural killer (NK) cell development. These data revealed the importance of NK cells in rejecting human xenografts and suggested that cancer stem cells should not be considered "rare" a priori unless proven experimentally in the most stringent immunocompromised models available.

The implications of the cancer stem cell hypothesis raise several questions about glioma cell lines used for brain tumor research: Do glioma cell lines contain bonafide cancer stem cells? If so, how does culture condition affect the frequency of cancer stem cells? What cell lines and culture conditions most faithfully recapitulate the proposed hierarchical organization of gliomas? The focus of this chapter is to relate current concepts in cancer stem cell biology to the use of primary and long-established glioma cell lines. We briefly review how cell culture conditions influence tumor genetics, gene expression, immunogenicity, and differentiation status. Understanding these features of experimental cell cultures is important to generate in vitro and in vivo preclinical models that are better able to predict human responses.

Cancer Stem Cells in Traditional Glioma Lines

Glioma cell lines are among the most commonly used tools for basic and translational brain tumor research. In practice, it may be impossible to demonstrate that the majority of traditional cell lines in culture are capable of generating a transplanted tumor that can phenocopy the original tumor because the primary tumor is unlikely to be available for study. Therefore, many long-established cell lines do not meet the operational definition of a cancer stem cell. Nonetheless, the ability to self-renew and initiate tumors has been demonstrated in numerous traditionally cultured glioma cell lines and these lines often exhibit phenotypic and functional heterogeneity. For instance, most of the long-established lines have maintained a rare (0.1–10%) subset of cells that are within the "side population"

(SP), as determined by flow cytometry for the ability to efflux Hoechst dye (Kondo et al., 2004; Patrawala et al., 2005; Wu et al., 2008). This feature is relevant when implanted tumor models are treated with drugs that are substrates for efflux transporters that "pump" drugs out of the cell similar to the Hoechst dye. In addition, murine glioma cells can be enriched for tumor initiation potential by selection of cells expressing stem cell markers discussed later in the chapter (Kondo et al., 2004; Wu et al., 2008). Intriguingly, these populations of cells are not always overlapping, exposing several populations within cell lines that have features ascribed to cancer stem cells. Despite the presence of cancer stem cell features in long-established cell lines, we argue below that primary tumor cell lines grown in conditions that preserve the genotype and phenotype of primary tumor should become the mainstream model system to study cancer stem cell biology.

Establishment of Glioma Stem Cell Lines

Glioma cancer stem cell lines can be derived from surgical resection of primary brain tumors through in vitro culture in stem cell selective conditions. Reynolds and Weiss (1992) published the first reports of a serum-free culture medium that allowed the isolation of neural stem cells (NSCs) from adult mouse striatum. The isolated normal NSCs proliferated as free-floating spheres (neurospheres) in the presence of epidermal growth factor (EGF) and basic fibroblast growth factor (bFGF). These cells expressed nestin, a neural precursor intermediate filament, and were capable of generating progeny with the morphology and phenotypes characteristic of differentiated neurons and astrocytes of the adult striatum. Based on the ability for extended self-renewal and multipotency, these isolated brain cells fulfilled the criteria for stem cells. The growth factor supplemented serum-free culture method has become the standard condition for isolation and rigorous characterization of NSCs.

Using the NSC culture condition, a fraction of dissociated primary brain tumor cells proliferate as non-adherent spheres, which have subsequently been referred to as tumorspheres. Brain tumor cells expanded as tumorspheres have been implanted into the brain of immunocompromised mice to generate tumors displaying the hallmark histopathological features of high-grade gliomas: areas of necrosis surrounded by pseudo-palisade structures, microvascular proliferation, and pleomorphic nuclei with mitotic figures (Galli et al., 2004). Such tumors were also shown to self-renew in serial transplantation assays. Additionally, high-grade gliomas display diffuse infiltration and often recur at distant sites from the primary tumor. Serum-free cultured tumor cells are highly motile and can infiltrate into the surrounding cerebral cortex, migrate across the corpus callosum, and even extend into the contralateral hemisphere (Galli et al., 2004; Lee et al., 2006). These reports demonstrated that glioma cells cultured in serum-free conditions retained the ability to self-renew and phenocopy the parental brain tumor after transplantation, thereby operationally defining them as brain tumor stem cells (BTSCs). In the presence of differentiation inducing conditions, normal NSCs can generate neurons, astrocytes, or oligodendrocytes. BTSCs are aberrant in their differentiation, however, and are capable of generating progeny expressing markers of all brain lineages within a single tumor cell (Galli et al., 2004; Lee et al., 2006). While the stem cell associated feature of multipotency is retained by BTSCs, differentiation capacity alone is not sufficient to classify a tumor cell as a cancer stem cell.

Isolation and Enrichment of Glioma Stem Cells

Neurospheres and tumorspheres contain a heterogeneous population of cells due to two main factors: (i) short-lived immature progenitors also proliferate in serum-free media (Reynolds and Rietze, 2005; Suslov et al., 2002), (ii) the limited diffusion of nutrients and oxygen through the sphere results in spontaneous differentiation and apoptosis of cells near the core (Bez et al., 2003). Considerable attention has been directed at identifying cell surface markers that can be used to prospectively identify and select for true BTSCs from progenitors within the tumorspheres.

The first candidate cell surface marker identified for BTSCs was CD133, an epithelial and neural progenitor marker. Singh et al. (2004) reported that as few as 100 CD133$^+$ human brain tumor cells inoculated into immunocompromised mice were able to generate tumors with identical phenotypes to the

primary tumors. However, use of cell surface markers to enrich for BTSCs has been controversial since many exceptions, including CD15$^+$/CD133$^-$ BTSCs, have been isolated from primary human gliomas (Mao et al., 2009; Son et al., 2009). In addition, studies have shown that tissue culture conditions affect the expression of cell surface markers. Griguer et al. (2008) demonstrated that stable CD133$^-$ glioma cells become CD133$^+$ upon exposure to energetic stressors such as hypoxia or mitochondrial depletion. These results have further complicated the use of cell surface markers such as CD133 for enrichment of BTSCs.

In order to avoid the sole reliance on cell surface markers, BTSCs have also been identified using marker independent methods. The SP phenotype has been used to identify BTSCs enriched in drug efflux transporters (Bleau et al., 2009). Additionally, sorting of freshly isolated tumor cells based on autofluorescence in the FL1 channel has been proposed as method for purifying BTSCs (Clement et al., 2010). Furthermore, CD133$^+$, CD15$^+$, and FL1$^+$ cells are capable of generating CD133$^-$, CD15$^-$, and FL1$^-$ progeny, respectively. These observations supported a hierarchal model for these populations and suggested they had stem-cell properties originally attributed to leukemia stem cells. However, SP and non-SP populations in addition to FL1$^+$ and FL1$^-$ populations can contain CD133$^+$ cells (Bleau et al., 2009; Clement et al., 2010), suggesting that these methods do not isolate a homogenous population. A consistent immunophenotype that has been replicated by independent laboratories based on a cocktail of positive or negative selection markers that yields an unequivocally pure BTSC population has yet to be determined. Nonetheless, the neurosphere culture system is a viable approach to sustain BTSCs for experimentation.

Effect of Serum on Genetics, Gene Expression, and Phenotype

Analysis by multiple independent research groups has revealed significant differences between serum and serum-free cultured glioma cells. Cytogenetic analysis has demonstrated that long-term culturing of BTSCs (up to 70 passages) in serum-free conditions results in a relatively stable telomerase activity and karyotype

(Galli et al., 2004; Lee et al., 2006). In serum-free conditions, tumor cells remain relatively diploid except for glioma-specific gain or loss of chromosomes, e.g.: deletion of INK4a/ARF at chromosome 9, loss of chromosome 10q, and trisomy of chromosome 7. Global gene expression profiling revealed that tumorsphere cultures were remarkably similar to the parental tumors and normal NSCs and expressed high levels of stem cell/self-renewal associated genes, including Sox2, Oct4, Nanog, and Musashi family proteins (Lee et al., 2006). Interestingly, nervous system developmentally regulated genes (i.e.: HOX cluster, Hedgehog pathway, Notch pathway) are present across multiple tumorsphere-derived lines (Galli et al., 2004; Günther et al., 2008). These findings suggest that tumorsphere culture faithfully maintains glioma cells with a stem cell-like profile.

In stark contrast, current data suggests that exposure to serum rapidly and irreversibly changes the genotype and phenotype of the tumor cells in such a way that they no longer faithfully mimic the primary tumor. Global gene expression profiling revealed that serum-cultured primary tumor cells are more closely related to traditional serum cultured glioma lines (U87MG, U251), but markedly distinct from the parental tumors and matched serum-free cultured cells (Lee et al., 2006). It has also been reported that tumor cells maintained in serum initially lose telomerase activity, but regain high telomerase activity as cells adapt to culture in serum, typically occurring prior to 10 passage in vitro (Lee et al., 2006). In addition, serum-cultured glioma cells progressively undergo genomic rearrangements resulting in primarily polyploid cell lines. Unlike tumors formed upon transplantation of matched serum-free BTSCs, the tumors generated from primary cells cultured in serum did not phenocopy the array of histopathological features of the parental gliomas. Instead, serum cultured cells formed well circumscribed tumors that exhibited a "pushing" or mass effect growth pattern akin to brain metastases and established glioma cell lines such as U87MG (Lee et al., 2006). Since the ability to recapitulate the primary tumor is a pre-requisite criterion to be considered a cancer stem cell, it remains questionable if cell lines derived in serum should continue to be used in basic and preclinical research. The preferred use of serum-free culture systems offers a new avenue to generate biologically accurate models for interrogating cancer stem cell biology.

Requirements for Cytokines and Supplements in Tumorsphere Cultures

It is important to assess the requirements for cytokines and supplements in neurosphere cultures because these reagents add significant complexity and financial expenses relative to serum methods. Phillips et al. (2006) demonstrated the existence of a subclass of gliomas for which BTSCs proliferated in the absence of EGF and FGF. This proliferative subclass of gliomas (distinct from proneural and mesenchymal subclassifications) displays significantly higher PCNA and Ki67 immunohistological staining. BTSCs with the capacity for mitogen independent growth can form tumorspheres in serum-free media alone, but the addition of EGF and FGF increases the viability and number of tumorspheres (Kelly et al., 2009). Exogenous mitogen-independent BTSCs also initiated invasive high-grade gliomas in immunocompromised mice that were indistinguishable from EGF and FGF supplemented BTSCs. The absence of exogenous growth factors selects for the BTSC population that has acquired the genetic mutations for autocrine stimulation or constitutive activation of intracellular signaling pathways.

Similarly, we have investigated the requirement for commonly used supplements in the neurosphere system, namely B27 and N2. Results from human and mouse BTSCs cultured with EGF and FGF but without B27 demonstrated that B27 was not required for growth, but more than doubled growth rate in both systems (data not shown). Experiments performed to assess the requirement for N2 revealed similar trends. However, we did not determine what molecular subclass of glioma these lines were derived from and therefore these results are preliminary at best.

Modifications to the Serum-Free Tumorsphere Method

Although the tumorsphere method has allowed the prolonged culture of BTSCs, considerable emphasis has been placed on improving the serum-free culture condition. A major limitation to preclinical studies using the tumorsphere culture is that penetration of gene transfer reagents, antibodies, and drugs into the sphere is not homogenous. Furthermore, measurement of cell viability can be hampered by variable cell death within the necrotic core of the tumorsphere. One approach for eliminating the gradient of nutrients and therapeutics has been to promote cell proliferation as a monolayer on artificial extracellular matrix (ECM)/laminin coated plates. The utility of this method has been demonstrated with primary human glioma lines, but is equally appropriate for primary murine brain tumors (Fig. 21.1). This alternative method preserves the tumor-specific genomic abnormalities, nervous system developmental signaling, and stem cell associated profile of the primary tumors that is seen with the standard tumorsphere culture (Fael Al-Mayhani et al., 2009; Pollard et al., 2009). However, small changes in copy number of chromosomes can be detected at later passages (>50 passages in vitro). Despite minimal changes after extended monolayer culturing, the adherent serumfree culture condition has significant advantages and may prove to be better suited for high-throughput drug screening of BTSCs. From a practical stand point, media changes would be much faster if the cells were adherent, which is not a trivial consideration for large-scale drug screens or clinical tumor cell vaccine production.

In addition to adherence, recent studies suggest that oxygen, which is a master regulator of cell metabolism and gene expression, is an important variable in optimizing BTSC culture methodology. Oxygen levels in the mammalian brain range from 0.6 to 8% (Erecinska

and Silver, 2001). Similarly, oxygen concentrations are heterogeneous in the glioma microenvironment, ranging from 0.1 to 10% and trending towards lower oxygen tension as tumor grade increases (Evans et al., 2004). A desirable feature of tissue culture models is to mimic, as closely as possible, the in vivo tumor microenvironment so that experimentation is more likely yield answers that are relevant to tumor biology in situ. Therefore, the standard practice of culturing glioma cells at atmospheric oxygen ($\sim$20% O_2) is counterintuitive. In support of optimizing oxygen concentrations for BTSCs culture, glioma cells cultured in 1, 3, 5 or 7% O_2 exhibited increased expression of stem cell markers (Platet et al., 2007; Li et al., 2009; McCord et al., 2009) and in some cases enhanced selfrenewal and tumor initiation relative to cells cultured in 20% O_2 (Li et al., 2009; McCord et al., 2009).

Our laboratory has investigated the effect of oxygen levels on BTSC immunogenicity. We have demonstrated glioma cells grown in 5% O_2 are a superior source of vaccine antigen relative to cells grown in standard 20% O_2. Culture of glioma cells in tumor physiologic oxygen increased the activation, proliferation, and tumoricidal function of cytotoxic T lymphocytes through mechanisms requiring toll-like receptor two (Olin et al., 2010). In addition, we documented that glioma cells grown in 5% O_2 expressed higher levels of known glioma associated antigens such as Sox2 and IL-13Rα2. On the basis of these studies, we have initiated a clinical trial treating glioma patients with a BTSC vaccine produced in 5% O_2. Further studies

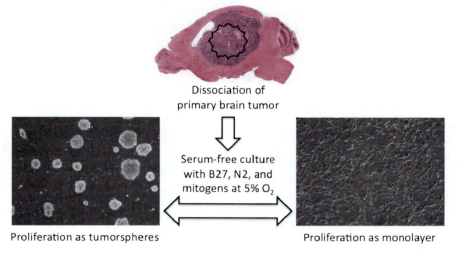

Dissociation of
primary brain tumor

Serum-free culture
with B27, N2, and
mitogens at 5% O_2

Proliferation as tumorspheres   Proliferation as monolayer

Fig. 21.1 Primary tumor cells have been isolated from a murine glioma and grown in complete stem cell media. These cell lines can be readily manipulated to expand as tumorspheres or as a monolayer culture on Matrigel

are warranted to better understand how tissue culture oxygen may change BTSC biology.

Discussion

Recent studies have demonstrated that the cancer stem cell model initially validated in leukemia may apply to solid tumors, including brain tumors. If indeed gliomas are propagated by a slowly dividing stem-like cell that gives rise to proliferative cells that propagate the disease, then only animal models that mimic this hierarchy will be predicative of treatment efficacy in the human disease. However, there has been a disconnect between the emerging view of cancer as a stem cell disease requiring therapeutic targeting of BTSCs and the standard practice of using of long-established serum-cultured lines in the laboratory. Pioneering studies have demonstrated that standard tissue culture conditions (e.g., animal serum and atmospheric oxygen) markedly change the genetics, gene expression, phenotype, differentiation, and immunogenicity of the cultured cells in a way that makes them less reflective of the primary tumor. As a result, transplantation of cell lines grown in serum does not faithfully recapitulate all the phenotypic features of heterogeneous tumors. It is worth considering how these standard xenograft models may contribute to "false positive" therapeutic responses in preclinical settings leading to minimal changes in the dismal prognosis for patients with malignant glioma. A paradigm shift in experimental therapeutics in which complete elimination of the stem cell compartment will be required to affect a cure is clearly warranted. Implementation of recent improvements in BTSC culture methodology as part of the mainstream system for basic research has great potential to enhance preclinical modeling.

One area of preclinical modeling that deserves attention is the relationship between invasive growth (or lack thereof) and drug delivery across the blood-brain barrier (BBB). The central core of tumors is highly angiogenic, containing new and leaky blood vessels, and this leakiness actually allows diagnosis via contrast-enhanced MRI using gadolinium. However, the disruption of brain vasculature is directly related to tumor size and the distance from the central core (Jain et al., 2007). Furthermore, the BBB is intact at the growing edge of the tumor, near diffusely infiltrating glioma cells, and early in the development

of the vascular niche of BTSCs (Gilbertson and Rich, 2007). Where the BBB is intact, systemically administered large and small molecule therapeutics must traverse the capillary membrane to obtain access to the brain. Fine et al. (2006) demonstrated that the concentration of paclitaxel in the central core of human brain tumors was twice as high as in the immediate tumor periphery and ten-fold higher than in the normal brain surrounding the tumor. The need for chemotherapeutics to reach the bulk tumor mass, the growing edge of the tumor, and invasive glioma cells lends credence to the optimization of systemic circulation for delivery of drug treatments.

An important feature of BTSC culture conditions is the ability to generate xenografts that can phenocopy the heterogeneity and infiltrative nature of the primary tumor. This heterogeneity, which may involve cells that differentially efflux drugs and intrinsically resist apoptosis, is one likely explanation for the failure of drugs that work by a single mechanism of action. Moreover, since a subpopulation of BTSCs are also resistant to radiation therapies (Bao et al., 2006), long-term efficacy of chemotherapeutics will depend upon drug delivery to the invasive glioma cells residing behind an intact, functional BBB throughout the entire brain. Unfortunately, the well-circumscribed tumors that arise when standard serum-cultured cell lines are inoculated into the rodent brain are likely to overestimate drug efficacy because these xenografts lack an appreciable tumor population protected by an intact BBB. In contrast, BTSC lines grown in serum-free conditions are capable of generating "whole-brain disease" illustrated by diffuse infiltration into normal brain structures. Therefore, BTSC culture conditions have the potential to facilitate major advances in preclinical evaluation of novel drugs by accurately modeling the impact of invasion on drug delivery. Widespread acceptance of these tissue culture protocols, including serum-free media, adherence, and tumor physiologic oxygen, should facilitate development of effective targeted therapies of glioma in the foreseeable future.

References

Bao S, Wu Q, McLendon RE, Hao Y, Shi Q, Hjelmeland AB, Dewhirst MW, Bigner DD, Rich JN (2006) Glioma stem cells promote radioresistance by preferential activation of the DNA damage response. Nature 444:756–760

Bez A, Corsini E, Curti D, Biggiogera M, Colombo A, Nicosia RF, Pagano SF, Parati EA (2003) Neurosphere and neurosphere-forming cells: morphological and ultrastructural characterization. Brain Res 993:18–29

Bleau A-M, Hambardzumyan D, Ozawa T, Fomchenko EI, Huse JT, Brennan CW, Holland EC (2009) PTEN/PI3K/akt pathway regulates the side population phenotype and ABCG2 activity in glioma tumor stem-like cells. Cell Stem Cell 4:226–235

Clarke MF, Dick JE, Dirks PB, Eaves C, Jamieson C, Jones D, Visvader J, Weissman IL, Wahl G (2006) Cancer stem cells–perspectives on current status and future directions: AACR workshop on cancer stem cells. Cancer Res 66:9339–9344

Clement V, Marino D, Cudalbu C, Hamou M-F, Mlynarik V, de Tribolet N, Dietrich P-Y, Gruetter R, Hegi ME, Radovanovic I (2010) Marker-independent identification of glioma-initiating cells. Nat Methods 7:224–228

Erecinska M, Silver IA (2001) Tissue oxygen tension and brain sensitivity to hypoxia. Respir Physiol 128:263–276

Evans SM, Judy KD, Dunphy I, Jenkins WT, Hwang WT, Nelson PT, Lustig RA, Jenkins K, Magarelli DP, Hahn SM, Collins RA, Grady MS, Koch CJ (2004) Hypoxia is important in the biology and aggression of human glial brain tumors. Clin Cancer Res 10:8177–8184

Fael Al-Mayhani TM, Ball SLR, Zhao J-W, Fawcett J, Ichimura K, Collins PV, Watts C (2009) An efficient method for derivation and propagation of glioblastoma cell lines that conserves the molecular profile of their original tumours. J Neurosci Methods 176:192–199

Fine RL, Chen J, Balmaceda C, Bruce JN, Huang M, Desai M, Sisti MB, McKhann GM, Goodman RR, Bertino JS Jr., Nafziger AN, Fetell MR (2006) Randomized study of paclitaxel and tamoxifen deposition into human brain tumors: implications for the treatment of metastatic brain tumors. Clin Cancer Res 12:5770–5776

Galli R, Binda E, Orfanelli U, Cipelletti B, Gritti A, De Vitis S, Fiocco R, Foroni C, Dimeco F, Vescovi AL (2004) Isolation and characterization of tumorigenic, stem-like neural precursors from human glioblastoma. Cancer Res 64:7011–7021

Gilbertson RJ, Rich JN (2007) Making a tumour's bed: glioblastoma stem cells and the vascular niche. Nat Rev Cancer 7:733–736

Griguer CE, Oliva CR, Gobin E, Marcorelles P, Benos DJ, Lancaster JR Jr, Gillespie GY (2008) CD133 is a marker of bioenergetic stress in human glioma. PLoS One 3:e3655

Günther HS, Schmidt NO, Phillips HS, Kemming D, Kharbanda S, Soriano R, Modrusan Z, Meissner H, Westphal M, Lamszus K (2008) Glioblastoma-derived stem cell-enriched cultures form distinct subgroups according to molecular and phenotypic criteria. Oncogene 27:2897–2909

Hope KJ, Jin L, Dick JE (2004) Acute myeloid leukemia originates from a hierarchy of leukemic stem cell classes that differ in self-renewal capacity. Nat Immunol 5:738–743

Jain RK, di Tomaso E, Duda DG, Loeffler JS, Sorensen AG, Batchelor TT (2007) Angiogenesis in brain tumours. Nat Rev Neurosci 8:610–622

Kelly JJP, Stechishin O, Chojnacki A, Lun X, Sun B, Senger DL, Forsyth P, Auer RN, Dunn JF, Cairncross JG, Parney IF, Weiss S (2009) Proliferation of human glioblastoma stem cells occurs independently of exogenous mitogens. Stem Cells 27:1722–1733

Kondo T, Setoguchi T, Taga T (2004) Persistence of a small subpopulation of cancer stem-like cells in the C6 glioma cell line. Proc Natl Acad Sci 101:781–786

Lapidot T, Sirard C, Vormoor J, Murdoch B, Hoang T, Caceres-Cortes J, Minden M, Paterson B, Caligiuri MA, Dick JE (1994) A cell initiating human acute myeloid leukaemia after transplantation into SCID mice. Nature 367:645–648

Lee J, Kotliarova S, Kotliarov Y, Li A, Su Q, Donin NM, Pastorino S, Purow BW, Christopher N, Zhang W, Park JK, Fine HA (2006) Tumor stem cells derived from glioblastomas cultured in bFGF and EGF more closely mirror the phenotype and genotype of primary tumors than do serum-cultured cell lines. Cancer Cell 9:391–403

Li Z, Bao S, Wu Q, Wang H, Eyler C, Sathornsumetee S, Shi Q, Cao Y, Lathia J, McLendon RE, Hjelmeland AB, Rich JN (2009) Hypoxia-inducible factors regulate tumorigenic capacity of glioma stem cells. Cancer Cell 15:501–513

Mao X-G, Zhang X, Xue X-Y, Guo G, Wang P, Zhang W, Fei Z, Zhen H-N, You S-W, Yang H (2009) Brain tumor stem-like cells identified by neural stem cell marker CD15. Transl Oncol 2:247–257

McCord AM, Jamal M, Shankavarum UT, Lang FF, Camphausen K, Tofilon PJ (2009) Physiologic oxygen concentration enhances the stem-like properties of CD133+ human glioblastoma cells in vitro. Mol Cancer Res 7:489–497

Olin MR, Andersen BM, Zellmer DM, Grogan PT, Popescu FE, Xiong Z, Forster CL, Seiler C, SantaCruz KS, Chen W, Blazar BR, Ohlfest JR (2010) Superior efficacy of tumor cell vaccines grown in physiologic oxygen. Clin Cancer Res 16:4800–4808

Patrawala L, Calhoun T, Schneider-Broussard R, Zhou J, Claypool K, Tang DG (2005) Side population is enriched in tumorigenic, stem-like cancer cells, whereas ABCG2+ and ABCG2- cancer cells are similarly tumorigenic. Cancer Res 65:6207–6219

Phillips HS, Kharbanda S, Chen R, Forrest WF, Soriano RH, Wu TD, Misra A, Nigro JM, Colman H, Soroceanu L, Williams PM, Modrusan Z, Feuerstein BG, Aldape KD (2006) Molecular subclasses of high-grade glioma predict prognosis, delineate a pattern of disease progression, and resemble stages in neurogenesis. Cancer Cell 9:157–173

Platet N, Liu SY, Atifi ME, Oliver L, Vallette FM, Berger F, Wion D (2007) Influence of oxygen tension on CD133 phenotype in human glioma cell cultures. Cancer Lett 258:286–290

Pollard SM, Yoshikawa K, Clarke ID, Danovi D, Stricker S, Russell R, Bayani J, Head R, Lee M, Bernstein M, Squire JA, Smith A, Dirks P (2009) Glioma stem cell lines expanded in adherent culture have tumor-specific phenotypes and are suitable for chemical and genetic screens. Cell Stem Cell 4:568–580

Quintana E, Shackleton M, Sabel MS, Fullen DR, Johnson TM, Morrison SJ (2008) Efficient tumour formation by single human melanoma cells. Nature 456:593–598

Reynolds BA, Rietze RL (2005) Neural stem cells and neurospheres–re-evaluating the relationship. Nat Methods 2:333–336

Reynolds BA, Weiss S (1992) Generation of neurons and astrocytes from isolated cells of the adult mammalian central nervous system. Science 255:1707–1710

Singh SK, Hawkins C, Clarke ID, Squire J, Bayani J, Hide T, Henkelman R, Cusimano M, Dirks PB (2004) Identification of human brain tumour initiating cells. Nature 432: 396–401

Son MJ, Woolard K, Nam D-H, Lee J, Fine HA (2009) SSEA-1 is an enrichment marker for tumor-initiating cells in human glioblastoma. Cell Stem Cell 4:440–452

Suslov ON, Kukekov VG, Ignatova TN, Steindler DA (2002) Neural stem cell heterogeneity demonstrated by molecular phenotyping of clonal neurospheres. Proc Natl Acad Sci USA 99:14506–14511

Wu A, Oh S, Wiesner SM, Ericson K, Chen L, Hall WA, Champoux PE, Low WC, Ohlfest JR (2008) Persistence of CD133+ cells in human and mouse glioma cell lines: detailed characterization of GL261 glioma cells with cancer stem cell-like properties. Stem Cells Dev 17: 173–184

Chapter 22

Glioblastoma Cancer Stem Cells: Response to Epidermal Growth Factor Receptor Kinase Inhibitors

Federica Barbieri, Adriana Bajetto, Alessandra Pattarozzi, Monica Gatti, Roberto Würth, Carola Porcile, Antonio Daga, Roberto E. Favoni, Giorgio Corte, and Tullio Florio

Abstract Glioblastoma (GBM) is the most common and aggressive neoplasia of the central nervous system in adults. Despite continued improvements in surgery, chemotherapy, and radiotherapy, clinical outcome is still dismal and better understanding of GBM biology is needed to develop novel therapies. Recent studies have demonstrated the existence of a small subpopulation of cells with stem-like features termed cancer stem cells (CSCs) in several human cancers, including GBM. CSCs are slow growing, self-renewable and highly tumorigenic, give rise to progeny of multiple lineages, and are chemo-radio-resistant, often expressing high levels of multidrug resistance and drug efflux genes. According to CSC hypothesis, current therapies are cytotoxic to the bulk of highly proliferative tumor cells but fail to kill the relatively quiescent and resistant CSC subpopulation, thus allowing these cells to survive and induce tumor recurrence. These characteristics allow GBM CSCs to survive cytotoxic therapies and drive tumor recurrence. The epidermal growth factor receptor (EGFR/HER1) belongs to the receptor tyrosine kinase (TK) family that regulates cell proliferation, survival, differentiation and motility. Overexpression of EGFR occurs in several tumors, including GBM, correlates with increased cell proliferation, decreased apoptosis, and a poorer prognosis, sustaining cancer development and progression. Small-molecules targeting EGFR-TK (TK inhibitors, TKIs) are the most clinically developed EGFR targeted-therapies for the treatment of GBM. We reported that cultures enriched in CSC isolated from human GBMs undergo growth arrest and cell death in the presence of EGFR-TKIs. The high incidence of EGFR overexpression, amplification or co-expression of the mutated, constitutively active EGFRvIII in GBMs raised expectations that treatment with EGFR TKIs, such as gefitinib or erlotinib, would have significant positive effects. This review summarizes current knowledge regarding EGFR molecular abnormalities and dysregulation in high-grade gliomas, the role of CSCs in GBM, and discusses the implications of the CSC hypothesis for the development of future EGFR-targeted therapies for brain tumors.

Keywords Glioblastoma · Cancer stem cells · Tyrosine kinase inhibitors · ERK1/2 · Akt

Introduction

EGFR and Molecular Signaling Pathways

Epidermal growth factor receptor (EGFR/HER1) is a well-characterized, widely expressed 170 KDa single-chain transmembrane glycoprotein (Mendelsohn and Baselga, 2006), belonging to the human epidermal growth factor receptor (HER) family, composed of four members (HER1-4). EGFR is structured in four functional domains: an extracellular ligand-binding domain, a hydrophobic transmembrane domain, an intracellular tyrosine kinase (TK) domain ending with a C-terminus regulatory domain. EGFR, whose gene is located on chromosome 7p12-13, shares a high degree of amino-acid sequence homology with the avian erythroblastosis virus, v-erbB (Gschwind et al., 2004)

T. Florio (✉)
Laboratory of Pharmacology, Department of Oncology, Biology and Genetics, University of Genova, 16132 Genova, Italy
e-mail: Tullio.florio@unige.it

M.A. Hayat (ed.), *Tumors of the Central Nervous System, Volume 1*,
DOI 10.1007/978-94-007-0344-5_22, © Springer Science+Business Media B.V. 2011

Several ligands bind to HER receptor family; in particular EGF, TGF-α, epigen and amphiregulin specifically bind to EGFR, other related proteins (beta-cellulin, epiregulin, heparin-binding EGF) bind both EGFR and HER4. The binding of ligands to EGFR induces homo- or hetero-dimerization among the HER family, and the activation of the TK domain that, in turn, triggers trans/autophosphorylation of multiple tyrosines located on the receptor itself. This activates a series of intracellular signaling cascades to affect cytosolic tyrosine kinase activity and gene transcription, which cause cell proliferation, inhibition of apoptosis, invasion and metastasis and also stimulates angiogenesis. It was shown that EGFR may also exist as preformed dimers in the cell membrane and a ligand-induced conformational change stimulates its intrinsic kinase activity (Yarden, 2001).

Three major EGFR intracellular signalling pathways have been identified. The first one involves Ras-Raf-mitogen-activated protein kinase (MAPK, mainly ERK1/2) signalling, in which phosphorylated EGFR activates the small G protein Ras. Activated, GTP-bound, Ras stimulates the Raf-MEK-MAPK cascade to affect gene transcription, G1/S cell-cycle progression, and cell proliferation. The second pathway involves the phosphoinositol 3-kinase (PI3-K)-Akt-mammalian target of rapamycin (mTOR) cascade, which modulates the major cellular survival and anti-apoptosic signals via the activation of transcription factors, such as NFkB.

Other downstream targets of EGFR are the phospholipase C/protein kinase C (PKC) and the Janus kinase/signal transducers (JAK) and activators of transcription (STAT) pathways. Phospholipase C cleaves phosphatidyl inositol 4, 5,-bisphosphate (PIP2) to inositol 3-phosphate, which leads to the release of Ca^{++} from intracellular stores and, in concert with diacyl glycerol, the activation of PKC. PKC, in turn, can cross-talk with the Raf-MEK-MAPK pathway, via the direct phosphorylation and activation of Raf-1 (Yarden, 2001). STATs stimulate transcription of factors that promote cell survival and oncogenesis, and are activated by EGFR signaling either directly, by EGFR mediated JAK activation, or indirectly through Src kinase family. As the known cellular processes influenced by EGFR signaling continue to grow, the effects of the complete biochemical network associated to EGFR activation could involve further, not entirely known, actors. Inactivation of the EGFR can

be mediated either by receptor dephosphorylation by phosphotyrosine phosphatases (Pan et al., 1992) or receptor downregulation. Receptor downregulation is the most prominent regulator of EGFR signal attenuation and involves the internalization and subsequent degradation of the activated receptor in the lysosomes (Yarden, 2001).

Glioblastoma and EGFR

GBM is an aggressive, primary tumor of the central nervous system that follows a rapidly letal clinical course mainly because of its highly infiltrative nature. Classified as World Health Organization grade IV astrocytic tumors, GBMs have a pronounced mitotic activity, marked tendency toward microvascular proliferation, necrosis, and high proliferative rates. Despite the survival advantage provided by recently developed protocols of concurrent radio-therapy and adjuvant alkylating chemotherapy with temozolomide, the prognosis of patients with GBM remains poor, with median overall survival of about 12 months and 2-year survival rates of 26%, in the most favorable subgroup (Furnari et al., 2007).

The clinical course of the vast majority of GBMs is characterized by rapid development without clinical, radiological or morphologic evidence of a less malignant precursor lesion (primary or de novo GBMs), in contrast to secondary GBMs that develop by progression from lower-grade astrocytomas. At molecular level, EGFR amplification and overexpression is more frequent in primary than in secondary GBMs. The observation that EGFR gene is often amplified in GBM supports its potential role as a therapeutic target, since its activation modulates cell proliferation, motility and survival, and imbalance in the EGFR-ligand system leading to an increase in EGFR signaling, gives rise to neoplastic transformation.

Independent or combined mechanisms can lead to EGFR oncogenic activity: increased autocrine levels of the ligands (mainly EGF and TGFα), overexpression of EGFR protein (found in 40–50% of GBMs), cross-talk with heterologous receptor systems, and EGFR mutations producing defective or constitutively active variants of the receptor. In clinical oncology, deregulation of EGFR activity leads to chemo- and radio-resistance, disease progression and poor overall survival. Beside GBM, EGFR function is dysregulated in other human cancers including lung, head and neck, breast, colon and bladder malignancies (Citri and Yarden, 2006) in which several deletions and mutations of EGFR were described that result in increased catalytic TK activity (Mendelsohn and Baselga, 2003).

In GBM, overexpression and constitutive activation, via genomic alterations of EGFR, occur almost exclusively in primary tumors. Many intrinsic alterations of the receptor structure have been described such as the extracellular domain deletions of the EGFR gene (named EGFR vI, vII and vIII) frequently detected in GBMs. EGFRvIII is the most common mutant form (occurring in 30% of all GBM and in 50% of those with amplified wild type EGFR), which encoded for protein called Δ-EGFR, that lacks the exons 2–7 of the extracellular ligand-binding domain and displays ligand-independent constitutive activation of the tyrosine kinase domain (Furnari et al., 2007; Mendelsohn and Baselga, 2003). EGFRvIII variant has been found, although less frequently, in breast cancer and NSCLC but, in contrast to w.t. EGFR, it is not expressed in normal tissues. The sustained oncogenic signal increases cell proliferation and reduces apoptosis, leading to enhanced tumorigenic behavior of human GBM cells (Narita et al., 2002). Recently, novel missense mutations have been also identified in the intracellular domain of about 13% of GBM and GBM cell lines studied (Lee et al., 2006) providing alternative mechanism of EGFR activation in this tumor. On the contrary, mutations of EGFR TK domain occur almost exclusively in non-small lung cancer (Pao et al., 2004).

EGFRvIII activates canonical EGF-dependent signal transduction cascades to promote tumor growth. The Ras/MEK/MAPK signalling pathway, involved in proliferation and cell-cycle progression and the PI3-K/Akt/mTOR cascade, inhibiting apoptosis, emerged as central players in GBM pathogenesis by promoting proliferation, tumorigenesis, migration, invasion, tumor-induced neovascularization and impairing apoptosis. In addition, PTEN (phosphatase and tensin homolog on chromosome 10), a tumor suppressor gene, negatively regulating the PI3-K pathway, is mutated and inactivated in almost half gliomas (Furnari et al., 2007). Expression of EGFRvIII in gliomas was demonstrated to promote tumor formation and growth, and it has been suggested that this occurs through constitutively active PI3-K/Akt pathway and

through the MAPK pathway. Patients with EGFRvIII-expressing tumors have a shorter interval to clinical recurrence after treatment and poorer survival times than patients with EGFRvIII-negative tumors (Bax et al., 2009).

Thus, molecular profiling of GBM may enable the identification of subgroups among phenotypically homogeneous tumors, as far as PI3K activation status, PTEN loss and EGFRvIII expression could be particularly helpful for the optimal use of EGFR-TKI in GBM patients. Indeed, a correlation between co-expression of EGFRvIII and PTEN has been shown in recurrent GBMs samples from patients who have been treated with EGFR-TKI, influencing drug responsiveness (Mellinghoff et al., 2005). Moreover, the combined treatment with the EGFR-TKI erlotinib and rapamycin (mTOR inhibitor) has been shown to increase the response of PTEN-deficient GBM cells (Wang et al., 2006). Activated EGFR (EGFRvIII) has also been shown to be responsible of the radio and chemoresistance of GBM cells through the enhancement of resistance to apoptosis. In addition to EGFR signaling pathway, other receptor TKs (such as PDGFR, VEGFR and MET) that are simultaneously activated in GBMs, should be included in the detail of tumor molecular profile, since these receptors frequently cooperate in tumor cell signaling. The cross-talk between receptor TKs may be targeted with multiple kinase inhibitors or combined regimens, to enhance cytotoxicity and to achieve a better management of the disease (Furnari et al., 2007).

Anticancer Drugs Targeting EGFR

A number of strategies have been developed to specifically target EGFR, including small-molecule targeting EGFR TK (TK inhibitors, TKIs) that inactivate the tyrosine kinase domain, anti-EGFR mAbs that can target directly to extracellular epitopes, peptide vaccination therapy, conjugates of toxins to anti-EGFR antibodies and EGFR ligands, radio-immuno-conjugates and RNA based therapies.

Some of these are now being used clinically including monoclonal Abs, EGFR-TKI and ligand conjugates (Sharma et al., 2009). Monoclonal antibodies (i.e. cetuximab and panitumumab) mainly act through the binding to the extracellular domain of the EGFR competing with its natural ligands and/or provoking the internalization of Ab/EGFR complex, thus preventing receptor phosphorylation. On the other hand, EGFR TKIs competitively bind to the ATP-binding pocket of the intracellular EGFR catalytic domain, reversibly blocking the catalytic activity and inhibiting the receptor autophosphorylation and downstream signaling. EGFR-TKIs are generally less specific than Ab, since their molecular target, the EGFR-ATP-binding site, is similar among TKs, thus in many cases they may inhibit various growth factor TK receptors, such as other EGFR family members or PDGFR and VEGFR (Karaman et al., 2008).

Gefitinib (Iressa) and erlotinib (Tarceva) are two orally active quinazoline derivatives EGFR TKIs that share very similar physico-chemical and pharmacological features.

Both drugs affect cell growth and survival through the inhibition of ERK1/2 and Akt pathways as a consequence of EGFR-TK blockade. Indeed, Akt may represent a molecular determinant for gefitinib responsiveness since Akt activation is down-regulated in response to this drug in NSCLC cell lines. In addition apoptosis is considered a relevant mechanism for EGFR-TKI-mediated anticancer effects, following the disruption of the balance between anti- and pro-apoptotic Bcl-2 family proteins. Accordingly to the multiple EGFR mediated biological activities, EGFR-TKIs induce both pro-apoptotic and antiproliferative activity. In particular, in in vitro cancer models, these molecules induce cell cycle arrest in the G1-S phase transition, a critical step in cell cycle regulation, up-regulation of p27^{KIP1}, p21^{WAF1} and p15^{INK4b} (cyclin-dependent kinase inhibitor proteins) leading to growth inhibition. In normal cells EGFR participates to the control of cytoskeleton organization and cell morphology while in cancer cells this regulation is disrupted leading to the malignant phenotype. EGFR-TKIs, such as gefitinib have been shown to block EGF-dependent cytoskeleton re-organization and cell invasiveness (Barnes et al., 2003).

Other clinically approved EGFR inhibitors active on multiple TKs and under investigation for the therapy of GBM include lapatinib (Tykerb, inhibitor of EGFR, and HER2) and vandetanib (Zactima, active on EGF and VEGFR). Investigational combination therapies include erlotinib and gefitinib in association with the mTOR inhibitors everolimus (Afinitor), and temsirolimus (Torisel) (Loew et al., 2009).

Current Status of EGFR-TKIs in Clinical Trials for Glioblastoma

The current standard treatment for patients with high-grade gliomas is multi-modal, including maximal safe surgical resection, followed by a combination of radiation and chemotherapy with temozolomide, followed by adjuvant chemotherapy with temozolomide (Temodar). Adjuvant chemotherapy with procarbazine, lomustine and vincristine (PCV regimen) has failed to improve survival in prospective randomized studies, both in grade IV and in grade III tumors. Nevertheless, based on a large meta-analysis nitrosourea-based chemotherapy may marginally improve survival in selected patients. Implantation of chemotherapy-impregnated wafers (carmustine polymer, Gliadel) into the resection cavity before radiotherapy has shown to improve marginally the median survival compared with radiotherapy alone.

The introduction of temozolomide in combination with radiotherapy increased 2-year survival rate from 10 to 26% and the median survival of patients with GBM by 3 months when compared with radiotherapy alone (Stupp et al., 2005). Also, epigenetic silencing of the O6-methylguanine-DNA methyltransferase (MGMT) DNA repair gene by methylation causes impairment of DNA repair and has been associated with increased patient survival. In fact, it was showed that GBM patients treated with a methylated MGMT promoter together with temozolomide and radiotherapy resulted in a median survival of 21.7 months (Hegi et al., 2005). However, the constant recurrence of GBM makes the continuous search for more effective treatments both for initial therapy and at the time of relapse an unavoidable goal for the pharmacological research.

Among new drugs designed to interfere with specific cellular targets in cancer cells, EGFR-TKIs have produced interesting response in NSCLC patients. Since EGFR represents a particularly selective target in malignant gliomas and the intracranial delivery of standard anticancer agents is limited, the small molecules EGFR-TKI may represent an innovative therapeutic approach for brain tumors and metastases. Several clinical trials report the use of gefitinib and erlotinib in brain malignancies, but, despite many pre-clinical studies evidenced EGFR as an important target in GBM tumorigenesis, in vivo studies did not meet the expectations and only modest antitumoral activity has been reported among recurrent GBM patients treated with erlotinib or gefitinib (Raizer et al., 2010). In addition, a phase II trial evaluating the efficacy of gefitinib monotherapy in recurrent GBMs did not show improvement in progression-free survival at 6 months being not different from historical controls (Rich et al., 2004). The analysis of both wild type and constitutively active mutant EGFR forms in patients treated with gefitinib revealed the lack of association of either form with sensitivity to gefitinib.

Although EGFR TKIs show insufficient activity in unselected patients with GBM, these drugs may be efficacious in selected groups of patients bearing particular biomarkers. The molecular analysis of tissue derived from clinical trials may help to understand the failure of in vivo treatments. To determine whether molecular effects of erlotinib or gefitinib were associated with clinical responses, EGFR signalling was investigated at molecular level in vivo, in tissue derived from patients enrolled in the North American Brain Tumor Consortium (NABTC) multicenter phase I/II clinical trial 01–03. This study showed no obvious association between erlotinib/gefitinib sensitivity and effects on EGFR expression and phosphorylation, or with the activation of downstream signalling (RAS/MAPK or PI3-K/AKT). Similarly, the analysis of EGFR mutations did not evidence any correlation with EGFR TKI treatment (Lassman et al., 2005). Two retrospective studies identified PTEN and EGFR as molecular determinants of response to erlotinib treatment. The co-expression of EGFRvIII and PTEN was significantly associated with clinical response to erlotinib treatment (Mellinghoff et al., 2005) and a better response to erlotinib was observed in patients with GBM bearing high levels of EGFR expression and low levels of phosphorylated Akt (Haas-Kogan et al., 2005). However, a recent European randomized phase II study compared erlotinib administered alone or with either temozolomide or carmustine, as standard treatments, describing opposite results. No response with erlotinib treatment, or EGFR overexpression was observed. In addition, all patients that co-expressed PTEN and EGFRvIII, rapidly progress after erlotinib treatment (van den Bent et al., 2009). These findings, being still contradictory, rise the obvious question why these drugs failed to produce clinical results despite EGFR signalling is activated in almost 50% of GBMs. The insufficient correlation between inhibitions of EGFR signalling may reflect an insufficient drug penetration into tumor or may be do to a limited tumor dependence on EGFR pathway. Both erlotinib and gefitinib are relatively polar and have low molecular weight allowing a good penetration of the blood-brain barrier. However, tumor tissue penetration of erlotinib corresponds to 6–8% of the plasma concentration reflecting an insufficient drug delivery (Lassman et al., 2005; Karpel-Massler et al., 2009). Moreover, even in the presence of altered expression of EGFR, growth and migration of tumor cells may depend on other growth factors that act independently or together with EGF. In this hypothesis, it is clear that a single target therapy is unlikely to control the complex biology of GBM and the use of erlotinib or gefitinib in combination with other target therapy, radiation and chemotherapy, may improve the clinical effect.

The EGF growth dependency of tumors may be linked to the grade or the origin. Low and high-grade glioma have distinct, albeit overlapping genetic alterations. EGFR gene amplification and PTEN mutations are common in de novo GBMs and both of these alterations are infrequent in secondary GBMs that commonly contain TP53 mutations and PDGFR gene amplifications. Radiotherapy may increase EGFR activation and EGFR over-expression in pre-clinical models to increase resistance to that treatment (Prados et al., 2008). EGFR amplification confers resistance to alkylating-based treatments, including temozolomide. Early inhibition of EGFR may give better response and potentially improve the radiotherapy and chemotherapy response. The combined treatment of erlotinib and temozolomide during and following radiotherapy had better survival than historical controls (Prados et al., 2009). However, a very similar study conducted in North Central Cancer Treatment Group Study N0177 led to different conclusions. Likely differences in survival after similar pharmacological treatment should reflect differences in patient characteristics (Brown et al., 2008).

Among the possible factors limiting EGFR TKIs clinical benefit, the activation of downstream pathway component or alternative intracellular pathway by additional growth factor receptors may counterbalance the inhibition of EGFR activation. Preclinical studies have shown that the antitumor activity of EGFR TKIs can be enhanced by the combination with mTOR inhibitor. mTOR is a downstream target of the PI3-K pathway on which converges also the signalling generated by the loss of PTEN. The simultaneous targeting of upstream and downstream mediator of PI3-K signal may produce greater antitumor activity. Based on this rationale phase II clinical trials using gefitinib and sirolimus have been developed and are currently in progress (Karpel-Massler et al., 2009).

Cancer Stem Cells and Glioblastoma

One of the most attracting concepts in cancer research today is the cancer stem cell (CSC) hypothesis. It was proposed that a minority of transformed progenitors or stem cells, with deregulated self-renewal properties, is the source of tumor cell renewal and may influence tumor behavior, including proliferation, response to chemo- and radio-therapy and metastatic spreading. Indeed, cancers, like normal tissues, are composed of phenotypically and morphologically heterogeneous cell populations (Hanahan and Weinberg, 2000) but with a homogenous genetic background, suggesting that they might derive from a rare CSC population. Thereby, two cell populations can be identified in cancers: CSCs a minority of undifferentiated, limitless self-renewing and slow-cycling cells, and a larger population of differentiated tumor cells fast growing but with proliferative capacity restricted only to few cycles (Reya et al., 2001). CSCs share some fundamental properties with normal stem cells: self-renewal, ability to multilineage differentiation and expression of distinctive stem biomarkers (Fig. 22.1). In operational terms, the CSCs are the only cancer cells able to initiate a tumor when xenotransplanted in immunocompromised mice, so that they are also called tumor initiating cells (TICs) to highliglht their tumorigenic potential.

Till now, potential CSCs have been identified in hematologic malignancies and solid tumors such as breast, prostate, pancreas, head and neck, colon and primary GBMs (Reya et al., 2001). Several pathways (i.e. Wnt, Notch and Sonic Hedgehog), known to regulate normal stem cell fate and self-renewal are beginning to be elucidated also in CSC. Furthermore, tumor suppressor genes such as PTEN and TP53 (tumor protein p53) have also been implicated in the regulation of CSC self-renewal, and their deregulation leads to uncontrolled self-renewal and tumorigenesis.

CSCs have been isolated from different CNS tumors, such as adult and pediatric gliomas, anaplastic olidendrogliomas, medulloblastomas and ependymomas (Hadjipanayis and Van Meir, 2009). The identification of CSCs (or TICs) in GBM may explain, at least in part, some biological and clinical evidence of GBMs, such as cell type heterogeneity and resistance to radiation and chemotherapy. In fact, due to their potential capability to recapitulate an entire tumor, these cancer stem or progenitor cells have been hypothesized to be responsible for the relapse and chemo- and radio-resistance. GBMs are known for resistance to therapy, which has been attributed to DNA-repair ability (Bao et al., 2006), a number of deregulated molecular pathways (elongated cell cycle and enhanced basal activation of checkpoint proteins) and, more recently, to the particular biological behavior of tumor stem-like cells. Different mechanisms have been detected in GBM CSCs that make them a difficult target for antineoplastic agents: the expression of HOX genes, encoding homeodomain transcription factors, the elevated expression of anti-apoptotic and multidrug resistance-associated protein (MRP), overexpression of multiple ion channels (i.e. chloride intracellular channel 1, CLIC1) (Stiles and Rowitch, 2008). In addition, CSCs express antigens specific for neural progenitor and stem cells including nestin, a neurofilament protein, the glycoprotein CD133 (prominin-1), identified as a prognostic factor for poor survival in glioma patients treated with concomitant chemoradiotherapy, Musashi-1 and BMI-1. Clearly implicated in the genesis of GBM, also EGFR expression plays a role in neural progenitor development and is speculated to contribute directly to CSC maintenance.

In fact, EGF plays a pivotal role in the self-renewal and multilineage differentiation of normal neural stem cells in combination with the basic fibroblast growth factor (bFGF), vascular-endothelial growth factor (VEGF) and platelet-derived growth factor (PDGF). Different studies evaluated the importance of these growth factors and their receptors in glioma growth and maintenance, demonstrating that these factors are also involved in proliferation, tumorigenicity and malignancy of the tumor. CSCs are highly resistant to radiotherapy and to many cytotoxic drugs, likely due to increased DNA repair activity, and overexpression of ATP-dependent efflux pumps. Indeed, as normal stem cells are resistant to the induction of apoptosis by cytotoxic agents and radiation therapy, CSCs display

CANCER STEM CELLS CHARACTERISTICS

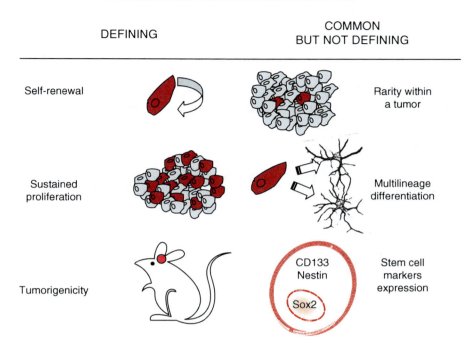

Fig. 22.1 Brain cancer stem cells are identified by both functional defining characteristics and features that are often detected but not necessarily present within the tumor stem cell subpopulation

increased resistance to these agents as compared with the more differentiated cancer cells that constitute the mass of the tumor. Furthermore, the activation of several signalling cascades including EGF/EGFR, sonic Hedgehog, Notch, and Wnt/β-catenin combined with the increased DNA repair mechanisms and ABC transporter-mediated drug efflux in cancer stem cells may be responsible for their resistance to standard therapies.

Moreover, alterations of CSC microenvironment may influence their biological and molecular behavior and, as a consequence, tumor development or growth. Thus, the molecular targeting of this cancer cell subpopulation must be considered for improving the efficacy of the current anti-cancer strategies with the aim to sensitize tumors toward conventional therapies and effectively abrogate tumorigenesis. Targeting CSCs is particularly interesting considering the high rate of recurrence in GBMs. Surgery can often remove over 90% of the tumor bulk, but the cells that have migrated away from the visible tumor in the infiltrated brain parenchyma, will proliferate and lead to the relapse (Stiles and Rowitch, 2008).

Glioblastoma Cancer Stem Cells: Response to EGFR-TKIs

Notwithstanding unsatisfactory results in the initial clinical trials, the possible EGFR targeting for GBM treatment is still a reasonable hypothesis. Moreover, the relevance of EGFR signalling in CSC proliferation and self-renewal, the possible efficacy of EGFR-TKIs on this tumor cell subpopulation is an extremely relevant question as a proof of principle to better tuning anti GBM therapies. In particular, considering CSC role in development, progression and recurrence of GBMs, we evaluated the in vitro sensitivity of human GBM CSC-enriched cultures to gefitinib and erlotinib, as proof of principle for the potential efficacy of EGFR-TKIs to target GBM CSCs (Griffero et al., 2009). To accomplish this task, we studied GBM CSCs from seven fresh human GBMs tissues derived from patients that underwent surgery for the first time and never received chemotherapy or radiotherapy. Cells were expanded in vitro in a CSC selection-permissive medium and the expression of different stem cell markers, multilineage differentiation and tumorigenicity in immunodeficient mice was evaluated to define their CSC nature. After this characterization, GBM CSCs have been tested for their sensitivity to the antiproliferative activity of erlotinib and gefitinib and for the identification of the molecular determinants of the observed effects.

The first critical step in CSC research is the isolation of human GBM cancer stem cells from post-surgical explants. This can be obtained plating single cells obtained after dissociation of the tumors at clonal density in a stem cell permissive medium containing EGF and bFGF, adopting conditions widely described for the propagation of neural stem cells. Under these culture conditions, primary GBM cells grow in vitro as floating sphere-like aggregates (neurospheres) that are formed within 1–2 weeks of culture and continuously proliferate for several weeks by replenish fresh medium. However, to obtain more experimentally manageable cultures we developed a protocol to grow CSC as attached monolayer using matrigel-coated dishes. We demonstrated that under these conditions CSCs retain stemness properties including self-renewal, multilineage differentiation and tumorigenic potential. We obtained 7 different CSC cultures from 7 high grade gliomas, named GBM 1–7 that have been deeply characterized to ensure the reliability of our CSC culture model before analyze their pharmacological properties. Among CSC characteristics the central features are their relatively unlimited self-renewal capacity, the expression of stem markers and the differentiation capacity. The formation of neurospheres in limiting dilution experiments is one of the parameters to control the in vitro ability of self-renewal that in our study has been verified throughout the experiments. Moreover, GBM CSCs have been characterized and isolated on the basis of their expression of various cell surface molecules such as CD133 and nestin (Table 22.1), specific markers for both neural stem cells and brain tumor CSCs that were quantitatively and qualitatively similar in non-adherent or monolayer cultures. All the isolated GBM CSCs displayed the potential for multilineage differentiation as verified by culturing the cells under differentiating conditions (removal of growth factors and addition of fetal calf serum in the medium) that resulted in the acquisition of typical astroglial morphology and high expression of differentiation markers as microtubule-associated protein 2 (Map2: neuronal marker) and

glial fibrillary acidic protein (GFAP: astroglial marker) within 2 weeks.

However, to date, the only definite proof able to discriminate CSCs from differentiated non-tumorigenic cancer cells is the in vivo tumorigenicity that is detected in CSCs while the bulk of cells in the tumor lacks this capacity. All GBMs, when orthotopically xenografted into immune-compromised mice formed tumors (after about 2–6 months) (Table 22.1), with highly invasive properties and histopathological properties of the parental neoplasia, thus confirming that our cultures are enriched in CSCs, retaining the potential for developing brain tumors. Again, the monolayer culture on matrigel preserved the tumorigenic properties. Moreover, the experimental tumors generated by intracranial injection of CSC cultures recapitulated the phenotype of the original human tumor, demonstrating various grades of infiltration into the surrounding cerebral cortex and GBM cells showed a propensity to migrate along the *corpus callosum* or other mice brain structures: this indicates that our CSC culture protocol allows the isolation of CSCs from human GBM and that these CSCs can retain after prolonged culture timing defined features such as tumorigenicity, long-term self renewing and multipotency (Fig. 22.2).

Importantly, we were able to re-obtain neurospheres re-culturing our GBM CSCs under non-adherent stem cells conditions (Fig. 22.2). This observation strongly supports the relevance of the cell culturing model we developed, to evaluate the biological characteristics and pharmacological responsiveness of human GBM cells. Once validated GBM CSC culture model, we used this innovative model for pharmacological studies focusing on the evaluation of the sensitivity to gefitinib and erlotinib. CSC cultures were treated with increasing concentrations (0.5, 1 and 5 μM) of erlotinib and gefitinib and their survival was evaluated and compared to vehicle-treated cells at different time points (time 0, and after 1–4 days of treatment). Significant cell toxicity was observed in five out of seven CSC cultures. Only one CSC culture, named GBM2 was completely insensitive to both drugs and another, GBM7, was responsive only to the highest concentrations tested.

In details, erlotinib caused a time- and dose-dependent inhibition of cell survival at the concentration of 5 μM in GBM1, 3, 4, 5, 6 and 7, reaching, as maximal inhibition, a reduction of cell survival ranging from 40 to 62%. Lower effects were observed with

Table 22.1 Charcterization of glioblastoma CSC culture and biological and molecular effects of EGFR-TKIs

Tumor code	In vitro expression of stem markers % of positive cells		In vivo tumorigenicity (Days survival, median)[c]	EGFRTKIs sensitivity Inhibition of proliferation % Maximal inhibition at 5 μM (time)		Effects of EGFR-TKIs on EGFR activation % of residual EGFR, ERK1/2 and Akt activation[d]						PTEN expression
	CD133[a]	Nestin[b]		Gefitinib	Erlotinib	Gefitinib			Erlotinib			mRNA
						pEGFR	pERK 1/2	PAkT	pEGFR	PERK 1/2	PAkT	
GBM1	3 ± 1.5	93 ± 2	165	63 (72 h)	62 (96 h)	16 ± 2	45 ± 6	34 ± 7	8 ± 1	18 ± 5	9 ± 3	+
GBM2	1.8 ± 0.8	78 ± 2.5	85	3 (48 h)	2 (96 h)	3 ± 1	3 ± 1	105 ± 9	10 ± 3	15 ± 4	101 ± 12	–
GBM3	4.5 ± 1.5	95 ± 3.5	80	55 (48 h)	68 (96 h)	21 ± 4	28 ± 4	28 ± 6	41 ± 7	32 ± 3	42 ± 5	+
GBM4	83 ± 3	76 ± 2.5	110	70 (96 h)	43 (96 h)	8 ± 2	18 ± 3	37 ± 11	3 ± 2	35 ± 8	12 ± 3	+
GBM5	85 ± 4.5	40 ± 6	75	38 (96 h)	35 (96 h)	12 ± 2	42 ± 11	43 ± 9	46 ± 9	43 ± 11	39 ± 9	+
GBM6	2.5 ± 1	69 ± 3	145	79 (72 h)	46 (96 h)	9 ± 2	39 ± 9	40 ± 7	15 ± 4	16 ± 3	34 ± 12	+
GBM7	1.8 ± 0.5	93 ± 2	87	35 (72 h)	41 (72 h)	98 ± 13	90 ± 12	102 ± 10	48 ± 6	9 ± 2	38 ± 8	+

[a]Immunocytochemistry
[b]Flow cytometry
[c]Data represent range of time in which brain tumors reach a mass that required the sacrifice of mice after injection of 10^5 cells
[d]Densitometric values ±%S.E. of the maximal inhibition observed of the EGF-induced protein phosphorylation (set as 100%)
Data from Griffero et al. (2009)

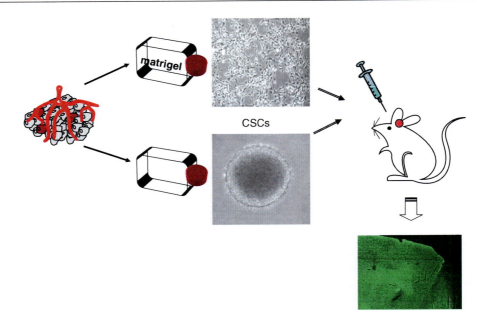

Fig. 22.2 Isolated cancer stem cells (CSCs) obtained from mechanical dissociation brain tumor specimens can be cultured as non-adherent neurospheres (**a**) or on matrigel-coated flask as monolayers (**b**), without modify their stem potential. Indeed, both types of culture are enriched in CSCs, being capable to recapitulate original tumors when orthotopically xenografted into nude mice (**c**), representative immunofluorescence of mouse brain cryosection labeled with anti-human nestin antibody, showing the diffuse infiltration of the brain parenchyma derived from GBM CSC injection

lower doses of erlotinib (0.5–1 μM) in the GBM CSC cultures, while no statistically significant effects were observed in GBM7 cells. Interestingly, GBM2 CSCs were completely insensitive to all drug concentrations tested, even after 4 days of treatment. Similar but not completely super-imposable results were obtained after treatment with gefitinib. In fact, while GBM3 displayed a high sensitivity to gefitinib that was comparable to what observed with erlotinib, GBM1 and 4 showed an increased responsiveness as compared to erlotinib: –73% and –62% cell survival, after 3 days of treatment with 5 μM, and a statistically significant inhibition already after 24 h of treatment with 1 and 0.5 μM gefitinib, respectively. GBM5 and GBM6 showed maximal inhibition similar to that observed after erlotinib treatment and the antiproliferative effect was statistically significant already at the concentration of 0.5 μM after 72 h of treatment.

GBM2 confirmed the absolute insensibility to EGFR inhibition, while as far as GBM7 is concerned low concentrations of gefitinib were completely ineffective and a moderate reduction in the proliferation rate was observed only at highest concentration (5 μM) and for prolonged times of treatment (up to 4 days). Results are summarized in Table 22.1.

In agreement with our results, a recent paper (Soeda et al., 2008) underlying the essential role of EGFR in mitogenic regulation of human brain tumor stem cells, reports that gefitinib affects self-renewal, survival and proliferation in three CSC enriched cultures.

The observation that different responsiveness to drugs are displayed by individual GBM CSCs cultures (Table 22.1), as observed for the variability of clinical outcomes in different patients, is relevant to identify GBM-specific responses and possible molecular determinants for such unsatisfactory effects in this subset of tumors.

To better understand the molecular determinants of the differential response to erlotinib and gefitinib, we first measured EGFR expression by competitive binding of EGF to its specific transmembrane cell receptor in all the cultures. A partial correlation between the receptor number and the responsiveness to EGFR TKIs antiproliferative effects was observed: the more responsive GBM CSCs (GBM 1, 3 and 4) displayed the highest number of EGFR site/cell, while the less responsive GBM 2 and 7 showed low levels of expression of the receptor. However, GBM 5 and 6 combined a small number of binding sites with a significant inhibition of cell proliferation, excluding that the lack of response to the drugs may depend on low EGFR expression levels.

Thus, a more precise correlation with cytotoxic effects of erlotinib and gefitinib should be due to other mechanisms that EGFR expression levels and possibly to the signal transduction mechanisms activated by EGFR. First, the specificity of the effects of erlotinib and gefitinib on the proliferation rate of human glioma CSCs was evaluated by testing their effects on EGFR phosphorylation/activation induced by EGF (40 ng/ml). EGF induced activation of EGFR in all CSC cultures while in the presence of erlotinib, EGF-induced EGFR phosphorylation was completely inhibited in all CSC cultures. Similarly, gefitinib pre-treatment affected EGF-induced EGFR phosphorylation in all the cell lines with GBM 7 cells showing low sensitivity (Table 22.1). Interestingly, comparable results were recently reported in which EGFR phosphorylation was inhibited by gefitinib in a concentration-dependent manner in 3 GBM CSC cultures (Soeda et al., 2008).

EGFR activation triggers three major intracellular signalling cascades: the Ras-Raf-MEK-ERK, the PI-3 K/Akt and the STAT3-dependent signalling events. Previous studies report, that gefitinib suppressed phosphorylation of both ERK1/2 and Akt in CSC isolated from human gliomas while STAT-3 activation levels were not affected by the treatment (Soeda et al., 2008). To assess a possible role for EGFR activation of the MAP kinase cascade in our CSC cultures, the potential modulation of ERK1/2 activation by EGFR-TK inhibitors was evaluated (Table 22.1). Erlotinib treatment caused a significant reduction of ERK1/2 phosphorylation induced by EGF in all CSCs that almost completely matched with the effects on EGFR phosphorylation. A significant inhibition of ERK1/2 phosphorylation was also observed after gefitinib treatment in all CSCs even if a lower effect was shown in GBM 7 cells with a barely detectable reduction of ERK1/2 phosphorylation only at the highest concentration tested. Interestingly, in GBM2 derived CSC cultures significant effects of erlotinib and gefitinib on EGFR and ERK1/2 activation were observed although the drug lacks cytotoxic effects. Thus, a different mechanism should be responsible for the resistance of these drugs.

It was reported that the effects of EGFR, as a key mediator of oncogenesis in human tumors, are mediated not only through ERK1/2 signalling, but also PI-3K/Akt signalling plays a relevant role in cell survival and proliferation. Furthermore, constitutively activated Akt pathway is often associated to lack of tumor response to EGFR inhibitors. In order to study this downstream pathway, we analyzed Akt phosphorylation in basal or EGF-treated conditions, in the presence or absence of erlotinib and gefitinib. Erlotinib pretreatment caused a significant reduction of the kinase activation in all CSCs but had no effect either on basal or EGF-induced Akt phosphorylation of GBM2 cells. Gefitinib also powerfully inhibited the activation of Akt by EGF while lacking efficacy in GBM2 and GBM7. Moreover, in GBM2 CSCs, Akt was already maximally phosphorylated already in basal conditions. Collectively these data suggest the evidence of possible tumor-related specific responses related to Akt activation status as a possible molecular determinant of EGFR TKI sensitivity (Table 22.1). This hypothesis was examined through the analysis of the mRNA expression of the main intracellular inhibitor of the PI-3K/Akt pathway PTEN, that was significantly expressed amounts in CSCs derived from all the GBM analyzed, with only GBM2 cells that showed downregulation of PTEN mRNA (Table 22.1). Thus, the constitutive activation of Akt was likely dependent on the low expression of PTEN as observed in GBM2 cells and the inhibition of Akt activation was required for the antiproliferative effects of EGFR TKI in GBM CSC-enriched cultures, as already shown for human GBM in vivo (Mellinghoff et al., 2005). The presence of EGFR activation has been shown to be associated to EGFR-TKI sensitivity particularly in tumors with EGFR-dependent activation of the anti-apoptotic PI3K/Akt pathway as observed in GBM (Haas-Kogan et al., 2005) and NSCLC (Cappuzzo, 2005) even if a conclusive association of EGFR gene amplification and expression in response to EGFR TKIs, (i.e. erlotinib) in GBM has not been assessed.

Our study clearly revealed different and individual responsiveness to EGFR TKI in a significant series of GBM CSC cultures that on one hand reflects the possibility that only small fraction of GBMs respond to treatment to this drugs (for example only those in which an inhibition of Akt may be induced) and, on the other, underlines the necessity of further studies to identify more predictive and specific markers for EGFR TKI sensitivity in glioma CSCs able to identify subgroups of patients that may be responsive to these class of drugs.

Conclusions and Future Perspectives

Advances have been made in the understanding the genetic, molecular and biological mechanisms responsible for brain tumor development and these progresses are exploited for the development of novel treatment strategies targeting the key molecules of tumorigenic pathways. The main goal of anticancer strategies is to design therapies able to reflect the unique biological features of individual tumors, reaching a personalized drug treatment. Regarding GBM, a more comprehensive knowledge of the molecular and biological characteristics of EGFR, together with other molecules involved in its signalling network, will contribute to the successful therapeutic targeting of EGFR (Karpel-Massler et al., 2009). Therefore, the first option in designing new generation of clinical trials in oncology may be to analyze tumor tissues to identify genetic and biochemical features that distinguish responders and non-responders, so that both groups of patients may receive optimal therapy. The tumor biological and molecular characterization includes the possible detection of CSCs, since one of the most interesting

implications of CSC hypothesis is the future potential to improve cancer treatment. In particular, it is essential to design strategies based upon a better understanding of the signaling pathways that control aspects of self-renewal and survival in CSCs, to identify novel therapeutic targets in these cells.

As evidenced from the studies reported in this review, some discrepancies arise between the promising pre-clinical in vitro data, also on GBM cancer stem cells, and the not completely convincing clinical results on the benefit of EGFR TKIs. An obvious explanation for these observations is the difficulty encountered in extrapolating in vitro studies on tumor cell lines, although GBM CSCs may represent an innovative powerful model for pre-clinical drug testing for in vivo and clinical applications. Moreover, it should be taken into account, as emerged from our in vitro study, the relatively high percentage of CSCs in GBM that are significantly affected by EGFR-TKI treatment but not completely eradicated, thus leading to possible re-growth capability of these cells. Thus, combination treatments (EGFR TKI in association with PDGFR or mTOR inhibitors, for example) should provide more complete cytotoxic results (Fig. 22.3). On the other

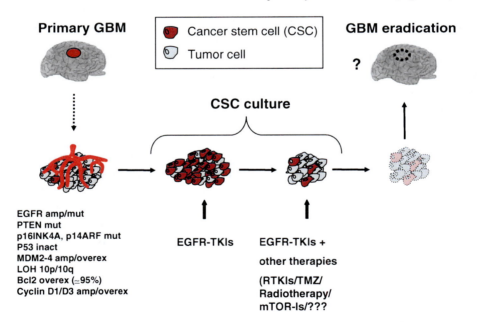

Fig. 22.3 Eradication of tumors requires successful targeting of all cancer cells likely using a combination of drugs active against all cancer cell subpopulations (including CSCs) and different molecular targets. Tumor biological and molecular characterization of GBMs by in vitro and in vivo studies identified several molecules and pathways altered in GBMs. A relatively

high percentage of CSCs in GBM are significantly affected by EGFR TKIs treatment but not completely, thus leading to possible re-growth capability of these cells. A multiple approach including several drugs targeting EGFR and other RTKs or their related intracellular transducers may lead to complete ridding of all cancer cells and tumor eradication

hand the assumption of the rarity of cancer stem cell within malignancies could not be correct for all cancer types, especially in high grade and poorly differentiated tumors as GBM, that recent studies did not limit to the CD133+ subpopulation (Kern and Shibata, 2007). Thus GBM can be successfully treated impairing the survival not only of the bulk of the differentiated tumor mass but also all or the vast majority of CSCs that preferentially escape therapy (Kern and Shibata, 2007).

Although CSCs exist in probably all tumor histotypes and this subpopulation is endowed of high tumorigenic potential in mice xenografts, we still have little knowledge of their behavior within the tumor (in patients) to definitely identify their relevance in cancer therapy. Further studies are needed to characterize CSCs in greater details, to define their distinctive features and to put therapies that specifically target CSCs into practice. However, since GBM shows aggressive development and highly malignant phenotype, including very low differentiated and highly deregulated cancer cells with extensive necrosis and angiogenesis, the distinction between the cancer stem cells and the bulk of the tumor might be reduced. These features may influence therapeutic response and prevent satisfactory cure of GBM patients.

In conclusion, from a clinical point of view the concept that GBM and other cancers could be treated by selectively targeting CSCs is one of the most exciting implications of CSC hypothesis but at present it represents only an intriguing potentiality.

Thus, eradication of tumors still requires both the successful targeting of all cancer cells likely using a combination of drugs active against all cancer cell subpopulation and *vs.* different molecular targets. Therefore, a multiple approach including several drugs that target EGFR and/or other receptor TKs or their related intracellular effectors, may represent an optimal future treatment modality for GBM, integrating CSCs in the view of both tumorigenesis and cancer treatment.

References

Bao S, Wu Q, Mclendon RE, Hao Y, Shi Q, Hjelmeland AB, Dewhirst MW, Bigner DD, Rich JN (2006) Glioma stem cells promote radioresistance by preferential activation of the DNA damage response. Nature 444:756–760

Barnes CJ, Bagheri-Yarmand R, Mandal M, Yang Z, Clayman GL, Hong WK, Kumar R (2003) Suppression of epidermal growth factor receptor, mitogen-activated protein kinase, and pak1 pathways and invasiveness of human cutaneous squamous cancer cells by the tyrosine kinase inhibitor ZD1839 (iressa). Mol Cancer 2:345–351

Bax DA, Gaspar N, Little SE, Marshall L, Perryman L, Regairaz M, Viana-Pereira M, Vuononvirta R, Sharp SY, Reis-Filho JS, Stavale JN, Al-Sarraj S, Reis RM, Vassal G, Pearson AD, Hargrave D, Ellison DW, Workman P, Jones C (2009) Egfrviii deletion mutations in pediatric high-grade glioma and response to targeted therapy in pediatric glioma cell lines. Clin Cancer Res 15:5753–5761

Brown PD, Krishnan S, Sarkaria JN, Wu W, Jaeckle KA, Uhm JH, Geoffroy FJ, Arusell R, Kitange G, Jenkins RB, Kugler JW, Morton RF, Rowland KM, Buckner JC (2008) Phase I/II trial of erlotinib and temozolomide with radiation therapy in the treatment of newly diagnosed glioblastoma multiforme: north central cancer treatment group study N0177. J Clin Oncol 26:5603–5609

Cappuzzo F (2005) Erlotinib in gliomas: should selection be based on EGFR and akt analyses?. J Natl Cancer Inst 97:868–869

Citri A, Yarden Y (2006) EGF-ERBB signalling: towards the systems level. Nat Rev Mol Cell Biol 7:505–516

Furnari FB, Fenton T, Bachoo RM, Mukasa A, Stommel JM, Stegh A, Hahn WC, Ligon KL, Louis DN, Brennan C, Chin L, Depinho RA, Cavenee WK (2007) Malignant astrocytic glioma: genetics, biology, and paths to treatment. Genes Dev 21:2683–2710

Griffero F, Daga A, Marubbi D, Capra MC, Melotti A, Pattarozzi A, Gatti M, Bajetto A, Porcile C, Barbieri F, Favoni RE, Lo Casto M, Zona G, Spaziante R, Florio T, Corte G (2009) Different response of human glioma tumor-initiating cells to epidermal growth factor receptor kinase inhibitors. J Biol Chem 284:7138–7148

Gschwind A, Fischer OM, Ullrich A (2004) The discovery of receptor tyrosine kinases: targets for cancer therapy. Nat Rev Cancer 4:361–370

Haas-Kogan DA, Prados MD, Tihan T, Eberhard DA, Jelluma N, Arvold ND, Baumber R, Lamborn KR, Kapadia A, Malec M, Berger MS, Stokoe D (2005) Epidermal growth factor receptor, protein kinase B/akt, and glioma response to erlotinib. J Natl Cancer Inst 97:880–887

Hadjipanayis CG, Van Meir EG (2009) Tumor initiating cells in malignant gliomas: biology and implications for therapy. J Mol Med 87:363–374

Hanahan D, Weinberg RA (2000) The hallmarks of cancer. Cell 100:57–70

Hegi ME, Diserens AC, Gorlia T, Hamou MF, De Tribolet N, Weller M, Kros JM, Hainfellner JA, Mason W, Mariani L, Bromberg JE, Hau P, Mirimanoff RO, Cairncross JG, Janzer RC, Stupp R (2005) MGMT gene silencing and benefit from temozolomide in glioblastoma. N Engl J Med 352:997–1003

Karaman MW, Herrgard S, Treiber DK, Gallant P, Atteridge CE, Campbell BT, Chan KW, Ciceri P, Davis MI, Edeen PT, Faraoni R, Floyd M, Hunt JP, Lockhart DJ, Milanov ZV, Morrison MJ, Pallares G, Patel HK, Pritchard S, Wodicka LM, Zarrinkar PP (2008) A quantitative analysis of kinase inhibitor selectivity. Nat Biotechnol 26:127–132

Karpel-Massler G, Schmidt U, Unterberg A, Halatsch ME (2009) Therapeutic inhibition of the epidermal growth factor receptor in high-grade gliomas: where do we stand?. Mol Cancer Res 7:1000–1012

Kern SE, Shibata D (2007) The fuzzy math of solid tumor stem cells: a perspective. Cancer Res 67:8985–8988

Lassman AB, Rossi MR, Raizer JJ, Abrey LE, Lieberman FS, Grefe CN, Lamborn K, Pao W, Shih AH, Kuhn JG, Wilson R, Nowak NJ, Cowell JK, Deangelis LM, Wen P, Gilbert MR, Chang S, Yung WA, Prados M, Holland EC (2005) Molecular study of malignant gliomas treated with epidermal growth factor receptor inhibitors: tissue analysis from north american brain tumor consortium trials 01-03 and 00-01. Clin Cancer Res 11:7841–7850

Lee JC, Vivanco I, Beroukhim R, Huang JH, Feng WL, Debiasi RM, Yoshimoto K, King JC, Nghiemphu P, Yuza Y, Xu Q, Greulich H, Thomas RK, Paez JG, Peck TC, Linhart DJ, Glatt KA, Getz G, Onofrio R, Ziaugra L, Levine RL, Gabriel S, Kawaguchi T, O'neill K, Khan H, Liau LM, Nelson SF, Rao PN, Mischel P, Pieper RO, Cloughesy T, Leahy DJ, Sellers WR, Sawyers CL, Meyerson M, Mellinghoff IK (2006) Epidermal growth factor receptor activation in glioblastoma through novel missense mutations in the extracellular domain. PLoS Med 3:e485

Loew S, Schmidt U, Unterberg A, Halatsch ME (2009) The epidermal growth factor receptor as a therapeutic target in glioblastoma multiforme and other malignant neoplasms. Anticancer Agents Med Chem 9:703–715

Mellinghoff IK, Wang MY, Vivanco I, Haas-Kogan DA, Zhu S, Dia EQ, Lu KV, Yoshimoto K, Huang JH, Chute DJ, Riggs BL, Horvath S, Liau LM, Cavenee WK, Rao PN, Beroukhim R, Peck TC, Lee JC, Sellers WR, Stokoe D, Prados M, Cloughesy TF, Sawyers CL, Mischel PS (2005) Molecular determinants of the response of glioblastomas to EGFR kinase inhibitors. N Engl J Med 353:2012–2024

Mendelsohn J, Baselga J (2003) Status of epidermal growth factor receptor antagonists in the biology and treatment of cancer. J Clin Oncol 21:2787–2799

Mendelsohn J, Baselga J (2006) Epidermal growth factor receptor targeting in cancer. Semin Oncol 33:369–385

Narita Y, Nagane M, Mishima K, Huang HJ, Furnari FB, Cavenee WK (2002) Mutant epidermal growth factor receptor signaling down-regulates P27 through activation of the phosphatidylinositol 3-kinase/akt pathway in glioblastomas. Cancer Res 62:6764–6769

Pan MG, Florio T, Stork PJ (1992) G protein activation of a hormone-stimulated phosphatase in human tumor cells. Science 256:1215–1217

Pao W, Miller V, Zakowski M, Doherty J, Politi K, Sarkaria I, Singh B, Heelan R, Rusch V, Fulton L, Mardis E, Kupfer D, Wilson R, Kris M, Varmus H (2004) EGF receptor gene mutations are common in lung cancers from "never smokers" and are associated with sensitivity of tumors to gefitinib and erlotinib. Proc Natl Acad Sci USA 101:13306–13311

Prados MD, Chang SM, Butowski N, Deboer R, Parvataneni R, Carliner H, Kabuubi P, Ayers-Ringler J, Rabbitt J, Page M, Fedoroff A, Sneed PK, Berger MS, Mcdermott MW,

Parsa AT, Vandenberg S, James CD, Lamborn KR, Stokoe D, Haas-Kogan DA (2009) Phase II study of erlotinib plus temozolomide during and after radiation therapy in patients with newly diagnosed glioblastoma multiforme or gliosarcoma. J Clin Oncol 27:579–584

Prados MD, Yung WK, Wen PY, Junck L, Cloughesy T, Fink K, Chang S, Robins HI, Dancey J, Kuhn J (2008) Phase-1 trial of gefitinib and temozolomide in patients with malignant glioma: a north american brain tumor consortium study. Cancer Chemother Pharmacol 61:1059–1067

Raizer JJ, Abrey LE, Lassman AB, Chang SM, Lamborn KR, Kuhn JG, Yung WK, Gilbert MR, Aldape KA, Wen PY, Fine HA, Mehta M, Deangelis LM, Lieberman F, Cloughesy TF, Robins HI, Dancey J, Prados MD (2001) A phase II trial of erlotinib in patients with recurrent malignant gliomas and nonprogressive glioblastoma multiforme postradiation therapy. Neurooncol 12:95–103

Reya T, Morrison SJ, Clarke MF, Weissman IL (2001) Stem cells, cancer, and cancer stem cells. Nature 414:105–111

Rich JN, Reardon DA, Peery T, Dowell JM, Quinn JA, Penne KL, Wikstrand CJ, Van Duyn LB, Dancey JE, Mclendon RE, Kao JC, Stenzel TT, Ahmed Rasheed BK, Tourt-Uhlig SE, Herndon JE 2nd, Vredenburgh JJ, Sampson JH, Friedman AH, Bigner DD, Friedman HS (2004) Phase II trial of gefitinib in recurrent glioblastoma. J Clin Oncol 22:133–142

Sharma PS, Sharma R, Tyagi T (2009) Receptor tyrosine kinase inhibitors as potent weapons in war against cancers. Curr Pharm Des 15:758–776

Soeda A, Inagaki A, Oka N, Ikegame Y, Aoki H, Yoshimura S, Nakashima S, Kunisada T, Iwama T (2008) Epidermal growth factor plays a crucial role in mitogenic regulation of human brain tumor stem cells. J Biol Chem 283:10958–10966

Stiles CD, Rowitch DH (2008) Glioma stem cells: a midterm exam. Neuron 58:832–846

Stupp R, Mason WP, Van Den Bent MJ, Weller M, Fisher B, Taphoorn MJ, Belanger K, Brandes AA, Marosi C, Bogdahn U, Curschmann J, Janzer RC, Ludwin SK, Gorlia T, Allgeier A, Lacombe D, Cairncross JG, Eisenhauer E, Mirimanoff RO (2005) Radiotherapy plus concomitant and adjuvant temozolomide for glioblastoma. N Engl J Med 352:987–996

Van Den Bent MJ, Brandes AA, Rampling R, Kouwenhoven MC, Kros JM, Carpentier AF, Clement PM, Frenay M, Campone M, Baurain JF, Armand JP, Taphoorn MJ, Tosoni A, Kletzl H, Klughammer B, Lacombe D, Gorlia T (2009) Randomized phase II trial of erlotinib versus temozolomide or carmustine in recurrent glioblastoma: EORTC brain tumor group study 26034. J Clin Oncol 27:1268–1274

Wang MY, Lu KV, Zhu S, Dia EQ, Vivanco I, Shackleford GM, Cavenee WK, Mellinghoff IK, Cloughesy TF, Sawyers CL, Mischel PS (2006) Mammalian target of rapamycin inhibition promotes response to epidermal growth factor receptor kinase inhibitors in PTEN-deficient and PTEN-intact glioblastoma cells. Cancer Res 66:7864–7869

Yarden Y (2001) The EGFR family and its ligands in human cancer. Signalling mechanisms and therapeutic opportunities. Eur J Cancer 37(Suppl 4):S3–S8

Part IV
Therapy

Chapter 23

Low- and High-Grade Gliomas: Extensive Surgical Resection

Nader Sanai and Mitchel S. Berger

Keywords Glioma · Extent of resection · Low-grade · High-grade

Introduction

Central nervous system (CNS) tumors are a major cause of morbidity and mortality with ~18,000 new cases of primary intracranial tumors diagnosed each year in the United States. This represents ~2% of all adult tumors in this country. More than half of these are high-grade gliomas. These lesions are very aggressive and the vast majority of patients invariably have tumor recurrence, with the median survival period ranging from 1 to 3 years after initial diagnosis. Despite facing a better prognosis when compared to higher grade glial tumors, 50–75% of patients harboring low-grade gliomas eventually die of their disease. Median survival durations have been reported to range between 5 and 10 years, and estimates of 10-year survival rates range from 5 to 50%.

Although a primary tenet of neurosurgical oncology is that survival can improve with greater tumor resection, this principle must be tempered by the potential for functional loss following a radical removal. Current neurosurgical innovations aim to improve our anatomic, physiologic, and functional understanding of the surgical region of interest in order to prevent potential neurological morbidity during resection. Emerging imaging technologies, as well as state-of-the-art intraoperative techniques, can facilitate extent of resection while minimizing the associated morbidity profile. Specifically, the value of mapping motor and language pathways is well-established for the safe resection of intrinsic tumors.

Interestingly, controversy persists regarding prognostic factors and treatment options for both low- and high-grade hemispheric gliomas. Among the various tumor- and treatment-related parameters, including tumor volume, neurological status, timing of surgical intervention, and the use of adjuvant therapy, only age and tumor histology have been identified as reliable predictors of patient prognosis. Importantly, despite significant advances in operative techniques and pre-operative planning, the effect of glioma extent of resection in prolonging tumor-free progression and/or survival remains unknown. While the importance of glioma resection in obtaining tissue diagnosis and decompressing mass effect are unquestionable, a lack of Class I evidence prevents similar certainty in assessing the influence of extent of resection. Even though low-grade and high-grade gliomas are distinct in their biology, clinical behaviors, and outcomes, understanding the effect of surgery remains equally important for both.

The Evolution of Cortical Mapping Strategies

Direct cortical stimulation has been employed in neurosurgery since 1930, first by Foerster (Foerster, 1931), and then later by Penfield (Penfield and Bolchey, 1937). In recent years, the technique of intraoperative

N. Sanai (✉)
Department of Neurological Surgery, Barrow Neurological Institute, Phoenix, AZ 85013, USA
e-mail: nader.sanai@bnaneuro.net

cortical stimulation has been adopted for the identification and preservation of language function and motor pathways. Stimulation depolarizes a very focal area of cortex which, in turn, evokes certain responses. Although the mechanism of stimulation effects on language are poorly understood, the principle is based on the depolarization of local neurons and also on passing pathways, inducing local excitation or inhibition, as well as possible diffusion to more distant areas by way of orthodromic or antidromic propagation. Studies employing optical imaging of bipolar cortical stimulation in monkey and human cortex have shown precise local changes, within 2–3 mm, after the activation of cortical tissue (Haglund et al., 1993). With the advent of the bipolar probe, avoidance of local diffusion and more precise mapping have been enabled with an accuracy of ~5 mm (Haglund et al., 1993).

Language mapping techniques were historically developed in the context of epilepsy surgery, where large craniotomies exposed the brain well beyond the region of surgical interest in order to localize multiple cortical regions containing stimulation-induced language and motor function, i.e., "positive" sites, prior to resection. Until recently, it has been thought that such positive site controls must be established during language mapping before any other cortical area could be safely resected. Using this approach, awake craniotomies traditionally identify positive language sites in 95% of the operative exposures. Brain tumor surgeons, however, are now evolving towards a different standard of language mapping, where smaller, tailored craniotomies often expose no positive sites. Tumor resection is, therefore, directed by the localization of cortical regions that contain no stimulation-induced language or motor function, i.e., "negative" sites. This "negative mapping" strategy represents a paradigm shift in language mapping technique by eliminating the neurosurgeon's reliance on the positive site control in the operative exposure, thereby, allowing for minimal cortical exposure overlying the tumor, less extensive intraoperative mapping, and a more time-efficient neurosurgical procedure.

Variability in Cortical Language Localization

Prediction of cortical language sites through classic anatomical criteria is inadequate in light of the significant individual variability of cortical organization (Ojemann et al., 1989), the distortion of cerebral topography from tumor mass effect, and the possibility of functional reorganization through plasticity mechanisms (Seitz et al., 1995). A consistent finding of language stimulation studies has been the identification of significant individual variability among patients (Ojemann et al., 1989). Speech arrest is variably located and can exceed beyond the classic anatomical boundaries of Broca's area for motor speech. It typically involves an area contiguous with the face-motor cortex and, yet, in some cases is seen several centimeters from the sylvian fissure. This variability has also been suggested by studies designed to preoperatively predict the location of speech arrest based upon the type of frontal opercular anatomy (Quinones-Hinojosa et al., 2003) or using functional neuroimaging. Similarly, for temporal lobe language sites, one study of temporal lobe resections assisted by subdural grids demonstrated that the distance from the temporal pole to the area of language function varied from 3 to 9 cm (Davies et al., 1994). Functional imaging studies have also corroborated such variability (FitzGerald et al., 1997). Furthermore, because functional tissue can be located within the tumor nidus, the standard surgical principle of debulking tumor from within to avoid neurologic deficits is not always safe. Consequently, the use of intraoperative cortical and subcortical stimulation to accurately detect functional regions and pathways is essential for safely removing dominant hemisphere gliomas to the greatest extent possible.

Avoidance of Functional Language Deficits Following Awake Mapping

Intraoperative cortical stimulation has yielded critical data regarding essential language sites, which seem to be organized in discrete mosaics that occupy a much smaller area of cortex than described by traditional language maps (Ojemann et al., 1989). Interestingly, the majority of these language sites are surrounded by cortex that, when stimulated, produce no language errors. In the temporal lobe, identification of speech areas within the superior and middle temporal gyri have been documented within 3 cm of the temporal lobe tip (Ojemann et al., 1989). In this region, the distance of the resection margin from the nearest language site is the most important variable in predicting the improvement of preoperative language deficits. Accordingly, if the distance of the resection margin from the nearest language site is > 1 cm, significantly fewer permanent language deficits occur (Haglund et al., 1994). Strict adherence to this principle when operating in any region of the dominant hemisphere can substantially reduce the risk of inadvertently resection functional tissue.

Patient Selection and the Role of Functional Imaging for Language Localization

Because the need to preserve cortical language function must be balanced with the goal of maximal tumor resection, intraoperative language mapping is advocated by some as the rule, rather than the exception (Taylor and Bernstein, 1999). The greatest risk of tumor recurrence is located within 2 cm of the contrast enhancing rim on imaging studies, supporting the concept that the resection should ideally go beyond the gross tumor margin apparent on preoperative imaging. However, because of the infiltrating nature of gliomas, it is more than likely that a portion of the mass will occupy, or be continuous with, functional tissue. This, again, emphasizes the need for cortical stimulation mapping to avoid injuring these critical areas, particularly language pathways. Although it is classically thought that patients who are neurologically intact or minimally affected preoperatively have their functional pathways either displaced or obliterated by infiltrative tumors, we now know that normally functioning language, motor, or sensory tissue can blend with tumor. Therefore, it is not only patients with tumors located within the frontal operculum that benefit from intraoperative language mapping, but also those with lesions in proximity to this region, as there is significant variability in this region's anatomical and functional organization (Quinones-Hinojosa et al., 2003).

Functional imaging has experienced considerable advances in both technology and availability, raising the question of whether it may supplant intraoperative cortical stimulation mapping. Devices such as functional magnetic resonance imaging (fMRI), positron emission tomography (PET), and magnetoencephelography (MEG) may aid in the preoperative planning of the surgical resection strategy, but these techniques remain too imprecise to delineate complex functions such as language mapping: their sensitivity (PET, 75%; fMRI, 81%) and specificity (PET, 81%; fMRI, 53%) are suboptimal (FitzGerald et al., 1997; Herholz et al., 1997). These modalities highlight language-associated areas of indeterminate significance, and they do not offer real-time information intraoperatively. Consequently, for the identification of functional language pathways and guidance of safe tumor removal, these diagnostic imaging tools are still only supplements, not substitutes, for direct intraoperative stimulation mapping.

Specialized Neuroanesthesia for the Awake Craniotomy

An experienced neuroanesthesia team is of paramount importance in not only achieving an accurate intraoperative language map, but in assuring a short and uncomplicated postoperative recovery. As compared to asleep craniotomies, awake craniotomies are associated with less procedural morbidity and fewer postoperative complications (Taylor and Bernstein, 1999) a testimony to the safety of the neuroanesthetic regimen for awake mapping.

In our practice, patients are premedicated with midazolam and monitoring, including a blood pressure cuff, and an axillary temperature probe is applied prior to positioning. Sedation is achieved with propofol (up to 100 μg/kg/min) and remifentanil (0.05 μg/kg/min and higher). Propofol/remifentanil boluses are also used for foley insertion and Mayfield head holder pin application. As an additional measure, the neurosurgeon provides scalp analgesia with generous injection of lidocaine/marcaine. Once the bone flap is removed, all sedatives are discontinued and the patient is asked to hyperventilate prior to dural opening. The dura is then infiltrated with lidocaine around the middle meningeal artery to avoid the discomfort associated with dural opening. No sedatives are administered during mapping and IV methohexital (10 mg/ml) as well as topical ice cold Ringer's solution is available for seizure suppression. Once mapping is complete, sedation is achieved with dexmedetomidine (up to 1 μg/kg/min) and remifentanil (0.05 μg/kg/min and higher).

Current Intraoperative Language Mapping Techniques

In general, a limited craniotomy should expose the tumor and up to 2 cm of surrounding brain. Using bipolar electrodes, cortical mapping is started at a low stimulus (1.5 mA) and increased to a maximum of 6 mA, if necessary. A constant-current generator delivers biphasic square wave pulses (each phase, 1.25 ms) in 4-s trains at 60 Hz across 1-mm bipolar electrodes separated by 5 mm. Stimulation sites (~10–20 per subject) can be marked with sterile numbered tickets. Throughout language mapping, continuous electrocorticography should be used to monitor afterdischarge potentials and, therefore, eliminate the chance that speech or naming errors are caused by subclinical seizure activity. Some groups also advocate the use of language mapping along subcortical white matter pathways (Duffau et al., 2003).

Speech arrest is based upon blocking number counting without simultaneous motor response in the mouth or pharynx. Dysarthria can be distinguished from speech arrest by the absence of perceived or visible involuntary muscle contraction affecting speech. For naming or reading sites, cortical stimulation is applied for 3 s at sequential cortical sites during a slide presentation of line drawings or words, respectively. All tested language sites should be repeatedly stimulated at least three times. A positive essential site can be defined as an inability to name objects or read words in 66% or greater of the testing per site. In all cases, a 1 cm margin of tissue should be measured and preserved around each positive language site in order to protect functional tissue from the resection (Lacroix et al., 2001). The extent of resection is directed by targeting contrast-enhancing regions for high-grade lesions and T2-hyperintense areas for low-grade lesions.

Functional Outcome Following Language Mapping for Dominant Hemisphere Gliomas

Despite the considerable evidence supporting the use of intraoperative cortical stimulation mapping of language function, the efficacy of this technique

in preserving functional outcome following aggressive glioma resection remains poorly understood. Nevertheless, the long-term neurological effects after using this technique for large, dominant-hemisphere gliomas are important to define in order to accurately advocate its use (Sanai and Berger, 2008).

Our experience with 250 consecutive dominant hemisphere glioma patients (WHO grades II–IV) suggests that functional language outcome following awake mapping can be favorable, even in the setting of an aggressive resection (Sanai and Berger, 2008). Overall, 159 of these 250 patients (63.6%) had intact speech preoperatively. At 1 week postoperatively, 194 (77.6%) remained at their baseline language function while 21 (8.4%) worsened and 35 (14.0%) had new speech deficits. However, by 6 months, 52 (92.8%) of 56 patients with new or worsened language deficits returned to baseline or better and the remaining 4 (7.1%) were left with a permanent deficit. Interestingly, among these patients, any additional language deficit incurred as a result of the surgery improved by 3 months or not all (Fig. 23.1). Thus, using language mapping, only 1.6% (4 of 243 surviving patients) of all glioma patients develop a permanent postoperative language deficit. One explanation for this favorable postoperative language profile may be our strict adherence to the "one-centimeter rule", first described by Haglund et al. (1993) which demonstrated that, for temporal lobe tumors, a resection margin of one centimeter or more from a language site significantly reduces postoperative language deficits.

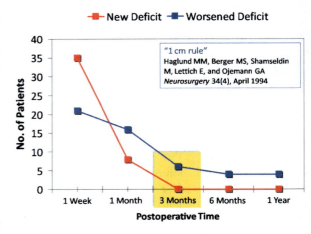

Fig. 23.1 Temporal profile of language deficit resolution following resection of dominant hemisphere gliomas

Tailored Craniotomies and the Value of Negative Language Mapping

In contrast to the classic mapping principles practiced in epilepsy surgery, where 95% of operative fields contain a positive language site, a paradigm shift is emerging in brain tumor language mapping, where positive language sites are not always found prior to resection (Fig. 23.2). In our practice, because of our use of tailored cortical exposures, < 58% of patients have essential language sites localized within the operative field. Our experience suggests that it is safe to employ a minimal exposure of the tumor and resect based upon a negative language map, rather than rely upon a wide craniotomy to find positive language sites well beyond the lesion.

Negative language mapping, however, does not necessarily guarantee the absence of eloquent sites. Despite negative brain mapping, permanent postoperative neurologic deficits have been reported (Taylor and Bernstein, 1999). In our experience with 250 consecutive dominant hemisphere glioma patients,

all 4 of our patients with permanent postoperative neurologic deficits had no positive sites detected prior to their resections. Other cases of unexpected postoperative deficits have also been attributed to progressive tumor infiltration into functional areas. Furthermore, both intraoperative stimulation and functional imaging techniques have provided evidence for redistribution of functional neural networks in cases of stroke (Seitz et al., 1995), congenital malformations (Maldjian et al., 1996), brain injury (Grady et al., 1989), and tumor progression (Seitz et al., 1995). Not surprisingly, it has been hypothesized that brain infiltration by gliomas leads to reshaping or local reorganization of functional networks as well as neosynaptogenesis (Duffau et al., 2003). This would explain the frequent lack of clinical deficit despite glioma growth into eloquent brain areas (Duffau et al., 2001; Seitz et al., 1995), as well as the transient nature of many postoperative deficits. In the case of language function located in the dominant insula, the brain's capacity for compensation of functional loss has also been associated with recruitment of the left superior temporal gyrus and left putamen (Duffau et al., 2001).

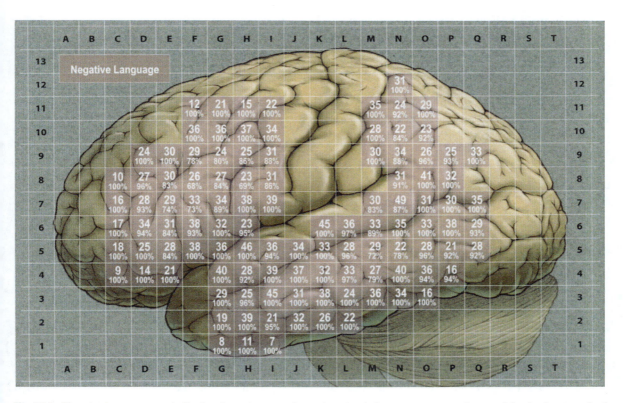

Fig. 23.2 Negative language map indicating the percentage of negative stimulations per square centimeter of the dominant cerebral hemisphere

An Evidence-Based Approach to Understanding the Value of Extent of Resection

Microsurgical resection remains a critical therapeutic modality for all gliomas. However, there remains no general consensus in the literature regarding the efficacy of extent of resection in improving patient outcome. With the exception of WHO Grade I tumors, gliomas are difficult to cure with surgery alone, and the majority of patients will experience some form of tumor recurrence. Patients with glioblastomas have median survival rates of 12.2–18.2 months (Hegi et al., 2005), while those with anaplastic astrocytomas can expect to survive 41 months on average (Keles et al., 2006). Low-grade gliomas carry a better prognosis, though the vast majority of patients eventually die of their disease and 5-year survival percentages range from 42 to 92% in the literature (Philippon et al., 1993; Rajan et al., 1994; Shaw et al., 2002; Yeh et al., 2005).

For all gliomas, the identification of universally-applicable prognostic factors and treatment options remains a great challenge. Among the many tumor- and treatment-related parameters, only patient age and tumor histology have been identified as reliable predictors of patient prognosis, although functional status can also be statistically significant. Suprisingly, despite significant advances in brain tumor imaging and intraoperative technology during the last 15 years, the effect of glioma resection in extending tumor-free progression and patient survival remains unknown.

Although low-grade and high-grade gliomas are distinct in their biology, clinical behavior, and outcome, understanding the efficacy of surgery remains equally important for each. With this in mind, an examination of the modern neurosurgical literature (1990 to present) reveals clues as to the role of extent of resection in glioma patient outcome (Fig. 23.3).

Low-Grade Glioma Extent of Resection Studies

Several studies (Claus et al., 2005; Haglund et al., 1994; Karim et al., 1996; Philippon et al., 1993; Rajan et al., 1994; Shaw et al., 2002; Shibamoto et al., 1993;

van Veelen et al., 1998; Yeh et al., 2005) since 1990 have applied statistical analysis to examine the efficacy of extent of resection in improving survival and delaying tumor progression among low-grade glioma patients. Five of these studies included volumetric analysis of extent of resection (Claus et al., 2005; Karim et al., 1996; Shibamoto et al., 1993; Smith et al., 2008; van Veelen et al., 1998). Of the nonvolumetric studies, 12 demonstrated evidence supporting extent of resection as a statistically significant predictor of either 5-year survival or 5-year progression-free survival. These studies were published from 1990 to 2005 and most commonly employed a combination of multivariate and univariate analyses to determine statistical significance. In most instances, extent of resection was defined on the basis of gross-total versus subtotal resection. Interestingly, only 3 nonvolumetric studies did not support extent of resection as a predictor of patient outcome. However, none of these reports evaluated progression-free survival, but instead focused solely on 5-year survival. Of the 5 volumetric low-grade glioma studies reviewed, 4 demonstrated statistical significance based upon 5-year survival. For their statistical analyses, each study divided the extent of resection percentages into two categories, although the cutoff threshold was different in each publication and varied from 75 to 100%.

High-Grade Glioma Extent of Resection Studies

Twenty-seven studies since 1990 have applied statistical analysis to examine the efficacy of extent of resection in improving survival and delaying tumor progression among high-grade glioma patients. Four of these studies included volumetric analysis of extent of resection (Keles et al., 1999; Keles et al., 2006; Lacroix et al., 2001; Pope et al., 2005). Of the nonvolumetric studies, 13 demonstrated evidence supporting extent of resection as a statistically significant predictor of either time to tumor progression or overall survival. Although some of these reports showed extent of resection to significantly affect both tumor progression and overall survival, every study showed a survival benefit. Ten studies, however, demonstrated no significant benefit based upon extent of resection.

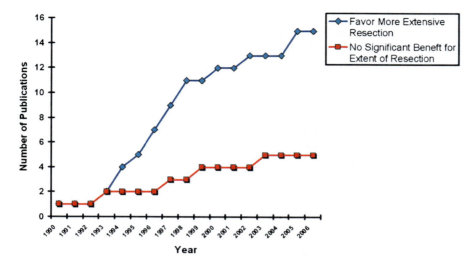

Fig. 23.3 Trends in the relative numbers of studies in the neurosurgical literature since 1990 statistically examining the impact of extent of resection on patient survival

Notably, the distribution of adjuvant chemotherapy and radiation treatment was comparable among all high-grade glioma extent of resection studies. Echoing the nonvolumetric study results, half of all high-grade volumetric studies showed a significant survival advantage with greater extent of resection.

Although the high-grade studies reviewed were all modern series conducted by expert neurosurgeons with access to comparable operative technologies, it remains difficult to define the many inherent disparities between the cases described that may have biased the reported findings. One factor that may distinguish various high-grade glioma studies from one another is the distribution of WHO Grade III and IV histologies among the study patients. After quantifying this parameter in each publication, it remains difficult to draw any firm conclusions regarding causality. Another dimension of extent of resection analysis that can greatly affect the reported findings is the method with which the extent of resection is calculated. Although volumetric MRI analysis is now the gold-standard, many centers still rely upon the surgeon's report or two-dimensional analysis based upon postoperative MR imaging. However, in examining the distribution of extent of resection methodologies and comparing them to the findings for both low-grade and high-grade gliomas, there appears to be a relatively even distribution of techniques for each study category.

Quantification of Improvement in Patient Outcome

For both low- and high-grade gliomas, one can define the mean survival time associated with subtotal versus gross-total resection in the modern neurosurgical literature. Although the level of evidence available for each tumor category does not permit a statistical meta-analysis, this measurement provides an overall estimation of the additional survival time these studies suggest may be gained through a greater extent of resection. Not surprisingly, the effect of a greater extent of resection was more pronounced in the low-grade glioma studies, where the mean survival was extended from 61.1 to 90 months. Among the high-grade gliomas, the improvement was more modest, with an increase from 64.9 to 75.2 months in WHO Grade III gliomas and from 11.3 to 14.5 months.

In conclusion, stimulation mapping is a reliable, robust method to maximize resection and minimize morbidity, even when removing gliomas within or near adjacent language pathways. Unlike motor function, speech and language are variably distributed and widely represented; thus, emphasizing the utility of language mapping in this particular patient population. Using modern language mapping techniques, in conjunction with standardized neuroanesthesia and neuromonitoring, the postoperative language resolution profile following glioma resection may be predictable. Specifically, in our experience, any additional language deficit incurred as a result of the surgery will improve by 3 months or not at all. Our experience also emphasizes the value of negative language mapping in the setting of a tailored cortical exposure. The value of extent of resection, however, remains less clear. Based upon the available studies for both low-grade and high-grade hemispheric gliomas in the literature, there is growing evidence, however, that a more extensive surgical resection may be associated with a more favorable life expectancy for both low-grade and high-grade glioma patients. Because no Class I evidence exists to support a particular management paradigm, the optimal combination of surgery, a chemotherapeutic agent, and radiation therapy remains unknown. Because it is unlikely that a prospective, randomized study will be designed to address these issues, retrospective, matched studies or prospective observational trials may be a more practical solution.

References

Claus EB, Horlacher A, Hsu L, Schwartz RB, Dello-Iacono D, Talos F, Jolesz FA, Black PM (2005) Survival rates in patients with low-grade glioma after intraoperative magnetic resonance image guidance. Cancer 103:1227–1233

Davies KG, Maxwell RE, Jennum P, Dhuna A, Beniak TE, Destafney E, Gates JR, Fiol ME (1994) Language function following subdural grid-directed temporal lobectomy. Acta Neurol Scand 90:201–206

Duffau H, Bauchet L, Lehericy S, Capelle L (2001) Functional compensation of the left dominant insula for language. Neuroreport 12:2159–2163

Duffau H, Capelle L, Denvil D, Sichez N, Gatignol P, Taillandier L, Lopes M, Mitchell MC, Roche S, Muller JC, Bitar A, Sichez JP, van Effenterre R (2003) Usefulness of intraoperative electrical subcortical mapping during surgery for low-grade gliomas located within eloquent brain regions: functional results in a consecutive series of 103 patients. J Neurosurg 98:764–778

FitzGerald DB, Cosgrove GR, Ronner S, Jiang H, Buchbinder BR, Belliveau JW, Rosen BR, Benson RR (1997) Location of language in the cortex: a comparison between functional mr imaging and electrocortical stimulation. Ajnr Am J Neuroradiol 18:1529–1539

Foerster O (1931) The cerebral cortex of man. Lancet 2:309–312

Grady MS, Jane JA, Steward O (1989) Synaptic reorganization within the human central nervous system following injury. J Neurosurg 71:534–537

Haglund MM, Berger MS, Shamseldin M, Lettich E, Ojemann GA (1994) Cortical localization of temporal lobe language sites in patients with gliomas. Neurosurgery 34:567–576. discussion 576

Haglund MM, Ojemann GA, Blasdel GG (1993) Optical imaging of bipolar cortical stimulation. J Neurosurg 78:785–793

Hegi ME, Diserens AC, Gorlia T, Hamou MF, de Tribolet N, Weller M, Kros JM, Hainfellner JA, Mason W, Mariani L, Bromberg JE, Hau P, Mirimanoff RO, Cairncross JG, Janzer RC, Stupp R (2005) Mgmt gene silencing and benefit from temozolomide in glioblastoma. N Engl J Med 352: 997–1003

Herholz K, Reulen HJ, von Stockhausen HM, Thiel A, Ilmberger J, Kessler J, Eisner W, Yousry TA,, Heiss WD (1997) Preoperative activation and intraoperative stimulation of language-related areas in patients with glioma. Neurosurgery 41:1253–1260. discussion 1260–1252

Karim AB, Maat B, Hatlevoll R, Menten J, Rutten EH, Thomas DG, Mascarenhas F, Horiot JC, Parvinen LM, van Reijn M, Jager JJ, Fabrini MG, van Alphen AM, Hamers HP, Gaspar L, Noordman E, Pierart M, van Glabbeke M (1996) A randomized trial on dose-response in radiation therapy of low-grade cerebral glioma: European organization for research and treatment of cancer (eortc) study 22844. Int J Radiat Oncol Biol Phys 36:549–556

Keles GE, Anderson B, Berger MS (1999) The effect of extent of resection on time to tumor progression and survival in patients with glioblastoma multiforme of the cerebral hemisphere. Surg Neurol 52:371–379

Keles GE, Chang EF, Lamborn KR, Tihan T, Chang CJ, Chang SM, Berger MS (2006) Volumetric extent of resection and residual contrast enhancement on initial surgery as predictors of outcome in adult patients with hemispheric anaplastic astrocytoma. J Neurosurg 105:34–40

Lacroix M, Abi-Said D, Fourney DR, Gokaslan ZL, Shi W, DeMonte F, Lang FF, McCutcheon IE, Hassenbusch SJ, Holland E, Hess K, Michael C, Miller D, Sawaya R (2001) A multivariate analysis of 416 patients with glioblastoma multiforme: prognosis, extent of resection, and survival. J Neurosurg 95:190–198

Maldjian J, Atlas SW, Howard RS 2nd, Greenstein E, Alsop D, Detre JA, Listerud J, D'Esposito M, Flamm ES (1996) Functional magnetic resonance imaging of regional brain activity in patients with intracerebral arteriovenous malformations before surgical or endovascular therapy. J Neurosurg 84:477–483

Ojemann G, Ojemann J, Lettich E, Berger M (1989) Cortical language localization in left, dominant hemisphere. An electrical stimulation mapping investigation in 117 patients. J Neurosurg 71:316–326

Penfield W, Bolchey E (1937) Somatic motor and sensory representation in the cerebral cortex of man as studied by electrical stimulation. Brain 60:389–443

Philippon JH, Clemenceau SH, Fauchon FH, Foncin JF (1993) Supratentorial low-grade astrocytomas in adults. Neurosurgery 32:554–559

Pope WB, Sayre J, Perlina A, Villablanca JP, Mischel PS, Cloughesy TF (2005) Mr imaging correlates of survival in patients with high-grade gliomas. AJNR 26:2466–2474

Quinones-Hinojosa A, Ojemann SG, Sanai N, Dillon WP, Berger MS (2003) Preoperative correlation of intraoperative cortical mapping with magnetic resonance imaging landmarks to predict localization of the broca area. J Neurosurg 99: 311–318

Rajan B, Pickuth D, Ashley S, Traish D, Monro P, Elyan S, Brada M (1994) The management of histologically unverified presumed cerebral gliomas with radiotherapy. Int J Radiat Oncol Biol Phys 28:405–413

Sanai N, Berger MS (2008) Mapping the horizon: techniques to optimize tumor resection before and during surgery. Clin Neurosurg 55:14–19

Seitz RJ, Huang Y, Knorr U, Tellmann L, Herzog H, Freund HJ (1995) Large-scale plasticity of the human motor cortex. Neuroreport 6:742–744

Shaw E, Arusell R, Scheithauer B, O'Fallon J, O'Neill B, Dinapoli R, Nelson D, Earle J, Jones C, Cascino T, Nichols D, Ivnik R, Hellman R, Curran W, Abrams R (2002) Prospective randomized trial of low- versus high-dose radiation therapy in adults with supratentorial low-grade glioma: initial report of a north central cancer treatment group/radiation therapy oncology group/eastern cooperative oncology group study. J Clin Oncol 20: 2267–2276

Shibamoto Y, Kitakabu Y, Takahashi M, Yamashita J, Oda Y, Kikuchi H, Abe M (1993) Supratentorial low-grade astrocytoma. Correlation of computed tomography findings with effect of radiation therapy and prognostic variables. Cancer 72:190–195

Smith JS, Chang EF, Lamborn KR, Chang SM, Prados MD, Cha S, Tihan T, Vandenberg S, McDermott MW, Berger MS (2008) Role of extent of resection in the long-term outcome of low-grade hemispheric gliomas. J Clin Oncol 26:1338–1345

Taylor MD, Bernstein M (1999) Awake craniotomy with brain mapping as the routine surgical approach to treating patients with supratentorial intraaxial tumors: a prospective trial of 200 cases. J Neurosurg 90:35–41

van Veelen ML, Avezaat CJ, Kros JM, van Putten W, Vecht C (1998) Supratentorial low grade astrocytoma: prognostic factors, dedifferentiation, and the issue of early versus late surgery. J Neurol Neurosurg Psychiatry 64:581–587

Yeh SA, Ho JT, Lui CC, Huang YJ, Hsiung CY, Huang EY (2005) Treatment outcomes and prognostic factors in patients with supratentorial low-grade gliomas. Br J Radiol 78: 230–235

Chapter 24

Brainstem Gangliogliomas: Total Resection and Close Follow-Up

George A. Alexiou and Neofytos Prodromou

Abstract Gangliogliomas are mixed glioneuronal tumors with two histological features: atypical ganglion cells and neoplastic glial cells. They comprise approximately 0.4% of all central nervous system tumors and less than 2% of all intracranial tumors. Gangliogliomas are usually located in temporal lobe. Brainstem gangliogliomas are unusual tumors and only few cases have been reported in the literature. Complete tumor resection if feasible, is usually associated with good prognosis. The surgical management of these tumors depends on their location. The definitive role of radiotherapy and chemotherapy has not yet been established. Even after resection a close long-term follow-up is mandatory for these patients.

Keywords Ganglioglioma · Brainstem · Treatment

Introduction

Gangliogliomas are mixed glioneuronal tumors with two histological features: atypical ganglion cells and neoplastic glial cells. They comprise approximately 0.4% of all central nervous system tumors and less than 2% of all intracranial tumors. They are usually low-grade tumors, but anaplastic variants have also been reported (Karremann et al., 2009; Zentner et al., 1994). Gangliogliomas have been reported to arise in every part of the neuraxis, the most common site being the temporal lobe and they have been associated with medically refractory epilepsy (Alexiou et al., 2009). The

G.A. Alexiou (✉)
Department of Neurosurgery, Children's Hospital "Agia Sofia",
Athens, Attikis 11561, Greece
e-mail: alexiougrg@yahoo.gr

patient's age range from 4 to 26 years and there is no sex predilection (Lagares et al., 2001). Brainstem gangliogliomas are unusual tumors and only few cases have been reported in the literature.

Clinical Presentation and Imaging Characteristics

Brainstem gangliogliomas usually have an indolent course due to their general benign nature. Nevertheless, cases of anaplastic tumors with shorter clinical history have been described (Hirose et al., 1992). The symptomatology depends on tumor size and location. Midbrain tumors may cause obstructive hydrocephalus and oculomotor nerve palsy. Pontine lesions can cause facial paresis or long-tract findings. Tumors in the medulla oblongata usually present with lower cranial nerve deficits.

Brainstem tumors are usually classified by means of MRI as diffuse and focal tumors (Jallo et al., 2004). Diffuse tumors are usually high grade whereas focal lesions are low grade. Brainstem gangliogliomas are usually focal lesions and their characteristics on radiological investigation are variable. They may be solid, cystic-solid or solid. Nevertheless, the majority of brainstem gangliogliomas are usually solid and well demarcated (Zentner et al., 1994). Calcifications may also be present. MRI is more sensitive than CT, not only for tumor detection but also for lesion delineation. On MRI they usually are iso or hypointense on T1-weighted images and hyperintense on T2-weighted images. Areas of contrast enhancement may be observed after gadolinium administration (Lagares et al., 2001). However, an accurate

M.A. Hayat (ed.), *Tumors of the Central Nervous System, Volume 1*,
DOI 10.1007/978-94-007-0344-5_24, © Springer Science+Business Media B.V. 2011

preoperative diagnosis and differentiation from other types of gliomas is unfeasible by conventional MRI. Perfusion MRI and MR spectroscopy can be potentially used to differentiate gangliogliomas from gliomas (Im et al., 2002; Law et al., 2004). Tumor dissemination into the subarachnoid space has also been reported (Hukin et al., 2002).

Management

Surgery

Surgery is the treatment of choice for supratentorial gangliogliomas and complete resection has been associated with favorable prognosis. Nevertheless, in brainstem lesions surgery is usually limited to tumors that appear well circumscribed or exophytic. Hydrocephalus that requires treatment, may coexist at the time of diagnosis or can develop postoperative due to blood and tumoral debris. Endoscopic third ventriculostomy or ventriculo-peritoneal shunt placement are viable treatment options of hydrocephalus.

Careful patient selection is of paramount importance for treatment decision-making. The goal of surgery is to operate before there is significant disability, to establish a definitive diagnosis and to decrease as much as tumor burden without causing significant neurological damage (Jallo et al., 2003). In several cases neurological deficits occurred after an effort for total resection (Lagares et al., 2001). The latest advantages in microsurgical techniques, neuroimaging, neurophysiological monitoring and neuroanaesthesia allowed for more aggressive approaches.

Surgical approaches to the brainstem are mainly through the posterior fossa. If the tumor is focal and endophytic then an excision can be performed since the low grade nature of ganglioglioma's usually displaces rather than infiltrates neural structures. Although in other pathologies the presence of a distinct plane of gliotic tissue between the tumor and adjacent brain tissue can allow a maximal excision, in gangliogliomas usually there is no clear tumor demarcation from the surrounding brain. For that reason, a complete resection may be impossible and should not be attempted because it has been associated with high morbidity (Jallo et al., 2003). In difficult to treat

endophytic tumors, stereotactic image-guided biopsy is an alternative and can provide help to establish an accurate diagnosis.

Gangliogliomas in the quadrigeminal plate are usually associated with trivenricular hydrocephalus without brainstem signs. In this location the tumor can be approached via an infratentorial supracerebellar route. The anatomy of the quadrigeminal plate may be unclear because of the tumor. Identification of the fourth cranial nerve origin has been advocated as a useful landmark for orientation (Cultrera et al., 2006). If the tumor is focal and well demarcated a gross total excision can be performed (Jallo et al., 2004).

Gangliogliomas with a dorsally exophytic component, that may extend into the 4th ventricle or cerebellopontine angle, are more frequent and can be more easily approached (Mpairamidis et al., 2008; Milligan et al., 2007). The greatest part of these tumors is usually located outside the brainstem. When located in the 4th ventricle they usually cause obstructive hydrocephalus and tumor removal restores the potency of the 4th ventricle. The approach usually involves a suboccipital craniotomy. After dura opening the 4th ventricle can be reached after splitting the vermis or by opening the tela choroidea and inferior medullary velum. The later approach has been associated with fewer postoperative complications (Mussi and Rhoton, 2000). Tumor is then excised with minimal retraction. During excision special care should be given to the floor of the 4th ventricle. Invasion towards the floor of the 4th ventricle has been associated with high morbidity due to the neighboring 6th and 7th nerve nuclei and other vital structures (Jallo et al., 2003).

Cervicomedullary gangliogliomas can be approached via a suboccipital craniotomy. A cervical laminotomy or laminectomy may be also needed. These tumors are usually endophytic and superficial and a careful resection can be performed via a median myelotomy of the caudal half of the medulla.

Intraoperative neurophysiological monitoring can improve surgical results while minimizing morbidity. Because brainstem tumors usually displace normal landmarks and the safe entry zones into the brainstem, mapping techniques can allow the identification of cranial nerves, their motor nuclei and corticospinal or corticobulbar pathways. Motor-evoked potentials of the corticobulbar tract can provide monitoring of the cranial motor nerves' functional integrity (Morota et al., 2010; Sala et al., 2007). Muscle motor-evoked potentials evaluate the pyramidal motor pathways and in combination with free-running electromyography provide an immediate and conclusive feedback of motor tract integrity (Sala et al., 2007). Apart from that, special microsurgical adjuncts such as cavitron ultrasonic aspirator and surgical laser can provide great help for tumor resection.

Radiotherapy and Chemotherapy

Postoperative conventional radiotherapy should be used in cases of subtotal excised tumors because it improves the local control (Rades et al., 2010). Furthermore, radiotherapy is also reserved for relapse or regrowth after surgery and for anaplastic tumors (Liauw et al., 2007). Nevertheless malignant degeneration of gangliogliomas after radiotherapy has also been reported (Rumana and Valadka, 1998). Hyperfractionated radiotherapy has also been used but with no improvement in overall survival. Radiosurgery has been also employed. Nevertheless, the radiation tolerance of the brainstem remains controversial (Sharma et al., 2008). The role of chemotherapy has not yet been established because of the tumor rarity. Chemotherapy regimens with vincristine, thiotepa and lomustine have been administered but with no clear benefit.

Prognosis

Total resection of brainstem ganglioglioma has been associated with favorable overall prognosis. However in the majority of cases the prognosis may not be optimal because of the difficulty in achieving a complete resection. In general, exophytic and cervicomedullary tumors usually have a better prognosis (Epstein and Farmer, 1993). Diffuse pontine tumors have the worst prognosis. For subtotally excised low grade gangliogliomas, close follow-up is mandatory for these patients because of the risk of regrowth (Luyken et al., 2004). In a series of 9 patients with brainstem gangliogliomas the 5-year survival rate was 73% and the 3-year event-free survival rate was 53% (Lang et al., 1993).

References

Alexiou GA, Varela M, Sfakianos G, Prodromou N (2009) Benign lesions accompanied by intractable epilepsy in children. J Child Neurol 24:697–700

Cultrera F, Guiducci G, Nasi MT, Paioli G, Frattarelli M (2006) Two-stage treatment of a tectal ganglioglioma: endoscopic third ventriculostomy followed by surgical resection. J Clin Neurosci 13:963–965

Epstein FJ, Farmer JP (1993) Brain-stem glioma growth patterns. J Neurosurg 78:408–412

Hirose T, Kannuki S, Nishida K, Matsumoto K, Sano T, Hizawa K (1992) Anaplastic ganglioglioma of the brain stem demonstrating active neurosecretory features of neoplastic neuronal cells. Acta Neuropathol 83:365–370

Hukin J, Siffert J, Velasquez L, Zagzag D, Allen J (2002) Leptomeningeal dissemination in children with progressive low-grade neuroepithelial tumors. Neurooncol 4: 253–260

Im SH, Chung CK, Cho BK, Wang KC, Yu IK, Song IC, Cheon GJ, Lee DS, Kim NR, Chi JG (2002) Intracranial ganglioglioma: preoperative characteristics and oncologic outcome after surgery. J Neurooncol 59:173–183

Jallo GI, Biser-Rohrbaugh A, Freed D (2004) Brainstem gliomas. Childs Nerv Syst 20:143–153

Jallo GI, Freed D, Roonprapunt C, Epstein F (2003) Current management of brainstem gliomas. Ann Neurosurg 3:1–17

Karremann M, Pietsch T, Janssen G, Kramm CM, Wolff JE (2009) Anaplastic ganglioglioma in children. J Neurooncol 92:157–163

Lagares A, Gómez PA, Lobato RD, Ricoy JR, Ramos A, de la Lama A (2001) Ganglioglioma of the brainstem: report of three cases and review of the literature. Surg Neurol 56: 315–322

Lang FF, Epstein FJ, Ransohoff J, Allen JC, Wisoff J, Abbott R, Miller DC (1993) Central nervous system gangliogliomas part 2: clinical outcome. J Neurosurg 79:867–873

Law M, Meltzer DE, Wetzel SG, Yang S, Knopp EA, Golfinos J, Johnson G (2004) Conventional MR imaging with simultaneous measurements of cerebral blood volume and vascular permeability in ganglioglioma. Magn Reson Imaging 22:599–606

Liauw SL, Byer JE, Yachnis AT, Amdur RJ, Mendenhall WM (2007) Radiotherapy after subtotally resected or recurrent ganglioglioma. Int J Radiat Oncol Biol Phys 67: 244–247

Luyken C, Blumcke I, Fimmers R, Urbach H, Wiestler OD, Schramm J (2004) Supratentorial gangliogliomas: histopatholic grading and tumor recurrence in 184 patients with a median follow-up of 8 years. Cancer 101:146–155

Milligan BD, Giannini C, Link MJ (2007) Ganglioglioma in the cerebellopontine angle in a child. Case report and review of the literature. J Neurosurg 107:292–296

Morota N, Ihara S, Deletis V (2010) Intraoperative neurophysiology for surgery in and around the brainstem: role of brainstem mapping and corticobulbar tract motor-evoked potential monitoring. Childs Nerv Syst 26:513–521

Mpairamidis E, Alexiou GA, Stefanaki K, Sfakianos G, Prodromou N (2008) Brainstem ganglioglioma. J Child Neurol 23:1481–1483

Mussi AC, Rhoton AL Jr. (2000) Telovelar approach to the fourth ventricle: microsurgical anatomy. J Neurosurg 92:812–823

Rades D, Zwick L, Leppert J, Bonsanto MM, Tronnier V, Dunst J, Schild SE (2010) The role of postoperative radiotherapy for the treatment of gangliogliomas. Cancer 116:432–442

Rumana CS, Valadka AB (1998) Radiation therapy and malignant degeneration of benign supra-tentorial gangliogliomas. Neurosurgery 42:1038–1043

Sala F, Manganotti P, Tramontano V, Bricolo A, Gerosa M (2007) Monitoring of motor pathways during brain stem surgery: what we have achieved and what we still miss?. Neurophysiol Clin 37:399–406

Sharma MS, Kondziolka D, Khan A, Kano H, Niranjan A, Flickinger JC, Lunsford LD (2008) Radiation tolerance limits of the brainstem. Neurosurgery 63:728–732

Zentner J, Wolf HK, Ostertun B, Hufnagel A, Campos MG, Solymosi L, Schramm J (1994) Gangliogliomas: clinical, radiological, and histopathological findings in 51 patients. J Neurol Neurosurg Psychiatry 57:1497–1502

Chapter 25

Glioblastoma: Temozolomide-Based Chemotherapy

Dagmar Beier and Christoph P. Beier

Abstract   During the last decade, radiotherapy in addition to chemotherapy with temozolomide became the gold standard for the therapy of malignant glioma. The authors summarize the current knowledge on the mechanism of action of temozolomide and mechanisms for chemoresistance. In addition, they describe today's standard of care and future directions for the therapy of glial tumors with a special focus on temozolomide-based therapies (incl. temozolomide rechallenge).

Keywords Temozolomide · Glioblastoma · Cancer stem cell · Glioma · Rechallenge · Pseudoprogression

Temozolomide: A New Alkylating Agent

The role of chemotherapy in the treatment of glioblastoma (GBM) has changed during the last two decades. Although alkylating substances such as ACNU, BCNU, and CCNU have been used since the late 1970s, it took until 2005 to prove that patients diagnosed with GBM benefit from chemotherapy in addition to radiotherapy and surgical resection. Here, the new alkylating agent temozolomide (TMZ) in addition to radiotherapy and surgical resection improved both, the overall survival and the progression-free survival of patients with newly diagnosed GBM (Stupp et al., 2005).

Temozolomide: Mechanism of Action

TMZ, (8-Carbamoyl-3-methylimidazo (5, 1-d)-1, 2, 3, 5-tetrazin-4(3H)-one, is not active by itself but undergoes rapid nonenzymatic conversion at physiologic pH to its active compound 5-3-(methyl)-1-(triazen-1-yl) imidazole-4-carboxamide (MTIC). MTIC causes DNA damage mainly by methylating the O^6-position of guanine (primary lesion) which then mismatches with thymine in double-stranded DNA (O^6G-T) in the first cell cycle after treatment. This mismatch induces futile cycles of mismatch repair triggered by recurrent GT-mismatches resulting in either double strand breaks or a critical recombinogenic secondary lesion. This secondary lesion is assumed to be a apurinic/athymidinic site formed during faulty mismatch repair that blocks replication, resulting in either DNA double strand breaks (tertiary lesion), sister chromatid exchange, or other aberrations (Roos and Kaina, 2006). Thus, not the primary lesions directly caused by TMZ but the tertiary lesions formed during faulty mismatch repair induce apoptosis or senescence (Hirose et al., 2001). Although intensively investigated, there is no agreement how TMZ actually accomplishes its antitumor activity. In addition to apoptosis, cell cycle arrest in the G2/M phase (Hirose et al., 2001), and autophagy (Kanzawa et al., 2004) mediated by TMZ have been described.

Due to the experimental uncertainties, the actual mechanism of action in the patient is controversially discussed. It is unclear if TMZ is effective in the patient on its own or if TMZ mainly increases the activity of radiotherapy and thereby improves the patient's outcome. Neither the study published by Stupp et al. (2005) nor other published investigations provide a

C.P. Beier (✉)
Department of Neurology, RWTH Aachen, Medical School,
Pauwelsstrasse 30, 52073 Aachen, Germany
e-mail: Christoph.beier@gmx.de

sound answer to this question. Unfortunately, there is no ongoing phase III clinical trial to investigate this question in GBM. Still, for anaplastic astrocytomas without LOH 1p19q, the EORTC initiated a multinational phase III trial (CATNON) that will provide an answer to this question by stratifying patients into four arms: radiotherapy alone, radiotherapy with concomitant application of TMZ, radiotherapy with adjuvant application of TMZ, and radiotherapy with concomitant and adjuvant application of TMZ.

Temozolomide: Evidence for Efficacy

The first phase I/II trial for TMZ in GBM was published by Yung et al. (2000) indicating the favourable tolerability of TMZ. A pharmacokinetic study by Brada et al. (1999) comparing the side effects of different serum concentrations achieved when 100–250 mg/m^2 TMZ were administered 5 days every 28 days, concluded that 200 mg/m^2 TMZ given 5 days every 28 days results in optimal serum concentrations and acceptable side effects. Using this scheme, TMZ showed promising results in patients with recurrent GBM as compared to historical controls and to procarbacine, suggesting that TMZ was effective in GBM (Brada et al., 2001; Yung et al., 2000).

The final proof of efficacy was provided by a large, randomised multicenter study initiated by the EORTC and the NCI (Stupp et al., 2005). In this trial, 573 patients were either treated with radiotherapy alone (60 Gy) or with combined radiochemotherapy (comprising 60 Gy and 75 mg/m^2 TMZ administered daily during radiotherapy) followed by a maintenance therapy with TMZ alone (150–200 mg/m^2 given 5 days every 28 days). The overall survival was increased from 12.1 months with radiotherapy alone to 14.6 months for patients who received radiotherapy with concomitant and adjuvant application of TMZ. Although these results were statistically significant, they appear disappointing at first glance. But two additional results of this study strongly favored the use of TMZ for first-line therapy. First, rescue therapy with TMZ in patients treated with radiotherapy alone only moderately improves survival, and patients performed worse as compared to those treated with the combined regimen directly after diagnosis. Second, patients in the TMZ group showed a meaningful increased 2 year

overall survival rate of 26.5% as compared to 10.4% in the radiotherapy group. Recent follow-up data indicate that TMZ also increases the proportion of long-term survival of 3 years or more, a 5 year survival of up to 15% was achieved in patients with very favourable prognostic factors (Stupp et al., 2009).

Overcoming the Resistance to Temozolomide

The good performance of a subgroup of patients raised the question for molecular prognostic factors. MGMT (O6-Methyl-Guanidine Methyl Transferase) removes O6-guanidine adducts induced by TMZ and thereby protects the tumor cell against TMZ. Hegi et al. (2005) showed that the methylation status of the MGMT promoter was a highly significant prognostic factor. Among patients treated with TMZ, those with methylated MGMT promoter survived 21.7 months as compared to 15.3 months in the group with unmethylated promoter. Although the latter group also significantly benefited from TMZ therapy due to an increased 6 months progression-free survival (PFS-6), the overall survival as compared to radiotherapy alone did not reach statistical significance. These findings question if TMZ according to the EORTC study (Stupp et al., 2005) should be given to patients with unmethylated MGMT promoter as well. A possible approach to overcome MGMT mediated resistance to TMZ is the kinetic of MGMT that detoxifies only one methylated O6-guanidine. This suggests that a more prolonged schedule of TMZ might result in an exhaustion of the MGMT activity and thus in an improved activity of TMZ. Multiple alternative dosing schemes have been evaluated and published. Brandes et al. (2006) reported that 75 mg/m^2 TMZ given for 21 days (followed by a 7 days break) to chemo-naive patients with recurrent GBM resulted in a PFS-6 of 30.3%. These results exceeded the results reported by Brada et al. (2001) for a similar patient population by far. Here, a PFS-6 of 18% was reported. No difference between MGMT methylated and unmethylated patients was seen. Unfortunately, the study was not powered enough to allow a final conclusion that the dosing scheme actually overcomes MGMT mediated TMZ resistance. Tuettenberg et al. (2005) treated 13 patients with newly diagnosed GBM with up to 10 mg/m^2 TMZ and the COX-2 inhibitor rofecoxib. The overall survival was 16 months, the PFS was 8 months. This schedule aimed at the tumor vessels, and the efficacy was thereby independent of the MGMT methylation status.

Wick et al. (2007) recently reported on very promising results using the "1 week on/1 week off" scheme consisting of 150 mg/m^2 for 7 days every other week. In this study, 90 patients with recurrent GBM were treated achieving a PFS-6 of 43.8%. Importantly, the schedule was active irrespective of the MGMT promoter status, indicating some activity in patients with unmethylated MGMT promoter. In addition to improved TMZ dosing schemes, new substances with synergistic activity are sought for and many efforts have been made to improve today's standard of care by adding other therapeutic agents. Encouraging results have recently been published by Prados et al. (2008). Sixty-five patients with newly diagnosed GBM or gliosarcoma were treated with Erlotinib – a EGFR tyrosine kinase inhibitor – during and after radiotherapy as add-on to today's standard of care. Median survival of patients with methylated MGMT promoter was 25.5 months compared to 14.6 months for patients with unmethylated MGMT promoter. Nevertheless, although many different therapeutic approaches have been under evaluation, none of them has proven to be more effective than today's standard of care for first-line therapy of GBM in a randomized phase III trial.

Adjuvant Temozolomide and Temozolomide Rechallenge

The profile of TMZ side effects is very favourable given its good clinical efficacy. It includes mainly haematological side effects. In the study by Stupp et al. (2005) only 14 of 287 patients (i.e., 5%) discontinued therapy due to therapy-related side effects (mainly CTC °III and °IV leuko- and thrombopenia). Additionally mainly gastrointestinal side effects occurred including nausea and vomitus. Fortunately, they responded well to antiemetic treatment by e.g., 5-HT3-receptor antagonists. Knowing that TMZ is effective against GBM and considering that viable tumor cells persist in the brain, clinical neurooncologists tend to administer TMZ for more than 6 cycles (Hau et al., 2007). In a German survey by these authors, 50 centers admitted to prescribe TMZ longer

than the 6 cycles recommended, a proportion that may be representative for western countries. Although even long-term administration for more than 12 cycles (i.e., > 63 weeks after diagnosis) was well tolerated, there is hardly any evidence suggesting an improved activity of long-term TMZ. In addition to the work by Hau et al. (2007), who found a trend towards a more favourable outcome of patients treated with long-term TMZ, Colman et al. (2002) presented their work from the M.D. Anderson Cancer Center at the meeting of the American Society for Neurooncology in 2002, indicating that patients might benefit from long-term use longer than 18 cycles. A phase I/II trial using long-term TMZ combined with pegylated liposomal doxorubicin did not detect a statistical significant improvement of patients treated with long-term TMZ and pegylated liposomal doxorubicin in addition to resection and standard radiotherapy (Beier et al., 2009). Notably, the study was powered to detect a 20% increase of the PFS-12 supporting the overall validity of these data. Still, a randomised trial answering this highly relevant question is lacking. In recurrent GBM, TMZ is the only chemotherapeutic agent so far proven effective. Although other drugs that are commonly used (BCNU, CCNU, ACNU, Procarbacin, and Irinotecan) have been shown to have promising effects in non-randomised phase II trials, widely accepted evidence for the activity of these drugs is lacking. Therefore, the use of TMZ after tumor recurrence is obvious ("TMZ Rechallenge"). While the use of TMZ in patients with tumor recurrences after having finished 6 cycles of TMZ is plausible, there is increasing evidence that the change of the TMZ dosing schedule and an increase in the concentration of this drug might also be effective. Indeed, Perry et al. (2008) reported on a PFS-6 of 17% and overall response rate of 47% in patients who received 50 mg/m^2 daily TMZ after progressing under ongoing therapy with TMZ. In patients that had discontinued therapy with TMZ without tumor progression, the recurrent tumor was stable for at least 6 months in 57% of all patients.

At the moment, there is no additional evidence published so far. A trial initiated by the German Neurooncological Working Group investigating the efficacy of dose-intensified TMZ for tumor recurrence after therapy with TMZ will start to recruit patients in 2009. In this trial, two different schedules (1-week on/1 week off and 3 weeks on/1 week off) will be compared in patients that progressed under ongoing treatment with TMZ. Based on the available evidence and knowing the limited efficacy of other drugs used in the therapy of GBM, the compassionate use of TMZ with increased doses (e.g., 1 week on/1 week off) may be warranted in selected patients until the results of clinical trials become available.

Pseudoprogression

An increase of the contrast-enhancing lesion in the MRI without actual tumor growth is referred to as pseudoprogression. Brandes et al. (2008) reported that in a series of 50 patients showing "tumor progression" according to standard criteria (Macdonald et al., 1990) 4 weeks after completion of the combined radiochemotherapy: 32 patients showed pseudoprogression while only 18 patients actually progressed. Importantly, patients with methylated MGMT promoter showed significantly more often pseudoprogression as compared to patients with unmethylated promoter. In the latter group, the increase of the lesion most likely indicated actual tumor progression. In a second report, Brandsma et al. (2008) have reported similar rates of pseudoprogression. Although the phenomenon itself is not controversially discussed, its incidence is unknown. Several clinical neurooncologists feel that the actual rate of pseudoprogression is far below the 50% published by Brandes et al. (2008) and Brandsma et al. (2008). Still, there is a consensus that pseudoprogression is a serious problem because it might prompt the treating physician to stop the actually effective therapy with TMZ. Conversely, if TMZ is no more effective, other alkylating agents or new targeted therapies applied in clinical trials might be more beneficial for the patients. New imaging methods are currently under investigation and help to guide the physician. Especially positron emission tomography (PET) has been thoroughly investigated and is already used routinely in committed neurooncological centers. FDG-PET distinguish between necrosis and viable tumor and FET-PET indicates viable tumor tissue (e.g., Popperl et al., 2004). Still, both PET modalities are expensive and not available on a routine base in all neurooncological centers. In addition, it is unclear if pseudoprogression may also occur under treatment with TMZ. Although there are no reports focussing on this issue, the clinical experience and a recent publication on the susceptibility of GBM cancer stem cells suggests that this may be possible (Beier et al., 2008).

Cancer Stem Cells: Resistance Against Temozolomide

Cancer stem cells (CSC) are frequently thought to mediate tumor resistance to different therapeutic modalities. The underlying CSC hypothesis states that only a rare subpopulation of tumor cells, the so-called CSC, are able to maintain tumor growth. In addition, CSC later differentiate into progenitor-like or differentiated tumor cells that define the histological features of the entity (Reya et al., 2001). For several different brain tumors CD133$^+$ but not CD133$^-$ tumor cells were able to reconstitute the initial tumor in vivo when injected into immune-deficient nude mice (Singh et al., 2004). The CSC hypothesis also states that tumor relapses are driven by CSC having escaped multimodal therapy. It predicts that only therapies that efficiently eliminate the CSC fraction of a tumor are able to induce long-term responses and thereby cure the tumor.

It was recently shown that TMZ selectively depleted GBM CSC in a dose-dependent manner, whereas it affected little overall viability. When CD133$^+$ CSC lines were treated with up to 500 μM TMZ during different periods of time, there was a dose-dependent reduction of CD133$^+$ cells (by 80%), cell proliferation (by up to 100%), as well as of clonogenicity (by up to 100%), whereas cell death did not exceed 6%. Irrespective of pulse-treatment or long-term treatment, stem cell-like properties were selectively dose-dependently depleted. In addition, when tumor cells that had been treated with doses of TMZ corresponding to the doses that completely abrogated clonogenicity were injected into immune-deficient nude mice, they only built up scar-like lesions that did not contain any proliferating tumor cells. In contrast, untreated tumor cells formed invasively growing lesions (Beier et al., 2008). The concentrations required to eliminate CSC in vitro can be reached in the plasma of patients but not in the cerebrospinal fluid due to the incomplete penetration of TMZ through the blood-brain barrier. This may explain why on the one hand CSC are susceptible to TMZ, but on the other hand patients die despite treatment with TMZ. Based on the cumulative data, there is no convincing evidence that the increased chemoresistance of CSC mediates the poor overall response of GBM to chemotherapy. In contrast, experimental evidence suggests that TMZ may actually deplete CSC and thereby improve the patients' overall survival.

Summary

Although today's standard of care, TMZ, administered concomitant with radiotherapy and adjuvant, according to the EORTC trial by Stupp et al. (2005), has improved the patients PFS and overall survival, still patients inevitably die within a few years and long-term survival is rare. Referring to the actual state of knowledge, treatment of GBM patients with methylated MGMT promoter according to the EORTC trial by Stupp et al. (2005) is obligatory. Although overall survival of patients with unmethylated MGMT promoter was not significantly improved, they benefited from TMZ therapy due to an increased PFS-6 (Hegi et al., 2005). Thus, patients with an unmethylated MGMT promoter should be treated with TMZ as long as no therapeutical approach showing more efficacy has been introduced. Alternative dosing schemes that may overcome MGMT-mediated resistance to TMZ require intensive study before they can replace or complement today's standard of care. Unfortunately, no new chemotherapeutic agent showing comparable efficacy with TMZ has been identified so far. Still, there is hope that future innovative therapeutic approaches that may focus on CSC will substantially improve the dismal prognosis of patients diagnosed with GBM.

References

Beier D, Rohrl S, Pillai DR, Schwarz S, Kunz-Schughart LA, Leukel P, Proescholdt M, Brawanski A, Bogdahn U, Trampe-Kieslich A, Giebel B, Wischhusen J, Reifenberger G, Hau P, Beier CP (2008) Temozolomide preferentially depletes cancer stem cells in glioblastoma. Cancer Res 68: 5706–5715

Beier CP, Schmid C, Gorlia T, Kleinletzenberger C, Beier D, Grauer O, Steinbrecher A, Hirschmann B, Brawanski A, Dietmaier C, Jauch-Worley T, Pietsch T, Proescholdt M, Rummele P, Muigg A, Stockhammer G, Hegi M, Bogdahn U, Hau P (2009) RNOP-09: pegylated liposomal doxorubicine and prolonged temozolomide in addition to radiotherapy in newly diagnosed glioblastoma – a phase II study. BMC Cancer 9:308

Brada M, Hoang-Xuan K, Rampling R, Dietrich PY, Dirix LY, Macdonald D, Heimans JJ, Zonnenberg BA, Bravo-Marques JM, Henriksson R, Stupp R, Yue N, Bruner J, Dugan M, Rao S, Zaknoen S (2001) Multicenter phase II trial of temozolomide in patients with glioblastoma multiforme at first relapse. Ann Oncol 12:259–266

Brada M, Judson I, Beale P, Moore S, Reidenberg P, Statkevich P, Dugan M, Batra V, Cutler D (1999) Phase i dose-escalation and pharmacokinetic study of temozolomide (SCH 52365) for refractory or relapsing malignancies. Br J Cancer 81:1022–1030

Brandes AA, Franceschi E, Tosoni A, Blatt V, Pession A, Tallini G, Bertorelle R, Bartolini S, Calbucci F, Andreoli A, Frezza G, Leonardi M, Spagnolli F, Ermani M (2008) MGMT promoter methylation status can predict the incidence and outcome of pseudoprogression after concomitant radiochemotherapy in newly diagnosed glioblastoma patients. J Clin Oncol 26:2192–2197

Brandes AA, Tosoni A, Cavallo G, Bertorelle R, Gioia V, Franceschi E, Biscuola M, Blatt V, Crino L, Ermani M (2006) Temozolomide 3 weeks on and 1 week off as first-line therapy for recurrent glioblastoma: phase II study from gruppo italiano cooperativo di neuro-oncologia (GICNO). Br J Cancer 95:1155–1160

Brandsma D, Stalpers L, Taal W, Sminia P, van den Bent MJ (2008) Clinical features, mechanisms, and management of pseudoprogression in malignant gliomas. Lancet Oncol 9:453–461

Colman H, Hess KR, Turner MC, Puduvalli VK, Gilbert MR (2002) Impact of duration of temozolomide therapy on progression-free survival in recurrent malignant glioma. Neurooncol 4:308–381

Hau P, Koch D, Hundsberger T, Marg E, Bauer B, Rudolph R, Rauch M, Brenner A, Rieckmann P, Schuth J, Jauch T, Koch H, Bogdahn U (2007) Safety and feasibility of long-term temozolomide treatment in patients with high-grade glioma. Neurology 68:688–690

Hegi ME, Diserens AC, Gorlia T, Hamou MF, de Tribolet N, Weller M, Kros JM, Hainfellner JA, Mason W, Mariani L, Bromberg JE, Hau P, Mirimanoff RO, Cairncross JG, Janzer RC, Stupp R (2005) MGMT gene silencing and benefit from temozolomide in glioblastoma. N Engl J Med 352: 997–1003

Hirose Y, Berger MS, Pieper RO (2001) P53 effects both the duration of G2/m arrest and the fate of temozolomide-treated human glioblastoma cells. Cancer Res 61:1957–1963

Kanzawa T, Germano IM, Komata T, Ito H, Kondo Y, Kondo S (2004) Role of autophagy in temozolomide-induced cytotoxicity for malignant glioma cells. Cell Death Differ 11: 448–457

Macdonald DR, Cascino TL, Schold SC Jr, Cairncross JG (1990) Response criteria for phase II studies of supratentorial malignant glioma. J Clin Oncol 8:1277–1280

Perry JR, Rizek P, Cashman R, Morrison M, Morrison T (2008) Temozolomide rechallenge in recurrent malignant glioma by using a continuous temozolomide schedule: the "rescue" approach. Cancer 113:2152–2157

Popperl G, Gotz C, Rachinger W, Gildehaus FJ, Tonn JC, Tatsch K (2004) Value of O-(2-[18f]fluoroethyl)-L-tyrosine PET for the diagnosis of recurrent glioma. Eur J Nucl Med Mol Imaging 31:1464–1470

Prados MD, Chang SM, Butowski N, DeBoer R, Parvataneni R, Carliner H, Kabuubi P, Ayers-Ringler J, Rabbitt J, Page M, Fedoroff A, Sneed PK, Berger MS, McDermott MW, Parsa AT, Vandenberg S, James CD, Lamborn KR, Stokoe D, Haas-Kogan DA (2009) Phase II study of erlotinib plus temozolomide during and after radiation therapy in patients with newly diagnosed glioblastoma multiforme or gliosarcoma. J Clin Oncol 27:579–584

Reya T, Morrison SJ, Clarke MF, Weissman IL (2001) Stem cells, cancer, and cancer stem cells. Nature 414:105–111

Roos WP, Kaina B (2006) DNA damage-induced cell death by apoptosis. Trends Mol Med 12:440–450

Singh SK, Hawkins C, Clarke ID, Squire JA, Bayani J, Hide T, Henkelman RM, Cusimano MD, Dirks PB (2004) Identification of human brain tumour initiating cells. Nature 432:396–401

Stupp R, Hegi ME, Mason WP, van den Bent MJ, Taphoorn MJ, Janzer RC, Ludwin SK, Allgeier A, Fisher B, Belanger K, Hau P, Brandes AA, Gijtenbeek J, Marosi C, Vecht CJ, Mokhtari K, Wesseling P, Villa S, Eisenhauer E, Gorlia T, Weller M, Lacombe D, Cairncross JG, Mirimanoff RO (2009) Effects of radiotherapy with concomitant and adjuvant temozolomide versus radiotherapy alone on survival in glioblastoma in a randomised phase III study: 5-year analysis of the EORTC-NCIC trial. Lancet Oncol 10: 459–466

Stupp R, Mason WP, van den Bent MJ, Weller M, Fisher B, Taphoorn MJ, Belanger K, Brandes AA, Marosi C, Bogdahn U, Curschmann J, Janzer RC, Ludwin SK, Gorlia T, Allgeier A, Lacombe D, Cairncross JG, Eisenhauer E, Mirimanoff RO (2005) Radiotherapy plus concomitant and adjuvant temozolomide for glioblastoma. N Engl J Med 352:987–996

Tuettenberg J, Grobholz R, Korn T, Wenz F, Erber R, Vajkoczy P (2005) Continuous low-dose chemotherapy plus inhibition of cyclooxygenase-2 as an antiangiogenic therapy of glioblastoma multiforme. J Cancer Res Clin Oncol 131:31–40

Wick A, Felsberg J, Steinbach JP, Herrlinger U, Platten M, Blaschke B, Meyermann R, Reifenberger G, Weller M, Wick W (2007) Efficacy and tolerability of temozolomide in an alternating weekly regimen in patients with recurrent glioma. J Clin Oncol 25:3357–3361

Yung WK, Albright RE, Olson J, Fredericks R, Fink K, Prados MD, Brada M, Spence A, Hohl RJ, Shapiro W, Glantz M, Greenberg H, Selker RG, Vick NA, Rampling R, Friedman H, Phillips P, Bruner J, Yue N, Osoba D, Zaknoen S, Levin VA (2000) A phase II study of temozolomide vs. Procarbazine in patients with glioblastoma multiforme at first relapse. Br J Cancer 83:588–593

Chapter 26

Drug-Resistant Glioma: Treatment with Imatinib Mesylate and Chlorimipramine

Ayhan Bilir and Mine Erguven

Abstract Glioblastoma (GBM) is the most common and malignant primary brain tumor. Despite recent advances in treatment regimens, the prognosis of patients remains poor. Although different combined therapies of surgery, radiation and chemotherapy are being essayed in order to cope with resistance and relapse to prolong survival time and reach complete remission, these have still demonstrated equivocal significant benefit. In chemotherapy era, this shortcoming lead investigators to design new antineoplastic agents. Although most of them reached their aim, one side of the coin shows that this process from bench to in vivo and phase trials take a lot of time and money resulting in more death and the formation and/or incidence of economic crisis. Another side of the coin is lack of stability and/or quality of patients' social life during chemotheraphy due to psychiatric disorders. Two parts of the coin are apart so they are not valuable. Consequently, investigators start to search whether commonly and effectively used non antineoplastic drugs for a long time in clinic has anti-neoplastic effects and/or has ability to potentiate antineoplastic drugs cytotoxicity or not. An antidepressant chlorimipramine (CIMP) has been being involved in these trials and proposed as a promising antineoplastic agent. In addition, investigators chose to experience current antineoplastic agents which their success were proved at specific cancer types for another cancer types such as an antileukemic agent imatinib mesylate (IM) in GBM.

This chapter focuses on GBM, and the roles of IM and CIMP in the treatment of GBM.

Keywords Imanib mesylate · Chlorimipramine · Glioblastoma

Introduction

Glioblastoma is the most common and malignant primary brain tumor. Despite recent advances in treatment regimens, the prognosis of patients remains poor. The majority of the patients die within a year of diagnosis, and the 5 year survival of patients worldwide with glioma is only 10%. Although different combined therapies of surgery, radiation, and chemotherapy are being essayed in order to cope with the obstacles as resistance and relapse to prolong survival time and reach complete remission, these have still demonstrated equivocal significant benefit (Furnari et al., 2007; Raguz and Yagüe, 2008). In the chemotherapy era, this shortcoming lead investigators to design new antineoplastic agents, and to use them alone or in combination with the old ones (Zhou and Gallo, 2008). Although these advances achieved same success, this process from bench to in vivo and phase trials took considerable time and financial resources, resulting in more deaths. We are still suffering from a lack of stability and/or quality of patients' social life during chemotheraphy, due to psychiatric disorders such as depression. Consequently, investigators started to search whether or not commonly and effectively used nonantineoplastic drugs for a long time in clinic has antineoplastic effects and/or has ability to potentiate antineoplastic drugs cytotoxicity (Daley et al., 2005).

A. Bilir (✉)
Istanbul Faculty of Medicine, Department of Histology and Embryology, Istanbul University, 34390 Istanbul, Turkey
e-mail: aybilir@gmail.com; bilira@istanbul.edu.tr

An antidepressant chlorimipramine was used in these trials and was proposed as a promising antineoplastic agent. In addition, investigators chose to experiment with current antineoplastic agents which have proven successful for specific cancer types and for another cancer types. These antineoplastic agents target same pathways but are effected negatively by different mutations such as imatinib mesylate in chronic myeloid leukemia and imatinib mesylate in glioblastoma. This chapter focuses on glioblastoma and the roles of imatinib mesylate and chlorimipramine in the treatment of glioblastoma.

Glioblastoma

The incidence of primary brain tumors worldwide is approximately 7 per 100.000 individuals per year, acoounting for 2% of the primary tumors, and 7% of the years of life lost due to this cancer before the age of 70. Gliomas are the most common tumors of the human brain. Approximately, half of all primary brain tumors are collectively known as gliomas. Gliomas arise from glial cells, the building-block cells of the connective and supportive, tissues in the central nervous system (CNS). The common gliomas are diffuse gliomas which infiltrate throughout the brain parenchyma. These are classified histologically and/or ultrastructurally as astrocytomas, oligodendrogliomas, and oligoastrocytomas. They are graded on a World Health Organization (WHO) classification system scale of I to IV according to their degree of malignancy based on different histological features and genetic alterations. Grade I tumors are benign and can be cured if they can be surgically resected; grade II tumors are incurable with surgery because of their early diffuse infiltration of the surrounding brain, and long treatment regimens are needed to treat this disease completely; grade III tumors have increased anaplasia and proliferate over grade IV tumors and are more rapidly fatal; grade IV tumors possess advanced features of malignancy, and are resistant to radio/chemotherapy. Hence, they are characterized with poor prognosis resulting in the death within ~9–12 months. Grade I, II, III, and IV designation is reserved for pilocytic astrocytoma, low grade astrocytoma (LGA), anaplastic astrocytoma, and glioblastoma multiforme (GBM), respectively. The most frequent subtypes are glioblastoma (47%) and

grade II–III astrocytoma (23%), followed by oligodendroglioma and mixed glioma (Furnari et al., 2007).

Glioblastoma patients generally have a dismal prognosis, with an average survival time of only 9–12 months from their diagnosis, and thus they can be named as "terminator". GBM accounts for ~50% of adult gliomas; and up to 10% of pediatric gliomas are either anaplastic astrocytomas or GBMs. GBM occurs with at an incidence of 3 per 100,000 per year, producing ~9,000 cases annually in the United States. Cases of GBMs are distributed over a broad range of ages, with an average age of 53 years at diagnosis. Prognosis factors include age and post-operative physical performance status. The tumors of older patients are more aggressive and more resistant to treatment. The patients who are alive 3–5 years following diagnosis are defined as "long-term survivors" and are very rare. Younger age than the average of 53 years is usually the only common feature of long-term survivors (Furnari et al., 2007).

Important characteristics of GBMs are aberrant cellular proliferation, diffuse infiltration, prospensity for necrosis, robust angiogenesis, high resistance to apoptosis, and genomic instability. The intratumoral heterogenity combined with a putative cancer stem cell (CSC) subpopulation and incomplete atlas of epigenetic lesions are the reasons of poor prognosis/high tumoral resistance against chemotherapeutics and recurrence. GBMs have been subdivided into the primary (de novo) and secondary (progessive) GBMs according to their clinical evaluation. Primary GBMs are commonly detected as subtypes, and tend to occur in older patients above the age of 45 years. Primary GBMs presents in an acute de novo manner without any evidence of prior clinical disease. In contrast, secondary GBMs are quite rare and commonly detected in younger patients below the age of 45 years. In addition, the latter initially present with lower grade astrocytomas and latterly ~70% of grade II gliomas transform into GBMs within 5–10 years of the initial diagnosis, regardless of prior therapy. Primary and secondary GBMs show differences in their clinical characteristics and genetic profiles (different transcriptional patterns and frequency of specific mutations as the mutations of tumour supressor genes retinoblastoma [Rb] and p53 result in DNA copy number aberrations). However, they also have similarities, which are morphologically indistinguishable and show poor prognosis (Furnari et al., 2007).

Glioblastomas circumvent the blockage of tumour supressor genes (p53, phosphatase and tensin homolog deleted on choromosome 10 [PTEN], and [Rb]) on positive regulators of cell division, survival and motility. These positive regulators are receptor tyrosine kinases [RTKs, i.e. Platelet derived growth factor receptor (PDGFR), Epidermal growth factor receptor (EGFR), Vascular endothelial growth factor receptor (VEGFR)], growth factors [i.e. platelet derived growth factor (PDGF), vascular endothelial growth factor (VEGF)], cell adhesion molecules (i.e. integrins) and their two major downstream signaling pathways [i.e. mitogen activated protein kinase (MAPK), phosphoinositide-3 kinases (PI3Ks)]. Molecular pathogenesis of primary GBMs present (1) mutations of INK4aARF, PTEN, EGFR, loss of heterozygosity (LOH) of chromosome 10p and 10q, (2) amplications of EGFR, Cyclin D1/3, murine double minute 2 and 4 (MDM2 and MDM4), and (3) overexpressions of Bcl2-like-12 (Bcl2L 12) ($\sim$95%), cyclin D 1/3, MDM2 or MDM4. In contrast, molecular pathogenesis of secondary GBMs present (1) mutations of tumor supressors p53, Rb, PTEN ($\sim$10%), loss of chromosomes 10q, 11p, 19q, (2) amplications of cyclin dependent kinases 4/6 (CDK4/6), and (3) overexpressions of PDGFR, PDGF, CDK4/6.

Glioblastomas, the most highly vascular of all solid tumors and microvascular hyperplasia, define both the histological phenotype of primary and secondary GBM. Although primary and secondary GBMs possess different genomic profiles, they form a final common angiogenesis pathway involving hypoxia inhibitory factor (HIF) and non-HIF-dependent downstream effectors such as VEGF, PDGF, stromal cell-derived factor-1 (SDF-1), endostatin, and thrompospondin 1 and 2 (TSP-1 and TSP-2). Because of their significant roles in GBMs' molecular pathogenesis, these molecules/pathways are accepted as "magic bullets" for the treatment of GBMs (Furnari et al., 2007).

Imatinib Mesylate: From Leukemia to Glioblastoma

Imatinib mesylate (IM; STI-571, Gleevec®) is a 2-phenylaminopyrimidine derivative small molecule ATP analogue. IM is a potent and selective inhibitor of several protein tyrosine kinases of the receptors for PDGF, breakpoint-cluster region-Abelson leukaemia virus protein (bcr-abl), stem cell factor (SCF), and c-kit by interacting with the adenosine triphosphate (ATP)-binding site. Thus, IM blocks the ability of these factors to use ATP (O'Reilly et al., 2005; Bilir et al., 2008). It has been reported that mitochondria and telomerase are also targets of IM. IM induces apoptosis through its mitochondrial uncoupling effect, resulting in the induction of reactive oxygen species (ROS), the decrease of membrane potential, mitochondrial permeability transition pore (MPTP) formation, cytochrome C release, activation of caspase-3 and endonuclease G, which result in DNA degradation (O'Reilly et al., 2005; Bilir et al., 2008). IM reduces human telomerase reverse transcriptase (hTERT) expression, and down regulates telomerase activity (Bilir et al., 2008). IM was initially used to treat CML, but it is also currently the drug of choice for the treatment of metastatic gastrointestinal stromal tumors (GISTs) (O'Reilly et al., 2005). The success of this compound in the treatment of CML and GISTs has led to the broader application in the treatment of other tumors, such as small lung cancer, anaplastic thyroid cancer, prostate cancer, and GBM (Kilic et al., 2000; O'Reilly et al., 2005; Bilir et al., 2008).

Previous reports demonstrated that monotherapy by using IM is efficacious in in vitro models of GBM because of its potency to inhibit the signaling pathway of PDGFR (Kilic et al., 2000). Although it was shown that monotherapy with IM is also effective in in vivo models of GBM, IM could not achieve the same success as in in vitro models because of its poor brain distribution (Bihorel et al., 2007; Declèves et al., 2008). Unfortunately, in accordance with in vivo studies, monotherapy with IM has minimal activity in Phase II studies of GBM. IM has not provided the dramatic results sometimes seen with other targeted therapies such as IM in CML (Reardon et al., 2005; Wen et al., 2006). Previous studies showed that IM is a substrate of ATP-binding cassette (ABC) transportes which are excreted by the drug from the cell and expressed at the blood-brain barrier (BBB). It was shown that two efflux pumps P-glycoprotein (p-gp or multidrug resistance protein Mdr1a) and breast cancer resistance protein (Bcrp1) have a significant role in the restriction of IM to brain among ABC transporters (Bihorel et al., 2007; Declèves et al., 2008).

Although IM has minimal activity, when combined with an alkylating agent temozolamid (TMZ; Temodar®) in Phase I trial (Reardon et al., 2008) and a ribonucleotide reductase inhibitor hydroxyurea in Phase II trial (Reardon et al., 2005), this combined therapies improved patient's quality of life and outcome. In addition, Ziegler et al. (2008) combined IM with an inhibitor of apoptosis proteins (IAPs) blocker in human GBM cells in vitro, effects in orthotopic mouse models of GBM and in primary human GBM neurospheres. They induced apoptosis human GBM cells in vitro and had synergistic antitumor effect in animal models and neurospheres. These authors demonstrated that concomitant inhibition of IAPs can overcome resistance to RTK inhibitors in human malignant glioblastoma cells. Radiotherapy is an important treatment option for the treatment of GBMs, combined effects of IM and radiation were also investigated in human GBM cells in vitro and in mouse models by Oertel et al. (2006) and in patients by Scheda et al. (2007). Oertal et al. (2006) showed that IM can enhance the tumor growth reduction induced by radiotherapy in GBM models. However, Scheda et al. (2007) reported unsatisfactory results of radiotherapy plus IM in comparison to low dose TMZ plus radiation, and they proposed that a high prevalence of unfavorable prognostic factors in the respective patients might be the reason of this failure.

Chlorimipramine

Chlorimipramine (CIMP; clomipramine or Anafranil®) is the tricyclic anti-depressant that has been in clinical use for over 30 years, and shows its effect through the competitive inhibition of the serotonin and norepinephrine transporters. CIMP belongs to the dibenzazepine class of pharmacologic agents (Nadgir and Malviya, 2008). Previous studies which were made on various types of cancer cells, including drug-resistant human leukemias, human renal cancer cells, solid murine tumors, non-Hodkin's lymphoma cells, and a wide range of cell cultures derived from brain tumor (e.g., astrocytomas, mixed oligo-astrocytomas, GBM, and menningiomas) revealed the novel effect of CIMP as an antineoplastic agent (Daley et al., 2005). CIMP has an advantage over other antineoplastic

agents because it is strongly lipophilic; thus, CIMP crosses easily the membranes of mitochondria and BBB (Levkovitz et al., 2005; Rooprai et al., 2003), and selectively kils tumor cells without damaging normal cells (Daley et al., 2005).

Chlorimipramine blocks oxygen consumption by inhibiting complex-III of the mitochondrial respiratory chain, resulting in the initiation of cascade started with the induction of reactive oxygen species (ROS), the decrease of membrane potential, mitochondrial permeability transition pore (MPTP) formation, cytochrome C release, activation of caspase-3 and endonuclease G, and ended with DNA degradation, and finally apoptotic cell death (Daley et al., 2005; Levkovitz et al., 2005). Interestingly, Merry et al. (1991) showed that CIMP also causes irreversible DNA damage in both normal and neoplastic cells, but mitochondrial damage has only been observed in neoplastic cells. In other studies proposed that CIMP selectively damages tumor cells (Daley et al., 2005).

In spite of many reports suggesting that CIMP exerts apoptotic cell death, as mentioned earlier, only one report by us has proposed for the first time that autophagy is also involved in the mode of CIMPs' antineoplastic action. In our study, we investigated the therapeutic potential of CIMP used in combination with IM using monolayers and spheroid cultures of malignant C6 glioma cells in vitro. We showed CIMP potentiates the cytotoxicity of IM with few exceptions. A striking result of this study was obtained by using an electron microscope at 24 and 96 h of incubation times (Figs. 26.1 and 26.2). Although previous studies have shown that both IM (Figs. 26.1b and 26.2b, and CIMP (Figs. 26.1c and 26.2c, induced severe mitochondria damage and IM induced autophagic vacuoles, they also showed that CIMP induced autophagic vacuoles and the increase in number of autophagic vacuoles when used with IM (Figs. 26.1d and 26.2d. We also evaluated the percentage of apoptosis by using Annexin-V-FITC/PI dual staining. The results of apoptosis were consistent with the electron microscope results in that the increase in percentage of apoptosis by CIMP increase in the combination group where the increase in number of autophagic vacuoles was observed (Figs. 26.1c and 26.2c (Bilir et al., 2008). Moreover, CIMP has been demonstrated to reverse multidrug resistance (MDR) to conventional antineoplastic agents, such as doxorubicin (Pommerenke and Volm, 1995).

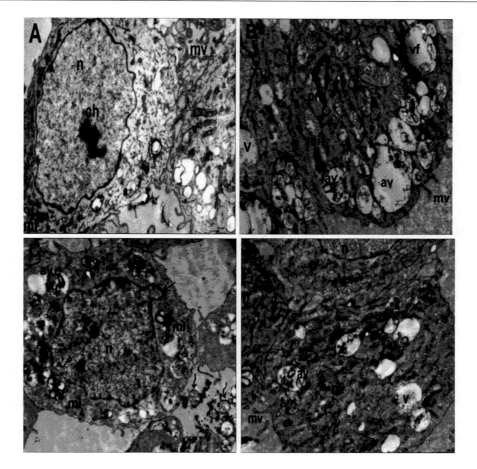

Fig. 26.1 Transmission electron microscopy views of C6 glioma spheroids at 24th h: (**a**) Control group (Original magnification of ×7,500), (**b**) Imatinib group (Original magnification of × 12,000), (**c**) Chlorimipramine group (Original magnification of ×15,000). One *arrow* represents the extention of nucleus to cytoplasm like a pseudopod, and wavy arrows represent presumably apoptotic bodies, (**d**) Imatinib with chlorimipramine. One *arrow* represents mitochondria with disrupted outer membrane and two *arrows* represent mitochondria swelling with criastae damage. (Original magnification of × 12,000). *av*: autophagic vacuole, *ch*: chromatin, *n*: nucleus, *mi*: mitochondria, *mv*: microvillus, *pn*: pyknotic nucleus, *v*: vacuole, *vf*: vacuole fusion, *vp*: package of vacuoles. (Bilir et al., 2008)

Discussion

Several therapeutic strategies including surgery, chemotherapy, radiotherapy, and their combinations, have been used to treat GBMs. According to a Pubmed search, 13773 manuscripts were published from 1940s to 2008 for defining this illness and finding cure. Although novel therapeutic approaches were developed, the active and quick evolutionary process of GBMs' cell machinery has created difficulty for these therapies. Especially chemotherapy, one of the main therapeutic strategies, has encountered a resistance problem since its introduction at the end of the Second World War. Raguz and Yagüe (2008) defined resistance accurately as a faithful shadow which has been following the chemotherapy.

Many factors contribute to the development of drug resistance, including pharmacological and physiological factors such as drug metabolism, inadequate entry of the drug into the tumor, infusion rate and route of delivery, and GBM specific factors. Tumor specific factors such as mutations in tumor supressor genes and mitogenes as growth factor receptors (PDGFR, EGFR), and their ligands resulting in the activation of downstream signaling pathways (mainly through PI3K and MAPK). These downstream pathways will affect

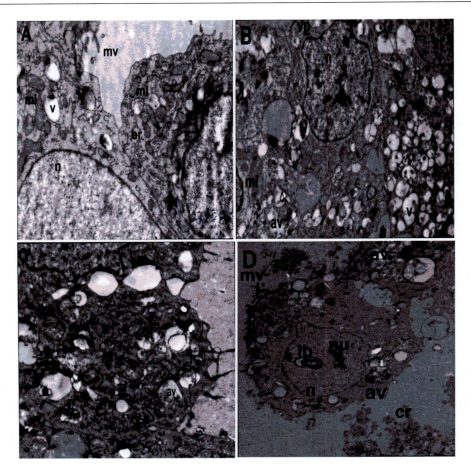

Fig. 26.2 Transmission electron microscopy views of C6 glioma spheroids at 96th h: (**a**) Control group (Original magnification of × 15,000), (**b**) Imatinib group (Original magnification of × 6,000), (**c**) Chlorimipramine group (Original magnification of ×12,000) *arrows* represents the separation point of cell from the proliferation zone of spheroid, (**d**) Imatinib with chlorimipramine. (Original magnification of ×4,000). *av*: autophagic vacuole, *er*: endoplasmic reticulum, *n*: nucleus, *nu*: nucleolus, *mi*: mitochondria, *mv*: microvillus, *v*: vacuole, *vp*: package of vacuoles, *cr*: remnants of cell, *lb*: lamellar body. (Bilir et al., 2008)

activation of DNA repair systems [O6-methylguanine-DNA methyltransferase (MGMT) and telomerase] and cell cycle. Overexpressed membrane proteins such as drug efflux pumps ABC transporters (p-gp and Bcrp1), and overexpressed cell to cell/cell to ECM proteins (integrins) have all demonstrated to play an important role in GBMs' drug resistance. Due to their significant roles in forming GBM resistance, these molecular pathways seemed to represent ideal therapeutic targets, as previous studies showed that their antagonism leads to an improvement in the therapeutic ratio of chemotherapy (Furnari et al., 2007).

In order to overcome resistance and reach a complete response, new drugs are needed for main therapy and/or adjuvant therapy. These antineoplastic agents target the same pathways but are effected negatively by different mutations such as IM in CML and IM in GBM. IM alone showed minimal activity, but IM combined with radiotherapy and other drugs such as hydroxyurea and TMZ showed increased activity to treat GBM (Reardon et al., 2005; Reardon et al., 2008). IM is transported by human and rodent ATP-binding cassette (ABC) transporters such as P-gp and Bcrp (Breedveld et al., 2005; Declèves et al., 2008). Bihorel et al. (2007) used in situ brain perfusion to investigate the mechanisms of IM transport across the mouse BBB. They used the p-gp inhibitors valspodar and zosuquidar and the p-gp/Bcrp1 inhibitor, elacridar in order to increase IM and its active metabolit accumulation in the brain. They increased IM uptake (2.5-fold), as did the deficiency of p-gp in Mdr1a/1b (–/–) mice (5.5-fold). They perfused imatinib with elacridar and enhanced the brain uptake of IM in wild-type (4.1-fold) and Mdr1a/1b (–/–) mice (1.2-fold). However, the brain uptake of IM was similar in wild-type and Bcrp1 (–/–) mice when it was perfused at a non-saturating concentration. The brain uptake of CGP74588, an active metabolite of IM, was also low. These authors concluded that IM transport at the mouse BBB is limited by p-gp and probably by Bcrp1, and that CGP74588 transport is restricted by Bcrp1. In contrast, Declèves et al. (2008) found new data which raised the question of the role of p-gp in the resistance of recurrent GBMs to IM. They also investigated whether ABC transporters determine the pharmacokinetics of IM and its pharmacological active metabolite CGP74588 in rat C6 glioma cells, and although they used same inhibitors as those by Bihorel et al. (2007), the accumulation of IM into C6 cells increased linearly with the extracellular concentration of IM (0.5–50 μM) not by these drug efflux pump inhibitors. Declèves et al. (2008), in addition, found that there was less CGP74588 than IM in C6 cells, and its concentration increased with the extracellular concentration in a sigmoid fashion. Furthermore, when combined with an alkylating agent TMZ, in a Phase I trial and a ribonucleotide reductase inhibitor hydroxyurea in a Phase II trial, the combined therapies improved patient's quality of life and outcome. The combination of IM with a IAPs in human glioblastoma cells in vitro, in orthotopic mouse models of GBM and in primary human GBM neurospheres, also overcome resistance. These drugs are also substrates for ABC transporters, and the mechanisms of their action are independent from direct p-gp inhibition, but they have been successful.

In our study, we combined IM with an antidepressant CIMP in 10 μM concentration to increase IM-induced cytotoxicity in rat C6 glioma cells and spheroids (three dimensional (3D) cell culture) (Bilir et al., 2008). We found that treatment with IM and CIMP in combination was slightly better than single agents using both monolayers and spheroid cultures of malignant C6 glioma cells. The results of this study did not fully support the hypothesis that CIMP could induce a synergistic effect on IM-induced cytotoxicity. By using a number of different techniques to evaluate the effect of the combination group on cell proliferation index, apoptosis index, cyclic adenosine monophosphate (cAMP) levels, and bromodeoxyuridine labeling index (BrDU-LI), the following results were obtained: (i) cell proliferation was synergistic at 96 h; (ii) the cell viability results were additive only at 48 h; (iii) the decrease of BrDU-LI represented a synergistic effect at 24 and 72 h; (iv) decrease in the percentage of spheroid culture cells in S-phase; (v) reduced cAMP levels; (vi) both IM and CIMP induced autophagy that was detected mainly through the presence of autophagic vacuoles with multilamellar bodies with the electron microscope (Figs. 26.1 and 26.2), increase of autophagy represented a synergistic effect; and (vii) the combination group represented a synergistic effect in apoptosis.

Alterations of spheroid morphology revealed that both IM and CIMP induced the cellular autophagy machinery, and increased autophagy was observed in the combination group in our study. Ertmer et al. (2007) described, for the first time, the process of autophagy with the mode of action of IM. They considered that autophagy may promote apoptosis in cancer cells. They revealed that the IM dose-dependently activates the cellular autophagy machinery in mammalian cells, independently of tissue type, species origin, or the immortalization status of cells. In contrast to the study by Ertmer et al. (2007), Carew et al., 2007b) considered that autophagy may promote cancer cell survival and play important roles in chemoresistance of cancer to some therapeutic agents, which typically induce an apoptotic response. They showed that disrupting autophagy augmented the anticancer activity of the histone deacetylase (HDAC) inhibitor suberoylanilide hydroxamic acid (SAHA) in IM refractory CML and in IM-resistant primary CML cells from patients bearing mutations in Bcr-Abl, including the T315I mutation that causes resistance to currently utilized tyrosine kinase inhibitors and translates into a very poor clinical prognosis (Carew et al., 2007a; Ertmer et al., 2007). Mishima et al. (2008) used 12-O-tetradecanoyl-phorbol-13-acetate (TPA), an autophagy inducer, and chloroquine, an autophagy inhibitor, and IM in K562 cells. Ertmer et al. (2007) used IM to induce cell death in K562 cells in order to confirm that autophagy regulates the cell survival system in K562 cells. They found that autophagy has not been considered during IM treatment; nonetheless, co-treatment with IM and chloroquine markedly enhanced

IM-induced cell death, compared to K562 cells treated only with IM. They showed that autophagy deeply relates to the cell survival system and that inhibition of autophagy accelerates TPA- or IM-induced cell death. Thus, blocking of autophagy could be a new strategy in the treatment of CML.

In contrast, autophagy was also proposed to combat apoptosis-resistant cancers with a special emphasis on GBMs by Lefranc and coworkers (Lefranc and Kiss, 2006; Lefranc et al., 2007). Kanzawa et al. (2004) reported that TMZ induces autophagy and part of TMZ cytotoxic activity is exerted through proautophagic processes, at least in GBM cells, as a result of the formation of O^6-methylguanine in DNA. They demonstrated that glioma cells thus respond to TMZ by undergoing G_2/M arrest, but ultimately die from autophagy. Roos et al. (2007) showed that part of TMZ cytotoxic activity is also a result of the induction of late apoptosis. The data reported by Kanzawa et al. (2004) and Roos et al. (2007) are not contradictionary in that combined autophagy and apoptosis can be seen in the same cell, and in other instances cell can switch between two cell death mechanisms in a mutually exclusive manner. So, it is not surprising that IM has minimal activity, but when combined with an alkylating agent TMZ in Phase I trial, this combined therapy improved patient's quality of life and outcome.

Taken together, the results from Annexin-V-FITC/PI staining which evaluated apoptotic index, in concordance with Carew et al., 2007b), demonstrated that because low apoptotic index was seen for 96 h in IM-related group, autophagy seemed to take part in chemoresistance of C6 glioma cells. There are no previous reports on the effect of CIMP on autophagy and, the process of autophagy with the mode of action of CIMP. When we evaluated high apoptotic index in singly applied CIMP-treated group and increased apoptotic index in the combination group, autophagy seemed to be a step to go to cell death. In concordance with Kanzawa et al. (2004) and Roos et al. (2007), we can suggest that the action of CIMP is like TMZ in that one part of CIMP cytotoxic activity can be a result of autophagy, and another part is that the induction of late apoptosis or CIMP-treated cell could switch between two cell death mechanisms in a mutually exclusive manner.

During the chemotherapy process, it is important to target cancer cells and protect normal cells. Merry et al. (1991) showed that CIMP also causes irreversible

DNA damage and blocks oxygen consumption through the inhibition complex-III of the mitochondrial respiratory chain lines in both normal and neoplastic cells, but interestingly, mitochondria damage has only been observed in neoplastic cells (Merry et al., 1991). According to this manuscript, CIMP due to its ability to form DNA damage in both normal and neoplastic cells, does not seem to target only neoplastic cells. Further studies by Daley et al. (2005) showed that CIMP can cause cell death in human glioma cells in a caspase 3-dependent manner without affecting primary human glia. In contrast to Merry et al. (1991), Daley et al. (2005) showed that CIMP possesses a selective cytotoxic effect on all brain tumors (astrocytomas, mixed oligoastrocytomas, GBM and meningiomas) whereas normal human astrocytes were not affected. One of the most promising developments in chemotherapy has been to substitute cytotoxic agents that inhibit non-specific targets in cellular pathways which contribute to carcinogenesis and resistance (Sathornsumetee et al., 2007). It was shown that CIMP acts specifically on mitochondria, and consequently induces apoptosis and autophagy (Bilir et al., 2008; Daley et al., 2005).

In addition to the chemotherapeutic benefit as potentiation of cytotoxicity, Mumoli and Cei (2008) reported that CIMP induces diabetes. In contrast, Louvet et al. (2008) and Chodorowski et al. (2007) reported that treatment of prediabetic and new onset diabetic mice with IM prevented and reversed type 1 diabetes (T1D), but had no effect on type 2 diabetes (T2D). Interestingly, cross-talk of IM and CIMP in chemetherapy is based on the potentiation of IM-cytotoxicity by CIMP, but IM can prevent and reverse CIMP-induced complications during or after chemotherapy.

In our study, we used rat C6 glioma to evaluate the effects of IM with CIMP. C6 rat glioma is a chemo-resistant experimental brain tumor which is difficult to treat with a combination of drugs (Bilir et al., 2008; O'Reilly et al., 2005). Although, it was shown that this cell line has properties similar to human GBM and has been widely used as a model system for the investigation of human GBM (Grobben et al., 2002), further investigations which use human glioblastoma cell lines (T98G, U87MG etc.) are needed to evaluate the effects of CIMP on IM. In addition, we used spheroid culture (3D-cell culture) of C6 glioma cell line with monolayer culture of this cell line as it is difficult to extrapolate from in vitro findings to studies in vivo and in humans. In order to evaluate the alterations of the ultrastructure by IM, CIMP and the combination group, spheroid model of C6 glioma was used in our study. Multicellular tumor spheroids (MTS) is also an in vitro model, but represents an intermediary level between monolayer growing cells and tumors in animals and humans. The cytology and morphology of MTS are similar to experimental tumors in mice and human. Spheroids more closely mimic the real biologic environment by providing cell-to-cell adhesion and signalling. Due to these characteristics, spheroids quite realistically represent the results of the drug effects by including limitations in penetration, distribution, and feedback mechanisms in cell signaling (Monazzam et al., 2005). Our in vitro study could provide the basis for a possible use of these drug combinations for in vivo and various ongoing clinical trials in the treatment of GBM.

Conclusions and Future Prospects

Resistance of apoptosis is a characteristic of many different cancers including GBM. GBM usually escapes the most sophisticated combined radiotherapies and chemotherapies that target apoptosis. Autophagy is proposed as an alternative tumor-suppressing mechanism to overcome resistance to radio/chemotherapies. Lefranc et al. (2007) compared autophagy to a Trojan horse which combats GBMs. The most striking evidence for proautophagic chemotherapy is derived from the use of TMZ, a proautophagic cytotoxic drug that has demonstrated real therapeutic benefits in GBM patients (Lefranc et al., 2007). Although CIMP is not technically a chemotherapeutic agent, its ability to induce autophagy seems to play an important role in the treatment of GBM. In addition, its use in the combined treatment of patients may overcome IM resistance in the near future. Further investigations should be done to translate the proposed effectiveness of CIMP in vitro – in combination-to benefit patients suffering from GBM. Thus, this approach will meet the requirements of low toxic and cheap multitargeted therapies for the treatment of patients suffering from multiple illnesses at the same time, including leukemia and GBM and/or GIST, in addition to suffering from psychiatric disorders at the same time.

References

Bihorel S, Camenisch G, Lemaire M, Scherrmann JM (2007) Influence of breast cancer resistance protein (abcg2) and P-glycoprotein (abcb1a) on the transport of imatinib mesylate (gleevec) across the mouse blood-brain barrier. J Neurochem 102:1749–1757

Bilir A, Erguven M, Oktem G, Ozdemir A, Uslu A, Aktas E, Bonavida B (2008) Potentiation of cytotoxicity by combination of imatinib and chlorimipramine in glioma. Int J Oncol 32:829–839

Breedveld P, Pluim D, Cipriani G, Wielinga P, van Tellingen O, Schinkel AH, Schellens JH (2005) The effect of bcrp1 (abcg2) on the in vivo pharmacokinetics and brain penetration of imatinib mesylate (gleevec): implications for the use of breast cancer resistance protein and P-glycoprotein inhibitors to enable the brain penetration of imatinib in patients. Cancer Res 65:2577–2582

Carew JS, Nawrocki ST, Cleveland JL (2007a) Modulating autophagy for therapeutic benefit. Autophagy 3:464–467

Carew JS, Nawrocki ST, Kahue CN, Zhang H, Yang C, Chung L, Houghton JA, Huang P, Giles FJ, Cleveland JL (2007b) Targeting autophagy augments the anticancer activity of the histone deacetylase inhibitor SAHA to overcome bcr-abl-mediated drug resistance. Blood 110:313–322

Chodorowski Z, Sein Anand J, Hellmann A, Prejzner W (2007) No influence of imatinib on type 2 diabetes. Przegl Lek 64:370–371

Daley E, Wilkie D, Loesch A, Hargreaves IP, Kendall DA, Pilkington GJ, Bates TE (2005) Chlorimipramine: a novel anticancer agent with a mitochondrial target. Biochem Biophys Res Commun 328:623–632

Declèves X, Bihorel S, Debray M, Yousif S, Camenisch G, Scherrmann JM (2008) ABC transporters and the accumulation of imatinib and its active metabolite CGP74588 in rat C6 glioma cells. Pharmacol Res 57:214–222

Ertmer A, Huber V, Gilch S, Yoshimori T, Erfle V, Duyster J, Elsässer HP, Schätzl HM (2007) The anticancer drug imatinib induces cellular autophagy. Leukemia 21:936–942

Furnari FB, Fenton T, Bachoo RM, Mukasa A, Stommel JM, Stegh A, Hahn WC, Ligon KL, Louis DN, Brennan C, Chin L, DePinho RA, Cavenee WK (2007) Malignant astrocytic glioma: genetics, biology, and paths to treatment. Genes Dev 21:2683–2710

Grobben B, De Deyn PP, Slegers H (2002) Rat C6 glioma as experimental model system for the study of glioblastoma growth and invasion. Cell Tissue Res 310:257–270

Kanzawa T, Germano IM, Komata T, Ito H, Kondo Y, Kondo S (2004) Role of autophagy in temozolomide-induced cytotoxicity for malignant glioma cells. Cell Death Differ 11:448–457

Kilic T, Alberta JA, Zdunek PR, Acar M, Iannarelli P, O'Reilly T, Buchdunger E, Black PM, Stiles CD (2000) Intracranial inhibition of platelet-derived growth factor-mediated glioblastoma cell growth by an orally active kinase inhibitor of the 2-phenylaminopyrimidine class. Cancer Res 60:5143–5150

Lefranc F, Facchini V, Kiss R (2007) Proautophagic drugs: a novel means to combat apoptosis-resistant cancers, with a special emphasis on glioblastomas. Oncologist 12:1395–1403

Lefranc F, Kiss R (2006) Autophagy, the trojan horse to combat glioblastomas. Neurosurg Focus 20:E7

Levkovitz Y, Gil-Ad I, Zeldich E, Dayag M, Weizman A (2005) Differential induction of apoptosis by antidepressants in glioma and neuroblastoma cell lines: evidence for P-C-Jun, cytochrome C, and caspase-3 involvement. J Mol Neurosci 27:29–42

Louvet C, Szot GL, Lang J, Lee MR, Martinier N, Bollag G, Zhu S, Weiss A, Bluestone JA (2008) Tyrosine kinase inhibitors reverse type 1 diabetes in nonobese diabetic mice. Proc Natl Acad Sci U S A 105:18895–18900

Merry S, Hamilton TG, Flanigan P, Freshney RI, Kaye SB (1991) Circumvention of pleiotropic drug resistance in subcutaneous tumours in vivo with verapamil and clomipramine. Eur J Cancer 27:31–34

Mishima Y, Terui Y, Mishima Y, Taniyama A, Kuniyoshi R, Takizawa T, Kimura S, Ozawa K, Hatake K (2008) Autophagy and autophagic cell death are next targets for elimination of the resistance to tyrosine kinase inhibitors. Cancer Sci 99:2200–2208

Monazzam A, Razifar P, Lindhe O, Josephsson R, Långström B, Bergström M (2005) A new, fast and semi-automated size determination method (SASDM) for studying multicellular tumor spheroids. Cancer Cell Int 5:32

Mumoli N, Cei M (2008) Clomipramine-induced diabetes. Ann Intern Med 149:595–596

Nadgir SM, Malviya M (2008) In vivo effect of antidepressants on [3h]paroxetine binding to serotonin transporters in rat brain. Neurochem Res 33:2250–2256

Oertel S, Krempien R, Lindel K, Zabel A, Milker-Zabel S, Bischof M, Lipson KE, Peschke P, Debus J, Abdollahi A, Huber PE (2006) Human glioblastoma and carcinoma xenograft tumors treated by combined radiation and imatinib (gleevec). Strahlenther Onkol 182:400–407

O'Reilly T, Wartmann M, Maira SM, Hattenberger M, Vaxelaire J, Muller M, Ferretti S, Buchdunger E, Altmann KH, McSheehy PM (2005) Patupilone (epothilone B, EPO906) and imatinib (STI571, glivec) in combination display enhanced antitumour activity in vivo against experimental rat C6 glioma. Cancer Chemother Pharmacol 55:307–317

Pommerenke EW, Volm M (1995) Reversal of doxorubicin-resistance in solid tumors by clomipramine. In Vivo 9:99–101

Raguz S, Yagüe E (2008) Resistance to chemotherapy: new treatments and novel insights into an old problem. Br J Cancer 99:387–391

Reardon DA, Desjardins A, Vredenburgh JJ, Sathornsumetee S, Rich JN, Quinn JA, Lagattuta TF, Egorin MJ, Gururangan S, McLendon R, Herndon JE 2nd, Friedman AH, Salvado AJ, Friedman HS (2008) Safety and pharmacokinetics of dose-intensive imatinib mesylate plus temozolomide: phase 1 trial in adults with malignant glioma. Neurooncol 10:330–340

Reardon DA, Egorin MJ, Quinn JA, Rich JN, Gururangan S, Vredenburgh JJ, Desjardins A, Sathornsumetee S, Provenzale JM, Herndon JE 2nd, Dowell JM, Badruddoja MA, McLendon RE, Lagattuta TF, Kicielinski KP, Dresemann G, Sampson JH, Friedman AH, Salvado AJ, Friedman HS (2005) Phase II study of imatinib mesylate plus hydroxyurea in adults with recurrent glioblastoma multiforme. J Clin Oncol 23:9359–9368

Rooprai HK, Christidou M, Pilkington GJ (2003) The potential for strategies using micronutrients and heterocyclic drugs to treat invasive gliomas. Acta Neurochir (Wien) 145: 683–690

Roos WP, Batista LF, Naumann SC, Wick W, Weller M, Menck CF, Kaina B (2007) Apoptosis in malignant glioma cells triggered by the temozolomide-induced DNA lesion O6-methylguanine. Oncogene 26:186–197

Sathornsumetee S, Reardon DA, Desjardins A, Quinn JA, Vredenburgh JJ, Rich JN (2007) Molecularly targeted therapy for malignant glioma. Cancer 110:13–24

Scheda A, Finjap JK, Tuettenberg J, Brockmann MA, Hochhaus A, Hofheinz R, Lohr F,and, Wenz F (2007) Efficacy of different regimens of adjuvant radiochemotherapy for treatment of glioblastoma. Tumori 93:31–36

Wen PY, Yung WK, Lamborn KR, Dahia PL, Wang Y, Peng B, Abrey LE, Raizer J, Cloughesy TF, Fink K, Gilbert M, Chang S, Junck L, Schiff D, Lieberman F, Fine HA, Mehta M, Robins HI, DeAngelis LM, Groves MD, Puduvalli VK, Levin V, Conrad C, Maher EA, Aldape K, Hayes M, Letvak L, Egorin MJ, Capdeville R, Kaplan R, Murgo AJ, Stiles C, Prados MD (2006) Phase I/II study of imatinib mesylate for recurrent malignant gliomas: north american brain tumor consortium study 99–08. Clin Cancer Res 12:4899–4907

Zhou O, Gallo JM (2008) Differential effect of sunitinib on the distribution of temozolomide in an orthotopic glioma model. Neurooncol 11:301–310

Ziegler DS, Wright RD, Kesari S, Lemieux ME, Tran MA, Jain M, Zawel L, and, Kung AL (2008) Resistance of human glioblastoma multiforme cells to growth factor inhibitors is overcome by blockade of inhibitor of apoptosis proteins. J Clin Invest 118:3109–3122

Chapter 27

Glioblastoma Multiforme: Molecular Basis of Resistance to Erlotinib

Marc-Eric Halatsch and Georg Karpel-Massler

Abstract Erlotinib, an epidermal growth factor receptor (EGFR) tyrosine kinase inhibitor, exerts widely variable antiproliferative effects on human glioblastoma multiforme (GBM) cell lines in vitro and in vivo. Those effects are independent of EGFR baseline expression levels, raising the possibility that more complex genetic properties form the molecular basis of the erlotinib-sensitive and erlotinib-resistant GBM phenotypes. By analyzing gene expressions in cell lines with sensitive, intermediately responsive and resistant phenotypes, a recent study has proposed candidate genes for GBM response to erlotinib (J Neurosurg 111: 211–218, 2009). The ten gene candidates for conferring GBM resistance to erlotinib (*CACNG*4, *FGFR*4, *HSPA*1B, *HSPB*1, *NFATC*1, *NTRK*1, *RAC*1, *SMO*, *TCF*7L1, *TGFB*3) potentially represent therapeutic targets, interfering with which may enhance the efficacy of erlotinib against GBM. Five additional genes (*BDNF*, *CARD*6, *FOSL*1, *HSPA*9B, *MYC*) warrant further investigation regarding their roles as putative co-targets of erlotinib. The aim of the current chapter is to review the data based on which molecular determinants of the biological response of GBM cells to erlotinib have been proposed. In this regard, special emphasis is given to the concepts of oncogene addiction and oncogenic shock.

Keywords Glioblastoma multiforme · Epidermal growth factor receptor · Oncogene addiction · Oncogenic shock

Introduction

Quantitative and qualitative alterations of the epidermal growth factor receptor (EGFR) are a hallmark of primary glioblastoma multiforme (GBM) (Halatsch et al., 2000; 2006). We have previously reported that erlotinib, an EGFR tyrosine kinase inhibitor, exerts widely variable antiproliferative effects on nine human GBM cell lines in vitro and in vivo (Halatsch et al., 2004). Those effects were independent of EGFR baseline expression levels, raising the possibility that more complex gene expression profiles form the molecular basis of the erlotinib-sensitive and erlotinib-resistant GBM phenotypes. Recent research indicates that *EGFR* amplification and mutation in combination with maintenance of wild-type *phosphatase and tensin homolog deleted on chromosome 10* (*PTEN*) (Mellinghoff et al., 2005) and low levels of phosphorylated protein kinase B/Akt (Haas-Kogan et al., 2005) contribute to a molecular signature of a subgroup of GBM that is likely to respond to EGFR inhibition. However, any combination of these molecular alterations appears insufficient to confer obligate sensitivity of GBM towards erlotinib (Sarkaria et al., 2007). By analyzing a set of erlotinib-sensitive, intermediately responsive and erlotinib-resistant GBM cell lines, a recent study has set out to determine additional candidate genes mediating sensitivity or resistance of human GBM towards erlotinib (Halatsch et al., 2009).

M.-E. Halatsch (✉)
Department of Neurosurgery, University of Ulm School of Medicine, D-89075 Ulm, Germany
e-mail: marc-eric.halatsch@uniklinik-ulm.de

Biological Response of Glioblastoma Multiforme Cell lines to Erlotinib and Gene Expression Analysis: Methodology

Cell Lines

From nine established GBM cell lines previously described (Halatsch et al., 2004), four were selected to represent the erlotinib-sensitive (G-599GM), intermediately responsive (G-210GM and G-750GM) and erlotinib-resistant (G-1163GM) phenotypes, respectively. The proliferative properties, including response to erlotinib, of one additional cell line derived from a secondary GBM (H-199GM) were established as previously described (data not shown), and this cell line was assigned to group III, i.e., the erlotinib-sensitive phenotype (group I: inhibition of cellular proliferation after 10 days of continuous erlotinib exposure [3 μMol] $\leq$ 33.3% compared to control cells; group II: growth inhibition > 33.3% and $\leq$ 66.7%; group III: growth inhibition > 66.7%) (Halatsch et al., 2004). Cells were maintained in Roswell Park Memorial Institute 1640 cell culture medium (BioWhittaker, Walkersville, MD) supplemented with 10% heat-inactivated fetal calf serum and incubated in a humidified 5% carbon dioxide atmosphere at 37°C. Medium was exchanged twice weekly, and cells were passaged upon reaching subconfluence. At the beginning of the study, all cell lines were beyond their 20th passage. The neuropathological diagnoses of GBM were confirmed by immunocytochemical staining for glial fibrillary acidic protein and vimentin.

RNA Extraction

Total cellular RNAs were isolated in three biological replicates from the above cell lines using a spin column system (RNeasy Mini Kit, Qiagen, Hilden, Germany), quantitated using spectrophotometry, adjusted to equal concentrations, and treated with RNase-free DNase I (Promega, Madison, WI).

RNA Processing, Microarray Hybridization and Feature Extraction

For microarray target preparation and hybridization, 2 μg of total cellular RNAs were processed for each of the 15 samples. The Codelink Expression Array Reagent Kit (Applied Microarrays, Tempe, AZ) was used for cDNA synthesis and subsequent in vitro transcription with biotin-16-UTP (Roche Applied Science, Penzberg, Germany). The biotinylated cRNAs were recovered using the RNeasy Mini Kit (Qiagen), spectrophotometrically quantitated, and 10 μg per sample were fragmented and hybridized to Codelink Human Whole Genome Bioarrays according to the manufacturer's protocol (Applied Microarrays). After incubation at 37°C for 18 h, the arrays were washed, stained with Streptavidin-Cy5 (Applied Microarrays) and read using an Axon GenePix 4000B scanner as described in the manufacturer's manual (Molecular Devices, Sunnyvale, CA). The scanned image files were analyzed using the Codelink Expression Analysis software 4.0 (Applied Microarrays).

Statistical Analysis and Gene Annotation

Raw microarray intensity values were preprocessed by performing background correction and cyclic loess normalization using the software R (version 2.5.0.) (Diez et al., 2007). If applicable, up to two missing intensity values per gene were imputed using k-nearest neighbour averaging.

For each member of a preselected group of 814 genes involved in major proliferation and apoptosis signaling pathways relevant to cancer, intensity values were compared between the three different phenotypes (sensitive, intermediately responsive and resistant, respectively). Those values were tested for a monotone trend employing the non-parametric, two-sided Jonckheere-Terpstra test.

The Jonckheere-Terpstra test was implemented into a multiple test procedure (Van der Laan et al., 2004) included in the R software package. This procedure uses a bootstrapping approach to estimate the null distribution of the joint test statistics. The resulting gene-specific p-values were adjusted for multiplicity by controlling the family-wise type I error rate at the 5%-level. Genes with an adjusted $p < 0.05$ were referred to as statistically significant pre-candidate genes for response to erlotinib.

The list obtained by statistical analysis was submitted to the Database for Annotation, Visualization and Integrated Discovery (DAVID) (http://david.abcc.ncifcrf.gov/), and sublists were created using DAVID's functional annotation tools. During that process, obvious non-candidate genes were identified and removed from the analysis.

Confirmatory Quantitative Reverse Transcription-Polymerase Chain Reaction (qRT-PCR)

For complementary (c)DNA synthesis, 50 pg of total cellular RNA were processed for each of the samples according to the manufacturer's recommendations (QuantiTect Reverse Transcription, Qiagen). Aliquots of 3 μl of the obtained cDNA were added to the real-time PCR mix (17 μl) consisting of the respective gene-specific sense and antisense primers (final concentration of 0.5 pmol/μl per primer) and the PCR master mix (QuantiTect SYBR Green PCR, Qiagen). SYBR green I dye was used for real-time PCR on a 7500 Real-Time PCR System (Applied Biosystems, Darmstadt, Germany) with the following amplification conditions: 2 min at 50°C and 10 min at 95°C followed by 40 cycles of each 15 s at 95°C and 1 min at 60°C. The final cycle consisted of 15 s at 95°C, 1 min at 60°C, 15 s at 95°C and 15 s at 60°C. To design primer pairs for the candidate gene targets with a product size ranging from 60–131 bases, the Universal ProbeLibrary Assay Design Center (Roche Applied Science) and *Primer3* (http://primer3.sourceforge. net) were used. Primers (18-25-mers) were custom-synthesized by Sigma-Aldrich (Munich, Germany). The amount of cDNA was calculated by normalizing Ct values with those of previously chosen housekeeping genes (hypoxanthine-guanine phosporibosyltransferase 1, tyrosine 3-monooxygenase/tryptophan 5-monooxygenase activation protein zeta polypeptide, and peptidylprolyl isomerase A), expression of which was determined by parallel analysis.

Candidate Genes for GBM Response to Erlotinib

Expression analysis of prospectively selected 814 genes involved in major proliferation and apoptosis signaling pathways identified 19 genes the expression of which significantly correlated with phenotype. Of those 19 genes, 32%, 24% and 20% belonged to the MAPK, JNK and WNT signaling pathway while representation of these pathways within the source gene group was 45%, 5% and 9%, respectively. Expressions of seven candidate genes increased with cellular sensitivity towards erlotinib, and the opposite was observed for the remaining twelve genes (Fig. 27.1). *TGFB*3 was exceptional in that its relative range of expression among the different cellular phenotypes cumulatively exceeded one order of magnitude (Fig. 27.1). Functional annotation analysis revealed two (*DUSP*4, *STAT*1) and ten (*CACNG*4, *FGFR*4, *HSPA*1B, *HSPB*1, *NFATC*1, *NTRK*1, *RAC*1, *SMO*, *TCF*7L1, *TGFB*3) genes conclusively associated with sensitivity and resistance to erlotinib, respectively (Fig. 27.2). Moreover, five genes (*BDNF*, *CARD*6, *FOSL*1, *HSPA*9B, *MYC*) involved in antiapoptotic signaling pathways were unexpectedly found to be associated with sensitivity (Fig. 27.2). Two genes (*CASP*6, *CDK*5) were excluded from the candidate gene list because of obvious incongruency between their respective distribution of expression among the different erlotinib-related GBM cell line phenotypes (suggesting conferral of resistance against erlotinib) and their proposed proapoptotic function (Fig. 27.2).

Of the remaining 17 genes, four (*FGFR*4, *FOSL*1, *MYC* and *RAC*1) were found to play established roles in the pathogenesis, maintenance and/or progression of malignant glioma.

Next, the virtual localizations of individual prominent genes within the statistical distribution of correlation between gene expression and categories of cellular response to erlotinib were determined. Those individual prominent genes were either conjectured to be involved in modulating cellular response of GBM cells to erlotinib (i.e., *EGFR*, *PTEN* and *AKT*1) and/or to play a role in GBM pathogenesis. Within that data set, the expression of none of these genes correlated to the cellular phenotype under investigation.

In the final step of the analysis, it was examined whether any of the products of the 17 identified genes were arranged in a directly sequential or parallel manner within established signaling pathways. Noteworthy, *CACNG*4, *FGFR*4 and *NTRK*1 assume parallel roles at the beginning of the MAPK signaling pathway. The scopes of the products of these genes converge into the activation of rat sarcoma viral oncogene homolog (RAS) via growth factor

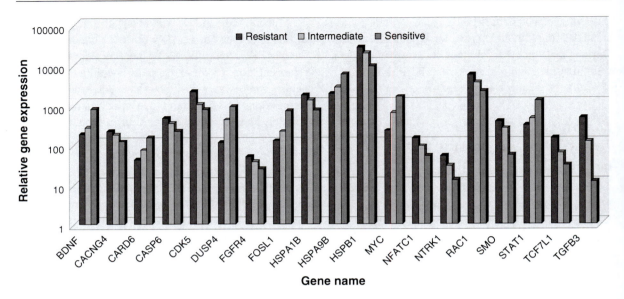

Fig. 27.1 Gene expressions with significant correlation to biological response of GBM cell lines towards erlotinib as determined by Jonckheere-Terpstra statistics from a group of 814 prospectively selected genes involved in major apoptosis and signaling pathways (Halatsch et al., 2009). Relative gene expressions are mean values of up to two cell lines per phenotype and three biological replicates per cell line

Fig. 27.2 Candidate genes for GBM response to erlotinib (Halatsch et al., 2009). Sublists were created using DAVID (see *Materials and Methods*). Based on the analysis, *CASP*6 and *CDK*5 were excluded from the candidate gene list (lower part of left box). Five genes (*BDNF*, *CARD*6, *FOSL*1, *HSPA*9B, *MYC*) involved in antiapoptotic signaling pathways were unexpectedly found to be associated with sensitivity (upper part of left box)

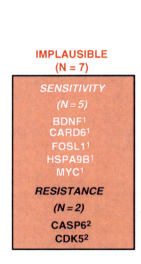

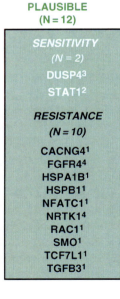

receptor-bound protein 2 (GRB2) and son of sevenless (SOS), a signaling pathway that is also utilized by EGFR.

Gene expressions were confirmed by qRT-PCR. With the exception of *HSPA*9B and *STAT*1, confirmation was unequivocal. For these genes, quantitative gene expression of the intermediately responsive group of cell lines expectedly was 4.84- and 8.61-fold below that of the erlotinib-sensitive phenotype, but also 1.03- and 1.36-fold below that of the erlotinib-resistant cell lines, respectively. However, because the differences between gene expressions of the erlotinib-resistant and intermediately responsive cell lines were small compared to gene expressions of the erlotinib-sensitive phenotype (i.e., ratio of 0.006 and 0.04, respectively), both genes were retained within the candidate gene list.

Discussion

Erlotinib-Related Pheno- and Genotypes

In a current study, by examining gene expression profiles in GBM cell lines with sensitivity, intermediate responsiveness and resistance towards erlotinib, the authors identified a total of twelve candidate genes for GBM response to erlotinib (Halatsch et al., 2009). Among those, the ten gene candidates for conferring GBM resistance to erlotinib potentially represent therapeutic targets, interfering with which may enhance the efficacy of erlotinib against GBM. Five additional genes involved in antiapoptotic signaling pathways were unexpectedly found to be associated with sensitivity. Based on this obvious contradiction, those genes qualify as putative co-targets of erlotinib.

With regard to the ten candidate resistance genes, previous studies have established absence of either expression, overexpression or constitutive activation of *FGFR*4, *HSPA*1B, *HSPB*1, *NFATC*1, *NTRK*1, *RAC*1, *SMO* and *TGFB*3 in normal glia, thus supporting feasibility of therapeutic targeting of these genes (Arion et al., 2007; Aronica et al., 2004; Charytoniuk et al., 2002; De Groot et al., 1999; Fuhrmann et al., 1999; Pérez-Ortiz et al., 2008; Senger et al., 2002; Villapol et al., 2008).

The implementation of the intermediately responsive cellular phenotype into the study design plausibly increased analytical precision, a feature that would have been difficult or even impossible to realize in other models and that may outweigh some of the well-known methodical limitations associated with cell culture studies.

While providing even a brief review on the 17 candidate genes is clearly beyond the scope of this chapter, eight of them deserve special consideration as they factually stand out compared to the remainder of genes. Firstly, the relative range of expression of *TGFB*3 among the different cellular phenotypes renders this gene a particularly clear-cut candidate.

Secondly, *FGFR*4, *FOSL*1, *MYC* and *RAC*1 assume established roles in the pathogenesis, maintenance and/or progression of malignant glioma. The expression of *FGFR*4, to begin with, has been shown to correlate with the histopathological grading of astrocytomas (Yamada et al., 2002); similarly, *FOSL*1 modulates

malignant features of glioma cells (Debinsky and Gibo, 2005; Koul et al., 2007). While MYC plays a well-known critical role in glioma cell proliferation (Barnett et al., 1998; Broaddus et al., 1997), RAC1 is a key contributor to glioma cell survival, probably via multiple signaling pathways including JNK (Senger et al., 2002). Interestingly, overexpression of EGFR variant (v)III, a naturally occurring, truncated and constitutively (ligand-independently) active receptor mutation found in a large subgroup of human GBM, results in an increase in basal JNK activity (Antonyak et al., 1998). In concordance with this observation, the relative overrepresentation of the JNK and WNT signaling pathways among the candidate genes identified in this study implies critical roles of these pathways in mediating biological response of GBM cells towards erlotinib. Moreover, DNA copy number gains for the 7p22 locus at which *RAC*1 resides are present in all of the human GBM cell lines used in this study (Ramirez et al., 2003), suggesting that "sensitivity" may already constitute "low-level resistance".

Thirdly, from a functional perspective, CACNG4, FGFR4 and NTRK1 are immediate neighbours within a wide distribution of 814 gene products across multiple signaling pathways; this "functional cluster" more strongly suggests a relationship between gene expression and erlotinib-related phenotype than "isolated" candidate genes do. Interestingly, the products of these functionally related genes join a signaling pathway that is also activated by EGFR.

In the analysis described above, no correlation was found between the expression of certain genes implied in modulating cellular response of GBM cells to erlotinib (i.e., *EGFR*, *PTEN* and *AKT*1) (Bianco et al., 2003; Haas-Kogan et al., 2005; Mellinghoff et al., 2005; Sarkaria et al., 2007) or proposed to play a role in GBM pathogenesis (Fischer et al., 1996; Lang et al., 1994; Reyes-Mugica et al., 1997; Von Deimling et al., 1995) on one hand and the erlotinib-related cellular phenotype on the other hand. While determination of protein phosphorylation was not the goal of that work, a putative role of these gene products for cellular response of GBM cells to erlotinib was not evident at the level of gene expression. However, reduction of the data set (e.g., to contain only genes involved in the primary and secondary GBM pathway) with concomitant diminution of multiplicity of hypothesis testing led to the identification of a few more candidate genes (Löw et al., 2009), consistent with the statistical significance level of these genes being closely below the current cut-off.

In view of the concept of "oncogene addiction" (Halatsch et al., 2000; Weinstein and Joe, 2006), the results described above provide some interesting insights. Obviously, each of the genes identified as potentially conferring resistance to erlotinib may provide "escape from oncogene addiction", i.e., a means for the GBM cell to circumvent otherwise critical EGFR inhibition and to maintain survival pathway signaling. Thus, the resistance candidate gene list may harbour members therapeutic co-targeting of which is essential for enhancing the efficacy of erlotinib against GBM. Conversely, the proliferation-enhancing effects of the EGFR likely activate negative feedback mechanisms involving increased expression of proliferation-inhibitory factors in order to maintain homeostasis (Weinstein, 2000). As a consequence of EGFR inhibition, the GBM cell might suffer a relative excess of the latter inhibitory factors and thus undergo apoptosis before a new level of homeostasis can be achieved. Based on the data summarized above, *DUSP4* and *STAT1* are candidate genes for encoding such factors. Interestingly, both of the cell lines representing the erlotinib-sensitive phenotype were derived from secondary GBMs. Future research must establish whether *DUSP4* and/or *STAT1* as well as any of the five additional genes involved in antiapoptotic signaling pathways that were unexpectedly found to be associated with sensitivity (*BDNF*, *CARD6*, *FOSL1*, *HSPA9B*, *MYC*) embody novel markers of secondary GBM pathogenesis.

While the hypotheses generated by the described study possess – as outlined above – a rational degree of both external and internal consistency, causative confirmation of the demonstrated statistical association between gene expressions and erlotibinib-related GBM phenotype (e.g., by transfection experiments) is warranted.

Oncogene Addiction Versus Oncogenic Shock

The transformation of a noncancerous cell into a malignant cell is attributed to the aquisition of multiple genetic alterations that account for characteristic phenotypic changes. However, despite the multitude of oncogenes present in tumor cells, it was shown that tumor cells can become dependent on the activity of only one single oncogene in order to maintain cellular proliferation or even survival. Acute deprivation from that specific oncogenic input may rapidly induce growth arrest or apoptosis. To concisely describe this phenomenon of dependency, the term "oncogene addiction" was coined (Weinstein, 2002). While the exact nature of the mechanisms leading to reprogramming of the cellular "circuitry" towards "oncogene addiction" remains unclear, it is presumed that the homeostasis of the transformed cell is maintained by concomitant upregulation of antiproliferative/proapoptotic signaling. Switching-off the proliferative signaling input from the addictive oncogene results in critical dysbalance, leading to growth arrest or apoptosis. Partly because the supposed change of the cell's "hardwiring" is central to the concept of oncogene addiction but difficult to define, a different concept has evolved to explain the cellular decay that follows acute disruption of oncogenic signaling. It was shown for many oncoproteins, including EGFR, that their activation effects both prosurvival and proapoptotic signaling (Johnson et al., 2000; Sordella et al., 2004). Experimental evidence suggests that proapoptotic factors have a longer half-life than the rather short-lived prosurvival factors, and sudden disruption of oncogene-mediated signaling changes the homeostasis of the cancer cell that usually is characterized by a predominance of prosurvival factors, to actually favor the proapoptotic side of the balance (Fig. 27.3). Sharma et al. (2006) showed a rapid decrease of the concentrations of downstream signaling regulators such as AKT, ERK1/2 or STAT3 and STAT5 (that are known to promote the prosurvival effects of EGFR, SRC or BCR-ABL) once the respective oncogene was inactivated. In contrast, proapoptotic regulators, including phosphorylated p38 MAPK, persisted significantly longer. Thus, acute inhibition of an oncogene may lead to a temporary predominance of oncogene-associated proapoptotic effectors, causing cell death. This phenomenon is referred to as "oncogenic shock". Unlike the concept of oncogene addiction, oncogenic shock implies that the oncogenic kinase is actively causing cell death by means of its residual, longer-lived proapoptotic signaling upon inactivation of the oncoprotein. Undefined changes of the cellular circuitry, as proposed by the addiction model, are not required within the concept of oncogenic shock, which

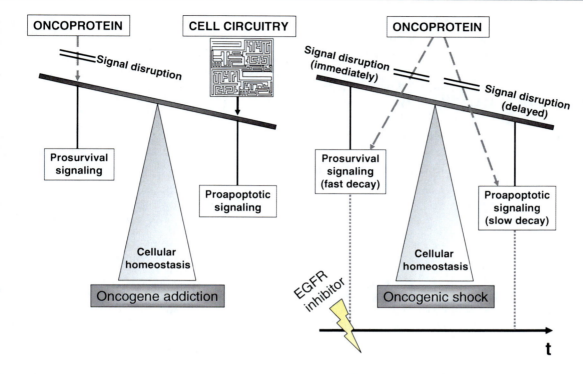

Fig. 27.3 Oncogene addiction versus oncogenic shock (Karpel-Massler et al., 2009). Disruption of specific oncogene signaling changes cancer cell homeostasis, shifting the balance toward proapoptotic signaling and subsequent cell cycle arrest or apoptosis. The addiction model postulates cellular reprogramming as a prerequisite for dependency on an oncogene. Cell death is caused by independent proapoptotic effectors from the cell circuitry. In contrast, the shock model hypothesizes that the oncogene's residual proapoptotic signaling suddenly predominates because of longer half-life of its constituents, leading to apoptosis

is experimentally supported by the observation that cells transfected with an active RAS oncogene containing an additional effector domain inhibiting the prosurvival PI3-K/AKT pathway undergo apoptosis, whereas cells without the additional domain do not (Sharma et al., 2006).

With regard to the problems encountered with EGFR inhibition in terms of therapeutic efficacy, some interesting aspects are added by the concept of oncogenic shock. Creation of an acute imbalance of the tumor cell homeostasis in favor of proapoptotic signaling would represent the key therapeutic goal. To reach that goal, targeting of one oncogene may not be sufficient, and identification of a relevant oncogene *pattern* may be the first step towards a more successful targeted therapy. The fact that in the first randomized, controlled phase II trial of erlotinib in recurrent glioblastoma neither sufficient activity of erlotinib nor a correlation of EGFRvIII expression and response were found supports the idea that a multitargeted therapeutic approach might be necessary. In addition, overexpression of a single receptor such as EGFR in an experimental setting may cause artificial addiction to that one gene, and its inhibition may result in apoptosis and impairment of malignant characteristics. However, such a model does not reflect the complexity encountered on the clinical level. Stommel et al. (2007) showed that even in glioblastoma cell lines a multitude of receptor TKs are simultaneously activated, and triple drug therapy was needed in order to completely inhibit downstream signaling. Thus, the concept of single-oncogene addiction probably will not apply to the majority of glioblastomas.

The antitumor effects of selective oncogene inhibition, e.g., by EGFR TK inhibitors, may be increased by concomitantly targeting multiple downstream prosurvival effectors. An additional important implication of the concept of oncogenic shock is that certain agents such as conventional chemotherapeutics that frequently cause DNA damage, cell cycle arrest and thereby inhibition of apoptosis, may not be candidates for a rational combination therapy with EGFR TK inhibitors.

The model of "oncogenic shock" provides a logical explanation for the biological response of tumor cells following oncogene inactivation and is supported by current experimental data. However, this concept needs to be further validated in the setting of drug development and subsequent clinical application (Karpel-Massler et al., 2009).

References

Antonyak MA, Moscatello DK, Wong AJ (1998) Constitutive activation of C-Jun N-terminal kinase by a mutant epidermal growth factor receptor. J Biol Chem 273: 2817–2822

Arion D, Unger T, Lewis DA, Levitt P, Mirnics K (2007) Molecular evidence for increased expression of genes related to immune and chaperone function in the prefrontal cortex in schizophrenia. Biol Psychiatry 62:711–721

Aronica E, Ozbas-Gerçeker F, Redeker S, Ramkema M, Spliet WG, van Rijen PC, Leenstra S, Gorter JA, Troost AJ (2004) Expression and cellular distribution of high- and low-affinity neurotrophin receptors in malformations of cortical development. Acta Neuropathol 108:422–434

Barnett SC, Robertson L, Graham D, Allan D, Rampling R (1998) Oligodendrocyte-type-2 astrocyte (O-2a) progenitor cells transformed with C-myc and H-ras form high-grade glioma after stereotactic injection into the rat brain. Carcinogenesis 19:1529–1537

Bianco R, Shin I, Ritter CA, Yakes FM, Basso A, Rosen N, Tsurutani J, Dennis PA, Mills GB, Arteaga CL (2003) Loss of PTEN/MMAC1/TEP in EGF receptor-expressing tumor cells counteracts the antitumor action of EGFR tyrosine kinase inhibitors. Oncogene 22:2812–2822

Broaddus WC, Chen ZJ, Prabhu SS, Loudon WG, Gillies GT, Phillips LL, Fillmore H (1997) Antiproliferative effect of C-myc antisense phosphorothioate oligodeoxynucleotides in malignant glioma cells. Neurosurgery 41:908–915

Charytoniuk D, Traifford E, Hantraye P, Hermel JM, Galdes A, Ruat M (2002) Intrastriatal sonic hedgehog injection increases patched transcript levels in the adult rat subventricular zone. Eur J Neurosci 16:2351–2357

Debinsky W, Gibo DM (2005) Fos-related antigen 1 modulates malignant features of glioma cells. Mol Cancer Res 3: 237–249

De Groot CJ, Montagne L, Barten AD, Sminia P, van der Valk P (1999) Expressions of transforming growth factor (TGF)-β1, -β2, and -β3 isoforms and TGF-β type I and type II receptors in multiple sclerosis lesions and human astrocyte cultures. J Neuropathol Exp Neurol 58: 174–187

Diez D, Alvarez R, Dopazo A (2007) Codelink: an r package for analysis of GE healthcare gene expression bioarrays. Bioinformatics 23:1168–1169

Fischer U, Meltzer P, Meese E (1996) Twelve amplified and expressed genes localized in a single domain in glioma. Hum Genet 98:625–628

Fuhrmann V, Kinkl N, Leveillard T, Sahel J, Hicks D (1999) Fibroblast growth factor receptor 4 (FGFR4) is expressed in adult rat and human retinal photoreceptors and neurons. J Mol Neurosci 13:187–197

Haas-Kogan DA, Prados MD, Tihan T, Eberhard DA, Jelluma N, Arvold ND, Baumber R, Lamborn KR, Kapadia A, Malec M, Berger MS, Stokoe D (2005) Epidermal growth factor receptor, protein kinase B/akt, and glioma response to erlotinib. J Natl Cancer Inst 97:880–887

Halatsch M-E, Gehrke E, Vougioukas VI, Bötefür IC, A.-Borhani F, Efferth T, Gebhart E, Domhof S, Schmidt U, Buchfelder M (2004) Inverse correlation of *epidermal growth factor receptor* (*EGFR*) mRNA induction and suppression of anchorage-independent growth by OSI-774, an EGFR tyrosine kinase inhibitor, in glioblastoma multiforme cell lines. J Neurosurg 100:523–533

Halatsch M-E, Löw S, Mursch K, Hielscher T, Schmidt U, Unterberg A, Feuerhake F (2009) Candidate genes for sensitivity and resistance of human glioblastoma multiforme cell lines to erlotinib. J Neurosurg 111:211–218

Halatsch M-E, Schmidt U, Bötefür IC, Holland JF, Ohnuma T (2000) Marked inhibition of glioblastoma target cell tumorigenicity in vitro by retrovirus-mediated transfer of a hairpin ribozyme against deletion-mutant *epidermal growth factor receptor* messenger RNA. J Neurosurg 92:297–305

Halatsch M-E, Schmidt U, Behnke-Mursch J, Unterberg A, Wirtz CR (2006) Epidermal growth factor receptor inhibition for the treatment of glioblastoma multiforme and other malignant brain tumours. Cancer Treat Rev 32:74–89

Johnson D, Agochiya M, Samejima K, Earnshaw W, Frame M, Wyke J (2000) Regulation of both apoptosis and cell survival by the V-src oncoprotein. Cell Death Differ 7: 685–696

Karpel-Massler G, Schmidt U, Unterberg A, Halatsch M-E (2009) Therapeutic inhibition of the epidermal growth factor receptor in malignant brain tumors – where do we stand? Mol Cancer Ther 7:1000–1012

Koul D, Shen R, Shishodia S, Takada Y, Bhat KP, Reddy SAG, Aggarwal BB, Yung WK (2007) PTEN down regulates AP-1 and targets c-fos in human glioma cells via PI3-kinase/Akt pathway. Mol Cell Biochem 300:77–87

Lang FF, Miller DC, Koslow M, Newcomb EW (1994) Pathways leading to glioblastoma multiforme: a molecular analysis of genetic alterations in 65 astrocytic tumors. J Neurosurg 81:427–436

Löw S, Vougioukas VI, Hielscher T, Schmidt U, Unterberg A, Halatsch M-E (2008) Pathogenetic pathways leading to glioblastoma multiforme: association between gene expressions and resistance to erlotinib. Anticancer Res 28: 3729–3732

Mellinghoff IK, Wang MY, Vivanco I, Haas-Kogan DA, Zhu S, Dia EQ, Lu KV, Yoshimoto K, Huang JH, Chute DJ, Riggs BL, Horvath S, Liau LM, Cavenee WK, Rao PN, Beroukhim R, Peck TC, Lee JC, Sellers WR, Stokoe D, Prados M, Cloughesy TF, Sawyers CL, Mischel PS (2005)

Molecular determinants of the response of glioblastomas to EGFR kinase inhibitors. N Engl J Med 353:2012–2024

Pérez-Ortiz JM, Serrano-Pérez MC, Pastor MD, Martín ED, Calvo S, Rincón M, Tranque P (2008) Mechanical lesion activates newly identified NFATC1 in primary astrocytes: implication of ATP and purinergic receptors. Eur J Neurosci 27:2453–2465

Ramirez T, Thoma K, Taja-Chayeb L, Efferth T, Herrera LA, Halatsch M-E, Gebhart E (2003) Specific patterns of DNA copy number gains and losses in eight new glioblastoma multiforme cell lines. Int J Oncol 23:453–460

Reyes-Mugica M, Rieger-Christ K, Ohgaki H, Ekstrand BC, Helie M, Kleinman G, Yahanda A, Fearon ER, Kleihues P, Reale MA (1997) Loss of DCC expression and glioma progression. Cancer Res 57:382–386

Sarkaria JN, Yang L, Grogan PT, Kitange GJ, Carlson BL, Schroeder MA, Galanis E, Giannini C, Wu W, Dinca EB, James CD (2007) Identification of molecular characteristics correlated with glioblastoma sensitivity to EGFR kinase inhibition through use of an intracranial xenograft test panel. Mol Cancer Ther 6:1167–1174

Senger DL, Tudan C, Guiot M-C, Mazzoni IE, Molenkamp G, LeBlanc R, Antel J, Olivier A, Snipes GJ, Kaplan DR (2002) Suppression of Rac activity induces apoptosis of human glioma cells but not normal human astrocytes. Cancer Res 62:2131–2140

Sharma S, Gajowniczek P, Way I, Lee DY, Jiang J, Yuza Y, Classon M, Haber DA, Settleman J (2006) A common signaling cascade may underlie "addiction" to the Src, BCR-ABL, and EGF receptor oncogenes. Cancer Cell 10:425–435

Sordella R, Bell D, Haber D, Settleman J (2004) Gefitinib-sensitizing EGFR mutations in lung cancer activate anti-apoptotic pathways. Science 305:1163–1167

Stommel J, Kimmelman A, Ying H, Nabioullin R, Ponugoti AH, Wiedemeyer R, Stegh AH, Bradner JE, Ligon KL, Brennan C, Chin L, DePinho RA (2007) Coactivation of receptor tyrosine kinases affects the response of tumor cells to targeted therapies. Science 318:287–290

Van der Laan MJ, Dudoit S, Pollard KS (2004) Part II. Stepdown procedures for control of the family-wise error rate. Stat Appl Genet Mol Biol 3(14) [Epub June 14]

Villapol S, Acarin L, Faiz M, Castellano B, Gonzalez B (2008) Survivin and heat shock protein 25/27 colocalize with cleaved caspase-3 in surviving reactive astrocytes following excitotoxicity to the immature brain. Neuroscience 153:108–119

Von Deimling A, Louis DN, Wiestler OD (1995) Molecular pathways in the formation of gliomas. Glia 15:328–338

Weinstein IB (2000) Disorders in cell circuitry during multistage carcinogenesis: the role of homeostasis. Carcinogenesis 21:857–864

Weinstein IB (2002) Cancer. Addiction to oncogenes – the achilles heal of cancer. Science 297:63–64

Weinstein IB, Joe AK (2006) Mechanisms of disease: oncogene addiction – a rationale for molecular targeting in cancer therapy. Nat Clin Pract Oncol 3:448–457

Yamada SM, Yamada S, Hayashi Y, Takahashi H, Teramoto A, Matsumoto K (2002) Fibroblast growth factor receptor (FGFR) 4 correlated with the malignancy of human astrocytomas. Neuro Res 24:244–248

Chapter 28

Enhanced Glioma Chemosensitivity

Rahima Patel, Leroy Shervington, and Amal Shervington

Abstract   Currently there is no cure for glioblastoma multiforme (GBM), and with chemotherapy compromised due to resistance, treatment of GBM is often difficult. Survival rates are generally poor, especially in older patients, this emphasizes the need for molecular targets designed to enhance efficiency of chemotherapy while limiting potential side effects. The development of combined therapy that ultimately incorporates molecular inhibition of immortalisation (telomerase), hsp90α, DNA repair (MGMT), EGFR, tumour suppressors, multi-drug resistance and cancer stem cell pathways is paramount to endeavour favourable innovative therapies, which in turn will help reduce the costs and ease the burden on health care.

Keywords Glioma · Chemosensitivity · Telomerase · MGMT · HSP90

Introduction

The most common primary tumour of the central nervous system (CNS) glioblastoma multiforme (GBM) inflicts a disproportional burden of mortality upon sufferers, with most patients succumbing to the disease within a year (Krex et al., 2007). Treatment strategies for GBMs include cytoreductive (debulking) surgery, external-beam radiation, and systemic chemotherapy. However, these approaches have limitations, the treatment is often compromised by the

A. Shervington (✉)
Brain Tumour North West, Faculty of Science, University of Central Lancashire, Preston, UK
e-mail: aashervington@googlemail.com

fact that GBMs are normally in close proximity to vital anatomical structures and lack a defined tumour edge. Chemotherapy was first introduced in the 1980s as part of the glioma treatment regime, with the most widely used class known as the alkylating agents (Krex et al., 2007). Despite the emergence of several anti-cancer agents, chemotherapeutic intervention has miserably failed with numerous GBM patients experiencing resistance and relapse. Efforts to develop strategies to overcome chemoresistance in GBM patients will help alleviate the cost of chemotherapy of health care. Furthermore, the development of effective treatment regimens with reduced side effects may lead to a satisfactory patient outcome. Several studies have focused on enhancing chemosensitivity using various targeted approaches. This review will focus on the following targets: immortalisation (telomerase), hsp90, DNA repair, EGFR, tumour suppressors, multi-drug resistance, and cancer stem cell pathways in glioma.

Inactivation of Telomerase

Telomerase (a ribonucleoprotein complex) allows cancer cells to overcome the Hayflick limitation that regulates their biological clock, maintains telomere length and subsequently prevents senescence. Telomeres are unique structures located at the terminal ends of each chromosome. The telomere repeats bind to sheltrin and function as caps, thus protects the ends of the DNA, preventing damage and promoting genomic stability and immortalisation (Wong et al., 2009). The active subunit of telomerase is found in cancer cells and tissues while it is generally absent in normal cells. Therefore, targeting hTERT (human telomerase reverse transcriptase) will subsequently affect telomere length and augment the likelihood of senescence, aiding chemotherapy while selectively sparing the normal brain cells. Cells with shorter dysfunctional telomeres are said to be more sensitive to chemotherapeutic agents due to induced fragmentation and multichromosomal fusions (Deng et al., 2009). The strategy of inhibiting telomerase has developed through basic research over the past decade, now providing potentially effective therapeutic targets for glioma. A reduction in telomerase activity through epigenetic inactivation of telomerase was shown to enhance glioma cell sensitivity to chemotherapeutic agents, cisplatin, taxol, and tamoxifen by approximately 2 fold (Patel et al., 2008). Inhibition of hTERT via RNA interference (RNAi) significantly inhibited the growth of subcutaneous tumours in nude mice models, and in comparison, xenographs that arose from telomerase inhibited GBM cells displayed a less aggressive phenotype and reduced angiogensis (Falchetti et al., 2006). 2-5 A(5′-phosphorylated 2′-5′-linked oligoadenylate)-linked antisense against human telomerase RNA component (2–5 A-anti-hTER) also inhibited the growth of glioma cells. Furthermore, combined 2–5 A-anti-hTER and cisplatin showed a synergistic effect, with a significant increase in apoptotic cells after therapy, making this a promising choice for future treatment (Iwado et al., 2007). Moreover, retroviral mediated inhibition of telomerase substantially decreased telomerase expression and subcutaneously grafted tumours from inhibited cells were significantly smaller in comparison (Zhao et al., 2007). Lentiviral vector encoding anti-hTERT siRNA reduced hTERT expression and telomerase activity to very low detectable levels in glioma cells; moreover, inhibition of hTERT reduced cell proliferation and migration prior to its effect on telomere length in vivo. Telomerase may play a role in the angiogenesis process (Zhao et al., 2007); thus, hTERT inhibition may improve the outcome of glioma patients when used in combination with standard routine therapy.

Indirect silencing of hTERT via DNA methyltransferase 1 (DNMT1) directed siRNA results in cell death and apoptosis, and when siRNA was combined with taxol or temozolomide, the concentration of the drugs used was substantially lower in comparison (up to 7 fold) (Shervington and Patel, 2008). Retinoid (a compound related to vitamin A) induced astrocytic differentiation and downregulated telomerase activity which enhanced the sensitivity to interferon-gamma (IFN-gamma) and increased apoptosis in human glioma cells (Das et al., 2009). Combining retinoid with conventional therapies such as temozolomide and cisplatin (Das et al., 2009) may further increase cell chemosensitivity.

In leukemia, telomerase was inhibited by a dominant-negative form of human telomerase (DN-hTERT), which sequentially enhanced chemosensitivity to doxorubicin and other related double-strand DNA break (DSB)-inducing agents (Tauchi et al., 2007). This could prove to be a successful approach for the treatment of glioma. Furthermore, inhibition of TFR2 (telomeric repeat binding factor 2) renders telomeres dysfunctional (Deng et al., 2009); thus, an enhanced effect would be observed if doxorubicin and (DSB)-inducing agents were used in combination with TRF2 inhibitors. Various natural products have been recognised for their chemo-preventive and anti-proliferative properties. Recently, polyphenol catechin, epigallocatechin-3-gallate (EGCG) the active ingredient found in green tea was shown to decrease hTERT expression in glioma cells. In addition, EGCG treated cells showed increased sensitivity to both cisplatin and tamoxifen (Shervington et al., 2009).

One of the major obstacles in enhancing brain cell chemosensitivity is the delivery system. An alternative approach that could be used to enhance chemosensitivity is intranasal delivery of telomerase inhibitor GRN163 which inhibits the growth of glioma cells through gradual reduction of telomeres followed by the onset of cellular senescence (Marian et al., 2010). Intranasal delivery of the inhibitor enables the compound to reach the intracerebral tumour without neurotoxic side effects, and hence, may provide a promising approach for targeted delivery of combined therapeutics. Furthermore, combined imetelstat (GRN163L, lipid conjugated antagonist) and temozolomide (8 μM) had a dramatic effect on cell survival and activated the DNA damage response pathways in primary human glioblastoma (GBM) tumour-initiating cells without shortening telomeres. This was due to increased induction of telomeric DNA breaks, which were not repaired in the absence of telomerase and/or elevated autophagy (Marian et al., 2010). Imetelstat treatment was shown to reduce tumour size in GBM xenografts propagated from patient samples. Furthermore, appropriate doses of imetelstat successfully crossed the blood brain barrier (Marian et al., 2010) hence may provide an encouraging therapy for GBM patients that does not require intranasal delivery and has no/limited known neurotoxic side effects. The effect of the telomerase inhibitor MST-312 (a synthetic telomerase inhibitor) on glioma cells was short term treatment induced DNA damage and ATM-dependent G2/M cell cycle arrest which decreased cell viability. However, this was more than just reducing the length of telomeres, MST-312 was able to exert its effects on cells which were only telomerase dependent those "with the crisis flagging signal" driving them to cell cycle arrest (Wong et al., 2009). Although further critical evaluation of telomerase inhibitors may be required, all the data discussed point to one fact and that is that hTERT, telomerase and telomere inhibition can sensitise gliomas to chemotherapeutic agents; thus, encouraging the development of combined therapies.

Targetting Hsp90α

For telomerase to be correctly folded and activated, heat shock protein 90 (Hsp90) must bind, along with co-chaperones p23, Hsp40, Hop and Hsp70 (referred to as a foldosome) (Panner et al., 2007). Hsp90 is the most abundant molecular chaperone within the cytosol, which forms an intracellular self-defence system prompting the refolding of proteins and preventing aggregation. The accumulation of mis-folded proteins may also contribute to chemoresistance. Hsp90α, an isoform of Hsp90, binds to proteins with unstable tertiary structures such as Akt and oncogenic forms of mutated epidermal growth factor receptor (EGFR) (Panner et al., 2007), both of which contribute to the growth of glioma cells. Furthermore, Hsp90α facilitates global inhibition of apoptosis, and is suggested to be a prerequisite for tumour formation by undoubtedly creating ideal cancer microenvironmental conditions. Most research on glioma is targeted towards hsp90α because only the induced hsp90α and not the constitutive hsp90β is upregulated in glioma (Panner et al., 2007). Hence, hsp90α could be an exciting therapeutic target in cancer because inhibition of this protein causes the simultaneous degradation of multiple oncoproteins and combinatorial blockade of numerous oncogenic pathways.

Inhibition of Hsp90α via 17-(allylamino)-17-demethoxygeldanamycin (17-AAG), a benzoquinone antibiotic derived from geldanamycin, was shown to reduce clonogenicity of glioma cells, and at low concentrations, potentiated the cytotoxicity of cisplatin and 1,3-bis(2-chloroethyl)-1-nitrosourea (Ohba et al., 2010). The enhanced cytotoxicity was a consequence of prolonged G(2)-M arrest accompanied by the suppression of cdc2 and cdc25C, and increased apoptotic cell death accompanied by the proteasomal degradation of the antiapoptosis proteins Akt and survivin (Hsp90 client proteins). Survivin has been shown to inhibit both caspase-dependent apoptosis and caspase-independent cell death in glioma. Given that survivin augments binding of Sp1 and c-Myc to the hTERT promoter (Endoh et al., 2005), suggests that 17-AAG indirectly targets other signalling processes/pathways (the six hallmark traits of cancer). Survivin knockdown by a siRNA decreased Sp1, and c-Myc phosphorylation proves that survivin participates not only in inhibiting apoptosis but also in prolonging the cellular lifespan by assisting cells to escape replicative senescence (Endoh et al., 2005). Inhibition of hsp90α by siRNA significantly decreased protein levels of hsp90α for up to 72 h following siRNA delivery, without altering the levels of hsp90β. The hsp90α inhibition helped localise FLIP, a protein that is a key suppressor of tumour necrosis factor-α-related apoptosis-inducing ligand (TRAIL) to its site of action in the DISC (death-inducing signalling complex) and sensitised otherwise resistant cells to chemotherapy (Panner et al., 2007). In addition, inhibiting hsp90α using siRNA in glioma increased cell sensitivity to temozolomide by almost 13 fold in comparison to scrambled siRNA treated cells. The reduction in hsp90α protein affected the expression of telomerase, confirming that hsp90 is involved in telomerase regulation through the folding of the holoenzyme complex (Cruickshanks et al., 2010).

Increased ERBB2 (a receptor tyrosine kinase belonging to the family of epidermal growth factor receptors, generally involved in cell differentiation, proliferation, and tumour growth) expression was responsible for paclitaxel resistance in ovarian cancer cells. However, when combined paclitaxel and non growth inhibitory concentrations of 17-AAG were administered, a sensitised effect was observed (Sauvageot et al., 2009). Not only was 17-AAG able to downregulate ERBB2 levels but also reduced endothelial cell migration. Moreover, given that ERBB2 levels in glioma are increasingly high in comparison to normal brain (Sauvageot et al., 2009), treatment with 17-AAG may facilitate the inhibition of ERBB2 and hsp90α which may benefit glioma patients. The binding affinity of hsp90 for 17-AAG is 100-fold higher in tumour cells compared to normal cells enabling selective drug targeting of tumour cells (Sauvageot et al., 2009). Interestingly, 17-AAG was not found to synergise with temozolomide but did act as a radio-sensitizer both in vitro and in vivo and thus, could potentially benefit temozolomide refractory patients. Furthermore, inhibition of hsp90α contributed to the DNA damage response in order to enhance radiation sensitivity through activation of the cell cycle checkpoint and double strand break repairs (Sauvageot et al., 2009). 17-AAG is potentially a promising candidate in the treatment of gliomas.

EGCG was shown to inhibit the transcriptional activity of the aryl hydrocarbon receptor (AhR) through a mechanism involving direct binding of EGCG to the C-terminus of hsp90 (Li et al., 2009); however, it is still unclear whether its direct binding had an effect on hsp90α expression. Pharmacological inhibition of AhR using novel AhR antagonists CH-223191 or AhR siRNA reduced clonogenic survival and reduced invasiveness of glioma cells (Gramatzki et al., 2009). AhR is associated with the folding of telomerase; thus, AhR inhibition may benefit glioma patients in the future. Combining Hsp90α and telomerase inhibitors with chemotherapeutic agents may further facilitate the enhancement of cancer therapies.

Inactivation of DNA Repair

O^6-methylguanine-DNA methyltransferase (MGMT) removes mutagenic and cytotoxic adducts from O^6 position in guanine, the preferred point of attack of many carcinogens specifically alkylating agents (Fukushima et al., 2009). In the absence of MGMT, these adducts are not removed, allowing the O^6-alkyl guanine to mispair with thymine during DNA replication and resulting in a G-to-A transition. If the mispairing is recognised by the post-replication mismatch repair system, the daughter strand along with the thymine will be removed, leaving the O^6- methylguanine to again pair with thymine during gap filling, and upon replication of the gapped structure double-strand breaks are formed (Fukushima et al., 2009). MGMT-deficient cells are more susceptible to spontaneous

mutations and polymorphisms, and thus MGMT inactivation leads to over whelming numbers of adducts driving cells to enter apoptosis.

Epigenetic inactivation of MGMT through methylation of the CpG island located in the promoter region has shown to enhance the sensitivity of cells to temozolomide and cisplatin (Krex et al., 2007) resulting in improved survival rates of GBM patients receiving alkylating agents as therapy. Molecular analysis of 55 primary GMB patients showed a higher proportion of MGMT hypermethylation in the long term survivor group, compared with a reference sample of unselected consecutive GBMs, further advocating that the inactivation of MGMT can be used to enhance chemosensitivity (Krex et al., 2007). Transcriptional silencing of MGMT in high grade oligodendroglial tumours has shown to contribute to chemosensitivity. Furthermore, MGMT gene promoter methylation status in 36 WHO (World Health Organisation) grade III gliomas revealed extensive epigenetic silencing of MGMT gene in high grade gliomas with an oligodendroglial component along with frequent 1p/19q co-deletion, which may contribute to the relative favourable prognosis of oligodendroglial tumours compared with pure astrocytic tumours (Yang et al., 2009).

Several substrates that inhibit MGMT include O^6-benzylguanine (BzG), O^6-4-bromothenylguanine (Patrin) and O^6-bromothenylguanine-C8-β-D-glucoside. Phase I and II studies have shown that combined MGMT inhibition and BCNU (carmustine) therapy, can enhance glioma sensitivity to BCNU. The inactivation of MGMT via siRNA increased sensitivity to BCNU (4 fold) in vitro, and a similar approach could be adapted for glioma patients. However, delivery is often a problem, with the most effective method of introducing siRNA or shRNAs being adenoviruses, which is often challenged by the medical profession. Nevertheless, phase I/II clinical studies with the E1B mutant oncolytic adenovirus ONYX-015 (p53 inhibitor) and cisplatin showed a favourable outcome and has been deemed relatively safe for gliomas (Jiang et al., 2006).

Given that p53 can regulate MGMT expression through a p53 binding site in the MGMT promoter, inhibition of p53 has been shown to enhance the effect of temozolomide in mice intracranial tumour implantation models (Dinca et al., 2008). This suggests that p53 may induce MGMT to negatively regulate temozolomide sensitivity, and that sequestration of Sp1 transcription factor could be one of the mechanisms by which p53 negatively regulates MGMT expression. In addition, p53 plays a protective role against cell death on treatment with chloroethylating agents, conversely this may not be the case when methylating agents are used in treatment strategies (Dinca et al., 2008). Interferon-β (IFN-β) administered in combination with nitrosourea, results in a marked enhancement in temozolomide sensitivity to human glioma cells. IFN-β acts as a drug sensitizer by downregulating MGMT transcription via p53 induction (Wakabayashi et al., 2008). Given that GBM patients with negative MGMT expression tend to have an overall better prognosis, combining IFN-β with chemotherapy may be a beneficial approach for glioma patients. All the evidence shows that MGMT inactivation can sensitise GBMs to alkylating agents, elevating the importance of MGMT in basic and translational cancer research. Methylation is the most common silencing mechanism of DNA repair genes, advocating the need to research and develop new demethylating agents. Other DNA repair pathways (mismatch repair (MMR) and base excision repair (BER)) may require inactivation or up regulation to further enhance the sensitivity of the chemotherapeutic agents used to treat glioma.

Targeting EGFR and Tumour Suppressors

Inhibition of receptor signalling via EGFR-specific tyrosine kinase inhibitor, AG1478, sensitised xenografts to cisplatin and significantly suppressed the growth of subcutaneous tumours in mice xenograft models in a synergistic manner (Huang et al., 2007). The combined AG1478 and cisplatin treatment further suppressed the growth of the tumour; and the silencing of EGFR and/or specific tyrosine kinase (c-Met) via siRNA in combination with standard chemotherapeutics could represent a new therapeutic approach to overcome resistance in gliomas that express high levels of EGFR. Given that Met receptor tyrosine kinase has an important role in regulating cell response to chemotherapy, combined inhibition of Met signalling in combination treatment regimens may benefit glioma patients in the future. Additionally, tamoxifen, a potent inhibitor, successfully crosses the blood brain barrier and inhibits the proliferation of glioma cells through the inhibition of protein tyrosine phosphorylation of the neu receptor (transmembrane glycoprotein) that resembles the EGFR (Gadji et al., 2009) and could be used as a potential agent in the treatment of GBMs.

Melanoma differentiation-associated gene-7/interleukin-24 (mda-7/IL-24), a tumour suppressor cytokine, induced apoptosis and cell cycle arrest, through specifically down regulating MGMT and activating p53; thus, advocating the use of mda-7/IL-24 as part of a novel approach to treat GMBs and to overcome temozolomide resistance (Yacoub et al., 2008). Inactivation of p53 sensitizes glioma cells to BCNU and temozolomide through G1 arrest and delays entry into S-phase. However, in contrast, p53 inactivation, renders glioma cells becoming significantly more resistant to cisplatin (Xu et al., 2005), indicating that p53 status may influence the chemosensitivity of glioma cells in a drug type specific manner. On the contrary, disruption of p53 by antisense oligos has been shown to sensitize wild type glioma cells to low doses of cisplatin and shifted the cellular response from G2/M arrest to apoptosis (Datta et al., 2004). Ectopic p16 (a tumour suppressor) expression has been shown to sensitize glioma cells towards vincristine and BCNU by approximately 1.5-2 fold; thus, modulating both radiotherapy and chemosensitivity of gliomas. Furthermore, p53 a down stream target of p16, plays a major role in apoptosis and cell cycle regulation and may contribute to the sensitivity of vincristine and BCNU. BRCA1, a tumour suppressor, has many roles in the DNA repair pathway, independent of p53. BRCA1 deficient breast cancer cells were found to be 5 times more sensitive to cisplatin and 25 times more sensitive to gemcitabine (Sharma et al., 2007). Targeting BRCA1 may prove to be a valuable target for gliomas given that BRCA1 is involved in brain tumour formation.

Targeting Multi Drug Resistance

Another major group of genes that deter treatment and sensitivity of chemotherapeutic drugs in gliomas are known as multidrug resistance (MDR) genes. They actively prevent chemotherapeutic drugs from entering the cell through efflux pumps on the membrane. These include the adenosine triophosphate binding cassette (ABC) super-family (mdr1, mrp1, ABCG2), vaults (lrp/mvp), and finally the anti-apoptotic gene

Bcl2 (Cui et al., 2010). Effective inhibition of these genes may also contribute to enhanced chemosensitivity of gliomas. Suppression of Gli1 (a key component of the hedgehog pathway) via cyclopamine enhanced chemosensitivity and increased apoptosis of glioma cells. The increased sensitivity, resulted in the downregulation of many drug resistant genes (mdr1, mrp1, mvp, MGMT, Bcl2 and survivin). Furthermore, lentiviral-short hairpin Gli1 (LV-shGli1) confirmed negative regulation of the hedgehog pathway and a decreased expression of these genes (Cui et al., 2010). The suppression of Gli1 may be a valid therapeutic option for overcoming MDR and may prevent the reoccurrence of glioma by increasing the success rate of chemotherapy.

Effective inhibition of Bcl2 protein in glioma cells markedly reduces cell proliferation, increases sensitivity to cisplatin, and leads to a complete loss of tumourigenicity through what may be described as marked morphological changes (Zhu et al., 2003). This suggests that targeting Bcl2 therapy does have the potential to enhance chemosensitivity of gliomas. Bcl2 levels in immortalised glioma cells are found to be moderately upregulated (Zhu et al., 2003), suggesting that these anti-apoptotic signals may play a role in the immortalisation, and therefore, the inhibition of Bcl2 may indirectly affect hTERT expression. Sequence specific mdr1 RNAi inhibits mRNA expression and affects P-gp protein in glioma cells, reversing the MDR phenotype, and providing a promising treatment strategy for human gliomas (Rittierodt et al., 2004). Furthermore, calcium antagonists have been used to reduce P-gp expression to enhance the effects of several chemotherapeutic agents used in the treatment of glioma.

Targeting Cancer Stem Cells

A small subpopulation of cells with stem-like properties/features called cancer stem cells (CSCs) are found in various cancer tissues and cell lines including glioma. They have been reported to contain a high expression level of MDR and drug transporter genes. Given that CSCs have unlimited proliferative potential (attributed to unlimited self-renewal capacity and multi linage differentiation), signifies the need to make them the primary target for potential

chemotherapy. Glioma CSCs are found to be resistant to various chemotherapeutic agents (etoposide, camptothecin, cisplatin, temozolomide, daunorubucin, doxorubicin, vincristine and methotrexate). This was not attributed to defective drug uptake or as a result of drug extrusion, but may be a consequence of abnormalities in the cell death pathway, specifically the over-expression of antiapoptotic factors and/or silencing of key death effectors (Eramo et al., 2006). Another approach that can be adapted to deplete the CSC pool in gliomas is to involve stimulating the cells to differentiate into mature cells; thus, inhibiting their proliferative potential. Previously, notch pathway (which controls specification, proliferation, and survival of non-neoplastic neural precursors), inhibition depleted CSCs and blocked engraftment in embryonic brain tumour (Fan et al., 2006). Inhibition of the notch pathway slowed the growth of tumour cells in vitro and in comparison the xenografts formed were relatively smaller in size due to the increase in apoptotic cells. The notch pathway inhibitors may be the first of a new class of chemotherapeutic agents that target CSCs, exploiting their unique molecular properties. It was found that HIF2α is essential for the maintenance of CSC phenotype, therefore, inhibiting HIF2α in combination with other conventional agents may prove to be a therapeutic approach that could possibly work, given that temozolomide induces a time-dependent decline of CSC subpopulation in glioma. High levels of EGFR and Akt have also been linked to CSCs (Gadji et al., 2009); thus, a multidirectional pathway inhibition may prove to be the best approach in eliminating the CSC population found in cancer.

Conclusion

Cancer is a multistep process, incorporating various defective pathways which is why a single approach is proving to be unsuccessful. This review provides an understanding of the numerous approaches taken in order to enhance the effects of chemotherapeutic agents used in the treatment of glioma. Emphasizing the need of developing new combined therapy that ultimately incorporates molecular inhibition of immortalisation (telomerase), hsp90α, DNA repair (MGMT), EGFR, tumour suppressors, multi-drug resistance, and cancer stem cell pathways. The ultimate strategy would be to eradicate gliomas completely. However, current research aims to develop novel combined therapies to improve the outcome of GBM patients, endeavouring to lead to favourable innovative therapies which in turn will help reduce the costs and ease the burden on health care.

References

Cruickshanks N, Shervington L, Patel R, Shervington A (2010) Can hsp90α siRNA combined with TMZ be a future therapy for gliomas? Cancer Invest 28(6):608–614

Cui D, Xu Q, Wang K, Che X (2010) Gli1 is a potential target for alleviating multidrug resistance of gliomas. J Neurol Sci 288:156–166

Das A, Banik NL, Ray SK (2009) Molecular mechanisms of the combination of retinoid and interferon-gamma for inducing differentiation and increasing apoptosis in human glioblastoma T98G and U87MG cells. Neurochem Res 34:87–101

Datta K, Shah P, Srivastava T, Mathur SG, Chattopadhyay P, Sinha S (2004) Sensitizing glioma cells to cisplatin by abrogating the P53 response with antisense oligonucleotides. Cancer Gene Ther 11:525–531

Deng Y, Guo X, Ferguson DO, Chang S (2009) Multiple roles for MRE11 at uncapped telomeres. Nature 460:914–918

Dinca EB, Lu KV, Sarkaria JN, Pieper RO, Prados MD, Haas-Kogan DA, Vandenberg SR, Berger MS, James CD (2008) P53 small-molecule inhibitor enhances temozolomide cytotoxic activity against intracranial glioblastoma xenografts. Cancer Res 68:10034–10039

Endoh T, Tsuji N, Asanuma K, Yagihashi A, Watanabe N (2005) Survivin enhances telomerase activity via up-regulation of specificity protein 1- and C-myc-mediated human telomerase reverse transcriptase gene transcription. Exp Cell Res 305:300–311

Eramo A, Ricci-Vitiani L, Zeuner A, Pallini R, Lotti F, Sette G, Pilozzi E, Larocca LM, Peschle C, De MR (2006) Chemotherapy resistance of glioblastoma stem cells. Cell Death Differ 13:1238–1241

Falchetti ML, Fiorenzo P, Mongiardi MP, Petrucci G, Montano N, Maira G, Pierconti F, Larocca LM, Levi A, Pallini R (2006) Telomerase inhibition impairs tumour growth in glioblastoma xenografts. Neurol Res 28:532–537

Fan X, Matsui W, Khaki L, Stearns D, Chun J, Li YM, Eberhart CG (2006) Notch pathway inhibition depletes stem-like cells and blocks engraftment in embryonal brain tumors. Cancer Res 66:7445–7452

Fukushima T, Takeshima H, Kataoka H (2009) Anti-glioma therapy with temozolomide and status of the DNA-repair gene MGMT. Anticancer Res 29:4845–4854

Gadji M, Crous AM, Fortin D, Krcek J, Torchia M, Mai S, Drouin R, Klonisch T (2009) EGF receptor inhibitors in the treatment of glioblastoma multiform: old clinical allies and newly emerging therapeutic concepts. Eur J Pharmacol 625:23–30

Gramatzki D, Pantazis G, Schittenhelm J, Tabatabai G, Kohle C, Wick W, Schwarz M, Weller M, Tritschler I (2009) Aryl

hydrocarbon receptor inhibition downregulates the TGF-beta/smad pathway in human glioblastoma cells. Oncogene 28:2593–2605

Huang PH, Mukasa A, Bonavia R, Flynn RA, Brewer ZE, Cavenee WK, Furnari FB, White FM (2007) Quantitative analysis of egfrviii cellular signaling networks reveals a combinatorial therapeutic strategy for glioblastoma. Proc Natl Acad Sci USA 104:12867–12872

Iwado E, Daido S, Kondo Y, Kondo S (2007) Combined effect of 2-5a-linked antisense against telomerase RNA and conventional therapies on human malignant glioma cells in vitro and in vivo. Int J Oncol 31:1087–1095

Jiang H, Alonso MM, Gomez-Manzano C, Piao Y, Fueyo J (2006) Oncolytic viruses and DNA-repair machinery: overcoming chemoresistance of gliomas. Expert Rev Anticancer Ther 6:1585–1592

Krex, D, Klink, B,, Hartmann, C, von DA, Pietsch T, Simon M, Sabel M, Steinbach JP, Heese O, Reifenberger G, Weller M, Schackert G (2007) Long-term survival with glioblastoma multiforme. Brain 130:2596–2606

Li Y, Zhang T, Schwartz SJ, Sun D (2009) New developments in hsp90 inhibitors as anti-cancer therapeutics: mechanisms, clinical perspective and more potential. Drug Resist Updat 12:17–27

Marian CO, Cho SK, McEllin BM, Maher EA, Hatanpaa KJ, Madden CJ, Mickey BE, Wright WE, Shay JW, Bachoo RM (2010) The telomerase antagonist, imetelstat, efficiently targets glioblastoma tumor-initiating cells leading to decreased proliferation and tumor growth. Clin Cancer Res 16:154–163

Ohba S, Hirose Y, Yoshida K, Yazaki T, Kawase T (2010) Inhibition of 90-kd heat shock protein potentiates the cytotoxicity of chemotherapeutic agents in human glioma cells. J Neurosurg 112:33–42

Panner A, Murray JC, Berger MS, Pieper RO (2007) Heat shock protein 90alpha recruits FLIPS to the death-inducing signaling complex and contributes to TRAIL resistance in human glioma. Cancer Res 67:9482–9489

Patel R, Shervington L, Lea R, Shervington A (2008) Epigenetic silencing of telomerase and a non-alkylating agent as a novel therapeutic approach for glioma. Brain Res 1188:173–181

Rittierodt M, Tschernig T, Harada K (2004) Modulation of multidrug-resistance-associated P-glycoprotein in human U-87 MG and HUV-ECC cells with antisense oligodeoxynucleotides to MDR1 mrna. Pathobiology 71:123–128

Sauvageot CM, Weatherbee JL, Kesari S, Winters SE, Barnes J, Dellagatta J, Ramakrishna NR, Stiles CD, Kung AL, Kieran MW, Wen PY (2009) Efficacy of the HSP90 inhibitor 17-AAG in human glioma cell lines and tumorigenic glioma stem cells. Neurooncol 11:109–121

Sharma VB, Kurian AW, Feldman A, Ford JM (2007) The role of BRCA1 in DNA repair and chemosensitivity. J Clin Oncol 25:18S

Shervington A, Patel R (2008) Silencing DNA methyltransferase (DNMT) enhances glioma chemosensitivity. Oligonucleotides 18:365–374

Shervington A, Pawar V, Menon S, Thakkar D, Patel R (2009) The sensitization of glioma cells to cisplatin and tamoxifen by the use of catechin. Mol Biol Rep 36:1181–1186

Tauchi T, Ohyashiki JH, Ohyashiki K (2007) Telomerase inhibition combined with other chemotherapeutic reagents to enhance anti-cancer effect. Methods Mol Biol 405:181–189

Wakabayashi T, Kayama T, Nishikawa R, Takahashi H, Yoshimine T, Hashimoto N, Aoki T, Kurisu K, Natsume A, Ogura M, Yoshida J (2008) A multicenter phase i trial of interferon-beta and temozolomide combination therapy for high-grade gliomas (INTEGRA study). Jpn J Clin Oncol 38:715–718

Wong VC, Ma J, Hawkins CE (2009) Telomerase inhibition induces acute ATM-dependent growth arrest in human astrocytomas. Cancer Lett 274:151–159

Xu GW, Mymryk JS, Cairncross JG (2005) Inactivation of P53 sensitizes astrocytic glioma cells to BCNU and temozolomide, but not cisplatin. J Neurooncol 74:141–149

Yacoub A, Park MA, Gupta P, Rahmani M, Zhang G, Hamed H, Hanna D, Sarkar D, Lebedeva IV, Emdad L, Sauane M, Vozhilla N, Spiegel S, Koumenis C, Graf M, Curiel DT, Grant S, Fisher PB, Dent P (2008) Caspase-, cathepsin-, and PERK-dependent regulation of MDA-7/IL-24-induced cell killing in primary human glioma cells. Mol Cancer Ther 7:297–313

Yang SH, Kim YH, Kim JW, Park CK, Park SH, Jung HW (2009) Methylation status of the O6-methylguanine-deoxyribonucleic acid methyltransferase gene promoter in world health organization grade III gliomas. J Korean Neurosurg Soc 46:385–388

Zhao P, Wang C, Fu Z, You Y, Cheng Y, Lu X, Lu A, Liu N, Pu P, Kang C, Salford LG, Fan X (2007) Lentiviral vector mediated sirna knock-down of htert results in diminished capacity in invasiveness and in vivo growth of human glioma cells in a telomere length-independent manner. Int J Oncol 31:361–368

Zhu CJ, Li YB, Wong MC (2003) Expression of antisense bcl-2 cdna abolishes tumorigenicity and enhances chemosensitivity of human malignant glioma cells. J Neurosci Res 74:60–66

Chapter 29

Malignant Glioma Patients: Anti-Vascular Endothelial Growth Factor Monoclonal Antibody, Bevacizumab

Richa Pandey and John F. de Groot

Abstract Malignant gliomas are the most common and the most devastating type of primary brain tumors in adults. Hence, the search for more effective treatments continues. Because a tumor's viability depends on its blood supply, antiangiogenic drugs are an attractive approach for treatment. The monoclonal antibody bevacizumab inhibits angiogenesis by blocking the binding of vascular endothelial growth factor (VEGF) to its receptors. Bevacizumab recently received accelerated approval for the treatment of recurrent glioblastoma. In this chapter, we first discuss antiangiogenic therapy and its mechanisms of action. We review the efficacy of bevacizumab as therapy for malignant glioma, as well as the drug's toxicity profile and ways of assessing response to therapy. Then we discuss mechanisms of resistance to anti-VEGF therapy. Finally, we present some ideas for future work.

Keywords Glioblastoma · Antiangiogenic therapy · Resistance · Myeloid cells

Introduction

Malignant gliomas are the most common and the most devastating type of primary brain tumors in adults. These highly vascularized tumors are associated with poor outcome because of their aggressive nature and high recurrence rate. The current standard of care for malignant gliomas is maximal safe resection followed by combination radiotherapy plus chemotherapy with temozolomide (TMZ) and then adjuvant TMZ (Stupp et al., 2005). The search for more effective treatments continues.

Key issues in the treatment of malignant gliomas are angiogenesis and tumor invasion as they promote tumor infiltration which prevents complete surgical resection and leads to tumor recurrence at distant sites. Because a tumor's viability depends on its blood supply, antiangiogenic drugs are an attractive approach for treatment. Here, we first discuss antiangiogenic therapy and its mechanisms of action. Then, we review the efficacy of the monoclonal antibody bevacizumab as therapy for different types of malignant glioma—glioblastoma and anaplastic glioma—as well as the drug's toxicity profile and ways of assessing response to therapy. Resistance to antiangiogenic therapy is a significant barrier to the long term effectiveness of this therapy and will be discussed. Finally, we present some ideas for future work.

Background

Angiogenesis in Malignant Gliomas

Angiogenesis, the physiologic process of the growth of new blood vessels from existing ones, is essential for tumor survival. Decades of research have confirmed that tumor growth and metastasis require angiogenesis to provide a constant supply of nutrients and oxygen. Viable tumor cells are typically located within 150 μm of vascular structures. Therefore, without angiogenesis, tumor growth becomes impaired when a tumor

J.F. de Groot (✉)
Department of Neuro-Oncology, Cancer Center, The University of Texas M.D. Anderson, Houstan, TX 77030, USA
e-mail: jdegroot@mdanderson.org

M.A. Hayat (ed.), *Tumors of the Central Nervous System, Volume 1*,
DOI 10.1007/978-94-007-0344-5_29, © Springer Science+Business Media B.V. 2011

expands beyond a diameter of 0.4–1 mm (Hanahan and Folkman, 1996). Without oxygen and nutrients, tumors develop hypoxia and necrosis, leading to the formation of new blood vessels.

Pathologic angiogenesis, or vascular proliferation, is a hallmark of glioblastomas and is critical for tumor development, maintenance and survival. Malignant gliomas have to maintain the delivery of nutrients and oxygen to support the rapidly dividing glioma cells, which is accomplished by co-opting existing host vessels or promoting the formation of new ones.

The initiation of tumor angiogenesis is a complex process whereby multiple molecules in normal and tumor tissues activate a series of signaling events that lead to the formation of new vessels. The recruitment of endothelial cells from the surrounding tissues requires pro-angiogenic growth factors, including vascular endothelial growth factor (VEGF), the related placental growth factor (PlGF), basic fibroblast growth factor (bFGF), and many others.

VEGF is a heparin-binding protein secreted by glioma cells near necrotic areas within the tumor. VEGF acts in a paracrine manner on two high-affinity transmembrane tyrosine kinase receptors present on endothelial cells: VEGFR-2 (KDR/Flk-1) and, less prominently, VEGFR-1 (Flt-1). Of the known pro-angiogenic factors, VEGF is one of the most important mediators of hypoxia-induced endothelial-cell proliferation, migration, and survival (Shweiki et al., 1992). VEGF is highly expressed in malignant gliomas because they have a poorly organized vascular bed, which leads to regions of inadequate blood flow and hypoxia. Elevated VEGF levels in glioblastomas have been correlated with high tumor blood-vessel density and increased tumor invasiveness, and a higher degree of vascularization has been linked to poor prognosis in patients with gliomas and other solid tumors (Zhou et al., 2003).

The importance of VEGF in the biology of anaplastic gliomas is less well established. Unlike glioblastomas, anaplastic astrocytomas do not have histologic evidence of necrosis or vascular proliferation, and thus these areas are not enhanced with the use of a contrast agent on magnetic resonance imaging (MRI). The lack of necrosis, potentially an indicator of tumor growth rate, may account for the lack of notable hypoxia-mediated VEGF expression in anaplastic gliomas. As part of their malignant transformation to higher-grade glioblastoma, anaplastic astrocytomas undergo the angiogenic switch–the process of induction of tumor vasculature–with evidence of abundant angiogenesis. This angiogenic switch is "off" when the effect of pro-angiogenic molecules is balanced by that of antiangiogenic molecules and is "on" when the net balance is tipped in favor of angiogenesis (Hanahan and Folkman, 1996). The blockade of VEGF, which is one of the primary pro-angiogenic molecules, may delay or interrupt the process of the angiogenic switch and thus may delay the transformation to a higher-grade tumor. VEGF blockade is thus an attractive therapeutic approach in this patient population.

Antiangiogenic Therapy

The discovery of the importance of angiogenesis in tumor growth and metastasis led to the use of drugs as inhibitors of angiogenesis. Multiple early-phase nonspecific or low-potency inhibitors of angiogenesis, such as thalidomide, have been tested in clinical trials in glioma, with little success. However, multiple new agents that potently inhibit VEGF receptors (VEGFRs) or the ligand VEGF are showing significant benefits in patients with malignant glioma. For example, the pan-VEGFR inhibitor cediranib (AZD2171) was shown to have a high radiographic response rate in patients with recurrent glioblastoma (Batchelor et al., 2007). Bevacizumab, which sequesters free VEGF, making it unavailable for the activation of VEGFRs, has also significantly improved response rates and prolonged progression-free survival (PFS). Bevacizumab recently obtained accelerated approval from the Food and Drug Administration (FDA) for the treatment of recurrent glioblastoma (Cohen et al., 2009).

Mechanisms of Action of Antiangiogenic Therapy

In contrast to cytotoxic chemotherapy, antiangiogenic therapy is likely to be cytostatic and will lead only indirectly to the death of tumor cells via the starvation of factors essential for cell survival. Marked structural and functional differences exist between the blood vessels newly formed within the tumor and normal blood vessels. VEGF, previously known as vascular permeability factor or VPF, mediates the permeability of the newly formed tumor vessels, making them tortuous and hyperpermeable (Dvorak et al., 1995). Such tumor vessels are poorly organized as a result of aberrant endothelial-cell proliferation and abnormal perivascular cells. These abnormalities and an increase in interstitial pressure from leaky vessels leads to compression of blood vessels by tumor cells impairing blood flow, which leads to hypoxia in the tumor microenvironment. This hypoxia may compromise the delivery and effectiveness of conventional cytotoxic, molecular targeted, and radiation therapies. Although one major rationale for the use of antiangiogenic therapy is to control this abnormal tumor vasculature, there are additional benefits. In addition to directly inhibiting tumor angiogenesis, antiangiogenic drugs may also provide a clinical benefit by normalizing the tumor vasculature, which improves drug delivery; providing a steroid-sparing effect, which improves quality of life; and specifically targeting glioma stem cells (GSCs) within the microvascular niche.

Normalization of Tumor Vasculature

The pruning of the abnormal tumor vessels and the reduction of abnormal permeability of the blood–brain barrier is called vascular normalization. Antiangiogenic agents, especially VEGF and VEGFR inhibitors, lead to apoptosis of endothelial cells and decrease vessel diameter, density, and permeability. These "normalized" vessels are still more permeable and less mature than their normal counterparts. However, the decrease in extracellular fluid pressure from permeable vessels reduces interstitial pressure. This improves oxygen delivery and is thought to lead to an improved metabolic tumor microenvironment, which creates opportunities for the use of combination treatments (Jain, 2001). In a study by Batchelor et al. (2007) using AZD2171, vascular normalization was observed to occur rapidly and to continue for 28 days with continuous treatment. This normalization was reproducible with re-challenge with the drug after "drug holidays" (Batchelor et al., 2007).

The functional implications of this normalization may depend on specific features of the tumor microenvironment. Anti-VEGF treatment of subcutaneous melanoma xenografts results in vessel normalization and concomitant better delivery of MRI contrast agents and oxygen to the tumor. In striking contrast,

similar treatment of brain tumors (both primary and metastatic) results in a reduction in contrast enhancement on MRI both in animal models and in human glioblastoma patients; this suggests that the brain microenvironment may be more sensitive to VEGF-targeted therapies (Bergers and Hanahan, 2008).

It is also becoming more apparent that the dose of an antiangiogenic agent is an important factor in modulating delivery of the drug to brain tumors. In an animal xenograft model study by Zhou and Gallo (2009), maximal intratumoral TMZ delivery was achieved in the group pretreated with low-dose sunitinib, as compared with high-dose and control groups. In that study, a vascular normalization index, which represents the fraction of the total tumor blood vessels that are functional, correlated significantly with the intratumoral TMZ concentration (Zhou and Gallo, 2009). Thus, the extent of vascular normalization and intratumoral adjuvant drug delivery may depend on the concentration of the antiangiogenic drug.

Steroid-Sparing Effect

VEGF-induced vasodilation and permeability are the cause of vasogenic edema in patients with malignant gliomas. Edema causes an increase in intracranial pressure and is one of the major factors contributing to the aggravation of neurologic symptoms in these patients. Corticosteroids are used to alleviate these symptoms. However, steroid use comes with an additional burden of toxicities, such as bone loss, hyperglycemia, hypertension, Cushing's syndrome, an increased risk of infection, steroid myopathy, and others. For patients with malignant gliomas, these toxicities present quality-of-life issues that are particularly important. The rapid normalization of vascular permeability by antiangiogenic drugs leads to reduced peritumoral edema and, eventually, to a reduced need for corticosteroid treatment in patients with malignant gliomas (Gerstner et al., 2009). The steroid-sparing action of anti-angiogenic drugs is an attractive approach to improving quality of life in these patients.

Activity Against the GSC Microvascular Niche

Glioma stem cells or GSCs are the self-renewing, multipotent cells that may contribute to the development of resistant phenotypes of tumors of the central nervous system. Studies have shown the presence of glioma cells that are similar to neural stem cells, called stem cell–like glioma cells (Bao et al., 2006). These multipotent tumor cells are CD133+, self-renewing, and relatively resistant to radiotherapy and chemotherapy. These cells are thought to thrive in the microvascular niche, and thus antiangiogenic drugs targeting endothelial cells may preferentially inhibit the growth or survival of GSCs. Bevacizumab (Bao et al., 2006) and VEGFR tyrosine kinase inhibitors (Fine, 2007) have been shown to have an effect against GSCs in animal models, and thus, one of the mechanisms of action of antiangiogenic drugs may be to inhibit these cells.

Bevacizumab

Bevacizumab is a humanized IgG1 monoclonal antibody with high affinity for the isoforms of VEGF-A. Its main mechanism of action is to sequester free VEGF, thus blocking the binding of VEGF to its receptors and thereby inhibiting angiogenesis. Bevacizumab is administered intravenously, typically at either 10 mg/kg every 2 weeks or 15 mg/kg every 3 weeks. The half-life of bevacizumab is approximately 21 days (range 11–50 days), and the predicted time to reach a steady-state concentration is about 100 days. When added to standard chemotherapy, bevacizumab showed significant clinical benefit, as measured by PFS at 6 months (PFS-6) and/or overall survival (OS) time, in patients with previously untreated or pretreated metastatic colorectal cancer (mCRC), advanced non–small cell lung cancer (NSCLC), and metastatic breast cancer (Chamberlain, 2010a). It has been approved as first- and second-line therapy for mCRC in combination with fluorouracil-based chemotherapy and as first-line therapy for unresectable, locally advanced, recurrent or metastatic non-squamous NSCLC in combination with carboplatin and paclitaxel.

The success of bevacizumab in the treatment of other solid tumors was a stimulus for the early trials of its use in patients with malignant gliomas. Although bevacizumab had undergone extensive clinical development, there was an initial reluctance to evaluate the drug in patients with tumors of the central nervous system, given the known risk of bevacizumab-induced

intratumoral hemorrhage. Indeed, some of the first observations demonstrating the risk of intratumoral hemorrhage with bevacizumab came from the discovery of underlying occult brain metastases in several patients with systemic tumors who presented with intracranial hemorrhage after treatment with bevacizumab (Chamberlain, 2010a).

Therapeutic Efficacy

The use of bevacizumab in patients with malignant gliomas has been extensively studied, with bevacizumab used both as a single agent and in combination with other chemotherapeutic agents, mostly irinotecan. Initial studies focused primarily on the use of bevacizumab in recurrent glioblastoma and anaplastic glioma, and many current studies are evaluating this agent in newly diagnosed glioblastoma. Historically, median survival is approximately 12–14 months for patients with glioblastoma and 2–3 years for patients with anaplastic astrocytoma. Patients with recurrent malignant gliomas respond to therapy less than 15% of the time and have median progression-free survival (PFS) times of 9 and 13 weeks for glioblastoma and anaplastic astrocytoma, respectively. A summary of the key clinical trial outcomes with bevacizumab-containing regimens in patients with recurrent glioblastoma and recurrent anaplastic glioma is shown in Table 29.1.

Combination Therapy for Recurrent Glioblastoma

In 2005, Stark-Vance conducted the first clinical study for the use of bevacizumab in combination with irinotecan for malignant glioma, after witnessing the favorable results of this regimen in metastatic colorectal cancer. Stark-Vance (Stark-Vance, 2005) treated 21 patients with recurrent glioblastoma with bevacizumab plus irinotecan and observed an overall response rate of 43%. These responses were evaluated using the Macdonald response criteria, which are based on changes in tumor enhancement as measured from T1-weighted post-gadolinium contrast scans (Macdonald et al., 1990). There were two treatment-related deaths, as a result of intracranial hemorrhage and intestinal perforation.

Reference	Tumor type (number of patients)	Drug regimen	Response rate (%)			Progression-free survival			Overall survival time (months)
			SD	PR	CR	Median (months)	6-Month rate (%)	12-Month rate (%)	
Recurrent GB (combination therapy)									
Stark-Vance (2005)	GB (11) Other HGG (10)	BV + irinotecan	52	38	5	NA	NA	NA	NA
Pope et al. (2006) (Pope et al., 2006)	GB (10) AG (4)	BV + etoposide or irinotecan	21	50	0	NA	NA	NA	NA
Vredenburgh et al. (2007b)	GB (23) AG (9)	BV + irinotecan	34	59	3	NA	GB: 38	NA	9.23
Vredenburgh et al. (2007a)	GB (35)	BV + irinotecan	24	57		5.5	46	20	9.7
Friedman et al. (2009)	GB (85) BV + irinotecan (82)	BV (85) BV + irinotecan (82)	NA	BV + irinotecan: 38		NA	BV + irinotecan:50.3	NA	BV + irinotecan:8.7
Norden et al. (2008)	GB (33)	BV + CT	NA	NA	NA	5.5	42	NA	8.2
Recurrent GB (single agent)									
Kreisl et al. (2009)	GB (48)	BV followed by BV + irinotecan	NA	35 (Macdonald criteria) 71 (Levin criteria)	NA	3.7	29	NA	7.2
Friedman et al. (2009)	GB (167)	BV (85) BV + irinotecan (82)	BV: 28	NA	NA	NA	BV: 42.6	NA	BV: 9.2
Chamberlain and Johnston (2010) (Chamberlain MC, 2010b)	GB (50)	BV	42	42		NA	42	22	8.5
Recurrent AG (combination therapy)									
Norden et al. (2008)	AG (21)	BV + CT	59	34		5.5	32	NA	8.2
Desjardins et al. (2008) (Desjardins A, 2008)	AG (33)	BV + irinotecan	33	52	9	8.1	55	39	15
Recurrent AG (single agent)									
Chamberlain and Johnston (2009b) (Chamberlain MC, 2009b)	AA (25)	BV	8	64	0	6.7	60	20	9
Chamberlain and Johnston (2009a) (Chamberlain MC, 2009a)	AO (22)	BV	5	68	0	6.75	68	23	8.5

Abbreviations: AA, anaplastic astrocytoma; AG, anaplastic glioma; AO, anaplastic oligodendroglioma; BV, bevacizumab; CR, complete response; CT, chemotherapy; GB, glioblastoma; HGG, high-grade glioma; NA, not available; PR, partial response; SD, stable disease

These exciting results led to the initiation of prospective clinical studies to test the bevacizumab-irinotecan combination in patients with recurrent malignant gliomas. Vredenburgh et al. (2007a) completed the first prospectively designed, single-institution, phase II trial of bevacizumab plus irinotecan for recurrent glioblastoma. In that study, 32 patients were treated with bevacizumab (10 mg/kg every 2 weeks) and 1 of 2 doses of irinotecan (340 mg/m^2 every 2 weeks for patients who received enzyme-inducing antiepileptic drugs [EIAEDs] and 125 mg/m^2 every 2 weeks for patients who did not receive EIAEDs). Vredenburgh et al. (2007b) observed an overall response rate of 63%; the response rate was 61% for patients with glioblastomas and 67% for patients with anaplastic gliomas, evaluated using the Macdonald criteria. The radiographic response rate and PFS-6 data might have been artificially elevated because the study included patients who had completed radiation therapy within 4 weeks of the study's initiation. The PFS-6 rate was 43% for patients with glioblastomas and 59% for patients with anaplastic gliomas (Vredenburgh et al., 2007a). These results compare favorably with data retrieved from the University of Texas M. D. Anderson Cancer Center database, which included 8 negative trials, with a PFS-6 rate of 15% for patients with glioblastomas and 31% for patients with anaplastic gliomas. The significant improvement in PFS rates for patients treated with bevacizumab compared to historical controls prompted additional studies using bevacizumab for the treatment of glioma. The toxicity of this regimen was brought to light when 28% of the patients were removed from the Vredenburgh et al. (2007b) trial because of potential drug-related adverse effects, 2 treatment-related deaths, and 4 venous and arterial thromboembolic events. Expanding their initial study, Vredenburgh et al. (2007b) treated 12 additional patients with an alternate bevacizumab schedule of 15 mg/kg every 3 weeks combined with irinotecan. They reported that the higher bevacizumab dose did not improve the PFS rate but that it carried significant toxicities (Vredenburgh et al., 2007b).

Norden et al. (2008) published the results of their single-institution experience using bevacizumab plus irinotecan. Their results mirrored those in other published reports (Macdonald et al., 1990; Stark-Vance, 2005) and further validated the potential of bevacizumab plus irinotecan in patients with recurrent malignant gliomas. Two key issues were highlighted in the study of Norden et al. (2008). First, patients who failed treatment with bevacizumab plus irinotecan were unlikely to have a radiographic response when the cytotoxic chemotherapy was changed to another cytotoxic agent while bevacizumab therapy was continued. In that study, in 23 patients for whom the cytotoxic drug was switched, the median time to radiographic progression was 7 weeks, and all but a few of those patients had unrelenting clinical deterioration and disease progression. Second, the authors demonstrated that patients who required anticoagulation for venous thrombotic events were safely anticoagulated without an elevated risk of hemorrhage (Norden et al., 2008).

Bevacizumab Monotherapy for Recurrent Glioblastoma

Two prospective randomized trials served as the basis for the subsequent FDA accelerated approval of bevacizumab for the treatment of recurrent glioblastoma. These studies highlighted an important distinction between gliomas and other solid tumors: namely, that in glioblastoma, bevacizumab appears to produce a clinical benefit even in the absence of concomitant chemotherapy, whereas in colorectal, lung, and breast cancers, bevacizumab appears to be effective only when combined with chemotherapy. This is not surprising given that the response rate of recurrent glioblastoma to irinotecan monotherapy is low (estimated to be <5%). This poor response rate and the suggestion that irinotecan increases toxicity led to two main studies designed to determine this agent's relative contribution to the overall effectiveness of bevacizumab-irinotecan combination therapy.

The first trial was the phase II BRAIN study (sponsored by Genentech), which further evaluated the use of bevacizumab alone for recurrent disease (Friedman et al., 2009). This multicenter, randomized, open-label, noncomparative study evaluated bevacizumab alone (10 mg/kg every 2 weeks) and bevacizumab plus irinotecan every 2 weeks (340 mg/m^2 for patients who received EIAEDs and 125 mg/m^2 for patients who did not receive EIAEDs) in patients with recurrent glioblastoma. The primary objective was to determine the efficacy of each regimen in improving PFS-6 rates compared with historical controls. Independent review of radiographic images demonstrated response rates of

28% for patients receiving bevacizumab alone versus 38% for patients receiving bevacizumab plus irinotecan. The PFS-6 rate was 43% for patients receiving bevacizumab alone and 50% for patients receiving bevacizumab plus irinotecan. The median OS time was 9.2 months for the bevacizumab-alone arm and 8.7 months for the combination arm. Neither of these median OS times was significantly different from published historical median OS time for patients receiving TMZ for recurrent glioblastoma (Lamborn et al., 2008). Thus, it is not clear that the short-term gain in PFS of bevacizumab containing therapy will translate into an improvement in OS time, although larger studies are needed to confirm these observations. However, most patients in the study by Friedman and colleagues reduced their steroid dose by 50% after starting bevacizumab (Friedman et al., 2009).

The second trial was the single-institution, phase II NCI 06-C-0064E study of 48 patients with recurrent glioblastoma treated with single-agent bevacizumab. In that study, 71 and 35% of the patients achieved radiographic response evaluated according to the Levin and Macdonald criteria, respectively (Kreisl et al., 2009). When radiographic criteria and stable or decreasing corticosteroid use were both used as measures of response, the objective response rate was 20%. The median duration of response was 3.9 months (Kreisl et al., 2009).

These two studies demonstrated an improved objective response rate relative to historical controls and led to the accelerated approval of bevacizumab monotherapy for progressive glioblastoma after prior up-front TMZ-based therapy. All these studies suggest that most of the radiographic response and clinical benefit may be attributable to bevacizumab and that eliminating irinotecan may improve the therapy's tolerability. The role of concurrent chemotherapy in combination with bevacizumab is unknown and is currently under investigation.

Bevacizumab for Recurrent Anaplastic Glioma

As discussed previously, VEGF blockade may delay or block the process of the angiogenic switch and hence the transformation of grade III brain tumors to a higher grade. Bevacizumab treatment in patients with recurrent anaplastic glioma has achieved favorable outcomes compared with historical controls; for those

treated with bevacizumab plus chemotherapy, response rates ranged from 34 to 68% and PFS-6 rates ranged from 32 to 68% (Chamberlain, 2010a).

Bevacizumab for Newly Diagnosed Glioblastoma

Favorable outcomes from using bevacizumab in the treatment of recurrent glioblastoma have led to studies examining the use of bevacizumab as first-line therapy for newly diagnosed glioblastoma. One phase II study has completed enrollment of patients for a trial of the combination of bevacizumab with the standard of care of radiotherapy plus TMZ for newly diagnosed glioblastoma. The observed toxicities of this regimen were acceptable and consistent with the typical on-target effects seen with antiangiogenic therapies. Preliminary analyses demonstrated that the efficacy of the regimen was encouraging (Lai et al., 2008). Although an apparent improvement was seen in the PFS endpoint, there was no significant difference between the overall survival rate for patients enrolled on the clinical trial and a historical control from the same institution with matching patient characteristics. Two large, ongoing phase III trials, RTOG 0825 (sponsored by the Radiation Therapy Oncology Group) and AVAGLIO (sponsored by Roche Pharmaceuticals), are currently evaluating the use of bevacizumab in patients with newly diagnosed glioblastoma.

Toxicity Profile

Overall, bevacizumab is well tolerated in patients with recurrent glioblastoma. The most common adverse effects with bevacizumab therapy are asthenia, pain, headache, diarrhea, dermatitis, impaired wound healing, low-grade bleeding (mostly epistaxis or other mucosal bleeding), hypertension, thromboembolic events, and proteinuria (Norden et al., 2008). Many of these toxicities are due to the inhibition of VEGF at sites other than the tumor. Although uncommon, higher grades of toxic effects, such as colon perforation, life-threatening central nervous system hemorrhages, and wound-healing complications, have also been reported (Chamberlain, 2010a; Norden et al., 2008). The toxicity associated with bevacizumab plus irinotecan was higher than that for bevacizumab alone in most studies (Friedman et al., 2009). A total of 66%

of the patients in the combination arm experienced toxicities of grade 3 or higher, compared with 46% of
the patients in the bevacizumab-alone arm. In addition,
43% of the patients in the combination arm experienced serious adverse events, compared with 26% in
the bevacizumab-alone arm. The toxicities of grade 3
or higher were mostly arterial and venous thrombotic
events and infection, although 2 central nervous system
hemorrhages and 1 gastrointestinal perforation were
observed in the combination arm. The therapy was
discontinued as a result of toxicities in 17.7% of the
patients in the combination arm, compared with 4.8%
of patients in the bevacizumab-alone arm (Friedman
et al., 2009). Clearly, the addition of irinotecan led
to more toxicity. Adverse effects such as bone marrow suppression, fatigue, and nausea were attributable
to the concurrently administered chemotherapy agent
irinotecan rather than to bevacizumab (Norden et al.,
2008). Indications for temporary suspension of bevacizumab therapy are moderate to severe proteinuria, uncontrolled hypertension, and the period within
4 weeks before any surgical procedure. Indications for
complete cessation of bevacizumab therapy are grade
3 or 4 intracranial hemorrhage, myocardial infarction,
bowel perforation, and wound dehiscence.

Biomarkers of Anti-Angiogenic Therapy

Given the prominent role that hypoxia plays in driving angiogenesis, invasion, and secretion of VEGF,
Sathornsumetee et al. (2008) evaluated the tissue
levels of VEGF and immunohistochemical markers
of hypoxia in patients with glioblastoma who were
treated with bevacizumab. These authors showed that
high tissue VEGF levels were correlated with radiographic response but not with OS time. They also
showed that tissue expression of the hypoxia marker
carbonic anhydrase IX (CA9) was associated with poor
outcome. Several ongoing studies are evaluating circulating biomarkers of response and of resistance to
antiangiogenic therapy.

Resistance to Anti-VEGF Therapy

Although bevacizumab has many benefits, the duration of benefit is not sustained in most patients.

Most preclinical and clinical data suggest that
antiangiogenic therapy delays or slows the rate of
progression of the tumor but that the tumor continues to progress after a short period of response.
Multiple mechanisms have been postulated to explain
the resistance of malignant gliomas to the antiangiogenic effects of bevacizumab treatment. Although
some tumors are intrinsically resistant, those tumors
that initially respond or are temporally stable eventually develop evasive (adaptive) resistance, an adaptation to overcome the effects of angiogenesis blockade (Casanovas et al., 2005). As discussed below,
there is experimental evidence for four main mechanisms of tumor adaptation to VEGF blockade: upregulation of non-VEGF-A pro-angiogenic molecular
signaling pathways; increasing infiltration of bone
marrow–derived pro-angiogenic cells; increasing vasculature integrity by increasing pericyte coverage,
hence obviating the need for VEGF-mediated survival signaling; and promoting invasion along existing vasculature (co-option), hence reducing a tumor's
dependence on neoangiogenesis for its survival
(see Fig. 29.1).

Upregulation of Non-VEGF-A Pro-angiogenic Molecular Signaling Pathways

VEGF is one of many mediators of angiogenesis in
tumors. Recent preclinical studies of glioma and of
pancreatic and other cancers have identified other pro-
angiogenic molecules that mediate blood vessel growth
as a replacement for VEGF (Casanovas et al., 2005;
Lucio-Eterovic et al., 2009). Antiangiogenic agents
lead to an initial response phase of decreased vascularity and tumor shrinkage (Fig. 29.1b). This transient
response phase is typically followed by restoration of
dense vascularization and tumor regrowth, likely indicating the establishment of VEGF-independent angiogenesis. Although multiple factors may be involved,
tumor cells subjected to acute hypoxia after loss of
perfusion lead to upregulation of genes responsible
for the production of other pro-angiogenic molecules
(Fig. 29.1c). Multiple factors may mediate this phenotype, including FGF1, FGF2, ephrin-A1, ephrin-
A2, angiopoietin 1 and others. In one study, patients
had higher levels of basic FGF or FGF2 (one of
the mediators of evasive resistance) at the time of
tumor recurrence than during the response phase

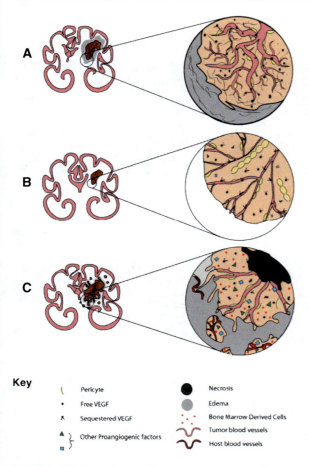

Key

Pericyte

Free VEGF

Sequestered VEGF

Other Proangiogenic factors

Necrosis

Edema

Bone Marrow Derived Cells

Tumor blood vessels

Host blood vessels

Fig. 29.1 Glioblastoma contain multiple cell types including tumor cells, pericytes, bone marrow derived cells and endothelial cells which are the main target of anti-VEGF therapy, as shown in (**a**). Following antiangiogenic therapy, there is a rapid reduction in cerebral edema (**b**). Potential mechanisms of resistance include increased pericyte coverage (**b**), the promotion of VEGF-independent angiogenesis via tumor and bone marrow cell angiogenic factor secretion and infiltration of tumor cells into normal brain via the process of vessel co-option (**c**)

Recruitment of Bone Marrow–Derived Pro-angiogenic Cells

Bone marrow–derived cells (BMDCs) such as endothelial cells and pericyte progenitors, tumor-associated macrophages, immature monocytic cells, and granulocytes can be attracted to sites of hypoxia, where they release pro-angiogenic factors. The vascular pruning by antiangiogenic therapy is thought to lead to intratumoral hypoxia and, hence, to increased expression of HIF-1α. Raised levels of HIF-1α induce an increase in levels of SDF-1α, which in turn recruits BMDCs to stimulate and maintain angiogenesis (Du et al., 2008). BMDCs such as endothelial cells and pericyte progenitors may contribute directly to neoangiogenesis, whereas vascular modulatory cells, predominantly CD45+ cells, may indirectly promote angiogenesis by secreting pro-angiogenic factors (Fig. 29.1c). Specific CD45+ vascular modulatory cells such as granulocytes are thought to express matrix metalloproteinase 9 (MMP9), which releases VEGF sequestered within the extracellular matrix, making it bioavailable to activate VEGFRs on endothelial cells (Bergers et al., 2000). MMP9 levels have been associated with tumor invasion and an increased risk of tumor progression. Thus, HIF-1α regulates VEGF activity in two ways: first, by increasing VEGF levels directly within the tumor and, second, by regulating mobilization of VEGF from the extracellular matrix by recruiting myeloid cells that release MMP9 at the tumor site (Du et al., 2008; Lucio-Eterovic et al., 2009). By carrying out the process of angiogenesis using upregulation of other pro-angiogenic pathways and increased recruitment of BMDCs, glioblastomas develop evasive resistance by finding a way to obviate the need for VEGF for angiogenesis.

(Batchelor et al., 2007). In a preclinical study by Lucio-Eterovic et al., bevacizumab-mediated blockade of VEGF in vitro was observed to lead to an increase in multiple pro-angiogenic factors, including FGF2 and angiogenin, which was one of the most-upregulated proteins after VEGF blockade (Lucio-Eterovic et al., 2009). An increase in contrast enhancement due to progressive angiogenesis associated with an increase in vascular permeability in a patient receiving continuous bevacizumab therapy is shown in Fig. 29.2a.

Increased Pericyte Coverage to Protect Tumor Blood Vessels

As discussed previously, tumor vasculature is nonuniform and aberrant. Pericytes, which are elongated, relatively undifferentiated peri-endothelial cells whose survival is promoted by platelet-derived growth factor (PDGF), are also an important part of the intratumoral vasculature. Some tumors are known to rely on pericytes to maintain a distinctively functional vascular

Fig. 29.2 Clinical examples of angiogenic progression (**a**) and diffuse and infiltrative non-enhancing tumor progression (**b**)

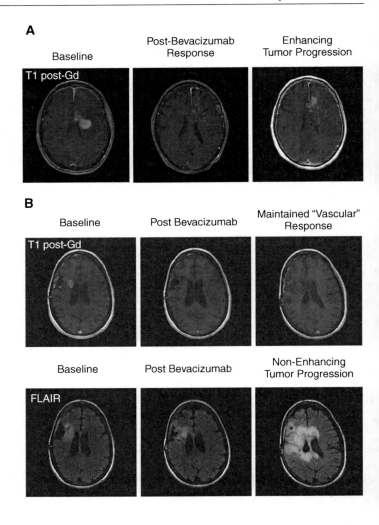

network tightly covered with pericytes during treatment with antiangiogenic agents (Bergers et al., 2003). These surviving tumor vessels are very different from the typical tortuous dilated vessels of the untreated tumor, which, by contrast, are less densely associated with pericyte coverage. The corollary to this statement is that endothelial cells can recruit pericytes to protect themselves from death after VEGF blockade. This observation is supported by studies showing that tumor vessels that lack adequate pericyte support are more vulnerable to VEGF inhibition (Benjamin et al., 1998; Bergers et al., 2003). So in treated tumors, blood vessels heavily surrounded by pericytes survive because pericytes can mediate endothelial-cell survival and quiescence (Fig. 29.1b). Recent studies aimed at an improved understanding of the importance

of pericytes in supporting tumor vasculature in a VEGF-A depletion state have targeted both pericytes and endothelial cells. These studies show an improved efficacy from the dual blockade of VEGFRs and PDGF receptors, which signal to endothelial cells and pericytes, respectively, as observed in animal models (Bergers et al., 2003). So, the concomitant use of a kinase inhibitor against PDGF receptors renders tumor endothelial cells more sensitive to VEGF inhibition.

Increased Tumor Capability for Invasion Without Angiogenesis

In 2000, Rubenstein et al. demonstrated that tumors may adapt to antiangiogenic therapy by increased invasiveness via co-option of host vessels. Using an anti-VEGFR antibody in a human glioblastoma xenograft model, they could slow bulk tumor growth using the VEGFR antibody, but, as a consequence, there was increased tumor infiltration and co-option of the host vasculature. This was associated with formation of multiple satellite tumors, many of which appeared beyond the margin of the primary tumor (Rubenstein et al., 2000). There is controversy about whether antiangiogenic therapy promotes tumor invasion itself or prolongs animal survival so that there is more time for tumors to invade. However, we recently demonstrated that noninvasive tumors in vivo can be forced to become invasive with prolonged suppression of VEGF using bevacizumab (Lucio-Eterovic et al., 2009). An example of a patient with non-enhancing tumor progression while on bevacizumab therapy is shown in Fig. 29.2b. There is an initial decrease in contrast enhancement which continues throughout the treatment duration. However, a progressive increase in FLAIR is seen and was coincident with the patient's clinical deterioration.

Similar to the animal models, observations were made in recent clinical studies to assess the patterns of glioblastoma recurrence during anti-VEGF therapy (Norden et al., 2008). It was noted that in some of the patients who had responded to bevacizumab therapy, the tumor progressed in an infiltrative and non-enhancing pattern. This appears to be a minority of patients since most patients have enhancing disease progression. This difference in progression pattern between responders and nonresponders suggests that the pro-infiltrative pattern may be directly related to the antiangiogenic effects of bevacizumab (Norden et al., 2008). By blocking neo-angiogenesis, bevacizumab creates changes in the tumor microenvironment. So we hypothesize that tumor infiltration may be induced by the hypoxia created by continuous antiangiogenic therapy, which may lead to activation of certain tissue factors and enzymes that promote infiltration. Because antiangiogenic therapy is known to reduce blood-vessel density to the point of inducing hypoxia, tumors treated with bevacizumab may develop a gradient of oxygen, glucose, and other growth factors between the primary tumor and distant brain endothelia, which are rich in these metabolites, and this gradient would promote a chemotactic response in the tumor cells (Rubenstein et al., 2000). Thus, tumor cells may migrate to more hospitable

areas of the brain, inducing a more "infiltrative" progression of the tumor. Unlike untreated malignant glioma cells, which appear to predominantly invade the brain parenchyma by infiltrating directly into neuropil and migrating along myelin fiber tracts, after treatment with antiangiogenic drugs, glioblastoma cells may be more likely to infiltrate as a multicellular sheet along the sides of existing blood vessels to distant parts of the brain parenchyma (Bergers and Hanahan, 2008).

Intrinsic Resistance to Antiangiogenic Therapy

Intrinsic resistance to antiangiogenic agents refers to the absence of any partial or complete radiographic response to treatment. Thus, a tumor is intrinsically resistant to antiangiogenic agents when tumor progression continues unabated in the face of antiangiogenic therapy. Intrinsic resistance of tumors to antiangiogenic drugs is a very intriguing concept, and there are many thoughts on why certain tumor types are indifferent to these agents. This type of resistance could be based on the fact that some tumors activate one of the aforementioned methods of evasive resistance to antiangiogenic agents even before the therapy is started, in response to selective pressures of the tumor microenvironment during malignant progression, for example, the presence of multiple pro-angiogenic signals other than VEGF. Other possible explanations may be related to the presence of high levels of inflammatory cells mediating vascular protection, such as CD11b+/Gr1+ myeloid cells, or to innate hypovascularity of the tumor, resulting in a lower dependence on angiogenesis for survival (Bergers and Hanahan, 2008).

Future Directions

Because of obvious improvement in PFS-6 in patients with malignant gliomas when bevacizumab is used, it has become an attractive agent for the treatment of these tumors. However, areas of uncertainty remain that require further study before we will know how to optimize anti-VEGF therapy.

Dosing and Administration

More studies need to be performed to provide guidance on the optimal dosing and administration schedule of bevacizumab to attain maximum efficacy and minimum toxicity. Ideally, the optimal dose that binds excess circulating VEGF molecules without adding any excess toxicity can be determined. Measuring levels of free VEGF molecules (unbound to bevacizumab) at different doses of the drug can tell us the lowest effective dose required for maximum sequestration of VEGF. Knowing the lowest effective dose of bevacizumab is also important for treatment combinations with other drugs, to maximize drug delivery and minimize the toxicities associated with the inhibition of multiple molecular targets. Given that the biologic half-life of bevacizumab is approximately 3 weeks, a less-frequent dosing schedule may be possible without compromising therapeutic efficacy (de Groot and Yung, 2008).

Response Criteria and Primary Endpoints

The assessment of response to antiangiogenic therapies is closely associated with the therapies' effects on vascular permeability. Currently, the Macdonald criteria are the most popular for assessing tumor response in patients with malignant gliomas. As mentioned previously, this approach uses standard MRI to measure changes in tumor size based on T1-weighted post-gadolinium images. Bevacizumab and other antiangiogenic agents normalize tumor vasculature and significantly reduce vascular permeability, thereby reducing vascular leakiness. As a direct result of this effect, there is reduced gadolinium enhancement, which is consistent with the Macdonal criteria (popular) definition of response.

PFS-6 has been the primary endpoint for most studies evaluating the use of bevacizumab in patients with glioblastoma. It is notable that even with evidence of tumor response on imaging studies and a considerable improvement in PFS, there has not been a significant change in the OS time of patients treated with bevacizumab. A reduction in contrast enhancement of the tumor has been noted in several studies within 24 h after a single dose of antiangiogenic drug treatment.

The paradox of a rapid response not translating into an improved OS time may be explained by the fact that a "vascular response" (or a decrease in contrast enhancement) may be independent of a true anti-tumor effect of these therapies.

To overcome these disparities, new response criteria and endpoints are being developed. Several ongoing and planned trials at various centers are studying the effect of bevacizumab on recurrent and newly diagnosed malignant gliomas, focusing on both PFS and OS endpoints. Recently, the Response Assessment in Neuro-Oncology (RANO) criteria (Wen et al., 2010) were developed to address some of the ongoing challenges facing neuro-oncologists who are evaluating new therapies for patients with malignant gliomas. The new criteria improve on the definitions of measurable disease, nonmeasurable lesions, multiple lesions, tumor response, disease progression, and other outcomes with less emphasis on contrast-enhanced imaging alone. In addition, advanced imaging techniques such as MR perfusion, diffusion-weighted imaging, and MR spectroscopy are being studied and evaluated as potential biomarkers of long-term tumor response.

Duration of Therapy

Like cediranib (AZD2171) and other antiangiogenic agents, bevacizumab may rapidly induce vascular normalization, leading to improved blood flow and oxygenation shortly after initiation of therapy (Batchelor et al., 2007; Jain, 2001). However, long-term anti-VEGF therapy may have the opposite effect. As discussed previously, hypoxia after VEGF blockade may cause other pro-angiogenic molecules to be upregulated. This adaptation causes restoration of the dense, tortuous, leaky tumor vasculature, which may then restrict drug delivery. Prolonged and continuous antiangiogenic therapy may lead to the opposite of the desired effect on tumor vasculature and drug delivery.

Treating the Non-enhancing, Infiltrative Glioma Phenotype

Finally, the long-term use of bevacizumab can lead to non-enhancing tumor infiltration via vessel co-option, which can occur in up to 25% of patients who initially have a radiographic response. This infiltrative pattern can spread throughout the brain, reaching a state similar to the disease extent seen with gliomatosis cerebri. This tumor phenotype is exceptionally difficult to treat, and at present no effective therapeutic strategies exist to rescue patients with this resistant phenotype. An in-depth understanding of the molecular mechanisms that promote this type of invasion is needed to help guide the development of new agents to prolong OS time in patients with malignant gliomas treated with antiangiogenic agents.

References

Bao S, Wu Q, Sathornsumetee S, Hao Y, Li Z, Hjelmeland AB, Shi Q, McLendon RE, Bigner DD, Rich JN (2006) Stem cell-like glioma cells promote tumor angiogenesis through vascular endothelial growth factor. Cancer Res 66: 7843–7848

Batchelor TT, Sorensen AG, di Tomaso E, Zhang WT, Duda DG, Cohen KS, Kozak KR, Cahill DP, Chen PJ, Zhu M, Ancukiewicz M, Mrugala MM, Plotkin S, Drappatz J, Louis DN, Ivy P, Scadden DT, Benner T, Loeffler JS, Wen PY, Jain RK (2007) AZD2171, a pan-VEGF receptor tyrosine kinase inhibitor, normalizes tumor vasculature and alleviates edema in glioblastoma patients. Cancer Cell 11: 83–95

Benjamin LE, Hemo I, Keshet. E (1998) A plasticity window for blood vessel remodelling is defined by pericyte coverage of the preformed endothelial network and is regulated by PDGF-B and VEGF. Development 125:1591–1598

Bergers G, Brekken R, McMahon G, Vu TH, Itoh T, Tamaki K, Tanzawa K, Thorpe P, Itohara S, Werb Z, Hanahan. D (2000) Matrix metalloproteinase-9 triggers the angiogenic switch during carcinogenesis. Nat Cell Biol 2: 737–744

Bergers G, Hanahan. D (2008) Modes of resistance to antiangiogenic therapy. Nat Rev Cancer 8:592–603

Bergers G, Song S, Meyer-Morse N, Bergsland E, Hanahan D (2003) Benefits of targeting both pericytes and endothelial cells in the tumor vasculature with kinase inhibitors. J Clin Invest 111:1287–1295

Casanovas O, Hicklin DJ, Bergers G, Hanahan. D (2005) Drug resistance by evasion of antiangiogenic targeting of VEGF signaling in late-stage pancreatic islet tumors. Cancer Cell 8:299–309

Chamberlain MC JS (2009a) Bevacizumab for recurrent alkylator-refractory anaplastic oligodendroglioma. Cancer 15:1734–1743

Chamberlain MC JS (2009b) Salvage chemotherapy with bevacizumab for recurrent alkylator-refractory anaplastic astrocytoma.. J Neurooncol 91:359–367

Chamberlain MC (2010a) 10 Questions about the use of bevacizumab in the management of recurrent malignant gliomas. Neurologist 16:56–60

Chamberlain MC JS (2010b) Salvage therapy with single agent bevacizumab for recurrent glioblastoma. J. Neurooncol 96:259–269

Cohen MH, Shen YL, Keegan P, Pazdur. R (2009) FDA drug approval summary: bevacizumab (avastin) as treatment of recurrent glioblastoma multiforme. Oncologist 14: 1131–1138

de Groot JF, Yung WK (2008) Bevacizumab and irinotecan in the treatment of recurrent malignant gliomas. Cancer J 14:279–285

Desjardins A, RD, Herndon JE 2nd, Marcello J, Quinn JA, Rich JN, Sathornsumetee S, Gururangan S, Sampson J, Bailey L, Bigner DD, Friedman AH, Friedman HS, Vredenburgh JJ (2008) Bevacizumab plus irinotecan followed by bevacizumab plus irinotecan at tumor progressionin recurrent glioblastoma. Clin Cancer Res 14:7068–7073

Du R, Lu KV, Petritsch C, Liu P, Ganss R, Passegue E, Song H, Vandenberg S, Johnson RS, Werb Z, Bergers G (2008) HIF1alpha induces the recruitment of bone marrow-derived vascular modulatory cells to regulate tumor angiogenesis and invasion. Cancer Cell 13:206–220

Dvorak HF, Brown LF, Detmar M, Dvorak AM (1995) Vascular permeability factor/vascular endothelial growth factor, microvascular hyperpermeability, and angiogenesis. Am J Pathol 146:1029–1039

Fine HA (2007) Promising new therapies for malignant gliomas. Cancer J 13:349–354

Friedman HS, Prados MD, Wen PY, Mikkelsen T, Schiff D, Abrey LE, Yung WK, Paleologos N, Nicholas MK, Jensen R, Vredenburgh J, Huang J, Zheng M, Cloughesy T (2009) Bevacizumab alone and in combination with irinotecan in recurrent glioblastoma. J Clin Oncol 27:4733–4740

Gerstner ER, Duda DG, di Tomaso E, Ryg PA, Loeffler JS, Sorensen AG, Ivy P, Jain, RK, Batchelor TT (2009) VEGF inhibitors in the treatment of cerebral edema in patients with brain cancer. Nat Rev Clin Oncol 6:229–236

Hanahan D, Folkman. J (1996) Patterns and emerging mechanisms of the angiogenic switch during tumorigenesis. Cell 86:353–364

Jain RK (2001) Normalizing tumor vasculature with antiangiogenic therapy: a new paradigm for combination therapy. Nat Med 7:987–989

Kreisl TN, Kim L, Moore K, Duic P, Royce C, Stroud I, Garren N, Mackey M, Butman JA, Camphausen K, Park J, Albert PS, Fine. HA (2009) Phase II trial of single-agent bevacizumab followed by bevacizumab plus irinotecan at tumor progression in recurrent glioblastoma. J Clin Oncol 27:740–745

Lai A, Filka E, McGibbon B, Nghiemphu PL, Graham C, Yong WH, Mischel P, Liau LM, Bergsneider M, Pope W, Selch M, Cloughesy. T (2008) Phase II pilot study of bevacizumab in combination with temozolomide and regional radiation therapy for up-front treatment of patients with newly diagnosed glioblastoma multiforme: interim analysis of safety and tolerability. Int J Radiat Oncol Biol Phys 71:1372–1380

Lamborn KR, Yung WK, Chang SM, Wen PY, Cloughesy TF, DeAngelis LM, Robins HI, Lieberman FS, Fine HA, Fink KL, Junck L, Abrey L, Gilbert MR, Mehta M, Kuhn JG, Aldape KD, Hibberts J, Peterson PM, Prados MD (2008)

Progression-free survival: an important end point in evaluating therapy for recurrent high-grade gliomas.. Neurooncol 10:162–170

Lucio-Eterovic AK, Piao Y, de Groot. JF (2009) Mediators of glioblastoma resistance and invasion during antivascular endothelial growth factor therapy. Clin Cancer Res 15: 4589–4599

Macdonald DR, Cascino TL, Schold SC Jr., Cairncross. JG (1990) Response criteria for phase II studies of supratentorial malignant glioma. J Clin Oncol 8:1277–1280

Norden AD, Young GS, Setayesh K, Muzikansky A, Klufas R, Ross GL, Ciampa AS, Ebbeling LG, Levy B, Drappatz J, Kesari S, Wen PY (2008) Bevacizumab for recurrent malignant gliomas: efficacy, toxicity, and patterns of recurrence. Neurology 70:779–787

Pope WB, Lai A, Nghiemphu P, Mischel P, Cloughesy TF (2006) MRI in patients with high-grade gliomas treated with bevacizumab and chemotherapy. Neurology 66:1258–1260

Rubenstein JL, Kim J, Ozawa T, Zhang M, Westphal M, Deen DF, Shuman MA (2000) Anti-VEGF antibody treatment of glioblastoma prolongs survival but results in increased vascular cooption. Neoplasia 2:306–314

Sathornsumetee S, Cao Y, Marcello JE, Herndon JE 2nd, McLendon RE, Desjardins A, Friedman HS, Dewhirst MW, Vredenburgh JJ, Rich JN (2008) Tumor angiogenic and hypoxic profiles predict radiographic response and survival in malignant astrocytoma patients treated with bevacizumab and irinotecan. J Clin Oncol 26:271–278

Shweiki D, Itin A, Soffer D, Keshet E (1992) Vascular endothelial growth factor induced by hypoxia May mediate hypoxia-initiated angiogenesis. Nature 359:843–845

Stark-Vance V (2005) Bevacizumab and CPT-11 in the treatment of relapsed malignant glioma.. In: World federation of neuro-oncology. Edinburgh, UK

Stupp R, Mason WP, van den Bent MJ, Weller M, Fisher B, Taphoorn MJ, Belanger K, Brandes AA, Marosi C, Bogdahn U, Curschmann J, Janzer RC, Ludwin SK, Gorlia T, Allgeier A, Lacombe D, Cairncross JG, Eisenhauer E, Mirimanoff RO (2005) Radiotherapy plus concomitant and adjuvant temozolomide for glioblastoma. N Engl J Med 352: 987–996

Vredenburgh JJ, Desjardins A, Herndon JE 2nd, Dowell JM, Reardon DA, Quinn JA, Rich JN, Sathornsumetee S, Gururangan S, Wagner M, Bigner DD, Friedman AH, Friedman HS (2007a) Phase II trial of bevacizumab and irinotecan in recurrent malignant glioma. Clin Cancer Res 13:1253–1259

Vredenburgh JJ, Desjardins A, Herndon JE 2nd, Marcello J, Reardon DA, Quinn JA, Rich JN, Sathornsumetee S, Gururangan S, Sampson J, Wagner M, Bailey L, Bigner DD, Friedman AH, Friedman HS (2007b) Bevacizumab plus irinotecan in recurrent glioblastoma multiforme. J Clin Oncol 25:4722–4729

Wen PY, Macdonald DR, Reardon DA, Cloughesy TF, Sorensen AG, Galanis E, Degroot J, Wick W, Gilbert MR, Lassman AB, Tsien C, Mikkelsen T, Wong ET, Chamberlain MC, Stupp R, Lamborn KR, Vogelbaum MA, van den Bent MJ, Chang SM (2010) Updated response assessment criteria for high-grade gliomas: response assessment in neuro-oncology working group. J Clin Oncol 28:1963–1972

Zhou Q, Gallo JM (2009) Differential effect of sunitinib on the distribution of temozolomide in an orthotopic glioma model. Neurooncol 11:301–310

Zhou YH, Tan F, Hess KR, Yung WK (2003) The expression of PAX6, PTEN, vascular endothelial growth factor, and epidermal growth factor receptor in gliomas: relationship to tumor grade and survival. Clin Cancer Res 9: 3369–3375

Chapter 30

Aggravating Endoplasmic Reticulum Stress by Combined Application of Bortezomib and Celecoxib as a Novel Therapeutic Strategy for Glioblastoma

Axel H. Schönthal

Abstract The endoplasmic reticulum (ER) stress response constitutes an adaptive mechanism that sustains cellular survival under adverse microenvironmental and other stress conditions, and thereby also supports chemoresistance of tumor cells. Due to their enhanced proliferation rate in combination with oftentimes limited blood supply, tumor cells frequently experience long-lasting, chronic ER stress conditions that set them apart from normal cells, and this differential may provide opportunities for pharmacologic intervention. The proteasome inhibitor bortezomib and the selective cyclooxygenase-2 (COX-2) inhibitor celecoxib have been shown to aggravate pre-existing ER stress in glioblastoma cells, and when combined exert synergistic tumoricidal effects in vivo. Thus, this particular drug combination may hold promise as a novel therapeutic strategy for glioblastoma.

Keywords Autophagy · CHOP · 2,5-dimethyl-celecoxib · GRP78 · Misfolded proteins · SERCA

Introduction

Similar to other tumor types, glioblastoma cells have undergone selective pressure and in the process have activated various molecular mechanisms that support

their proliferation and survival within a rather hostile microenvironment of hypoxia, low glucose conditions, acidity, and other adverse impacts. One of their defensive strategies is manifested through the chronic activation of the endoplasmic reticulum (ER) stress (ERS) response, also called the unfolded protein response (UPR). Low-level, chronic activation of the ERS response in glioblastoma cells represents an adaptive mechanism that not only supports tumor cell survival, but also enhances the chemoresistance of these cells. At the same time, however, the presence of chronic ERS sets tumor cells apart from normal cells and, therefore, provides a differential target, perhaps an Achilles' heel, that can be exploited for improved tumor therapy. This chapter will introduce the "yin-yang" principle of the ERS response, followed by a presentation of novel concepts that seek to exploit these processes pharmacologically in order to achieve improved therapeutic outcomes for glioblastoma patients.

The Endoplasmic Reticulum Stress Response

The ERS response is a cellular mechanism that is activated in response to various stressful stimuli, such as hypoxia, low glucose levels, misfolded proteins, disturbed calcium homeostasis, and others (Fig. 30.1). On the one hand, ERS can trigger defensive molecular mechanisms that adapt the cell to the stressful condition and consequently support increased cellular survival, but on the other hand it can initiate processes that lead to cell death. This opposing outcome is primarily determined by the intensity and duration of the ERS

A.H. Schönthal (✉)
Keck School of Medicine, University of Southern California, Los Angeles, CA 90033, USA
e-mail: schonthal@usc.edu

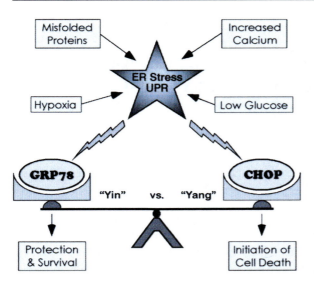

Fig. 30.1 Simplified depiction of the yin-yang balance of ER stress. ER stress (ERS) can be triggered by various unfavorable conditions, such as the accumulation of misfolded proteins, changes in the calcium balance between the ER and the cytosol, low levels of glucose, hypoxia, and others. The ERS response is also called the unfolded protein response (UPR), as some of the above stressors can impinge on proper protein folding. The mechanism of ERS/UPR involves the increased expression of GRP78 and CHOP, and—depending on the severity of the initial insult—one of these two master executors will gain dominance and decisively determine the resulting consequences, i.e., protection from stress or initiation of cell death. See text for further details

response and the respective molecular components that are involved. In this sense, this system follows a "yin-yang" principle, by which its low to moderate activity is cell protective and supports chemoresistance ("yin"), but where severe stress conditions will aggravate these processes to the point where they abandon their protective efforts and instead trigger cell death ("yang") (Boyce and Yuan, 2006; Marciniak and Ron, 2006).

The events of both modes, the defensive "yin" and the proapoptotic "yang", are executed through a series of orchestrated events that involve several molecular pathways and a number of individual proteins, whose expression and activities determine the respective outcome. Several recent review articles have provided comprehensive coverage of these complex mechanisms and the interested reader is referred to these reports for further details (Boyce and Yuan, 2006; Marciniak and Ron, 2006). For purposes of the therapeutic considerations presented here, the "yin-yang" principle of the ERS response can be reduced to the function of two of its critical executor proteins,

GRP78 and CHOP. Although many more components participate, these two proteins play decisive roles in properly executing the functions of the ERS response, and their activities form the basis of the respective "yin" or "yang" consequences (Fig. 30.1). Therefore, during the remainder of this discourse, the complex mechanisms of the ERS response will be simplified by primarily focusing on the involvement of GRP78 and CHOP as the major executors of this system.

GRP78 and Chop as Master Executors of the Endoplasmic Reticulum Stress Response

GRP78 (glucose regulated protein of molecular mass 78 kDa), also called BiP (immunoglobulin heavy chain binding protein), is a resident protein of the ER of all eukaryotic cells and belongs to the highly conserved heat shock protein (HSP) family (Li and Lee, 2006). It functions as a chaperone that is involved in polypeptide translocation, protein folding, and targeting of misfolded proteins for degradation. In addition, it has calcium-binding properties and controls the activation of three transmembrane ERS sensors involved in the control of translational and transcriptional regulation. For details on these three sensors (activating transcription factor-6, ATF6; inositol-requiring enzyme-1, IRE1; PKR-like ER kinase, PERK) and their associated functions, see (Boyce and Yuan, 2006).

In general, GRP78 expression is relatively low in normal, healthy cells, but its abundance will be greatly increased in response to various stressful challenges, such as hypoxia, low glucose levels, imbalance of intracellular calcium levels, or the accumulation of misfolded proteins. Increased expression of GRP78 is a generally accepted marker of ERS and UPR, and represents the adaptive effort of the stressed cell to neutralize potentially damaging consequences of the stressful insult and to reestablish homeostasis and proper cell functioning (Li and Lee, 2006). In this context, GRP78 can be viewed as the master executor of the protective "yin" module of the ERS response. In normal cells, the increased expression of GRP78 is generally transient, because reestablishing homeostasis terminates the cell's need for elevated amounts of GRP78 (Fig. 30.2).

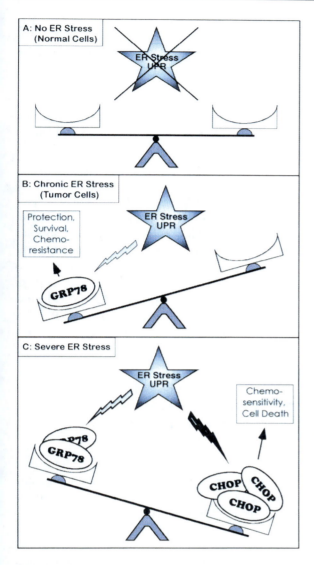

Fig. 30.2 Differential ER stress levels under different cellular conditions. There are three activity levels of the ER stress response system. (**a**) The "No ER Stress" condition is the default situation in normal cells. (**b**) In cancer cells, continuous, low-intensity stress generates the "Chronic ER Stress" condition, indicated by elevated levels of GRP78, which, among its various functions, suppresses pro-apoptotic components and thereby supports cellular survival and chemo-resistance. (**c**) Persistent, high level stress generates the "Severe ER Stress" situation, where pro-apoptotic components (such as CHOP) dominate and trigger cell death. The protective effort of GRP78 is overwhelmed, which contributes to the chemo-sensitization of tumor cells. Note that thickness of bolts corresponds to the intensity of stimulated expression of GRP78 and CHOP

Tumor cells frequently encounter stressful challenges, which are exacerbated by these cells' specific metabolic demands and permanent physiological changes, such as the Warburg effect, acidification

of the microenvironment, and expression of tumor-specific splice isoforms of pyruvate kinase (which is maintained even in cell culture, where growth conditions are usually plentiful) (Chen et al., 2007; Christofk et al., 2008). Not surprisingly, elevated levels of GRP78 can be frequently found in tumor tissues and in most cancer cell lines, and are viewed as an indicator of continuous, low level ERS (Li and Lee, 2006). Unlike the situation in most normal cells, increased levels of GRP78 in tumor cells remain elevated and are an expression of the chronic ERS situation of these cells (Fig. 30.2). As a consequence of this permanent increase, GRP78 not only serves to restore and protect certain basic cellular functions, but also, due to its anti-apoptotic properties, promotes tumor cell proliferation, survival, metastasis, and resistance to a wide variety of therapies. In this context, GRP78 expression may serve as a biomarker for tumor behavior and treatment response, and high levels of this protein have been associated with poor prognosis (Lee, 2007).

The prosurvival ("yin") function of GRP78 does not have unlimited capacity. If the stressful situation becomes too severe, the ERS response switches to its proapoptotic ("yang") function, which will overwhelm the protective effort of GRP78 and will initiate cell death. One of the decisive effectors of this switch is CHOP (CCAAT/enhancer binding protein homologous transcription factor), also called GADD153 (growth arrest and DNA damage-inducible gene 153), a proapoptotic transcription factor (Oyadomari and Mori, 2004). Normal, unstressed cells do not express appreciable amounts of this ERS-inducible protein, primarily because of the absence of the required stimuli. Tumor cells also do not express CHOP, despite the presence of chronic ERS because the dominant antiapoptotic function of GRP78 keeps CHOP transcription inactive (Suzuki et al., 2007). In response to acutely increased ER stress, however, both normal and tumor cells stimulate CHOP expression, and the duration and amount of elevated CHOP levels are a decisive factor in determining the cell's fate (Rutkowski et al., 2006). In case the protective "yin" components are able to regain control and subdue CHOP expression, the cell will survive. However, if severe ER stress persists, the proapoptotic "yang" module will attain dominance and will initiate cell death. Because of their relatively short-lived struggle for control, CHOP expression levels can be used as a convenient readout to reveal the acute phase of ER stress (Oyadomari and Mori, 2004; Rutkowski et al., 2006).

Chronic Endoplasmic Reticulum Stress as an Achilles' Heel of Cancer Cells

In its entirety, the ERS response musters substantial protective efforts in order to support cellular survival, yet also ensures controlled destruction of the cell when too much cellular damage threatens the organism as a whole. In the case of cancer cells, chronic ERS has shifted this balance towards increased survival and, as a direct consequence, provides for increased resistance against many commonly used chemotherapeutic agents. On the other hand, continuous engagement of the defensive module of this system distinguishes cancer cells from normal cells, and may provide an Achilles' heel that can be exploited by pharmacologic intervention aimed at the ERS response (Schönthal, 2008).

It is surmised that preexisting ERS in tumor cells restricts these cells' capacity to accommodate much additional ERS, whereas, normal cells harbor greater reserves to neutralize stressful insults targeted at the ER. Thus, pharmacologic intervention aimed at the ERS response would have to be relatively mild and controlled; as a result normal cells would remain able to tolerate and neutralize moderately increased ERS. However, at the same time aggravation of the preexisting ERS condition in tumor cells would suffice to force these cells into apoptosis. In essence, the tumor-specific therapeutic exploitation of the ERS response would entail the targeted aggravation of the preexisting ERS condition in tumor cells, i.e., a shift from "low/chronic ERS" (Fig. 30.2b) to "severe ERS" conditions (Fig. 30.2c), which would establish dominance of the proapoptotic "yang" module (in particular, CHOP) and resultant cell death. At the same time, normal cells would initiate their ERS response from its inactive state (Fig. 30.2a), and therefore enjoy more leeway to unfold the protective "yin" components. To achieve this differential outcome, the increase in ERS would have to be carefully modulated, rather than simply maximally exacerbated, because the latter condition would also be expected to damage normal cells, and therefore would likely generate serious unwanted side-effects during therapy.

Pharmacologic agents that maximally exacerbate ERS are known to be rather toxic, and therefore not suited for systemic delivery to cancer patients. For example, the naturally occurring sesquiterpene lactone thapsigargin is an exceptionally potent inducer of ERS, but at the same time is also very toxic to normal tissues (Treiman et al., 1998). Despite these drawbacks, direct delivery to the tumor tissue or the use of a tumor-activated prodrug could solve some of these problems. Such avenues of drug development are currently being pursued in the case of thapsigargin in order to harness its severe exacerbation of ERS for purposes of cancer therapy (Janssen et al., 2006).

In contrast to compounds that severely exacerbate ERS and whose pharmacologic activity needs to be strictly restricted to the tumor tissue, milder aggravators of ERS that are able to modulate this system in a controlled fashion might be better suitable for systemic delivery and fine-tuned applications, concomitant with reduced toxicity to normal tissues. Two such pharmacologic agents that appear to satisfy these requirements are bortezomib and celecoxib, and a few preclinical studies indicate that combined application of these compounds might be able to exploit ERS in a therapeutically beneficial fashion.

Bortezomib as an Aggravator of Endoplasmic Reticulum Stress

Bortezomib (PS-341; Velcade) is a proteasome inhibitor that has been clinically approved for treating multiple myeloma and mantle cell lymphoma (Adams and Kauffman, 2004). As shown in Fig. 30.3, blockage of proteasome function generates a backlog and accumulation of misfolded and other proteins destined for elimination by the ER associated degradation pathway (ERAD), and this represents a well-established signal for ERS (Fribley et al., 2004). Importantly, the retrograde jam of ERAD may increase the formation of aggresomes and may stimulate autophagic activity as a clearance alternative, thereby reducing the antitumor efficacy of bortezomib (Nawrocki et al., 2006). Therefore, blockage of aggresome formation with inhibitors of histone deacetylase-6 (HDAC6) (Kawaguchi et al., 2003), or inhibition of autophagy with the traditional antimalarial drug chloroquine (Carew et al., 2007) will close this outlet and further aggravate proapoptotic ERS (Fig. 30.3).

Several recently published studies are in agreement with the above model. For example, the antitumor cytotoxicity of bortezomib can be potentiated

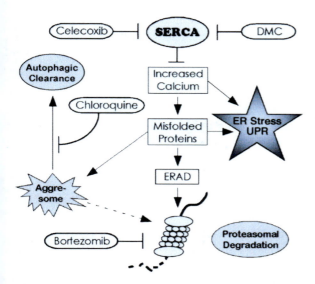

Fig. 30.3 Pharmacologic aggravation of ER stress. Celecoxib and its non-coxib analog 2,5-dimethyl-celecoxib (DMC) inhibit the function of SERCA (sarcoplasmic/ER calcium ATPase), resulting in the leakage of calcium from its ER storage space into the cytosol and acting as a potent trigger for ERS. Accumulating misfolded proteins are being disposed of via ER-associated degradation (ERAD) involving the proteasome, or via inclusion in aggresomes and removal through autophagy. Bortezomib inhibits the proteasome, causing a backlog of ERAD and thereby preventing relief from ER stress. Similarly, the autophagy inhibitor chloroquine prevents the elimination of aggresomes, thereby blocking another outlet for ER stress-triggering misfolded proteins. As a result, all these pharmacologic agents aggravate ER stress and are particularly effective when used in combination

when it is applied in combination with HDAC6 inhibitors (Hideshima et al., 2005; Nawrocki et al., 2006). Similarly, chloroquine, which has been shown to augment the chemosensitivity of tumor cells in vitro (Amaravadi et al., 2007; Carew et al., 2007), has yielded promising results in clinical trials with glioblastoma patients, where it displayed chemosensitizing effects when used as an adjuvant to the standard glioblastoma chemotherapeutic agent temozolomide (Briceno et al., 2007). Chemosensitization of glioblastoma cells towards temozolomide has also been achieved via the blockage of the major protective "yin" component of the ERS response, GRP78, with siRNA, further pointing to the critical relevance of these processes for cancer chemotherapy (Pyrko et al., 2007).

Presently, bortezomib has not received much attention with regard to its potential use in glioblastoma therapy, and this hesitation is primarily

grounded in the observation that this agent penetrates the blood brain barrier (BBB) very poorly (Hemeryck et al., 2007). However, in view of the available options to circumvent the BBB (which might be compromised due to extensive tumor expansion and "leaky" angiogenesis), the BBB as an obstacle might be manageable or indeed irrelevant in the case of intratumoral drug delivery, as can be accomplished, for example, via the Alzet mini-osmotic pump (Bittner et al., 2000).

Celecoxib as an Aggravator of Endoplasmic Reticulum Stress

Celecoxib (Celebrex) was developed as a selective inhibitor of cyclooxygenase 2 (COX-2) (Penning et al., 1997). However, over the years, it has become clear that this drug exerts additional pharmacologic activities, among them the ability to trigger ERS. The inhibition of COX-2 appears to play a prominent role in this drug's reported ability for the chemoprevention of colon carcinoma (Koki and Masferrer, 2002). However, the role of COX-2 inhibition has remained unclear in the case of celecoxib's potential therapeutic impact on advanced cancers, which instead may involve one or more of the drug's COX-2 independent activities (Grösch et al., 2006; Schönthal, 2007).

The search for COX-2 independent targets of celecoxib has yielded many candidates, although some of them may represent indirect consequences of other, further upstream events that are caused by this drug. For example, potent down-regulation of the essential cell cycle regulatory protein cyclin D in response to treatment of tumor cells with celecoxib has been explained by the drug's aggravation of ERS (Pyrko et al., 2008), where a major component of the ERS response is the transient inhibition of general protein synthesis. As a consequence, short-lived proteins, such as cyclin D, disappear from the cell's inventory. Several other intracellular targets of celecoxib have been identified, although in many cases it has remained unclear whether they represent direct or indirect responders and whether or not they are closely involved in mediating the drug's antitumor effects. However, in the case of ERS, accumulating evidence suggests that this cellular process might represent the critical effector of celecoxib's antitumor potency in advanced types of cancer cells (Schönthal et al., 2008).

The primary target of celecoxib that connects this drug to the aggravation of ERS is the sarcoplasmic/ER calcium ATPase (SERCA), an ER transmembrane protein that functions to pump calcium ions from the cytosol into the ER and thereby establishes the steep calcium gradient between these two cellular compartments. Inhibition of SERCA severely distorts calcium homeostasis and represents a well-known and efficient trigger of ERS (Denmeade and Isaacs, 2005) (Fig. 30.3). Inhibition of SERCA and resulting calcium spikes in the cytosol can be detected within minutes of applying celecoxib to cultured tumor cells and represent the earliest detectable effects of drug treatment. Importantly, resulting ERS has also been verified in tumors from celecoxib-treated animals, and in all cases the antitumor effects of celecoxib were found to closely correlate with the inhibition of SERCA, depletion of ER calcium stores, the appearance of markers of acute ERS (i.e., CHOP), and cell death (Schönthal, 2007).

Additional insight into the critical importance of ERS was provided by studies of close structural analogs of celecoxib with modified pharmacologic activities, where the apoptosis-inducing activity was separated from the COX-2 inhibitory activity. Two such analogs proved particularly useful in elucidating the role of COX-2 vs. ERS in tumor cell death. The first analog, 2,5-dimethyl-celecoxib (DMC) has lost COX-2 inhibitory function, yet has faithfully maintained antitumor and apoptosis-inducing potential (Schönthal, 2006; Zhu et al., 2002). Conversely, unmethylated celecoxib (UMC) harbors even more potent COX-2 inhibitory potency than celecoxib, but displays greatly reduced ability to inhibit tumor cell proliferation and to induce apoptosis (Chuang et al., 2008; Zhu et al., 2002). Like celecoxib, DMC is an inhibitor of SERCA and strong aggravator of ERS (Fig. 30.3), whereas UMC is comparatively weak and requires substantially higher concentrations to achieve similar effects, clearly revealing that the ability to aggravate ERS is entirely independent of COX-2 inhibitory activity (Chuang et al., 2008). This finding might be particularly relevant in view of celecoxib's recognized life-threatening side effects, which have been linked to the long-term inhibition of COX-2, and appear to represent a class effect of coxibs, such as celecoxib, rofecoxib (Vioxx), and valdecoxib (Bextra) (Dogne et al., 2006). In this regard, celecoxib analogs that exert potent antitumor activity but lack COX-2 inhibitory function, such as DMC, might be better suited for cancer therapeutic applications that involve long-term treatments at elevated dosages.

Combining Bortezomib and Celecoxib for Glioblastoma Therapy

The optimal antitumor efficacy of the above-mentioned pharmacologic agents might be realized in combination treatments, in particular when two or more of these agents are selected based on different molecular mechanisms to achieve aggravation of ERS (Fig. 30.3). In the case of bortezomib and celecoxib, such proof-of-principle has been provided by the demonstration that combination of these two compounds synergizes to aggravate ERS and achieves desirable antitumor outcomes (Kardosh et al., 2008).

When used by itself in the range of 5–10 nM, bortezomib effectively killed several genetically different glioblastoma cell lines, such as U87, LN229, T98G, and U251, and thus yielded a similar IC50 in glioblastoma cells as compared to multiple myeloma cells, which represent the current clinically relevant target of this agent (Kardosh et al., 2008; Mitsiades et al., 2002). Similarly, all these cell lines were sensitive to the cytotoxic effect of celecoxib and its non-coxib analog, DMC, when used in monotherapy fashion in vitro (Kang et al., 2007; Kardosh et al., 2004; 2007; Pyrko et al., 2006). However, when combined, substantially lower concentrations of the individual agents were required to achieve similar cytotoxicity (Kardosh et al., 2008). Importantly, the investigation of various markers of ERS revealed that combination drug treatment exerted potent aggravating effects on this stress system, and all tested ERS indicators (such as GRP78, CHOP) were elevated. These effects were closely aligned with the appearance of commonly known indicators (such as activated caspases 3, 4, 7, and 9) of apoptotic cell death, as well as cleavage of poly(ADP-ribose) polymerase-1 (PARP-1), a substrate of the terminal apoptosis executor, caspase 3 (Kardosh et al., 2008).

Not entirely unexpected, knock-down of GRP78 by siRNA further sensitized the glioblastoma cells to killing by the bortezomib plus celecoxib combination, further confirming the chemoprotective feature of GRP78 in these processes (Kardosh et al., 2008). Additionally, the non-coxib DMC was able to faithfully and potently mimic the enhancing effects of celecoxib in combination with bortezomib, and the critical contribution of the ERS response could also be established at the molecular and cellular levels. Most importantly, these ERS related cytotoxic drug combination effects could also be verified in a mouse xenograft tumor model, where the U87 glioblastoma cell line was implanted subcutaneously (Kardosh et al., 2008). Although intracranial tumor models have not yet been tested, these results are encouraging and strongly suggest that drug combinations (such as bortezomib plus celecoxib or bortezomib plus DMC) aimed at the ERS response should be investigated further and carefully evaluated for their potential clinical efficacy in brain cancer patients. Now that the pharmacologic exploitation of ERS has emerged as a novel strategy to combat cancer, it will be a matter of further characterizing the most potent cytotoxic or chemosensitizing drug combinations in vitro and *in vivo*, and subsequently establish their therapeutic efficacy in clinical trials.

Acknowledgements I am a grateful recipient of a grant from the National Brain Tumor Society (NBTS), and my research efforts are generously supported by NBTS's Mickey McDonald Welker Chair of Research.

References

Adams J, Kauffman M (2004) Development of the proteasome inhibitor velcade (bortezomib). Cancer Invest 22:304–311

Amaravadi RK, Yu D, Lum JJ, Bui T, Christophorou MA, Evan GI, Thomas-Tikhonenko A, Thompson CB (2007) Autophagy inhibition enhances therapy-induced apoptosis in a myc-induced model of lymphoma. J Clin Invest 117: 326–336

Bittner B, Thelly T, Isel H, Mountfield RJ (2000) The impact of co-solvents and the composition of experimental formulations on the pump rate of the ALZET osmotic pump. Int J Pharm 205:195–198

Boyce M, Yuan J (2006) Cellular response to endoplasmic reticulum stress: a matter of life or death. Cell Death Differ 13:363–373

Briceno E, Calderon A, Sotelo J (2007) Institutional experience with chloroquine as an adjuvant to the therapy for glioblastoma multiforme. Surg Neurol 67:388–391

Carew JS, Nawrocki ST, Kahue CN, Zhang H, Yang C, Chung L, Houghton JA, Huang P, Giles FJ, Cleveland JL (2007) Targeting autophagy augments the anticancer activity of the histone deacetylase inhibitor SAHA to overcome bcr-abl-mediated drug resistance. Blood 110:313–322

Chen Z, Lu W, Garcia-Prieto C, Huang P (2007) The warburg effect and its cancer therapeutic implications. J Bioenerg Biomembr 39:267–274

Christofk HR, Vander Heiden MG, Harris MH, Ramanathan A, Gerszten RE, Wei R, Fleming MD, Schreiber SL, Cantley LC (2008) The M2 splice isoform of pyruvate kinase is important for cancer metabolism and tumour growth. Nature 452: 230–233

Chuang H-C, Kardosh A, Gaffney KJ, Petasis NA, Schönthal AH (2008) COX-2 inhibition is neither necessary nor sufficient for celecoxib to suppress tumor cell proliferation and focus formation *in vitro*. Mol Cancer 38

Denmeade SR, Isaacs JT (2005) The SERCA pump as a therapeutic target: making a "smart bomb" for prostate cancer. Cancer Biol Ther 4:14–22

Dogne JM, Hanson J, Supuran C, Pratico D (2006) Coxibs and cardiovascular side-effects: from light to shadow. Curr Pharm Des 12:971–975

Fribley A, Zeng Q, Wang CY (2004) Proteasome inhibitor PS-341 induces apoptosis through induction of endoplasmic reticulum stress-reactive oxygen species in head and neck squamous cell carcinoma cells. Mol Cell Biol 24:9695–9704

Grösch S, Maier TJ, Schiffmann S, Geisslinger G (2006.) Cyclooxygenase-2 (COX-2)-independent anticarcinogenic effects of selective COX-2 inhibitors. J Natl Cancer Inst 98:736–747

Hemeryck A, Geerts R, Monbaliu J, Hassler S, Verhaeghe T, Diels L, Verluyten W, van Beijsterveldt L, Mamidi RN, Janssen C, De Coster R (2007) Tissue distribution and depletion kinetics of bortezomib and bortezomib-related radioactivity in male rats after single and repeated intravenous injection of 14 C-bortezomib. Cancer Chemother Pharmacol 60:777–787

Hideshima T, Bradner JE, Wong J, Chauhan D, Richardson P, Schreiber SL, Anderson KC (2005) Small-molecule inhibition of proteasome and aggresome function induces synergistic antitumor activity in multiple myeloma. Proc Natl Acad Sci USA 102:8567–8572

Janssen S, Rosen DM, Ricklis RM, Dionne CA, Lilja H, Christensen SB, Isaacs JT, Denmeade SR (2006) Pharmacokinetics, biodistribution, and antitumor efficacy of a human glandular kallikrein 2 (hK2)-activated thapsigargin prodrug. Prostate 66:358–368

Kang KB, Wang TT, Woon CT, Cheah ES, Moore XL, Zhu C, Wong MC (2007) Enhancement of glioblastoma radioresponse by a selective COX-2 inhibitor celecoxib: inhibition of tumor angiogenesis with extensive tumor necrosis. Int J Radiat Oncol Biol Phys 67:888–896

Kardosh A, Blumenthal M, Wang WJ, Chen TC, Schönthal AH (2004) Differential effects of selective COX-2 inhibitors on cell cycle regulation and proliferation of glioblastoma cell lines. Cancer Biol Ther 3:9–16

Kardosh A, Golden EB, Pyrko P, Uddin J, Hofman FM, Chen CT, Louie SG, Petasis NA, Schönthal AH (2008) Aggravated endoplasmic reticulum (ER) stress as a basis for enhanced glioblastoma cell killing by bortezomib in combination with celecoxib or its non-coxib analog, 2,5-dimethyl-celecoxib. Cancer Res 68:843–851

Kardosh A, Soriano N, Pyrko P, Liu YT, Jabbour M, Hofman FM, Schonthal AH (2007) Reduced survivin expression and tumor cell survival during chronic hypoxia and further cytotoxic enhancement by the cyclooxygenase-2 inhibitor celecoxib. J Biomed Sci 14:647–662

Kawaguchi Y, Kovacs JJ, McLaurin A, Vance JM, Ito A, Yao TP (2003.) The deacetylase HDAC6 regulates aggresome formation and cell viability in response to misfolded protein stress. Cell 115:727–738

Koki AT, Masferrer JL (2002) Celecoxib: a specific COX-2 inhibitor with anticancer properties. Cancer Control 9:28–35

Lee AS (2007) GRP78 induction in cancer: therapeutic and prognostic implications. Cancer Res 67:3496–3499

Li J, Lee AS (2006) Stress induction of GRP78/BiP and its role in cancer. Curr Mol Med 6:45–54

Marciniak SJ, Ron D (2006) Endoplasmic reticulum stress signaling in disease. Physiol Rev 86:1133–1149

Mitsiades N, Mitsiades CS, Poulaki V, Chauhan D, Fanourakis G, Gu X, Bailey C, Joseph M, Libermann TA, Treon SP, Munshi NC, Richardson PG, Hideshima T, Anderson KC (2002) Molecular sequelae of proteasome inhibition in human multiple myeloma cells. Proc Natl Acad Sci USA 99:14374–14379

Nawrocki ST, Carew JS, Pino MS, Highshaw RA, Andtbacka RH, Dunner K Jr., Pal A, Bornmann WG, Chiao PJ, Huang P, Xiong H, Abbruzzese JL, McConkey DJ (2006) Aggresome disruption: a novel strategy to enhance bortezomib-induced apoptosis in pancreatic cancer cells. Cancer Res 66: 3773–3781

Oyadomari S, Mori M (2004) Roles of CHOP/GADD153 in endoplasmic reticulum stress. Cell Death Differ 11:381–389

Penning TD, Talley JJ, Bertenshaw SR, Carter JS, Collins PW, Docter S, Graneto MJ, Lee LF, Malecha JW, Miyashiro JM, Rogers RS, Rogier DJ, Yu SS, Anderson Gd, Burton EG, Cogburn JN, Gregory SA, Koboldt CM, Perkins WE, Seibert K, Veenhuizen AW, Zhang YY, Isakson PC (1997) Synthesis and biological evaluation of the 1,5-diarylpyrazole class of cyclooxygenase-2 inhibitors: identification of 4-[5-(4-methylphenyl)-3-(trifluoromethyl)-1 h-pyrazol-1-yl]benze nesulfonamide (SC-58635, celecoxib). J Med Chem 40:1347–1365

Pyrko P, Kardosh A, Schönthal AH (2008) Celecoxib transiently inhibits protein synthesis. Biochem Pharmacol 75: 395–404

Pyrko P, Schönthal AH, Hofman FM, Chen TC, Lee AS (2007) The unfolded protein response regulator GRP78/BiP as a novel target for increasing chemosensitivity in malignant gliomas. Cancer Res 67:9809–9816

Pyrko P, Soriano N, Kardosh A, Liu YT, Uddin J, Petasis NA, Hofman FM, Chen CS, Chen TC, Schönthal AH (2006) Downregulation of survivin expression and concomitant induction of apoptosis by celecoxib and its non-cyclooxygenase-2-inhibitory analog, dimethyl-celecoxib (DMC), in tumor cells *in vitro* and *in vivo*. Mol Cancer 5(19)

Rutkowski DT, Arnold SM, Miller CN, Wu J, Li J, Gunnison KM, Mori K, Sadighi Akha AA, Raden D, Kaufman RJ (2006) Adaptation to ER stress is mediated by differential stabilities of pro-survival and pro-apoptotic mRNAs and proteins. PLoS Biol 4:e374

Schönthal AH (2006) Antitumor properties of dimethyl-celecoxib, a derivative of celecoxib that does not inhibit cyclooxygenase-2: implications for glioblastoma therapy. Neurosurg Focus 20(E21):1–10

Schönthal AH (2007) Direct non-cyclooxygenase-2 targets of celecoxib and their potential relevance for cancer therapy. Br J Cancer 97:1465–1468

Schönthal AH (2009) Endoplasmic reticulum stress and autophagy as targets for cancer therapy. Cancer Lett 275: 163–169

Schönthal AH, Chen TC, Hofman FM, Louie SG, Petasis NA (2008) Celecoxib analogs that lack COX-2 inhibitory function: preclinical development of novel anticancer drugs. Expert Opin Investig Drugs 17:197–208

Suzuki T, Lu J, Zahed M, Kita K, Suzuki N (2007) Reduction of GRP78 expression with siRNA activates unfolded protein response leading to apoptosis in HeLa cells. Arch Biochem Biophys 468:1–14

Treiman M, Caspersen C, Christensen SB (1998) A tool coming of age: thapsigargin as an inhibitor of sarco-endoplasmic reticulum ca(2+)-ATPases. Trends Pharmacol Sci 19: 131–135

Zhu J, Song X, Lin HP, Young DC, Yan S, Marquez VE, Chen CS (2002) Using cyclooxygenase-2 inhibitors as molecular platforms to develop a new class of apoptosis-inducing agents. J Natl Cancer Inst 94:1745–1757

Chapter 31

Targeted Therapy for Malignant Gliomas

Maame Dankwah-Quansah and Antonio M. Omuro

Abstract Malignant gliomas, including anaplastic astrocytomas, anaplastic oligodendrogliomas and glioblastomas are aggressive primary brain tumors and are associated with dismal prognosis. The standard treatment for glioblastomas consists of temozolomide and radiotherapy, but virtually all patients recur, with a fatal disease outcome. Molecular targeted therapy has been the focus of attention in the development of new treatments for malignant gliomas. Many signaling pathways that could potentially be targeted have been described, including P13k/Akt/mTOR, Ras/MAPK, and others. Unfortunately, the first generation of targeted therapy trials for malignant gliomas have been disappointing. While strategies targeting angiogenesis through VEFGR pathway inhibition have shown promising activity, results of single agent trials of several other drugs have been largely negative. Current research is focusing on the development of combination of different targeted agents and multi-targeted single agent treatments, as well as patient selection based on pre-existing molecular characteristics. In this chapter we review the development of targeted agents in malignant gliomas, with a focus on issues encountered in trials previously conducted, as well as future research venues.

Keywords Gliomas · Retinoblastoma · Rapamycin · Pathogenesis

A.M. Omuro (✉)
Department of Neurology, Memorial Sloan-Kettering Cancer Center, New York, NY 10021, USA
e-mail: omuroa@mskcc.org

Introduction

Malignant gliomas are the most common type of primary brain tumors. In the United States they account for about 70% of the 22,500 new cases of malignant primary brain tumors diagnosed in adults each year (CBTRUS, 2008). Malignant gliomas include World Health Organization (WHO) grade III and IV tumors. WHO grade III tumors include anaplastic forms of astrocytoma, oligodendroglioma, and oligoastrocytoma. WHO grade IV tumors include glioblastoma (GBM) and its variants. GBM is the most common glioma and is associated with a very aggressive course. Despite numerous clinical trials, minimal improvement in overall survival (OS) or progression-free survival (PFS) has been achieved in the past 20 years. The standard of care for newly diagnosed glioblastoma was established in a randomized trial conducted by the European Organization for Research and Treatment of Cancer (EORTC) (Stupp et al., 2005). In that study, radiotherapy with concomitant temozolomide followed by adjuvant temozolomide was tested against radiotherapy alone. The chemotherapy arm achieved improved OS (median, 15 vs., 12 months; 2 year OS, 27 vs., 10%) and PFS (median, 7 vs., 5 months). Retrospective tumor tissue analysis from patients in that trial showed that patients with tumor displaying MGMT (O6-methylguanine-DNA methyltransferase) promoter methylation benefitted most from the addition of the chemotherapy agent. However, even for those patients, the prognosis remained reserved (median OS: 21.7 months).

WHO grade III gliomas have a better prognosis than grade IV, with a median OS of 2–4 years for newly

M.A. Hayat (ed.), *Tumors of the Central Nervous System, Volume 1*,
DOI 10.1007/978-94-007-0344-5_31, © Springer Science+Business Media B.V. 2011

diagnosed anaplastic astrocytomas and 3–5 years for anaplastic oligodendrogliomas which are known to be chemosensitive. However, virtually all patients show recurrence, and disease follows a fatal course in almost all patients with malignant glioma. New approaches such as molecular targeted therapy are clearly needed. However, development of targeted agents has been challenging in malignant gliomas. Similar to other solid tumors, malignant gliomas are associated with highly heterogeneous molecular abnormalities. Many signaling pathways have been found to be differentially activated or silenced, with both parallel and converging complex interactions (Omuro et al., 2007; Wen and Kesari, 2008). It has been difficult to establish the most relevant targets, and to determine mechanisms of sensitivity and resistance to these drugs. This chapter summarizes the current status of the development of such targeted agents in gliomas.

Molecular Pathogenesis of Malignant Gliomas

Similar to other solid tumors, the pathogenesis of malignant gliomas involves molecular events resulting in deregulation of growth-factor signaling pathways and accumulation of genetic aberrations. GBMs can be grouped into two main subtypes on the basis of biologic and genetic differences. Primary GBMs usually develop in patients in the fifth decade of life. They are characterized by endothelial growth factor receptor (EGFR) amplification and mutations, loss of heterozygosity of chromosome 10q, deletion of the phosphatase and tensin homologue on chromosome 10 (PTEN), and p16 deletion (Furnari et al., 2007). Secondary GBMs are seen in younger patients as low grade or anaplastic astrocytomas. Over a period of several years, these tumors progress to higher grades, eventually transforming to GBMs. Secondary GBMs are less common than primary GBMs. They are morphologically indistinct and, to date, both types of GBMs have been treated with the same conventional therapies and included in the same studies with no distinction. However, secondary GBMs are molecularly distinct, and are characterized by mutations in p53 tumor suppressor gene (Watanabe et al., 1996), abnormalities in p16, retinoblastoma (Rb) pathway, overexpression of platelet derived growth factor receptor (PDGFR), and

loss of heterozygosity of chromosome 10q (Furnari et al., 2007; Ueki et al., 1996). Grade III astrocytomas usually have loss of heterozygosity of chromosome 19q and inactivation of retinoblastoma susceptibility locus 1 (RB1). Progression to GBM is associated with loss of chromosome 10. Low grade oligodendrogliomas are transformed to high grade when there are defects in PTEN, Rb, p53, and cell cycle pathways.

Deletion of 1p and 19q in gliomas is associated with an oligodendroglial phenotype (Bello et al., 1994; Ransom et al., 1992). Combined deletions of both arms are seen in up to 70% of oligodendrogliomas and 50% of mixed oligoastrocytomas (Felsberg et al., 2004; Okamoto et al., 2004; van den Bent et al., 2003). According to Jenkins et al., 2006, an unbalanced translocation mediates the combined 1p and 19q deletion in gliomas. This translocation is associated with a better prognosis and response to radiation therapy and chemotherapy, particularly gliomas with oligodendroglial components. Gliomas that have lost the entire short-arm of chromosome 1 (1p) and the entire long arm of chromosome 19 (19q) have two distinguishing features: they grow slowly, even those that are anaplastic and they respond to DNA damaging therapies. These characteristics distinguish 1p/19q codeleted gliomas from other low and high grade gliomas, including oligodendrogliomas with intact 1p and 19q alleles (Cairncross and Jenkins, 2008).

Targeting Receptor Tyrosine Kinases

The most important receptor tyrosine kinases that are targets for the development of molecular therapy for malignant gliomas have been EGFR, PDGFR, and vascular endothelial growth factor receptor (VEGFR). These growth factors initiate intracellular signaling mediated by tyrosine kinase activities. Tyrosine kinases act by phosphorylating tyrosine residues on proteins.

Epidermal Growth Factor Receptor

EGFR is abnormally activated in about 70% of solid cancers. The activation of EGFR pathways in cancer cells has been linked to increased motility, adhesion, invasion, and proliferation of tumor cells, as well as inhibition of apoptosis and induction of angiogenesis. EGFR transmembrane protein is made up of three domains: (1) an extracellular ligand-binding domain, (2) a transmembrane lipophilic region and, (3) an intracellular tyrosine kinase domain. Ligands bind to the extracellular domain of two receptors simultaneously resulting in two receptors bound together at the cell surface leading to modification of the three-dimensional structure of the receptor. This results in induction of intracellular cross-phosphorylation between the tyrosine kinase subunit of one receptor and the kinase subunit of the other. The activation of this process promotes signal transduction and gene activation mediated by several downstream signaling pathways, including the PI3K/AKT/mTOR, Ras/Raf/MAPK, and protein kinase C signaling pathways.

EGFR is amplified in the majority of GBMs, resulting in over-expression of EGFR. Mutations are frequent, particularly the EGFRvIII mutation, which correspond to a large deletion in exons 2 and 7, affecting the extracellular domain and resulting in a constitutively active receptor. Several strategies targeting EGFR and EGFRvIII in GBMs have been proposed, including the use of monoclonal antibodies against EGFR, bispecific antibodies, toxin-linked conjugates, vaccine therapies, and small molecule tyrosine kinase inhibitors (EGFR TKIs). The drugs that inhibit EGFR act by competing with adenosine triphosphate (ATP) for binding to the kinase pocket of the receptor. This leads to blockage of the receptor activation and transduction of post receptor signals. Several studies of the EGFR TKIs gefitinib and erlotinib have been conducted in GBM (Omuro et al., 2007). Most studies found very low response rates (0–13%), although one study utilizing erlotinib found 26% of responses (Vogelbaum et al., 2005). The median PFS was 2 and 3 months, and the median overall survival was 6 –10 months. Overall, results for both drugs do not seem to differ from historical controls. Presence of EGFR overexpression or amplification did not seem to predict clinical benefit from these drugs. However, some retrospective studies have suggested that patients with tumors with inactivated AKT, absence of *PTEN* loss, or presence of EGFRvIII are more likely to respond, although such findings have not been duplicated in other studies and have not been validated in a prospective setting. Therefore, in spite of a strong rationale, no role for EGFR inhibitors has been defined in gliomas to date, although results of further studies in selected populations are awaited.

Platelet-Derived Growth Factor Receptor

Platelet-derived growth factor receptors (PDGFs) consist of a group of four different polypeptide chains. These are PDGF-A, PDGF-B, PDGF-C, and PDGF-D. They exercise their cellular effects through two types of protein tyrosine kinase receptors: PDGF-alpha and PDGF-beta. Ligand binding induces receptor dimerization, activation, and autophosphorylation of the tyrosine kinase domain. This results in the activation of several signal transduction pathways, including Ras-MAPK, PI3k, the Src family kinase, signal transducers and activators of transcription factors (Stat), and phospholipase C gamma. The overexpression of PDGF and PDGFR has been shown to play an important role in the development of gliomas through autocrine stimulation of cancer cells, development of angiogenesis, and control of tumor interstitial pressure. PDGFR and PDGF are frequently expressed in secondary GBMs. This overexpression results from deregulated expression and is associated with loss of TP53 tumor suppressor gene.

The expression of PDGF and PDGFR are associated with a poorer prognosis in gliomas. A role for PDGFR as a potential target for the treatment of gliomas was suggested by the inhibition of growth in cell lines and xenograft models induced by PDGFR TKIs. Inhibition of PDGFR was correlated with decreased phosphorylated extracellular signal-regulated and pAKT levels, suggesting inhibition of MAPK and PI3K pathways.

The most studied PDGFR TKI is imatinib. It blocks the activity of Bcl-Abl, c-kit, and PDGFR. However, the use of imatinib in the treatment of malignant gliomas has not been successful (Raymond et al., 2008; Wen et al., 2006). Observed response rates were 4–6%, and median PFS has been 2–3 months. It is not known whether the lack of efficacy is due to poor tumor penetration or lack of a key role of PDGF pathways in such tumors. Some phase II studies suggested that the addition of hydroxyurea to imatinib could improve results, but a randomized trial was terminated early because of lack of efficacy for this combination. Ongoing studies are investigating whether new PDGFR TKIs with better brain penetration, such as tandutinib, may overcome resistance of gliomas to PDGFR inhibition.

Vascular Endothelial Growth Factor

VEGF has been shown to be a major regulator of tumor angiogenesis. The expression of VEGF has been correlated with increasing tumor grade in gliomas. VEGF is known to promote endothelial cell proliferation, migration, and tube formation. Approaches to block VEGF have been used in laboratory studies and have resulted in inhibition of tumor and new blood vessel growth in high grade astrocytic tumors (Cheng et al., 1996; Folkman et al., 1971; Stefanik et al., 2001). VEGF-A is a member of the VEGF family that acts as a key proangiogenic factor because of its specificity to endothelial cells and the multitude of responses it can elicit. The main receptors involved in relaying VEGF-A signaling are VEGFR-1 and VEGFR-2.

The most studied receptor is VEGFR-2, a potent tyrosine kinase that mediates endothelial cell signaling through the activation of Ras/Raf/MEK/MAPK, PI3K/AKT/PKB, and protein kinase C-beta pathways. Gliomas are highly vascularized tumors. They have been shown to overexpress VEGF-A, which has been linked to a poorer prognosis. Several studies have suggested that blocking VEGF pathways may normalize tumor vasculature and improve the delivery of chemotherapy, thus allowing higher drug concentrations. The proposed strategies for targeting VEGF include anti-VEGF-A and VEGFR-2 monoclonal antibodies, antisense oligonucleotides, ribozymes, and VEGFR TKI. Most VEGFR TKI drugs are not specific but act on other tyrosine kinase receptors. The best studied drugs for the treatment of gliomas have been vatalanib, sorafenib, sunitinib, and cediranib.

Vatalanib is a VEGFR-1 and VEGFR-2 TKI that has shown activity in glioma cell lines and xenograft models. It also binds to and inhibits related receptor tyrosine kinases, including PDGFR and c-kit. It is a multi-VEGFR inhibitor that blocks angiogenesis and lymphangiogenesis by binding the intracellular kinase domain of VEGFR. Conrad et al. (2004) conducted a phase I/II study of the effectiveness of vatalanib and found only modest efficacy. In that study, among the 47 evaluable patients treated with single-agent vatalanib, 4% achieved a partial response and 56% achieved disease stability for a median duration of stabilization of 3 months.

Sorafenib is a dual-action Raf and VEGFR receptor inhibitor. It blocks receptor phosphorylation and MAPK-mediated signaling. It is also known to inhibit growth in a number of tumor types. While single-agent efficacy data are lacking in gliomas, sorafenib is currently being investigated in combination with erlotinib, temsirolimus or tipifarnib in recurrent gliomas.

Sunitinib is a multi-targeted VEGFR-2 and PDGFR inhibitor, both of which play a role in tumor angiogenesis and cell proliferation. Simultaneously inhibiting VEGFR-2 and PDGFR leads to reduced tumor vascularization and death of cancer cells which ultimately leads to tumor shrinkage. This agent is currently being evaluated in a phase II trial in recurrent disease.

Cediranib is an oral pan-VEGFR TKI. A phase II study with cediranib in recurrent/progressive GBM found response rates of 56% (Gerstner et al., 2008). Twenty-six percent of patients were found to have no progression of disease at 6 months. The median PFS was 117 days and median OS was 227 days. In this study, cediranib was also shown to decrease vascular permeability as measured by MRI techniques resulting in a significant decrease in cerebral edema. As a result, a majority of patients were able to decrease or stop corticosteroids. A randomized study is ongoing to confirm these encouraging results.

In contrast to VEGFR TKIs, the humanized monoclonal antibody against VEGF Ferrara et al., (2004) is in advanced stage of development in gliomas. In a retrospective study Stark-Vance, (2005), 21 patients with malignant glioma were treated with a 6-week cycle of bevacizumab 5 mg/kg every other week and weekly irinotecan, 125 mg/m^2 for 4 weeks with 2 weeks of rest. This regimen was chosen based on safety data for colorectal cancer. There was one complete response and 8 partial responses, for an objective response rate of 43%. Eleven patients had stable disease and among those not meeting criteria for partial response, most of them had radiographic improvement consisting of reductions in peritumoral edema and contrast enhancement. These results were confirmed in a phase II study of bevacizumab and irinotecan in recurrent glioblastoma (Vredenburgh et al., 2007a, 2007b). The 6-month PFS among 35 patients was 46%, the 6-month OS was 77% and 20 of the 35 patients had at least a partial response. Given the impressive results in terms of response rates and PFS (and to a lesser extent, OS), this regimen is becoming a standard of treatment for recurrent glioblastoma. The major toxicity has been thromboembolic complications. Brain hemorrhages, a concern with the use of bevacizumab in brain tumors, have been rare and manageable, even in the setting of anticoagulation with low-weight heparin (frequently required due to thromboembolic complications). However, the relevance of irinotecan, an agent that is inactive in gliomas, has been questioned. Preliminary results of a randomized phase II study comparing single agent bevacizumab versus bevacizumab and irinotecan suggest no major differences in outcomes. Results in other types of cancer suggest that a combination with a cytotoxic agent is required for maximal bevacizumab activity, and that bevacizumab may be more active in newly-diagnosed disease. Therefore, results of studies investigating combinations with cytotoxic agents that are active in gliomas, such as an ongoing phase III study of bevacizumab and temozolomide for newly-diagnosed glioblastoma are eagerly awaited.

Targeting Downstream Cell Signaling Pathways in Gliomas

Downstream signaling pathways of receptor tyrosine kinases can serve as a possible target for the development of therapy for malignant gliomas. The most common deregulated pathways in malignant gliomas are Ras/MAPK and PI3K/Akt/mTOR.

PI3K/Akt/mTOR Pathway

In this pathway, receptor tyrosine kinases activate PI3K, which also generates phosphatidylinositol-3,4,5-triphosphate (PIP3), a lipid second messenger. PIP3 recruits phosphatidylinositol-dependant kinase-1 (PDK1) and Akt to the membrane, where Akt is phosphorylated and activated by PDK1. Akt will then phosphorylate different sets of substrates to mediate its effect. Akt can drive the proliferation of cells by inactivating glycogen synthase kinase-3 (GSK-3), which will inhibit cell cycle activators (e.g., cyclin D1 and Myc) and cell cycle inhibitor p27. Akt also promotes survival by inactivating proapoptotic protein BAD, NF-kB inhibitor IkB kinase (IKK), and FOXO family

of forkhead transcription factors (increases transcription of proptotic genes) (Chi and Wen, 2007).

Akt promotes cell growth through the inactivation of tumor suppressor tuberin (TSC2). Tuberin releases its inhibition on mTOR, which will phosphorylate eukaryotic initiation factor 4E binding protine-1 (4EBP1) and S6K. This will lead to increased translation. PI3K signaling is inhibited by PTEN lipid phosphatase, which inactivates PIP3. The PI3K-Akt pathway is upregulated in most malignancies, with mutations in its components found to be present in many types of cancers. Activation of this pathway in gliomas has been reported to be linked to poorer prognosis and more aggressive tumors. In malignant gliomas, this pathway is frequently activated through deletion of PTEN, overexpression of growth factor receptors, and PI3K mutations. This pathway is therefore of particular interest in gliomas, and potential downstream targets include Akt, mTOR and PI3K, as detailed below.

Mammalian Target of Rapamycin (mTOR)

Overactivation of the PI3K/Akt/mTOR pathway appears to play a key role in the downstream signaling pathways promoting growth and survival in several types of tumor cells, including glioma. mTOR plays a key role in the downstream signaling of the PI3K/Akt pathway through the regulation of cellular catabolism, anabolism, proliferation, cell cycle control, autophagy, angiogenesis, and apoptosis. In vitro studies have suggested that mTOR activity is highly activated in cells with deficient PTEN function, including glioma cell lines. Alterations of PTEN expression are frequent in high-grade gliomas, with PTEN mutations present in 15–40% of primary GBMs (Wang et al., 1997; Zhou et al., 1999).

Preclinical studies of gliomas have suggested that PTEN-deficient tumors show enhanced sensitivity to mTOR inhibition. This provided the rationale for clinical trials of mTOR inhibitors in GBMs. Phase II results of two studies using temsirolimus found that although drug metabolism was significantly affected by enzyme-inducing anticonvulsants, therapeutic serum levels could still be achieved with a dose of 250 mg/week. However, in terms of efficacy, results in unselected patients were disappointing, with no improvement in response rates, PFS, or OS. The

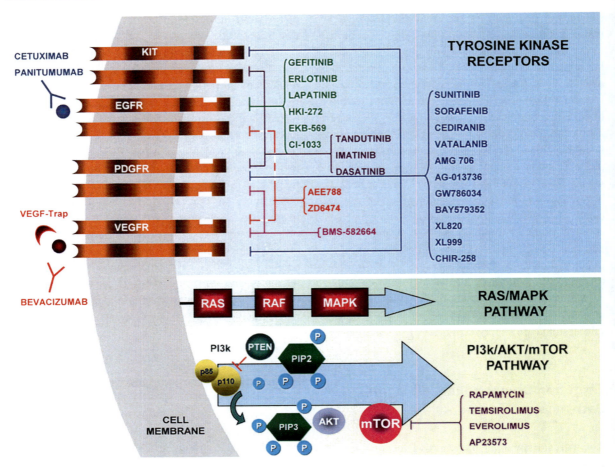

Fig. 31.1 Schematic representation of main oncogenetic signaling molecular pathways and corresponding single and multi-targeted drugs under development. Modified from Omuro et al., 2007, Molecular Cancer Therapeutics with permission

paucity of responses prevented adequate correlative studies in the search of markers of response (Chang et al., 2005; Galanis et al., 2005). One study suggested that grade 2 or higher hyperlipidemia and expression of p70s6k were predictors of clinical benefit (both $p = 0.04$), whereas EGFR amplification, PTEN deletion (fluorescence in situ hybridization), PTEN expression (immunohistochemistry), AKT, and pAKT were not (Galanis et al., 2005). However, those results were limited by the utilization of unconventional response criteria for the correlative analysis, and overall no current role for mTOR inhibition has been defined in gliomas. Kuhn et al. (2007) demonstrated that measurable intratumor concentrations of temsirolimus and sirolimus could be detected in GBMs after treatment with sirolimus, which suggests that tumor penetration

does not seem to play a major factor in drug resistance. Conversely, Cloughesy et al. (2008) suggested that mTOR inhibition with rapamycin in gliomas leads to a paradoxical activation of Akt through a loss of negative feedback, which may explain the lack of efficacy of this strategy. Other drugs such as PI3K inhibitors (XL765) and Akt inhibitors are now being tested in gliomas, and may provide a more attractive strategy to target the PI3K pathway than mTOR inhibition.

Ras/MAPK Pathway

This pathway plays an important role in cell proliferation and survival, as well as modulating cell adhesion and motility. It is triggered by activated receptor tyrosine kinase, which binds adaptor proteins that contain SH2 domains. Adaptor protein growth factor receptor-bound 2 (Grb2)/son of sevenless (SOS) facilitates the activation of Ras, which in turn activates Raf through a mechanism that is unknown. Activated Raf will then activate MEK, which activates MAPK. MAPK activates S6 kinase (S6K) and transcription factors (Fos, Myc, and Jun). This leads to transcription of genes that are associated with proliferation (Chi and Wen, 2007). Mutations in this pathway lead to increased signaling, which results in increased tumor growth, invasion, angiogenesis, and metastasis. Proteins in this pathway that constitute attractive targets for drug modulation include Ras, Raf, and MEK. Farnesyltransferase is involved with signal transduction in the Ras pathway; examples of farnesyltransferase inhibitors are tipifarnib and lonafarnib. Tipifarnib was found to have modest activity in gliomas as a single agent in phase I/II trials, but is now being evaluated in drug combinations such as with temozolomide and sorafenib. Drugs targeting the MAPK pathway are also being developed.

Multi-Targeted Therapy for Malignant Gliomas

As discussed earlier, the results of first generation targeted therapy trials for malignant gliomas have been disappointing. While strategies targeting angiogenesis through VEGFR pathway inhibition have shown promising activity, single agent trials on several other drugs have been largely negative. One strategy for improving outcomes is addressing multiple targets simultaneously. Possible strategies for such multi-targeted therapy include simultaneously targeting different parallel receptor tyrosine kinases pathways, targeting one specific pathway at more than one level, or blocking both upstream and downstream components. These strategies can be accomplished by combining two or more targeted drugs or through utilization of single-agent treatments with drugs that are less specific and that address multiple targets simultaneously.

Prompted by in vitro evidence of synergism between mTOR inhibitors and EGFR TKI, ongoing clinical research is testing such combinations, including trials of temsirolimus, everolimus, or sirolimus combined with gefitinib, erlotinib, or AEE788.

Although such studies have encountered minimal, or no drug-to-drug interaction, toxicity has been generally found to be significantly higher than that reported for single agents. As a result, defined maximum tolerated doses have been significantly lower for the combinations, in comparison to each single-agent doses, which may decrease both brain penetration and target modulation properties for each agent. A phase I study combining gefitinib and sirolimus in malignant gliomas found no significant pharmacokinetic interaction between the two drugs, but pharmacokinetics of both drugs were significantly affected by enzyme-inducing drugs. A partial response was seen in 2 of 34 patients and disease remained stable in 13 of 34 patients. No obvious molecular markers of response could be defined (Reardon et al., 2006). Results of a study using gefitinib and everolimus in the treatment of patients with recurrent GBMs have also been reported. Thirty-six percent of patients had stable disease and 14% had a partial response. Only one patient was reported to be progression-free at 6 months (Kreisl et al., 2009). Results of other studies are awaited.

Multi-targeted single-agent treatments are easier to develop as there is no need to evaluate drug-to-drug interactions or to manage potentially additive or unpredictable side effects of the combination of drugs. However, IC_{50} values for each of the intended targets can be very different, and concentrations achieved in vivo may not result in the same profile of target modulation as demonstrated in vitro. To date, the multi-targeted TKI tested in GBMs have all demonstrated minimal efficacy, including vandetanib, imatinib and vatalanib, with the exception of cediranib, which achieved promising results, as described earlier.

Conclusion

The development of targeted therapy for gliomas has been challenging. In addition to the complexity of the multiple pathways involved in solid tumor oncogenesis, which encompass intricate cross-talks and feedback loops, gliomas pose additional difficulties of their own, including necessity of developing drugs with adequate brain penetration, and with minimal interaction with anti-epileptic drugs. Yet, significant advances are being made. Based on the first trials, it became clear that seizure control could be achieved in most patients with non-enzyme inducing anti-epileptic drugs such as levetiracetam and lamotrigine, and patients could be safely switched to those drugs. This has allowed for expedited trials, with elimination of arms dedicated to patients on enzyme-inducing drugs. Moreover, surgical trials that evaluate drug penetration and target modulation in patients undergoing targeted agents have become increasingly common. This should improve our understanding of the mechanisms of drug resistance in gliomas, and eventually lead to development of more effective drugs or combinations.

References

Bello MJ, Vaquero J, de Campos JM, Kusak ME, Sarasa JL, Saez-Castresana J, Pestana A, Rey JA (1994) Molecular analysis of chromosome 1 abnormalities in human gliomas reveals frequent loss of 1p in oligodendroglial tumors. Int J Cancer 57:172–175

CBTRUS (2008) Statistical report: primary brain tumors in the United States, 1998–2002 Central Brain Tumor Registry of the United States, 2000–2004. http://www.cbtrus.org/reports/2007-2008/2007report.pdf. Accessed Jan 2009

Cairncross G, Jenkins R (2008) Gliomas with 1p/19q codeletion: A.K.A. oligodendroglioma. Cancer J 14:352–357

Chang SM, Wen P, Cloughessy T, Greenberg H, Schiff D, Conrad C, Fink K, Ian Robbins H, DeAngelis L, Raizer J, Hess K, Aldape K, Lamborn KR, Kuhn J, Dancey J, Prados MD (2005) for the North American Brain Tumor Consortium and the National Cancer Institute Phase II study of CCI-779 in patients with recurrent glioblastoma multiforme. Invest New Drugs 23:357–361

Cheng SY, Huang HJ, Nagane M, Ji. XD, Wang D, Shih CC, Arap W, Huang CM, Cavenee WK (1996) Suppression of glioblastoma angiogenicity and tumorigenicity by inhibition of endogenous expression of vascular endothelial growth factor. Proc Natl Acad Sci USA 93(16):8502–8507

Chi AS, Wen PY (2007) Inhibiting kinases in malignant gliomas. Exp Opin Ther Targets 11:473–496

Cloughesy TF, Yoshimoto K, Nghiemphu P, Brown K, Dang J, Zhu S, Hsueh T, Chen Y, Wang W, Youngkin D, Liau L, Martin N, Becker D, Bergsneider M, Lai A, Green R, Oglesby T, Koleto M, Trent J, Horvath S, Mischel PS, Mellinghoff IK, Sawyers CL (2008) Antitumor activity of rapamycin in a phase i trial for patients with recurrent PTEN-deficient glioblastoma. PLoS Med 5(1):e21

Conrad C, Friedman H, Reardon D, Provenzale J, Jackson E, Serajuddin D, Laurent D, Chen B, Yung WKA (2004) A phase I/II trial of single agent PTK 787/ZK 222584 (PTK/ZK), a novel, oral angiogenesis inhibitor in patients with recurrent glioblastoma multiforme (GBM). Am Soc Clin Oncol Annu Meet 22:1512

Felsberg J, Erkwoh A, Sabel MC, Kirsch L, Fimmers R, Blaschke B, Schlegel U, Schramm J, Wiestler OD, Reifenberger G (2004) Oligodendroglial tumors: refinement

of candidate regions on chromosome arm 1p and correlation of 1p/19q status with survival. Brain Pathol 14:121–130

Ferrara N, Hillan KJ, Gerber HP, Novotny W (2004) Discovery and development of bevacizumab, an anti-VEGF antibody for treating cancer. Nat Rev Drug Discov 3:391–400

Folkman J, Merler E, Abernathy C, Williams G (1971) Isolation of a tumor factor responsible for angiogenesis. J Exp Med 133:275–288

Furnari FB, Fenton T, Bachoo RM, Mukasa A, Stommel JM, Stegh A, Hahn WC, Ligon KL, Louis DN, Brennan C, Chin L, DePhino RA, Cavenee WK (2007) Malignant astrocytic glioma: genetics, biology, and paths to treatment. Genes Dev 21:2683–2710

Galanis E, Buckner JC, Maurer MJ, Kreisberg JI, Ballman K, Boni J, Peralba JM, Jenkins RB, Dakhil SR, Morton RF, Jaeckler KA, Scheithauer BW, Dancey J, Hidalgo M, Walsh DJ (2005) Phase II trial of temsirolimus (ccl-779) in recurrent glioblastoma multiforme: a north central cancer treatment group study. J Clin Oncol 23:5294–5304

Gerstner ER, Duda DG, di Tomaso E, Sorensen AG, Jain RK, Batchelor TT (2008) Cediranib, an oral pan-VEGF tyrosine kinase inhibitor in the treatment of glioblastoma. Curr Treat Opt Oncol 9:1–122

Jenkins RB, Blair H, Ballman KV, Giannini C, Arusell RM, Law M, Flynn H, Passe S, Felten S, Brown PD, Shaw EG, Buckner JC (2006) A T(1;19) (Q10;P10) mediates the combined deletions of 1p and 19q and predicts a better prognosis of patients with oligodendroglioma. Cancer Res 66:9852–9861

Kreisl TN, Lassman AB, Mischel PS, Scher HI, Teruya-Feldstein J, Shaffer D, Lis E, Abrey LE (2009) A pilot study of everolimus and gefitinib in the treatment of recurrent glioblastoma (GBM). J Neurooncol 92(1):99–105

Kuhn JG, Chang SM, Wen PY, Cloughesy TF, Greenberg H, Schiff D, Conrad C, Fink KL, Robins HI, Mehta M, DeAngelis L, Raizer J, Hess K, Lamborn KR, Dancey J, Prados MD (2007) Pharmacokinetic and tumor distribution characteristics of temsirolimus in patients with recurrent malignant glioma. Clin Cancer Res 13:7401–7406

Okamoto Y, DiPatre PL, Burkhard C, Horstmann S, Jourde B, Fahey M, Schuler D, Probst-Hensch NM, Yasargil MG, Yonekawa Y, Lutolf UM, Kleihues P, Ohgaki H (2004) Population -based study on incidence, survival rates, and genetic alterations of low-grade diffuse astrocytomas and oligodendrogliomas. Acta Neuropathol 108: 49–56

Omuro AMP, Faivre S, Raymond E (2007) Lessons learned in the development of targeted therapy for malignant gliomas. Mol Cancer Ther 6(7):1909–1919

Ransom DT, Ritland SR, Kimmel DW, Moertel CA, Dahl RJ, Scheithauer BW, Kelly PJ, Jenkins RB (1992) Cytogenetic and loss of heterozygosity studies in ependymomas, pilocytic astrocytomas, and oligodendrogliomas. Genes Chromosomes Cancer 5:348–356

Raymond E, Brandes AA, Dittrich C, Fumoleau P, Coudert B, Clement PMJ, Frenay M, Rampling R, Stupp R, Kros JM, Heinrich MC, Gorlia T, Lacombe D, van den Bent MJ (2008) Phase II study of imatinib in patients with recurrent gliomas of various histologies: a european organization for research and treatment of cancer brain tumor study group. J Clin Oncol 26:4659–4665

Reardon DA, Quinn JA, Vredenburgh JJ, Gururangan S, Friedman AH, Desjardins A, Sathornsumetee S, Herndon JE, Dowell JM, McLendon RE, Provenzale JM, Sampson JH, Smith RP, Swaisland AJ, Ochs JS, Lyons P, Tourt-Uhlig S, Bigner DD, Friedman HS, Rich JN (2006) Phase i trial of gefitinib plus sirolimus in adults with recurrent malignant glioma. Clin Cancer Res 12:860–868

Stark-Vance V (2005) Bevacizumab and CPT-11 in the treatment of relapsed malignant gliomas. Proc Soc Neurooncol 7:369

Stefanik DF, Fellows WK, Rizkalla LR, Rizkalla WM, Stefanik PP, Deleo AB, Welch WC (2001) Monoclonal antibodies to vascular endothelial growth factor (VEGF) and the VEGF receptor, FLT-1, inhibit the growth of C6 glioma in a mouse xenograft. J Neurooncol 55:91–100

Stupp R, Mason WP, van den Bent MJ, Weller M, Fisher B, Taphoorn MJ, Belanger K, Brandes AA, Marosi C, Bogdahn U, Curschmann J, Janzer RC, Ludwin SK, Gorlia T, Allgeier A, Lacombe D, Cairncross JG, Eisenhauer E, Mirimanoff RO (2005) Radiotherapy plus concomitant and adjuvant temozolomide for glioblastoma. N Engl J Med 352:987–999

Ueki K, Ono Y, Henson JW, Efird JT, von Deimling A, Louis DN (1996) CDKN2/P16 or RB alterations occur in the majority of glioblastomas and are inversely correlated. Cancer Res 56:150–153

Van den Bent MJ, Looijenga LH, Langenberg K, Dinjens W, Graveland W, Uytdewilligen L, Silevis Smith PA, Jenkins RB, Kros JM (2003) Chromosomal anomalies in oligodendroglial tumors are corrected with clinical features. Cancer 97:1276–1284

Vogelbaum M, Peereboom D, Stevens G, Barnett G, Brewer C (2005) Phase II study of erlotinib single agent therapy in recurrent glioblastoma multiforme. Eur J Cancer Suppl 3:135

Vredenburgh JJ, Desjardins A, Herndon II JE, Dowell JM, Reardon DA, Quinn JA, Rich JN, Sathornsumett S, Gururangan S, Wagner M, Bigner D, Friedman AH, Friedman HS (2007a) Phase II trial of bevacizumab and irinotecan in recurrent malignant glioblastoma. Clin Cancer Res 13:1253–1259

Vredenburgh JJ, Desjardins A, Herndon III JE, Marcello J, Reardon DA, Quinn JA, Rich JN, Sathornsumetee S, Gururangan S, Sampson J, Wagner M, Bailey L, Bigner DD, Friedman AH, Freidman HS (2007b) Bevacizumab plus irinotecan in recurrent glioblastoma multiforme. J Clin Oncol 25:4722–4729

Wang SI, Puc J, Li J, Bruce JN, Cairns P, Sidransky D, Parsons R (1997) Somatic mutations of PTEN in glioblastoma multiforme. Cancer Res 57:4183–4186

Watanabe K, Tachibana O, Sata K, Yonekawa Y, Kleihues P, Ohgaki H (1996) Overexpression of the EGF receptor and P53 mutations are mutually exclusive in the evolution of primary and secondary glioblastomas. Brain Pathol 6: 217–223

Wen PY, Kesari S (2008) Malignant gliomas in adults. N Engl J Med. 359:492–507

Wen PY, Yung WKA, Lamborn KR, Dahia PL, Wang Y, Pen B, Abrey LE, Raizer J, Cloughesy TF, Fink K, Gilbert M, Chang S, Junck L, Schiff D, Lieberman F, Fine HA, Mehta M, Robins HI, DeAngelis LM, Groves MD, Puduvalli VK, Levin V, Conrad C, Maher EA, Aldape K, Hayes M, Letvak L, Egorin MJ, Capdeville R, Kaplan R, Murgo AJ, Stiles C,, Prados MD (2006) Phase I/II Study of Imatinib Mesylate for Recurrent Malignant Gliomas: North American Brain Tumor Consortium Study 99–08.. Clin Cancer Res 12:4899–4907

Zhou XP, Li YJ, Hoang-Xuan K, Laurent-Puig P, Mokhtari K, Longy M, Sanson M, Delattre JY, Thomas G, Hamelin R (1999) Mutational analysis of the PTEN gene in gliomas: molecular and pathological correlations. Int J Cancer 20:150–154

Chapter 32

Glioblastomas: HER1/EGFR-Targeted Therapeutics

Georg Karpel-Massler and Marc-Eric Halatsch

Abstract The most common primary brain tumors are gliomas. Glioblastoma is the most malignant subtype and accounts for more than 50% of all gliomas. Patients with glioblastoma still face a poor prognosis, despite treatment according to the current standards of care. Thus, great effort is made to identify more successful therapeutic strategies. The epidermal growth factor receptor (HER1/EGFR) is one of the targets being in the focus of intense investigation. In 40–50% of glioblastoma dysregulation of HER1/EGFR is found and its overexpression represents one of the most common molecular abnormalities seen in high-grade gliomas. Various compounds have been developed to target HER1/EGFR or its mutant form, EGFRvIII. Clinical data is so far most advanced for tyrosine kinase (TK) inhibitors. But also radio-immuno conjugates, ligand-toxin conjugates, antibodies, RNA-based agents and vaccines have been developed and investigated on to a various extent. Unfortunately, the initial enthusiasm derived by promising results from experimental studies could not be confirmed by clinical studies. It seems that inhibition of solely HER1/EGFR is insufficient to provide a clinical benefit. Therefore, a multi-targeted approach tailored to the individual molecular pattern might be a more successful therapeutic strategy.

Keywords HER1/EGFR · Glioblastoma · Targeted therapy · Tyrosine kinase inhibitors · Multi-targeting

Introduction

The epidermal growth factor receptor (HER1/EGFR) belongs to the HER family of receptors and consists of an extracellular ligand-binding site, a transmembraneous part and an intracellular tyrosine kinase (TK) domain. Its most common ligands are epidermal growth factor (EGF) and transforming growth factor-α (TGF-α). Once ligands bind to their cognate HER family receptors, formation of HER receptor homodimers or heterodimers with a different HER family receptor occurs and activates the intrinsic TK. Subsequently, autophosphorylation of specific tyrosine residues within the cytoplasmic catalytic kinase domain of the receptor and initiation of cytoplasmic signaling cascades such as the ras-raf-mitogen-activated protein kinase (MAPK) pathway or the phosphatidylinositol 3-kinase (PI3-K)/Akt pathway occur (Fig. 32.1). The downstream signaling characteristics vary due to the different ligand-binding affinities of the HER family receptors and depend on how the homo- or heterodimer is composed. Receptors of the HER family are expressed on many cell types and initiate signal transduction from the cell surface to the intracellular compartment by which diverse cellular functions, including proliferation and differentiation, are regulated.

In more than 50% of various epithelial malignancies HER1/EGFR overexpression or activation was found. The causative relationship between dysregulation of the HER1/EGFR and neoplastic disorder is explained by the affection of downstream signal transduction resulting in impaired apoptosis and/or stimulation of proliferation, tumorigenesis, angiogenesis and invasion (Halatsch et al., 2006). Several mechanisms may lead to receptor dysregulation (Fig. 32.2). One of

G. Karpel-Massler (✉)
Department of Neurosurgery, University of Ulm School of Medicine, Steinhövelstraße 9, D-89075 Ulm, Germany
e-mail: georg.karpel@uniklinik-ulm.de

M.A. Hayat (ed.), *Tumors of the Central Nervous System, Volume 1*,
DOI 10.1007/978-94-007-0344-5_32, © Springer Science+Business Media B.V. 2011

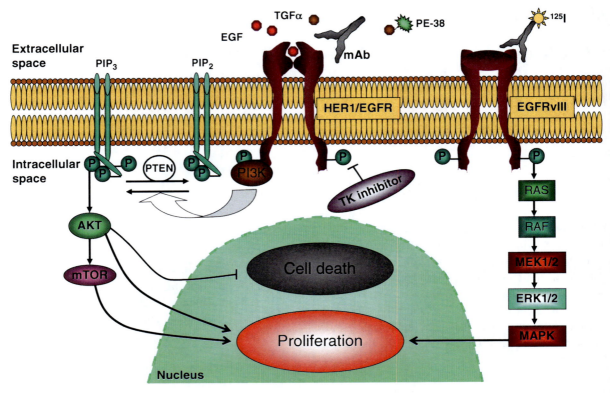

Fig. 32.1 Schematic representation of signal transduction and cellular effects due to activation of HER1/EGFR or its mutant forms. In addition, various HER1/EGFR-targeted therapeutic approaches are illustrated. Abbreviations: AKT, murine thymoma viral oncogene homolog; EGF, epidermal growth factor; HER1/EGFR, epidermal growth factor receptor; ^{125}I, iodine 125; mAb, monoclonal antibody; MAPK, mitogen-activated protein kinase; MEK, mitogen-activated protein kinase kinase; mTOR, mammalian target of rapamycin; PE-38, pseudomonas exotoxin 38; PI3-K, phosphatidylinositol 3-kinase; PIP$_2$, phosphatidylinositol 3,4 biphosphate; PIP$_3$, phosphatidylinositol 3,4,5 triphosphate; PTEN, phosphatase/tensin homolog on chromosome 10; RAF, murine leukemia viral oncogene homolog; RAS, rat sarcoma viral oncogene homolog; TGFα, transforming growth factor α; TK, tyrosine kinase (Karpel-Massler et al., 2009)

the possible mechanisms is gene amplification resulting in HER1/EGFR overexpression. It was shown that in glioblastoma 40–50% of the tumors overexpress HER1/EGFR. Another mechanism that may cause enhanced HER1/EGFR-mediated signaling is autocrine overproduction of HER1/EGFR ligands, leading to loss of external control of cell growth due to independent receptor activation. Mutational changes of the intrinsic receptor structure constitute a third mechanism that may lead to a pathologically altered HER1/EGFR signaling. The most interesting mutant form that accounts for approximately 60% of all mutants is EGFRvIII resulting from an in-frame deletion of 801 base pairs in the DNA sequence encoding

the extracellular ligand-binding domain. EGFRvIII is constitutively activated and its expression is related to cellular transformation and enhanced tumorigenicity (Nishikawa et al., 1994).

Current therapeutic measures have so far failed to substantially improve the poor outcome of patients with glioblastoma. Thus, new therapeutic approaches are urgently needed. Since evidence accumulates that HER1/EGFR is involved in the regulation of cellular differentiation and proliferation as well as promotion of tumor growth and malignant transformation, substantial interest in the creation of therapeutic strategies targeting HER1/EGFR and/or its mutant forms has been generated.

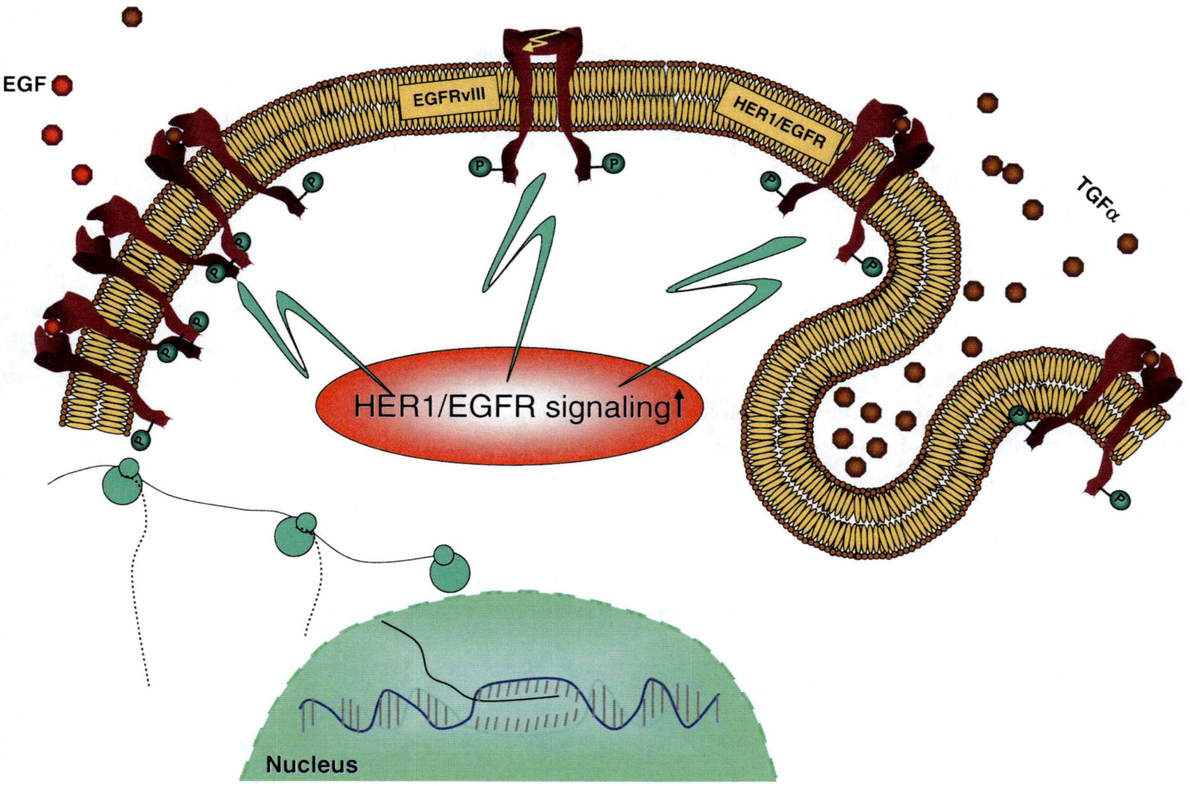

Fig. 32.2 Overview of potential mechanisms leading to dys-regulated HER1/EGFR signaling. Genetic amplification results in HER1/EGFR overexpression. EGFRvIII represents the most frequent mutant form and is characterized by continuous acti-vation independent of ligand-binding. Autocrine overproduction of HER1/EGFR ligands may also lead to independent receptor activation. Abbreviations: EGF, epidermal growth factor; HER1/EGFR, epidermal growth factor receptor; TGFα, trans-forming growth factor α

Therapeutic Options for the Treatment of Glioblastoma

Glioblastoma is the most common primary malignant brain tumor, accounts for more than 50% of all gliomas and is histologically characterized by a high prolif-eration rate, neo-angiogenesis and necrosis. Despite recent advances in diagnostic techniques and treat-ment, the clinical outcome of patients with glioblas-toma continues to be poor. Patients with glioblastoma typically encounter rapid tumor progression or recur-rence leading to death in 75% within 18 months of diagnosis (Gurney and Kadan-Lottick, 2001). The goal to attempt maximal safe surgical tumor resec-tion generally represents the first step in the treatment of glioblastoma according to the current standard of

care. However, maximal safe surgical resection means that the surgical procedure may have to be performed with limited radicality thus, sparing eloquent brain in order to avoid severe postoperative neurological deficits. Surgery is followed by radiotherapy com-bined with concomitant and subsequent chemotherapy with temozolomide (Temodar®/Temodal®, Schering Corporation, Kenilworth, NJ, USA.). Adjuvant admin-istration of 50–60 Gy of whole brain irradiation was shown by several randomized studies to increase survival by 14–36 weeks, irrespective of the extent of surgical tumor removal (Walker et al., 1980). Chemotherapy was initially found to provide only a modest therapeutic benefit. However, a new therapeu-tic standard of care was established when Stupp et al. showed in a randomized controlled trial that in patients with newly diagnosed glioblastoma administration of temozolomide given concomitantly with and subsequently to radiation therapy significantly increased 2-year survival from 10.4 to 26.5% and median survival from 12.1 to 14.6 months when compared to adjuvant radiation therapy alone (Stupp et al., 2005). But still, the prognosis of patients with glioblastoma remains grim as outlined by the fact that progression-free survival and overall survival were only 6.9 and 14.6 months, respectively.

Despite aggressive treatment only few patients are cured. Once tumors recur, life expectancy decreases drastically and therapeutic options are even more limited. If feasible, gross tumor resection should repeatedly be attempted. However, the risk of neurological deficits due to normal brain tissue injury increases significantly in face of progressive tumor invasion. Thus, repeated extensive tumor resection might not always be a reasonable approach. Local chemotherapy by placement of polifeprosan 20/carmustine (Gliadel Wafer, Guilford Pharmaceuticals, Baltimore, MD, USA.) implants at the site of tumor resection is associated with an increased survival of 2–3 months (Brem et al., 1995). For some patients stereotactic radiosurgery to focus radiation on the tumor bed to avoid damage to healthy surrounding tissue might be an option. However, for the most part survival is prolonged only modestly. Conventional chemotherapy does not provide significantly better outcome either, and resistance to chemotherapy is frequently encountered. Most published studies examining the effect of chemotherapy in recurrent glioblastoma were conducted prior to the introduction of temozolomide as a first-line therapeutic agent.

Nitrosoureas such as carmustine (BCNU) or lomustine (CCNU) were the most commonly used chemotherapeutics in the setting of recurrent glioblastoma, for more than three decades. Brandes et al. showed a response rate of 15% and a progression-free 6-months survival of 17.5% after adjuvant BCNU in a phase II clinical trial (Brandes et al., 2004). Another drug that has been frequently used for recurrent malignant glioma is procarbazine, an oral alkylating agent. A 30% response rate was reported for patients with recurrent malignant glioma receiving procarbazine in combination with CCNU and vincristine. Irinotecan (Camptosar®, Pfizer Pharmaceuticals, New York, NY, USA.), a topoisomerase I inhibitor, is one of the newer drugs that have been used in recurrent glioma. Response rates ranging from 2.2 to 16% were shown by several clinical studies and progression-free survival after 6 months was reported to be 25–43% (Raymond et al., 2003; Reardon et al., 2005).

Lately, anti-angiogenic agents were re-introduced for the treatment of recurrent malignant glioma. Application of bevacizumab (Avastin®, Genentech Inc., San Francisco, CA, USA.), a humanized monoclonal antibody targeted to vascular endothelial growth factor, showed promising clinical results. In a phase II study, 20 of 35 patients with recurrent glioblastoma who received a combined regimen of bevacizumab and irinotecan showed at least partial response. The 6-months overall survival rate was 77%, and the 6-months progression-free survival rate was 46%. In a randomized phase II trial comparing a larger population of patients with recurrent glioblastoma that received either bevacizumab without ($n = 85$) or with irinotecan ($n = 82$), response rates of 28.2–37.8% and 6-months progression-free survival rates of 42.6–50.3% with a median overall survival of approximately 9 months were achieved (Cloughesy et al., 2005).

In summary, despite vast progress in the medical field, no substantial improvement with regard to the clinical outcome of patients with glioblastoma was achieved over the last 50 years. However, growing knowledge about the biology of glioblastoma and its aberrant signaling pathways has revealed new promising targets for a possibly more successful therapy.

HER1/EGFR as a Target in the Treatment of Glioblastoma

There are two major subclasses of glioblastoma that are distinguished. Primary glioblastoma arise in a de novo fashion from normal glial cells or their precursors. Secondary glioblastoma are much less frequently encountered and develop by progression from a preexisting lower-grade glioma. Approximately 95% of all glioblastoma are estimated to be of primary origin, and only 5% may arise secondarily. On the molecular level, HER1/EGFR overexpression is found in about 60% of primary glioblastoma and in only 10% of secondary glioblastoma. Similarly, gene amplification of HER1/EGFR has been shown to be five times higher in primary glioblastoma when compared to secondary glioblastoma. In contrast, the frequency of inactivated p53 is significantly lower in primary glioblastoma than in secondary glioblastoma. Thus, amplification and overexpression of an oncogene versus inactivation of a tumor suppressor gene represents a major molecular difference between both glioblastoma subtypes. Dysregulation of multiple molecular pathways seems to be a prerequisite for the genesis of glial tumors. HER1/EGFR is the most frequently amplified gene in glioblastoma. Data from in vitro studies show that HER1/EGFR stimulates tumor growth, invasion and migration. Moreover, clinical data suggest that HER1/EGFR amplification is related to decreased overall survival and worse prognosis in patients with glioblastoma (Lund-Johansen et al., 1990; Shinojima et al., 2003).

EGFRvIII is the most common HER1/EGFR mutant form. Downstream signaling is enhanced due to constitutive TK activity in EGFRvIII. Data from bioptic glioblastoma specimens suggest concomitant overexpression of both EGFRvIII and HER1/EGFR in most of the tumors. However, in about 90% of glioblastoma, amplification and/or overexpression of EGFRvIII was exceeded by that of the wild-type receptor (Biernat et al., 2004). It was shown in a murine model of human glioma xenografts that EGFRvIII expression was related to increased proliferation, inhibition of apoptosis and tumor formation. These findings were confirmed by other studies which identified activation of the MAPK/ERK1/2 and PI3-K/Akt pathways as driving forces of cellular proliferation and tumor progression, thus explaining worse outcomes of patients with EGFRvIII-positive glioblastoma. In addition, in a murine model of intracranially xenografted glioblastoma cells, administration of a monoclonal antibody targeting EGFRvIII (mAb 806), resulted in a significant decrease of tumor growth, increase of apoptosis and prolongation of survival. In conclusion, the survival of glioblastoma cells overexpressing HER1/EGFR or EGFRvIII might depend on an enhanced HER1/EGFR-mediated downstream signaling and its interruption may cause cellular death or increase the cellular response towards other therapies. Therefore, different approaches have been developed to specifically inhibit dysregulated HER1/EGFR-mediated signaling at various levels. Such strategies include for example inhibition of ligand-binding to HER1/EGFR and subsequent TK activation by specific antibodies or targeting of regulatory elements in signal transduction by specific inhibitors.

Small-Molecule HER1/EGFR TK Inhibitors

HER1/EGFR TK inhibitors such as erlotinib (Tarceva®, Genentech Inc., San Francisco, CA, USA.) or gefitinib (Iressa®, AstraZeneca Pharmaceuticals, Wilmington, DE, USA.) are the most clinically advanced HER1/EGFR-targeted agents for the treatment of glioblastoma. These molecules compete reversibly with adenosine triposphate to bind to the intracellular catalytic TK domain of HER1/EGFR thus, inhibiting autophosphorylation of the receptor as well as further downstream signaling involving PI3-K/Akt and MAPK pathways. For the treatment of glioblastoma most experience exists for erlotinib and gefitinib. Both agents specifically inhibit HER1/EGFR, while erlotinib additionally inhibits EGFRvIII. In experimental studies, erlotinib was found to be more effective in the setting of glioblastoma than gefitinib. EGFRvIII expression in transformed glioblastoma cells was significantly diminished upon long-term exposure to erlotinib. In addition, induction of certain genes encoding pro-invasive proteins was inhibited. Experimental studies showed that the extent of erlotinib-mediated inhibition of anchorage-independent growth of glioblastoma-derived cell lines correlates inversely with the cellular capability to induce HER1/EGFR mRNA, emphasizing the important role of HER1/EGFR in the pathogenesis of glioblastoma (Halatsch et al., 2004). Gefitinib is most effective against tumors expressing HER1/EGFR with mutations in exons 19 and 21 of the TK domain, an alteration that is lacking in glioblastoma. This fact may partly explain why gefitinib exerts minor inhibitory effects on glioblastoma cells than erlotinib.

In the clinical setting, erlotinib as well as gefitinib were shown to fit a reasonable safety profile in phase I trials. Both drugs were generally well tolerated. In terms of clinical efficacy, Vogelbaum et al. showed in a phase II study examining 16 patients with recurrent glioblastoma combined partial response and stable disease rates of 25% (Vogelbaum et al., 2004). However, Raizer et al. reported in another phase II trial a median progression-free survival of only 12 weeks for patients receiving erlotinib monotherapy upon glioblastoma relapse. Similarly, hopes were disappointed by a randomized, controlled phase II trial published by van den Bent et al. Only 11.4% of the patients with recurrent glioblastoma treated with erlotinib were free of progression after 6 months compared to 24.1% of the patients treated with temozolomide or BCNU (van den Bent et al., 2007). Moreover, there was no significant difference in overall survival between the two treatment groups (7.7 months for the erlotinib group versus 7.3 months for the temozolomide/ BCNU group).

Clinical data on the efficacy of gefitinib in the setting of glioblastoma is even more controversial. In one phase II trial, 13% of the patients had a progression-free survival for more than 6 months (Rich et al., 2004). However, no objective response or significant increase in progression-free survival or median overall survival was found in comparison to historical controls. The North American Brain Tumor Consortium showed in another phase I/II trial a partial response in 13% of the patients with recurrent glioblastoma receiving prior radiotherapy (Lieberman et al., 2004). Noteworthy, to date neither for gefitinib nor for erlotinib clinical response could be correlated to HER1/EGFR gene amplification or EGFRvIII mutation.

Thus, a significant breakthrough in the treatment of glioblastoma is not obvious from the existing trials despite promising clinical findings with regard to response and stable disease rates in some trials especially for erlotinib. Changing the strategy towards a combined therapy of TK inhibitors and other targeted agents or conventional adjuvant therapies might increase the clinical benefit for patients suffering from glioblastoma. In a first phase I trial, simultaneous inhibition of upstream (HER1/EGFR) by erlotinib and downstream mediators of PI3-K signaling by sirolimus was examined in patients with recurrent high-grade glioma (Reardon et al., 2006). Thirty-eight percent of the patients showed stable disease, and 6% of the patients showed partial response within a median follow-up period of 35.2 weeks. In addition, identification of molecular signatures of yet unknown glioblastoma subgroups might lead to the identification of patients who will benefit most.

HER1/EGFR-Targeted Antibodies

Targeting antibodies to the extracellular domain of HER1/EGFR in order to prevent receptor-activating ligand binding represents a different strategy that is being studied for therapeutic use in glioblastoma. Cetuximab (Erbitux[TM], ImClone Systems Inc., New York, NY, USA. and Merck KGaA, Darmstadt, Germany) is one such specific antibody to HER1/EGFR under evaluation. In preclinical studies, systemic treatment with cetuximab was examined using intra- and extracranial xenograft models of highly HER1/EGFR-expressing human glioblastoma. For both intra- and extracranial xenografts, decreased proliferation and increased cell death were found. A phase I/II study combining cetuximab, radiotherapy and chemotherapy with temozolomide for the treatment of patients with primary glioblastoma is ongoing (Combs et al., 2006). TheraCim-hR3 (YM BioSciences Inc., Mississauga, Ontario, Canada), also refered to as nimotuzumab or Theraloc[®] (Oncoscience AG, Wedel, Germany) represents a different humanized antibody targeting HER1/EGFR that has been studied in the setting of malignant glioma. In a phase I/II clinical trial, 24 patients with newly diagnosed high-grade glioma were treated with TheraCim-hR3 in combination with radiotherapy. Complete response was observed in 16%, partial response in 21% and stable disease in 46% of the patients. The same research group reported a median survival of 17.47 months for 29 patients with malignant glioma, including 16 patients with glioblastoma and 13 patients with anaplastic astrocytoma who were treated concomitantly with radiotherapy and once-weekly 200 mg of hR3 intravenously. A multicenter, randomized phase III clinical study, currently evaluates the efficacy of adjuvant combined radiotherapy with concomitant and subsequent temozolomide alone compared to radiotherapy plus concomitant and subsequent temozolomide plus nimotuzumab (Theraloc[®]) in newly diagnosed glioblastoma.

Another therapeutic approach uses the specific binding properties of antibodies to direct noxious substances such as toxins or radioisotopes against HER1/EGFR-expressing tumors. ^{125}I-MAb 425 is a monoclonal antibody targeted against HER1/EGFR and labelled with iodine 125. It was shown in a phase I/II clinical trial that administration of ^{125}I-MAb 425 combined with radiotherapy resulted in a significantly increased median survival in patients with glioblastoma when compared to a control group receiving radiotherapy alone (Quang and Brady, 2004). Similar, conjugates of toxins such as Pseudomonas exotoxin A and HER1/EGFR-binding antibodies were shown to have good affinity, stability and cytotoxicity.

Antibodies represent molecules with high molecular weight. Thus, penetration of the blood-brain barrier

Fig. 32.3 Schematic illustration of convection enhanced delivery. Catheters are placed during surgery into the resection cavity. A perfusing system is connected to the intracranial catheters and delivers the drug to the site of tumor resection in order to maintain positive pressure. Thereby, drug distribution into the surrounding tissue is enhanced

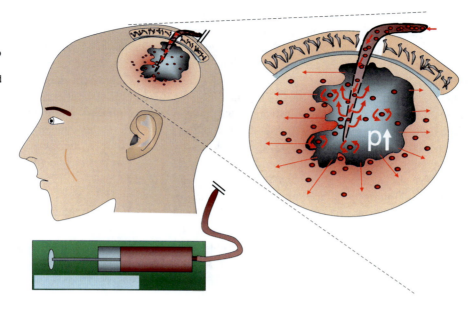

might not be sufficient to effectively treat brain tumors despite increased local permeability. The therapeutic concentrations in the tissue of interest are often insufficient, even when therapeutic agents are applied intra-operatively at the site of tumor resection. In order to overcome this problem, convection-enhanced delivery was developed (Fig. 32.3). This method is based on maintenance of positive pressure at the site of drug administration to enhance the spatial distribution of the drugs. The therapeutic agent is getting pumped into the site of tumor resection by surgically placed catheters. Preclinical evaluation of convection-enhanced delivery using immunotoxins in tumor models showed promising results (Hall et al., 2003). In clinical phase I and II studies, convection-enhanced delivery was shown to be efficient and well-tolerated by patients with glioblastoma. However, to date the clinical effect of this mode of delivery on disease control and outcome is not sufficiently evaluated.

RNA-Based Therapeutic Strategies

Several methods such as ribozymes, antisense RNA and RNA interference have been developed to interfere with genetic transcription or translation. Ribozymes are subsets of small RNA molecules that catalytically cleave certain RNA substrates in a site-specific manner. Sequence-specific recognition occurs through complementary flanking sequences whereas cleavage is mediated by a catalytic core. Hammerhead and hairpin ribozymes are the best characterized naturally occuring ribozyme types. Ribozymes can be delivered to tumor cells by means of a viral vector or by a plasmid. The advantage of using a retrovirus as a vector is that the ribozyme is integrated and expressed in proliferating tumor cells only. Thus, unwanted side-effects caused by inhibition of target gene expression in quiescent cells are avoided. In preclinical studies, the malignant phenotypes of transformed glioblastoma cells and fibroblasts were shown to be inhibited by EGFRvIII-targeted ribozymes. Retrovirus-mediated transfer of anti-EGFRvIII hairpin ribozymes into U87MG.EGFRvIII cells resulted in >90% reduction of EGFRvIII mRNA (Halatsch, 2001; Halatsch et al., 2000). In addition, anchorage-independent growth of U87MG.EGFRvIII cells was significantly inhibited.

Interference with translation and protein synthesis of HER1/EGFR can also be obtained by administration of antisense RNA. In preclinical studies, HER1/EGFR expression was shown to be reduced by HER1/EGFR antisense RNA which was associated with increased survival when compared to controls (Zhang et al., 2002). In addition, in an orthotopic murine xenograft model of human glioblastoma, injection of viral or plasmid vectors expressing EGFRvIII-targeted antisense RNA into the tumor yielded reduction of tumor volume (Shir and Levitzki, 2002).

RNA interference (RNAi) is another method to inhibit gene expression. This approach is based on suppression of homologous genes and induction of sequence-specific mRNA degradation by small interfering RNAs (siRNAs). In an experimental study, siRNAs targeting the intracellular TK domain of the human HER1/EGFR were transfected into human U251 glioma cells and produced 90% downregulation of the HER1/EGFR (Kang et al., 2006). Moreover, transfection with siRNA caused arrest of the cells in G2/M phase, delaying cell cycle progression and thereby inhibiting proliferation. In addition, an in vivo study using an U251 xenograft model showed that mice treated with in situ injections of siRNA had a 19% reduction in subcutaneous tumor volume and significantly decreased HER1/EGFR expression when compared to controls. In another murine model evaluating the effect of RNAi, targeting of HER1/EGFR in intracranial brain tumors resulted in extended survival by almost 90% (Zhang et al., 2004). However, conflicting data exist from an in vivo study of HER1/EGFR-targeted siRNA using U378MG and LN18 glioma cell lines. This approach resulted in specific down-regulation of HER1/EGFR mRNA and protein levels by 70–90% without exerting inhibitory effects on cell proliferation or migration, implying the presence of HER1/EGFR-independent proliferation (Vollmann et al., 2006). Thus, the potential value of RNAi as a therapeutic approach needs to be further explored.

EGFRvIII Targeted Vaccination Therapy

Based on the clinical observation that cerebral metastases were often resistant to immunotherapy despite good therapeutic response of certain extracerebral cancers, the brain was regarded as an immunologically privileged organ in the past. This postulate was supported in addition by experimental studies in rats showing that intracranially implanted tumors were much less frequently rejected in comparison to subcutaneously implanted tumors. However, the facts that gliomas are often infiltrated by inflammatory cells and that subcutaneous tumor implants can generate resistance to a subsequent intracranial tumor challenge show that the central nervous system is only partially privileged and rather immunologically highly active.

The concept of creating antitumor vaccines in order to allow immunologic recognition and subsequent elimination of malignant cells seems quite appealing. There is little data on HER1/EGFR-targeted vaccination therapy for the treatment of intracranial tumors. However, several experimental studies were conducted to examine if immunization against EGFRvIII may provide a benefit for the treatment of intracranial tumors. In a murine model, a conjugate of a peptide comprising the tumor-specific mutated segment of EGFRvIII (PEP-3) and keyhole limpet hemocyanin (KLH) was vaccinated (Heimberger et al., 2003). Mice intracerebrally injected with EGFRvIII-transfected murine melanoma cells (K1735EGFRvIII) and prior immunization with PEP-3-KLH showed a 173% increased median survival time when compared to controls. Moreover, vaccination with PEP-3-KLH in already established intracerebral tumors resulted in a 26% increase of median survival, thus demonstrating efficacy in a clinically more relevant setting. In another experimental study, Ashley et al. showed that immunization of mice with transfected allogenic 300.19/EGFRvIII cells induced a major histocompatibility complex class I-restricted response against EGFRvIII-bearing syngeneic B16-F10 melanoma or 560 astrocytoma cells that were implanted intracranially. In addition, median survival of vaccinated animals was significantly increased upon intracranial tumor challenge when compared to controls.

Clinical data about vaccination therapy in the setting of glioblastoma is sparse overall. In a phase II trial (ACTIVATE), 18 patients with newly diagnosed EGFRvIII-positive glioblastoma were treated with PEP-3-KLH (CDX-110, Celldex Therapeutics, Needham, MA, USA.) administered intradermally. Prior to vaccination, all patients underwent resection of at least 95% of the T1-gadolineum enhancing component of the tumor and chemoradiotherapy with concurrent temozolomide. Vaccination therapy was initiated by three doses given 2 weeks apart followed by monthly vaccinations for maintenance therapy. Median overall survival was shown to be 26 months (versus 15.2 months) and median time-to-progression 14.2 months (versus 6.3 months). In another phase II study (ACTII), patients underwent the same treatment regimen as mentioned before for the ACTIVATE trial but received in addition maintenance chemotherapy with temozolomide. Median overall survival was reported to be 23.2 months (versus 15.2 months) and median time-to-progression 15.2 months (versus 6.3 months). Unfortunately, both previously mentioned studies were compared to a historical control group. However, a randomized, controlled, multi-center phase II/III trial is being currently sponsored by Cellldex and evaluates the PEP-3-KLH (CDX-110) vaccination in a similar setting as the previous phase II studies. This study design may hopefully allow a better estimate of the real clinical benefit exerted by the PEP-3-KLH (CDX-110) vaccination.

Vaccination with oncolytic viruses targeting their deleterious potential to tumor cells seems like another intriguing approach. Attenuated vaccine strains of measles virus were shown to have potent antitumor activity against gliomas. In a murine xenograft model of EGFRvIII-overexpressing glioblastoma, intratumoral treatment with two EGFRvIII-retargeted measles virus strains resulted in tumor regression and a significant prolongation of median survival (Allen et al., 2006). In vitro assays confirmed specific binding and fusion of the viruses with tumor cells expressing EGFRvIII (U118-EGFRvIII, GBM6, GBM39), sparing non-EGFRvIII-expressing tumor cells (U118, GBM14) as well as normal human astrocytes and fibroblasts. Thus, a fundamental prerequisite for specific viral gene therapy targeted to EGFRvIII-expressing glioblastoma has been met. However, the safety and efficacy of virotherapy needs to be further evaluated by clinical studies in the setting of glioblastoma.

Factors Determining Response To HER1/EGFR TK Inhibitors

Despite the fact that the results from experimental studies examining the effect of HER1/EGFR TK inhibitors in glioblastoma were very promising, data from clinical studies were rather disappointing. A significant discrepancy was observed between HER1/EGFR overexpression (found in 40–50% of patients with glioblastoma) and the clinical response to TK inhibition (found in only 10–20% of the patients). This missing concordance between overexpression of HER1/EGFR and clinical response led to the hypothesis that susceptibility to HER1/EGFR TK inhibitors might depend on a multifactorial genetic predisposition.

A variety of clinical studies were set out to identify genetic markers that correlate to clinical response. Mellinghoff et al. conducted a retrospective clinical study examining expression of HER1/EGFR, EGFRvIII and phosphatase and tensin homolog deleted on chromosome 10 (PTEN), a tumor suppressor protein that negatively regulates the PI3-K pathway, in tumor specimens of patients with recurrent malignant glioma, previously treated with gefitinib or erlotinib (Mellinghoff et al., 2005). Coexpression of EGFRvIII and PTEN was significantly associated with clinical response to TK inhibitors. This finding was confirmed by in vitro experiments using human U87MG glioblastoma cell lines transfected with PTEN and EGFRvIII. In another study using an orthotopic xenograft model, eleven different patient-derived glioblastoma xenografts were injected intracranially into mice, followed by treatment with erlotinib at a dose of 100 or 150 mg/d. A survival benefit from erlotinib treatment was found for two xenografts (GBM12, GBM39). Both xenografts expressed aberrant HER1/EGFR along with wild-type PTEN. However, in one xenograft (GBM6) sharing identical HER1/EGFR and PTEN properties with GBM 39 response to erlotinib was missing. In addition, Brown et al. showed in a phase I/II trial of patients with newly diagnosed glioblastoma receiving erlotinib in combination with radiation therapy and temozolomide that concomitant presence of PTEN expression and HER1/EGFR amplification or EGFRvIII were not predictive for survival. Thus, coexpression of mutated HER1/EGFR and wild-type PTEN seems to be important for the responsiveness of glioblastoma to HER1/EGFR TK inhibition but its presence does not guarantee positive response. On the other hand, loss of PTEN seems to be associated with resistance to HER1/EGFR TK inhibitors. However, since only half of glioblastoma are expressing wild-type PTEN it seems likely that more complex molecular signatures are associated with response to HER1/EGFR TK inhibitors.

Experimental studies have examined the effects of inhibition of downstream key regulators such as mTOR and PI3-K in addition to the treatment with HER1/EGFR TK inhibitors. PTEN-deficient U87 and SF295 glioblastoma cells that were treated with rapamycin, an mTOR inhibitor and erlotinib showed significantly increased anti-proliferative effects when compared to cells receiving erlotinib alone (Wang et al., 2006). PTEN-deficient SF295 cells receiving dual therapy showed a 38% reduction in proliferation versus a 14% reduction in proliferation seen in cells treated with erlotinib alone. Monotherapy with rapamycin showed similar results as treatment with erlotinib alone. In a different study, a novel mTOR/PI3-K inhibitor (PI-103) was used allowing combined inhibition of both mTOR and PI3-K (Karpel-Massler et al., 2009). The antiproliferative effects of inhibition of mTOR and PI3-K in combination with erlotinib in PTEN-mutant glioma cells were even more pronounced when compared to erlotinib combined with either mTOR or PI3-K inhibition. In conclusion, multi-targeting might represent a key feature of a future therapeutic strategy to overcome resistance to HER1/EGFR TK inhibitors in the treatment of glioblastoma. Other studies will need to clarify whether additional, yet unidentified molecules within the signal transduction cascade further modulate clinical response to HER1/EGFR TK inhibitors.

Discussion

HER1/EGFR has been studied as a potential therapeutic target for the treatment of different human cancers for more than 20 years now. For glioblastoma there is striking evidence that dysregulated HER1/EGFR contributes to tumorigenesis. Thus, multiple strategies were developed to target HER1/EGFR or its mutant form EGFRvIII as antineoplastic measure including TK inhibitors, monoclonal antibodies, radio-immuno or ligand-toxin conjugates, RNA-based therapies and vaccines. The agents that are farthest along in research and clinical use are TK inhibitors such as erlotinib and gefitinib. Experimental and early clinical studies showed very promising results. However, translation into clinical practice failed. Van den Bent et al. showed in a first randomized, controlled clinical trial that, independent of HER1/EGFR expression status or presence of EGFRvIII, patients with recurrent glioblastoma had insufficient activity of erlotinib. Interestingly, there is a high variability in clinical response between individuals treated with HER1/EGFR TK inhibitors. Differences in the molecular biology of the individual tumors may partly explain this phenomenon and determine the extent of susceptibility towards HER1/EGFR TK inhibitors. Loss of PTEN is one such molecular

event that was shown to correlate to decreased response to treatment with HER1/EGFR TK inhibitors despite HER1/EGFR overexpression. Further identification of molecular determinants for susceptibility and resistance to HER1/EGFR TK inhibitors represents an inevitable prerequisite for the pursuit of this approach in order to achieve success.

More recent studies suggest that a multi-targeted approach directed at a combined inhibition of downstream molecular key factors such as PI3-K and/or additional inhibition of multiple PI3-K activating receptor tyrosine kinases (RTKs) may allow to overcome resistance towards a treatment with HER1/EGFR TK inhibitors alone. In an experimental setting, therapeutic response was significantly improved in PTEN-deficient cells that were treated with erlotinib and rapamycin (Wang et al., 2006). A different preclinical study showed co-activation of multiple RTKs for 19 out of 20 glioma cell lines. Downstream signaling was not influenced by specific inhibition of only one RTK. But concomitant inhibition of two RTKs caused a decrease in PI3-K activation and viability of U87MG.EGFRvIII cells. Data on clinical efficacy of a multi-targeted therapeutic approach are awaited.

An analysis of more than 80 brain tumor specimens including 40 WHO grade IV astrocytomas revealed a direct correlation between the extent of co-overexpression of HER1/EGFR, insulin-like growth factor-binding protein 2 (IGFBP2) and the hypoxia-induced transcription factor 2-alpha (HIF2A) and the histological grade as well as survival (Scrideli et al., 2007). It remains to be elucidated if the status of the EGFR/IGFBP2/HIF2A pathway might represent a useful indicator for clinical prognosis or if additional inhibition of the members of this pathway might prove a clinical benefit. Moreover, other HER1/EGFR-related pathways that are contributing to the dysregulated state of the tumor cell homeostasis might be discovered in the future and allow for the development of new therapeutic approaches.

From a current point of view, a combination therapy with different drugs targeting HER1/EGFR signaling at multiple levels appears to be most promising. An important focus of this multi-drug approach will be likely set on molecules causing resistance to HER1/EGFR-targeted agents.

Despite growing knowledge about the molecular mechanisms underlying resistance to HER1/EGFR-targeted therapeutics, the biological effects of

HER1/EGFR-inhibiting agents on glioblastoma cells are still only partially understood. Thus, manipulation of the molecular biology of the cancerous cell needs to be regarded as a sensitive issue and done with great care.

References

Allen C, Vongpunsawad S, Nakamura T, James C, Schroeder M, Cattaneo R, Giannini C, Krempski J, Peng K, Goble J, Uhm J, Russell S, Galanis E (2006) Retargeted oncolytic measles strains entering via the egfrviii receptor maintain significant antitumor activity against gliomas with increased tumor specificity. Cancer Res 66:11840–11850

Biernat W, Huang H, Yokoo H, Kleihues P, Ohgaki H (2004) Predominant expression of mutant EGFR (egfrviii) is rare in primary glioblastomas. Brain Pathol 14:131–136

Brandes A, Tosoni A, Amista P, Nicolardi L, Grosso D, Berti F, Ermani M (2004) How effective is BCNU in recurrent glioblastoma in the modern era? A phase II trial. Neurology 63:1281–1284

Brem H, Piantadosi S, Burger P, Walker M, Selker R, Vick N, Black K, Sisti M, Brem S, Mohr G (1995) Placebo-controlled trial of safety and efficacy of intraoperative controlled delivery by biodegradable polymers of chemotherapy for recurrent gliomas. The polymer-brain tumor treatment group. Lancet 345:1008–1012

Cloughesy T, Yung A, Vrendenberg J, Aldape K, Eberhard D, Prados M, Vandenberg S, Klencke B, Mischel P (2005) Phase II study of erlotinib in recurrent GBM: molecular predictors of outcome. J Clin Oncol 23:115s (Abs. 1507)

Combs S, Heeger S, Haselmann R, Edler L, Debus J, Huber P, Thilmann C (2006) Treatment of primary glioblastoma multiforme with cetuximab, radiotherapy, and temozolomide (GERT)-phase I/II trial study protocol. BMC Cancer 6:133

Gurney J, Kadan-Lottick N (2001) Brain and other central nervous system tumors: rates, trends, and epidemiology. Curr Opin Oncol 13:160–166

Halatsch M-E (2001) Selective ribozyme-mediated inhibition of 801-bp deletion-mutant *EGFR* mrna expression in human cancers. Signal 2:12–16

Halatsch M-E, Gehrke E, Vougioukas V, Bötefür I, Efferth T, Gebhardt E, Domhof S, Schmidt U, Buchfelder M (2004) Inverse correlation of *epidermal growth factor receptor* messenger RNA induction and suppression of anchorage-independent growth by OSI-774, an epidermal growth factor receptor tyrosine kinase inhibitor, in glioblastoma multiforme cell lines. J Neurosurg 100:523–533

Halatsch M-E, Schmidt U, Behnke-Mursch J, Unterberg A, Wirtz C (2006) Epidermal growth factor receptor inhibition for the treatment of glioblastoma multiforme and other malignant brain tumours. Cancer Treat Rev 32: 74–89

Halatsch M-E, Schmidt U, Bötefür I, Holland J, Ohnuma T (2000) Marked inhibition of glioblastoma target cell tumorigenicity in vitro by retrovirus-mediated transfer of a hairpin ribozyme against deletion-mutant epidermal growth factor receptor messenger RNA. J Neurosurg 92:297–305

Hall W, Rustamzadeh E, Asher A (2003) Convection-enhanced delivery in clinical trials. Neurosurg Focus 14:e2

Heimberger A, Crotty L, Archer G, Hess K, Wikstrand C, Friedman A, Friedman H, Bigner D, Sampson J (2003) Epidermal growth factor receptor III peptide vaccination is efficacious against established intracerebral tumors. Clin Cancer Res 9:4247–4254

Kang C, Zhang Z, Jia Z, Wang G, Qiu M, Zhou H, Yu S, Chang J, Jiang H, Pu P (2006) Suppression of EGFR expression by antisense or small interference RNA inhibits U251 glioma cell growth in vitro and in vivo. Cancer Gene Ther 13:530–538

Karpel-Massler G, Schmidt U, Unterberg A, Halatsch M (2009) Therapeutic inhibition of the epidermal growth factor receptor in high-grade gliomas – where do we stand? Mol Cancer Res 7:1000–1012

Lieberman F, Cloughesy T, Fine H, Kuhn J, Lamborn K, Malkin M, Robbins H, Yung W, Wen P, Prados M (2004) NABTC phase I/II trial of zd-1839 for recurrent malignant gliomas and unresectable meningiomas. J Clin Oncol 22:1510

Lund-Johansen M, Bjerkvig R, Humphrey P, Bigner S, Bigner D, Laerum O (1990) Effect of epidermal growth factor on glioma cell growth, migration, and invasion in vitro. Cancer Res 50:6039–6044

Mellinghoff IK, Wang MY, Vivanco I, Haas-Kogan DA, Zhu S, Dia EQ, Lu KV, Yoshimoto K, Huang JHY, Chute DJ, Riggs BL, Horvath S, Liau LM, Cavenee WK, Rao PN, Beroukhim R, Peck TC, Lee JC, Sellers WR, Stokoe D, Prados M, Cloughesy TF, Sawyers CL, Mischel PS (2005) Molecular determinants of the response of glioblastomas to EGFR kinase inhibitors. N Engl J Med 353:2012–2024

Nishikawa R, Ji X, Harmon R, Lazar C, Gill G, Cavenee W, Huang H (1994) A mutant epidermal growth factor receptor common in human glioma confers enhanced tumorigenicity. Proc Natl Acad Sci USA 91:7727–7731

Quang T, Brady L (2004) Radioimmunotherapy as a novel treatment regimen: ^{125}I-labeled monoclonal antibody 425 in the treatment of high-grade brain gliomas. Int J Radiat Oncol Biol Phys 58:972–975

Raymond E, Fabbro M, Boige V, Rixe O, Frenay M, Vassal G, Faivre S, Sicard E, Germa C, Rodier J, Vernillet L, Armand J (2003) Multicenter phase II study and pharmakokinetic analysis of irinotecan in chemotherapy-naive patients with glioblastoma. Ann Oncol 14:603–614

Reardon D, Quinn J, Vredenburgh J, Gururangan S, Friedman A, Desjardins A, Sathornsumetee S, Herndon Jn, Dowell J, McLendon R, Provenzale J, Sampson J, Smith R, Swaisland A, Ochs J, Lyons P, Tourt-Uhlig S, Bigner D, Friedman H, Rich J (2006) Phase I trial of gefitinib plus sirolimus in adults with recurrent malignant glioma. Clin Cancer Res 12:860–868

Reardon D, Quinn J, Vredenburgh J, Rich J, Gururangan S, Badruddoja M, Herndon Jn, Dowell J, Friedman A, Friedman H (2005) Phase II trial of irinotecan plus celecoxib in adults with recurrent malignant glioma. Cancer 103: 329–338

Rich J, Reardon D, Peery T, Dowell J, Quinn J, Penne K, Wikstrand C, VanDuyn L, Dancey J, McLendon R, Kao J, Stenzel T, Ahmed Rasheed B, Tourt-Uhlig S, Herndon Jn,

Vredenburgh J, Sampson J, Friedman A, Bigner D, Friedman H (2004) Phase II trial of gefitinib in recurrent glioblastoma. J Clin Oncol 22:133–142

Scrideli C, Carlotti C Jr, Mata J, Neder L, Machado H, Oba-Sinjo S, Rosemberg S, Marie S, Tone L (2007) Prognostic significance of co-overexpression of the EGFR/IGFBP-2/HIF-2a genes in astrocytomas. J Neurooncol 83:233–239

Shinojima N, Tada K, Shiraishi S, Kamiryo T, Kochi M, Nakamura H, Makino K, Saya H, Hirano H, Kuratsu J, Oka K, Ishimaru Y, Ushio Y (2003) Prognostic value of epidermal growth factor receptor in patients with glioblastoma multiforme. Cancer Res 63:6962–6970

Shir A, Levitzki A (2002) Inhibition of glioma growth by tumor-specific activation of double-stranded RNA-dependent protein kinase PKR. Nat Biotechnol 20:895–900

Stupp R, Mason W, van den Bent M, Weller M, Fisher B, Taphoom M, Belanger K, Brandes A, Marosi C, Bogdahn U, Curschmann J, Janzer R, Ludwin S, Gorlia T, Allgeier A, Lacombe D, Cairncross J, Eisenhauer E, Mirimanoff R (2005) Radiotherapy plus concomitant and adjuvant temozolomide for glioblastoma. N Engl J Med 352:987–996

van den Bent M, Brandes A, Rampling R, Kouwenhoven M, Kros J, Carpentier A, Clement P, Klughammer B, Gorlia T, Lacombe D (2007) Randomized phase II trial of erlotinib (E) versus temozolomide (TMZ) or BCNU in recurrent glioblastoma multiforme (GBM): EORTC 26034. J Clin Oncol 25:18S Abs. 2005

Vogelbaum M, Peereboom D, Stevens G (2004) Phase II trial of the EGFR tyrosine kinase inhibitor erlotinib for single agent therapy of recurrent glioblastoma multiforme: interim results. Proc Am Soc Clin Oncol 23:115

Vollmann A, Vornlocher H, Stempfl T, Brockhoff G, Apfel R, Bogdahn U (2006) Effective silencing of EGFR with rnai demonstrates non-EGFR dependent proliferation of glioma cells. Int J Oncol 28:1531–1542

Walker M, Green S, Byar D, Alexander EJ, Batzdorf U, Brooks W, Hunt W, MacCarty C, Mahaley MJ, Mealey JJ, Owens G, Ransohoff Jn, Robertson J, Shapiro W, Smith KJ, Wilson C, Strike T (1980) Randomized comparison of radiotherapy and nitrosoureas for the treatment of malignant glioma after surgery. N Engl J Med 303:1323–1329

Wang M, Lu K, Zhu S, Dia E, Vivanco I, Shackleford G, Cavanee W, Mellinghoff I, Cloughesy T, Sawyers C, Mischel P (2006) Mammalian target of rapamycin inhibition promotes response to epidermal growth factor receptor kinase inhibitors in PTEN-deficient and PTEN-intact glioblastoma cells. Cancer Res 66:7864–7869

Zhang Y, Zhang Y, Bryant J, Charles A, Boado R, Pardridge W (2004) Intravenous RNA interference gene therapy targeting the human epidermal growth factor receptor prolongs survival in intracranial brain cancer. Clin Cancer Res 10:3667–3677

Zhang Y, Zhu C, Pardridge W (2002) Antisense gene therapy of brain cancer with an artificial virus gene delivery system. Mol Ther 6:67–72

Chapter 33

Epidermal Growth Factor Receptor Inhibition as a Therapeutic Strategy for Glioblastoma Multiforme

Nikhil G. Thaker and Ian F. Pollack

Abstract Because of the poor responsiveness of glioblastoma multiforme to conventional therapies, there is a need to identify novel therapeutic strategies to improve patient survival. Growth factors, growth factor receptors, and their signal transduction pathways are normally implicated in cell survival and proliferation, and in tumor cells, aberrant regulation of these pathways is common and may effect tumorigenesis. Given the high frequency of mutations of the epidermal growth factor receptor (EGFR) and its downstream signaling pathways, including the phosphatidylinositol 3-kinase (PI3K) and the mammalian target of rapamycin (mTOR), several cell signaling pathways are being targeted by novel molecularly targeted therapies. In this chapter, we discuss the currently available therapeutic modalities targeting these pathways, including small molecule tyrosine kinase inhibitors, monoclonal antibodies, vaccines, ligand-toxin conjugates, radioimmunoconjugates, nuclear targeting through RNA-based therapies such as RNA interference, ribozymes, and antisense RNA, and inhibitors of intracellular signaling molecules, such as PI3K and mTOR inhibitors. Effective use of these therapies will likely necessitate combinatorial strategies of these agents and conventional therapies, which will ultimately rely on an understanding of the molecular features specific to the patient's tumor.

Keywords Epidermal growth factor · EGF receptor · Glioblastoma multiforme · Malignant glioma · Molecularly targeted therapeutics

Introduction

Glioblastoma multiforme (GBM) is a World Health Organization grade IV astrocytoma and is the most common primary malignant brain tumor in adults. GBM is characterized by a high degree of cellularity, necrosis, vascular proliferation, and anaplasia, and despite improvements in neuroimaging, surgery, and other therapeutic modalities, the prognosis for patients with GBM remains poor, with a median survival time of diagnosis of 14.6 months (Stupp et al., 2005).

Several cell signaling pathways have been implicated in tumorigenesis and glioma progression, and the epidermal growth factor receptor (EGFR), which is amplified and/or mutated in approximately 40 – 50% of GBM, may represent a particularly important contribution to this dysregulated proliferation. Given its high frequency alteration and association with a malignant phenotype, EGFR and its downstream signaling pathways, including the phosphatidylinositol 3-kinase (PI3K) and the mammalian target of rapamycin (mTOR), are being targeted by several novel therapeutic modalities, which have entered clinical trials. Because these therapies will likely be effective in only specific subsets of tumors, biological subgroups of glioma remain to be defined and

N.G. Thaker (✉)
Departments of Neurosurgery, Pharmacology and Chemical Biology, Children's Hospital of Pittsburgh, University of Pittsburgh School of Medicine, University of Medicine and Dentistry of New Jersey, New Jersey Medical School, Lyndhurst, NJ, USA
e-mail: thakerng@umdnj.edu

optimal combination therapy approaches need to be assessed and validated. In this chapter, we discuss the molecular biology and function of EGFR and its downstream signaling pathways in malignant glioma (MG) and the currently available therapeutic modalities targeting these signaling pathways. These novel therapies include tyrosine kinase inhibitors (TKI), monoclonal antibodies (mAb), vector-based therapy, vaccine therapy, and nuclear targeting through post-transcriptional/translational inhibition.

EGFR Family

EGFR is one of a family of tyrosine kinase (TK) receptors that belongs to the HER family, which includes EGFR (also known as erbB1, HER1, human EGFR-1, the cellular homolog of the v-erbB oncogene), erbB2 (HER2/neu), erbB3 (HER3), and erbB4 (HER4). EGFR is ubiquitously expressed in non-hematopoietic tissues and is the most common receptor in the EGFR family that is expressed in cancer cells. EGFR is a 170 kD cell-surface receptor that incorporates an extracellular domain that interacts with a ligand, a transmembrane domain that anchors the receptor to the cell membrane, and an intracellular TK domain that interacts with downstream signaling components. The TK is defective in erbB3/HER3, and erbB2/HER2 is an orphan receptor that does not activate with EGF family ligand binding. Dysregulation of these receptors is frequently seen in human cancers, and because of their pivotal role in tumorigenesis, they represent a promising anti-cancer target. Poor prognosis, tumor progression, and decreased sensitivity to chemotherapies have been associated with overexpression, amplification, or constitutive activation of EGFR. In theory, EGFR-targeted therapies may be more effective than conventional therapies because of their selective targeting of cancer cells compared to normal cells.

The ligands for these receptors include EGF, transforming growth factor-α (TGF-α), and amphiregulin, which all bind exclusively to EGFR; heparin-binding EGF and betacellulin, which both bind to EGFR and erbB4; heregulin, which binds to erbB3 and erbB4 and heterodimers with erbB2; and epiregulin, which binds to all receptors except erbB2 homodimers. HER2/neu is the only member of the EGFR/HER family that does not bind ligand. In general, ligands bind to two of the same receptors (homodimerization) or two different EGFR family receptors (heterodimerization) simultaneously, resulting in structural modification of the receptor molecule. This transmembrane protein is normally activated by ligand binding to its extracellular receptor domain, which subsequently allows intracellular cross phosphorylation of TK subunits of each receptor and activation of intracellular substrates, which contribute to signal transduction, cell proliferation, and invasion. Thus, ligand binding or constitutive signaling through EGFR can provide cells with a growth advantage under certain conditions. Three major pathways are activated by EGFR activation: Ras-Raf-mitogen-activated protein kinase (MAPK) pathway, phosphatidylinositol-3-kinase (PI3K)/Akt pathway, and the Janus kinase (JAK) and signal transducer and activator of transcription (STAT) pathway (Fig. 33.1), which will be described below.

EGFR and Malignant Glioma

GBM can be categorized into two groups based on clinical presentation. Primary, or "de novo", GBM represent 95% of all GBMs, present as advanced cancers that are histologically malignant at diagnosis, and generally arise in older patients. Secondary GBMs represent 5% of all GBM, show malignant progression from an antecedent lower-grade tumor, and are usually found in younger patients. Interestingly, these two subclassifications of GBM are associated with different sets of molecular alterations. Most primary GBM have genetic alterations in *EGFR*, phosphatase and tensin homolog deleted on chromosome 10 (*PTEN*), murine double minute 2 (*MDM2*), *p16INK4α*, and loss of chromosome 10. These mutations are less common in secondary glioblastomas, which have overexpression and amplification of platelet-derived growth factor receptor (*PDGFRα*), loss of chromosomes 19q and 9q, and mutations of *TP53* and *IDH1* or *IDH2*. However, the majority of secondary MG exhibit high levels of EGFR expression, despite the absence of gene amplification, which suggests that excessive EGFR

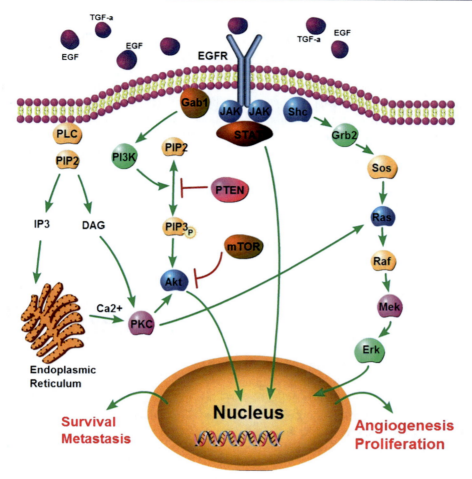

Fig. 33.1 Schematic depiction of receptor-mediated signaling and signal transduction in response to EGF/TGF-α binding to EGFR, highlighting the complexity of parallel pathways transmitting signals for growth, gene transcription, and survival, which are then mediated by effectors within the nucleus. EGF, epidermal growth factor; EGFR, epidermal growth factor receptor; Sos, son of sevenless; MEK, mitogen-activated protein kinase kinase; ERK, extracellular signal-related kinase; mTOR, mammalian target of rapamycin; PI3K, phosphatidylinositol-3-kinase; PKC, protein kinase C; PTEN, phosphatase and tensin homolog deleted on chromosome 10; STAT, signal transducer and activator of transcription protein; Raf, murine leukemia viral oncogene homolog; Ras, rat sarcoma viral oncogene homolog; AKT, protein kinase B; MAPK, mitogen activated protein kinase; PIP2, phosphatidylinositol 4,5-bisphosphate; PIP3, phosphatidylinositol (3,4,5)-trisphosphate

signaling may also contribute to proliferation, malignancy, and survival. Although EGFR amplification occurs in 40–50% of GBM, this alteration is present in only 10% of AA, suggesting that this change may contribute to the final stages of glioma progression by enhancing cell proliferation when substrate availability becomes limited in the tumor environment.

In some tumors with EGFR amplification, the *EGFR* gene is also rearranged, leading to constitutively active mutants. In approximately 40% of tumors with *EGFR* amplification, the gene has a deletion of exons 2–7 that causes a defect in the extracellular ligand binding domain, leading to ligand-independent constitutive activation. This truncated variant receptor, known as EGFRvIII, has a molecular mass of 145 kD versus 170 kD and may be an independent prognostic factor for poor survival outcome. This mutation frequently occurs in glioma, ovarian and breast carcinoma, non-small cell lung cancer (NSCLC), and other types of cancers. Other mutants have been described. For instance, mutations involving exons 18–21 effect increased sensitivity to TK inhibitors, while an amino acid change at codon 790 is associated with resistance to the small molecule TKI gefitinib.

Furthermore, the potential role of EGFR overexpression in gliomagenesis has been supported by several preclinical models. For instance, overexpression of mutant EGFR in neural progenitors or astrocytes induces the formation of tumors with histological features of GBM, and antibody-based therapies targeted at wild-type or mutant EGFR family members have shown efficacy in preclinical glioma models and have, therefore, provided a rationale for clinical translation of these targeted approaches.

Cell-Surface Interaction

The cellular response to ligand binding is mediated by cell-surface receptors. Binding of a ligand to the receptor induces conformational changes within the receptor, receptor cross-linking, and phosphorylation of intracellular tyrosine residues. Phosphorylation further activates the TK and exposes binding sites for intracellular adaptor molecules, such as Shc and Grb2 (growth factor receptor binding protein 2) (Fig. 33.1). These binding sites are Src homology 2 (SH2) domains that consist of phosphorylated tyrosine in the context of a longer amino acid motif. These adaptor molecules associate with exchange factors, such as Sos (son of sevenless), via Src homology 3 (SH3) domains. In turn, these exchange factors activate the Ras family by exchanging the nucleotide guanosine diphosphate (GDP) for guanosine triphosphate (GTP). For this to occur, Sos binds to GDP-Ras, which causes dissociation of GDP and binding of GTP to the Ras-Sos complex. Ras is active when GTP is bound. Excessive activation and signaling through this pathway has been implicated in the development of several human tumors, where mutation of a *RAS* gene results in a constitutively active protein. Although such activating mutations are rare in MG, Ras activity is markedly elevated due to dysregulation at the growth factor receptor level.

In addition to activation of the Ras pathway (above), growth factor receptors also activate several parallel signaling pathways (Fig. 33.1). For instance, PI3K and

phospholipase C-γ (PLCγ) are important molecules in phospholipid metabolism and are recruited to the activated TK receptor by adaptor proteins, such as Gab1. Activated PLCγ produces important intermediates such as diacylglycerol (DAG) and inositol 1,4,5-triphosphate (IP$_3$). IP$_3$ stimulates the release of intracellular calcium, which when combined with DAG, can activate protein kinase C (PKC). In turn, PKC may activate Ras, and therefore stimulate cell proliferation and survival through an alternative mechanism than that described above. Additionally, PI3K phosphorylates phosphatidylinositol 4,5-bisphosphate (PIP2) to phosphatidylinositol (3,4,5)-trisphosphate (PIP3), which then leads to activation of Akt and subsequent cell survival. Several of these pathways are described in detail below.

Signal Transduction

MAPK Cascade

Following the aforementioned cell-surface interactions, downstream signals can reach the nucleus through several mechanisms (Fig. 33.1). The MAPK cascade is one of the most important pathways that involves at least three separate kinases: Raf (MAPKKK), MEK (MAP/ERK kinase, also known as MAPKK), and ERK (MAPK, extracellular signal regulated kinase).

The most proximal kinase in the cascade is Raf, which includes at least three members. Raf is a serine/threonine kinase and is the cellular homolog of a viral oncogene that is capable of inducing transformation if overexpressed. Raf is activated by phosphorylation and in turn phosphorylates and activates MEK, which is a tyrosine and serine/threonine kinase. MEK subsequently activates ERK by phosphorylating tyrosine and threonine residues. Downstream effects of this cascade include activation of mediators that regulate transcription, translation, and cytoskeletal rearrangement, which has implications in cell motility. These mediators include other kinases that are grouped as MAPK-activated protein kinases (MAPKAPK), such as ribosomal S6 kinase. These mediators can directly modulate transcription by activation of the transcription regulatory factors Fos, Jun, Myc, and Elk-1 or activate translation by activating the ribosomal S6 protein. Furthermore, these mediators can also down-regulate transcription by activating glycogen synthase kinase 3 (GSK3).

Similar pathways exist in parallel with the MAPK pathway that conveys signals in response to stress or injury. One such pathway is the Jun terminal kinase (JNK) pathway, which may be activated by Ras-related G-proteins, such as Rac. This is followed by activation of p21Ras-related protein activated kinase (PAK), which in turn activates a cascade of intermediate signaling molecules that activate MAPKAPK-related kinases and nuclear effectors, such as Jun, to modulate DNA synthesis and transcription. Certain JNK isoforms are overexpressed and activated in glioma, implicating their role in glioma cell survival. In addition, the involvement of other Ras-activated G-proteins, such as Rac and Rho, may contribute to changes in cell motility.

Significant cross-talk may also exist between these signaling cascades. For example, several kinase constituents of the MAPK pathway can activate similar downstream targets, such as cytoplasmic kinases, transcription factors, and cell cycle checkpoint control elements. These pathways also interact with cAMP-dependent protein kinases, with cell cycle regulatory kinases, and with apoptotic signaling cascades to influence other regulators of cell homeostasis, proliferation, and death. Thus, the different cascades converge on similar downstream targets to regulate cell homeostasis, indicating that cellular response to stimuli may depend on the cell-type-specific profile of activated signaling elements.

Akt-Mediated Signaling

Another major downstream signaling pathway involves PI3K-induced activation of Akt (Fig. 33.1). PI3K are heterodimeric phospholipid kinases that comprise a regulatory subunit and a catalytic subunit. Upon activation, PI3K stimulates phosphorylation of phosphatidylinositol 4,5-bisphosphate (PIP2) to phosphatidylinositol (3,4,5)-trisphosphate (PIP3), which then leads to translocation of PDK1 and Akt. Akt is a serine/threonine kinase that is phosphorylated at a serine 473 and threonine 308 residues. Activated Akt phosphorylates several proteins involved in cell survival, such as Bad, glycogen synthase kinase,

mTOR, and forkhead transcription factor. The tumor suppressor PTEN normally negatively regulates the activation status of Akt by converting the active PIP3 to the inactive PIP2. Deactivating mutations or loss of *PTEN*, however, is common among primary GBM.

PLCγ/PKC-Mediated Signaling

Downstream activation of PKC via PLCγ-mediated production of calcium (Ca^{2+}) and DAG represents a third important signaling pathway (Fig. 33.1). PKC is a family of serine/threonine kinases that consists of approximately 10 isoenzymes, which can be further divided into three subgroups based upon their mechanisms of activation. The first group consists of four "conventional" or "classical" PKC isoenzymes (α, βI, βII, and γ), which require Ca^{2+}, a phospholipid such as phosphatidylserine (PS), and DAG for activation. The second group includes five "novel" PKC isoforms (δ, ε, η(L), θ, and μ). These isoforms lack the Ca^{2+}-binding domain and thus do not require Ca^{2+} for activation, although they do require DAG. The third group comprises two "atypical" PKC isoenzymes (ζ and ι), which require neither calcium nor DAG, but only PS for activation.

Depending upon the isoforms that are activated, PKC can lead to diverse cellular effects, such as cell proliferation and survival. For instance, intracellular effectors, such as Ras, Raf, and ERK, may be phosphorylated and activated by PKC to subsequently transduce a proliferative signal to the nucleus. Levels of PKC α and ε expression and activity, which may be several orders of magnitude greater in astrocytoma or MG than normal astrocytes, have been shown to correlate with the proliferative status of normal and neoplastic astrocytes. Not surprisingly, exposure of cells to EGF produces increased PKC activity that parallels increases in DNA synthesis, and pharmacological inhibition of PKC-mediated signaling blocks glioma proliferation and induces apoptosis.

Stat-Mediated Signaling

EGFR can also activate members of the signal transducers and activators of transcription (STAT) family, which translocate to the nucleus to directly influence transcription, the cell cycle, and cell survival (Fig. 33.1). STATs can be activated by a variety of intermediates, including receptors, Janus kinase (JAK), or other Src family members. In general, dysregulation of STAT-mediated signaling may lead to tumor survival and increased angiogenesis. Multiple isoforms of STAT proteins exist (STAT1, STAT2, STAT3, STAT4, STAT5A, STAT5B, and STAT6), which have diverse effects on cell growth, survival, and differentiation. For instance, STAT3 leads to proliferative and antiapoptotic effects, and its constitutive activation has been reported in glioma.

EGFR Inhibition as a Therapeutic Strategy for GBM

Cell survival, growth, and proliferation are normally regulated by growth factors, growth factor receptors, and multiple signal transduction pathways. However, in tumor cells, cell survival and growth may rely on constitutive activation of one or a few of these pathways as an indirect consequence of an abnormality in growth factor receptor signaling, which implies that greater selectivity and reduced therapeutic toxicity can potentially be achieved by direct inhibition of growth factor receptors and their downstream pathways. Thus, inhibition of EGFR activation or its downstream components, such as Ras, PI3K, PKC, and mTOR, is a promising strategy in glioma therapy. Several approaches exist for targeting EGFR/HER1, including small molecule TK inhibitors (TKIs), monoclonal antibodies (mAb), vaccines, ligand-toxin conjugates, radio-immunoconjugates, RNA-based therapies, and inhibitors of intracellular signaling, such as PI3K and mTOR inhibitors. A brief summary of several promising therapies is provided below and in Fig. 33.2.

Small Molecule EGFR TKI

A current approach for growth factor targeted inhibition involves a novel class of anti-cancer small molecule inhibitors that prevent activation of receptor TKs and their intracellular signaling pathways.

TKIs are low molecular weight compounds that competitively inhibit the ATP-binding sites involved in receptor activation. Initial applications of this approach used natural products, such as genistein or staurosporine, which were only minimally selective, and limited the clinical applicability of these agents. However, next-generation inhibitors have been developed from the quinazoline and pyrrolopyrimidine classes of chemicals to allow greater selectivity for one or more receptor TKs. This greater selectivity and low molecular weight have raised clinical expectations that systemic delivery of these agents could achieve blood-brain barrier penetrance and tumor-selective targeting. The most clinically advanced TKIs include gefitinib (Iressa, ZD1839, AstraZeneca) and erlotinib (Tarceva, OSI-774, Genentech), which are both reversible EGFR-targeting TKIs.

Gefitinib is currently approved for the treatment of advanced or metastatic NSCLC in patients who failed previous chemotherapy. This agent has been tested in MG and is effective in blocking EGFR-dependent cell signaling in cell lines that rely heavily on EGFR activation for proliferative stimulation and tumor growth. However, it has virtually no effect on EGFR-independent proliferation. Treatment with gefitinib is also associated with reduction in angiogenic factors, growth inhibition, and radiosensitization with traditional cytotoxic agents. It is well-absorbed orally and is active against EGFR at nanomolar concentrations, with significantly less activity against other EGFR members such as erbB2/HER2. This compound has also been shown to accumulate in GBM tissue at higher concentrations than plasma (Hofer et al., 2006).

Initial clinical studies reported that gefitinib was well-tolerated at effective doses, with common toxicities being an acneiform skin rash and diarrhea. Results from several clinical studies for non-central nervous system (CNS) solid tumors demonstrated activity of gefitinib as a single-agent (Fukuoka et al., 2003), although a phase III clinical study for advanced small-cell lung cancer failed to demonstrate a convincing benefit of adding this agent to conventional treatments (Herbst et al., 2004). Not surprisingly, recent reports have demonstrated that response to gefitinib is strongly influenced by tumor EGFR status, with a high percentage of objective responses among patients with EGFR mutations (Lynch et al., 2004), which confirms that this agent may well be a selective inhibitor in a subgroup of tumors. In several patients treated with

Fig. 33.2 Mechanisms of EGFR inhibition. EGFR inhibition occurs extracellularly through mAb binding, ligand binding, ligand-toxin conjugate binding, and vaccine therapy. Intracellular inhibition occurs through inhibition of tyrosine kinase phosphorylation by TK inhibitors. Nuclear targeting inhibits translation of EGFR mRNA through ribozyme and siRNA/antisense RNA therapies. mAb, monoclonal antibodies; siRNA, short interfering RNA; TK, tyrosine kinase; TGF-α, transforming growth factor – alpha; EGF, epidermal growth factor

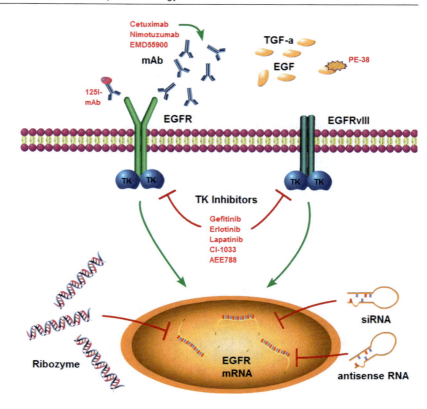

gefitinib who were noted to have objective therapeutic responses, mutational analysis showed that tumor specimens had mutations within the EGFR gene, generally involving gain-of-function changes close to the ATP-binding pocket of the TK domain (Lynch et al., 2004). These observations highlight the importance of determining the tumor genotype and phenotype for analyzing therapeutic responses and designing clinical trials.

Importantly, the type of receptor mutation may significantly influence the effect of gefitinib. Although increased therapeutic efficacy may be observed with specific types of mutations, the variant EGFRvIII may confer reduced sensitivity to gefitinib in in vivo brain tumor models (Heimberger et al., 2002), since this variant receptor is constitutively active independent of ligand binding. Additionally, alternative downstream signaling pathways that drive tumor proliferation may counteract the upstream inhibitory effect of these agents. For instance, *PTEN* mutations will counteract the effect of TKI due to sustained activity of downstream growth and survival signaling, which ultimately requires multiple signaling inhibitors to achieve an anti-tumor effect.

Several phase I/II studies of gefitinib have been initiated in patients with GBM and have included analysis of receptor expression and receptor mutational status to correlate with treatment responses. In a phase II study, 12.7% of patients had partial tumor regression, although the median times to progression were not better than historical controls (Lieberman et al., 2004). Furthermore, another phase II study by the North Central Cancer Treatment Group (NCCTG) had noted some radiographic responses but no superior survival benefits (Uhm et al., 2004). In another study for recurrent GBM, the median progression-free survival (PFS) was 2 months, the PFS at 6 months (PFS6) was 13%, and the median overall survival (OS) was 10 months, with no observed radiographic response (Rich et al., 2004). Studies are also in progress to determine whether combinations of gefitinib with conventional chemotherapeutic agents, such as temozolomide (TMZ), may enhance efficacy.

Erlotinib has also been tested in clinical trials for glioma. This agent inhibits EGFR autophosphorylation and cell growth at concentrations in the range of 20 nM, and higher concentrations are capable of inducing apoptosis. This agent is associated with a reasonable safety and toxicity profile that is comparable to gefitinib, and a phase II study in patients with NSCLC demonstrated tumor response (Perez-Soler, 2004). However, as with gefitinib, median PFS for these patients was no better than historical control data. Although Peereboom and colleagues (2010) found that the combination of erlotinib with TMZ and concurrent radiotherapy was well tolerated, it was unclear if outcomes improved.

Efforts have been made to determine whether a mutational profile could distinguish responders from non-responders. It has been noted that responses have been seen in tumors that had EGFR amplification and low levels of Akt or the variant EGFRvIII and preservation of PTEN, thereby suppressing constitutive Akt activation. In fact, long-term exposure to erlotinib may decrease expression of EGFRvIII in neoplastic cells. However, gefitinib had little to no activity against tumors expressing the EGFRvIII variant (Heimberger et al., 2002), though it may work best against tumors with a mutation in exons 18–21 of EGFR, which are more commonly found in NSCLC but lacking in glioma. Given the fact that responses were observed in only a subset of patients with gliomas, research efforts are in progress to determine whether a consistent molecular signaling profile exists to help distinguish responders from non-responders, and a more detailed analysis of receptor and signaling pathway mutations is necessary to identify a biologically relevant subset of patients for treatment.

Other Small Molecule EGFR TKI Inhibitors

A number of other small molecule inhibitors of EGFR are currently in soon to begin clinical trials in patients with brain tumors, including lapatinib (an EGFR/HER2 inhibitor), AEE788 (EGFR/ErbB2 and vascular endothelial growth factor receptor [VEGFR] inhibitor) and vandetanib (a VEGFR/EGFR inhibitor). Lapatinib (GW572016, GlaxoSmithKline) is a reversible EGFR inhibitor that has been well tolerated in phase I trials. It has demonstrated activity against erbB2-expressing tumors and distribution into glioma tissue and has recently been administered prior to surgical resection, with subsequent tumor analysis for suppression of EGFR and other downstream signaling molecules. CI-1033 (Pfizer Inc, Groton, CT)

and EKB-569 (Wyeth-Ayerst Laboratories, St. Davids, PA) are irreversible pan-EGFR inhibitors with activity against other erbB family members that may induce cell cycle arrest and apoptosis in EGFR-expressing cells. Toxicities have been identical to those of other EGFR inhibitors.

Antibody and Ligand-Based Therapy

Monoclonal antibodies (mAb) and ligand-based therapeutic modalities may prevent EGFR-activating ligand binding and subsequent downstream signaling. Several mAb targeting the extracellular domain of EGFR have been developed. Cetuximab (Erbitux, ImClone Systems, Inc) is a chimeric (mouse/human) monoclonal antibody against EGFR that has been approved for the treatment of patients with metastatic colorectal cancer who are refractory to irinotecan and patients with squamous cell cancer of the head and neck in combination with platinum-based chemotherapy, for first-line treatment of recurrent/metastatic disease, and in combination with radiation therapy when surgery is not possible. This agent has demonstrated pre-clinical antitumor activity in GBM and was effective when administered systemically in intracranial and extracranial models (Eller et al., 2002).

These results have encouraged further clinical development of this agent. A phase I/II clinical study combining cetuximab, TMZ, and radiotherapy (RT) in patients with primary GBM is currently ongoing. Additionally, the combination of cetuximab with either gefitinib or erlotinib yielded better results than with either agent alone and when patients were stratified according to EGFR gene amplification status, cetuximab was well tolerated but had limited activity in patients with recurrent high-grade glioma (Neyns et al., 2009).

Another humanized EGFR-targeted mAb is nimotuzumab (TheraCim-hR3, YM BioSciences Inc. or Theraloc, Oncoscience AG). This agent recognizes the extracellular domain of EGFR and inhibits TK activation. In a recent phase I/II trial, 29 patients with GBM, AA, and anaplastic oligodendroglioma underwent surgery and received nimotuzumab and RT. The antibody was well-tolerated, and there was no evidence of grade 3/4 adverse events. Seventeen percent of the patients had a complete response, 20.7% had a partial response, and 41.4% reached a stable disease. The median survival was 22 months for all patients, with a median survival time of 17 months for GBM (Ramos et al., 2006). A multicenter randomized phase III clinical trial is currently underway.

Another therapeutic approach to targeting EGFR-positive tumors utilizes EGFR-targeted mAbs that have been labeled with radioisotopes or toxic compounds. ^{125}I-mAb 425 is an EGFR-targeted mAb that is conjugated with a radiotherapeutic isotope [125]I. Preclinical studies have shown that ^{125}I-mAb 425 binds to the extracellular domain of EGFR receptors, is then internalized, and ultimately causes chromosomal breaks. In a phase I/II trial, combination therapy with ^{125}I-MAb 425 and RT demonstrated a significant increase in median survival in patients with GBM, when compared to patients treated with RT only (Quang and Brady, 2004).

Another EGFR-targeted approach has implemented immune-toxin conjugates, where specific receptor ligands are conjugated to a toxin gene, such as Pseudomonas exotoxin lacking the cell membrane translocation domain, to deliver targeting toxins to EGFR. The ligand interactions between TGF-α or EGF, for instance, and EGFR provide the basis for internalization of the toxin. TP-38 (IVAX Research, Inc.) is a ligand-conjugate that is composed of TGF-α and PE-38, a mutated Pseudomonas exotoxin. The EGFR receptor is used to selectively deliver this toxin to tumor cells. In a phase I study of 20 patients with recurrent malignant brain tumors, three patients demonstrated a radiographic response and one patient had a complete response with no evidence of tumor after 83 weeks (Sampson et al., 2003). DAB389EGF is another ligand-toxin conjugate that comprises a diphtheria toxin fused to EGF and is selectively toxic to cells that overexpress EGFR. Although this conjugate has shown efficacy in a murine glioma model, further detailed evaluation is awaited.

Compared to the low molecular weight TKI, antibodies are relatively high molecular weight agents that have limited penetration into the tumor due to the blood-brain barrier, which may limit the clinical efficacy of this therapeutic modality. Although blocking the EGFR pathway can interfere with cell proliferation in appropriately selected tumor cell lines and clinical situations, the blood-brain barrier remains a major obstacle to effective systemic administration of mAb and ligand-based therapies. Even direct injection

of these compounds results in slow diffusion through brain parenchyma at a rate that is inversely correlated to the size of the compound, which again severely limits drug distribution of high molecular weight agents. Convection-enhanced delivery (CED) is one strategy for circumventing these blood–brain barrier-related limitations. CED employs slow positive-pressure intraparenchymal infusion of microliter volumes to achieve bulk flow of a large molecular weight protein directly into the brain tumor or into its surrounding microenvironment. Tumor models with immunotoxins have shown improved spatial distribution, and clinical trials have reported that CED is efficient and well tolerated in patients with MG (Hall et al., 2003). However, further studies will be needed to identify the clinical relevance of this therapeutic delivery system.

Vaccine and Viral Therapy

Antitumor vaccines allow the immune system to recognize malignant cells and produce an immune response to eliminate them. The variant EGFRvIII has been an attractive target for vaccine therapy in MG. Ashley et al. (1997) demonstrated that immunization with allogeneic 300.19/EGFRvIII cells induced CD8[+] cytotoxic T-lymphocytes against EGFRvIII bearing syngeneic B16-F10 melanoma or 560 astrocytoma cells that had been injected intracranially. Overall, vaccination can generate a significant cytotoxic immune response, which is effective against intracranial tumors.

CDX-110 (PEP-3-KLH, Celldex Therapeutics) is a peptide vaccine that targets the constitutively active EGFRvIII by eliciting a cytotoxic T-cell immune response against tumor cells. In a recent phase II trial by Sampson et al. (2008), patients with newly diagnosed GBM who were EGFRvIII-positive received CDX-110 vaccine monotherapy as adjuvant therapy. Median overall survival was 26 months and the median time to progression was 14.2 months, which were more favorable than historical controls. Similarly, in the ACT II trial, where patients received combination CDX-110 and TMZ therapy, the median OS was 33.3 months and the median time to progression was 16.6 months. Although these results are promising, final results from both trials are eagerly awaited.

Oncolytic virus-based vaccines have also been used to target tumor cells. Attenuated strains of the measles virus have been shown to have anti-glioma effects.

Allen et al. (2006) demonstrated that EGFRvIII re-targeted oncolytic measles strains have significant antitumor activity, increased tumor specificity, and prolonged survival in a murine xenograft model of EGFRvIII-overexpressing GBM. EGFRvIII-retargeted viruses had significant antitumor activity against EGFRvIII-positive GBM but no toxic effect against normal cells. Although future research efforts will be needed to determine the efficacy and safety of this treatment, these preclinical results show significant promise for oncolytic virus-based therapies for glioma.

Inhibition of EGFR Synthesis

Several novel therapeutic strategies have been developed to inhibit the EGFR pathway at the post-transcriptional/translational level by degrading EGFR mRNA. These therapies include RNA interference (RNAi), ribozymes, and antisense RNA. RNAi with small interfering RNA (siRNA) can be used to inhibit gene expression. siRNA are short, double-stranded RNA molecules that induce sequence-specific mRNA transcript degradation and may inhibit cell proliferation by arresting cells in the G2/M phase. siRNA targeting the EGFR mRNA (siEGFR) yielded an 88% increase in survival time in an advanced intracranial brain cancer murine model, a 19% reduction in tumor volume, a decrease in EGFR/HER1 expression in a xenograft mouse model, and conferred cell cycle arrest and inhibition of cell growth and invasion (Kang et al., 2006; Zhang et al., 2004). However, in a study by Vollmann et al. (2006), although EGFR mRNA and protein expression were decreased by 70–90%, this agent did not confer an inhibitory effect on cell proliferation, migration, or activation status of EGFR-associated intracellular signaling cascades. These results demonstrate that glioma cells may continue to proliferate through non-EGFR dependent pathways and that a single-agent therapeutic approach may not be sufficient. Future research efforts will seek clarification of these contradictory studies and the clinical value of RNAi in glioma therapy.

Ribozymes are small RNA molecules that produce site-specific cleavage of RNA and subsequent abrogation of gene expression. Site-specific RNA recognition occurs through complementary flanking sequences, while RNA cleavage is conducted by a catalytic core. A major obstacle with this strategy, however, is delivery to the nucleus. Thus far, a viral-vector or plasmid has been used to deliver ribozymes to tumor cells. More specifically, a retrovirus has been preferably implemented, because this vector ensures that the ribozyme is integrated and subsequently expressed in proliferating cells only (i.e. tumor cells), thereby avoiding toxic effects to normal cells. EGFRvIII-targeted ribozymes can also induce significant reduction of EGFRvIII mRNA, inhibition of GBM tumorigenicity, and reduced proliferation of GBM-derived cell lines. However, given the low transduction efficiency associated with retroviral delivery, alternative nuclear delivery systems will be needed.

Another approach for inhibiting EGFR expression is the use of antisense RNA molecules, which are complementary RNA sequences that form complexes with mRNA to prevent translation and subsequent EGFR synthesis. Several delivery methods have been used, such as the intraoperative or intravenous administration of antisense EGFR RNA with a liposome vector. Zhang et al. (2002) implemented a unique vector for targeted delivery of an RNA-encoding plasmid that comprised a liposome tagged with (1) mAb against the mouse transferrin receptor (to allow transport across mouse tumor vasculature) and (2) mAb against the human insulin receptor (to allow transport across the human cancer cell plasma and nuclear membranes). Reduction of HER1/EGFR expression by HER1/EGFR antisense RNA was associated with increased survival and reduction of tumor volume.

mTOR and PI3K/Akt Inhibitors

Although a comprehensive discussion of intracellular signaling pathway inhibitors is beyond the scope of this chapter, we will briefly review several mTOR and PI3K inhibitors that have been preclinically and clinically developed, due to their increased interest as EGFR pathway-targeted single-agent and combination therapies.

Overexpression of growth factors or deletion of PTEN increases activation of the downstream mTOR. Several mTOR inhibitors are being investigated in clinical trials, including rapamycin (sirolimus, Rapamune, Wyeth), temsirolimus (CCI-779, Wyeth), AP23573 (Ariad), and everolimus (Rad-001, Certican, Novartis). These agents inhibit GBM proliferation in culture and in intracerebral xenografts and are able to penetrate the blood-brain barrier. Temsirolimus binds to the immunophilin FK-506 binding protein 12 (FKBP12) and forms a complex that inhibits mTOR, which results in inhibition of key signaling pathways and cell cycle arrest. This agent has demonstrated some activity as a single-agent and in combination with cisplatin in glioma, and in a recent phase II study, administration of temsirolimus to patients with GBM was well-tolerated and radiographic improvement was evident in some patients (Galanis et al., 2005).

Activation of Akt via PI3K is another major downstream intermediate in growth factor receptor-mediated signaling. Under normal conditions, Akt activation is inhibited by PTEN; however, *PTEN* is mutated in at least 40% of GBMs, which leads to constitutive activation of the PI3K pathway and Akt. The importance of this pathway is demonstrated by the fact that transfer of a wild-type *PTEN* gene to the PTEN-negative U87 glioma cell line suppresses tumor growth. Conversely, increased PI3K/Akt activity has been associated with radiation therapy resistance. Based on these observations, PI3K and Akt appear to be rational therapeutic targets for GBM, and perifosine (Keryx) is one such oral Akt inhibitor that is undergoing study in MG. Inhibitors of PI3K, such LY294002 and wortmannin, have demonstrated promising activity in pre-clinical models, but their toxicity profile or insolubility has precluded clinical use.

Multi-targeted single-agent therapies, however, may have improved pharmaceutical properties, and phase I clinical trials with these agents are currently in progress. NVP-BEZ235 is a novel dual PI3K/mTOR inhibitor that has shown promising inhibitory activity on tumor vasculature, breast cancer growth in cells with activating PI3K mutations, and primary human pancreatic cancer xenografts (Cao et al., 2009). In vivo glioma models treated with this agent have shown antiproliferative activity (Maira et al., 2008), and a phase I trial in patients with solid tumors is currently underway. Additionally, XL765 is a dual PI3K/mTOR inhibitor, and a phase I study in patients with recurrent MG is currently underway.

Inhibition of Angiogenesis and Tumor Invasion

There is growing evidence that EGFR-targeted inhibitors may also have indirect effects on the tumor microenvironment. Recent studies have demonstrated that secretion of VEGF, which is the most potent endothelial cell mitogen, by tumor cells depends significantly on EGFR-mediated signaling and that therapeutic efficacy of EGFR-targeting therapies may, in part, reflect this secondary effect. EGFR activation may up-regulate VEGF and matrix metalloproteinases (MMPs) in various cancers, including squamous cell cancers of the head and neck, malignant glioma, and human prostate, which may confer resistance to EGFR inhibition alone. Conversely, inhibition of EGFR-mediated signaling results in down-regulation of several angiogenic signaling mediators, including VEGFR, IL-8, bFGF, and MMP-9. Thus, an important part of evaluating the therapeutic efficacy of EGFR inhibition requires an understanding of the effects of these agents on the surrounding tumor vasculature.

Combination therapies targeting VEGFR and EGFR, therefore, hold promise for the treatment of glioma. Studies have suggested that combined inhibition of these receptors may be clinically efficacious in tumors where targeting either EGFR or VEGFR alone is ineffective, possibly due to interference of a molecular feedback loop responsible for acquired resistance to EGFR inhibitors. Simultaneous inhibition of these two pathways may also promote cell death through apoptosis, and may ablate tumor angiogenesis. The combination of bevacizumab and erlotinib was reasonably well-tolerated in recurrent MG, with radiographic responses reported in 12 of 25 patients, although it remains uncertain whether the combination offers an improved outcome to bevacizumab alone (Sathornsumetee et al., 2009). Another study has combined cetuximab with irinotecan and bevacizumab and results from this study and several others are eagerly awaited (Lassen, 2007).

EGFR-mediated signaling also has effects on invasion and motility, which may be effects of G-proteins, such as Rac, that influence cytoskeletal organization and MMPs. The variant receptor EGFRvIII has been associated with invasiveness, which is blocked by the

EGFR TKI erlotinib. These observations suggest that constitutive activation of this pathway is important for invasiveness and motility, and inhibition of this pathway with small molecule inhibitors or vector-based therapies may produce a significant reduction of this aggressive phenotype.

EGFR-Targeted Combination Chemotherapies

Given GBM heterogeneity and intrinsic resistance mechanisms to chemotherapeutics, EGFR-targeted single-agent molecularly targeted therapies have been unable to cure patients with MG, and first-generation clinical trials with these agents have fallen short of expectation. Redundancy and parallel processing of growth factor signaling pathways, loss of negative inhibition, mutations leading to the constitutively active EGFRvIII, co-activation of multiple TK receptors, including EGFR, PDGFR, and VEGFR, and limited intracranial drug delivery are the most notable mechanisms of in vitro and in vivo drug resistance. Understanding these major resistance mechanisms will facilitate the formation of rational combinatorial strategies with molecularly targeted therapies.

Given these therapeutic challenges and the multiple resistance mechanisms, combination therapies that target multiple signaling pathways or different components of the same pathway may prove more effective strategies. First, EGFR inhibitors can potentiate the activity of cytotoxic drugs, such as cisplatin, topotecan, gemcitabine, and taxol, and radiation therapy. The application of such combinatorial approaches in brain tumor therapeutics is already under way. In addition to the applicability of combining growth factor receptor-targeted strategies with conventional chemotherapy, recent studies indicate that combinations of growth factor receptor inhibitors with other molecularly targeted approaches may dramatically potentiate efficacy by circumventing intrinsic resistance mechanisms. These therapies include multi-targeting single-agent therapies or multi-targeting multi-agent therapies, both of which are being tested in MG.

Multi-targeting single-agent kinase inhibition is a promising strategy for the treatment of glioma, as discussed above. Targeting multiple signaling pathways in addition to EGFR with multi-targeted single-agent

kinase inhibitors may prove more efficacious than highly specific agents. Of note, AEE788 (EGFR and VEGFR-2 inhibitor, Novartis), vandetanib (EGFR and VEGFR-2, ZD6474, Zactima, AstraZeneca), lapatinib (EGFR/HER1 and HER2/Neu inhibitor), and NVP-BEZ235 (PI3K and mTOR inhibitor) are multi-targeting single-agent molecularly targeted therapies that are in various phases of preclinical and clinical development.

Additionally, multi-targeting multi-agent drug combinations are also a promising strategy for anti-glioma therapy. A strategy for rational combinatorial therapies relies on targeting of downstream intracellular effectors of the EGFR signaling pathway, such as PI3K and mTOR. Rapamycin has a sensitizing effect on EGFR inhibitors in PTEN-deficient and PTEN-intact GBM, and downregulation of Akt may be enhanced by EGFR blockade. However, EGFR may signal to mTOR through PKC, independently of Akt. Thus, inhibition of PKC may lead to decreased survival of glioma cells regardless of PTEN or EGFR status. A preliminary clinical trial with the combination of gefitinib and sirolimus suggested only a modest effect when combining these agents (Reardon et al., 2006), although additional studies are still in progress. In another study that combined gefitinib and everolimus, results were no better than historical controls (Nguyen et al., 2006). In fact, another study concluded that this combination had an increased incidence of toxicities and minimal activity in recurrent MG (Chang et al., 2009). mTOR inhibitors are also being combined with other targeted agents, including AEE788 (EGFR and VEGFR inhibitor), EKB569 (EGFR inhibitor), and sorafenib (VEGFR, PDGFR and Raf kinase inhibitor), and results from these studies are awaited.

An alternative strategy for improving the efficacy of EGFR inhibitors is to target and inhibit parallel signaling pathways, such as Raf, PDGFR, or VEGFR. A phase II study in patients with progressive or recurrent MG is currently underway that is assessing the combined inhibition of EGFR, PDGFR, VEGFR, and Raf with the combination of erlotinib and sorafenib (Peereboom, 2007), and a recent phase I/II study of this combination demonstrated modest response rates (Prados et al., 2009a).

EGFR targeting can also enhance alternative therapeutic modalities, including radiotherapy. Specifically, EGFR mAbs and EGFR-targeting TKIs, such as gefitinib and erlotinib, can effect marked radiosensitization. Increased signaling through the EGFR pathway may enhance resistance to the combination of radiotherapy and chemotherapy, and a rational strategy for overcoming this resistance focuses on the inhibition of the EGFR pathway. In recent phase I/II studies of erlotinib and TMZ with RT in newly diagnosed GBM, patients treated with the combination had better survival than historical controls in one study (Prados et al., 2009b) but no signs of benefit compared with TMZ controls in another study (Brown et al., 2008). In a phase I/II trial in newly diagnosed GBM, the combination of gefitinib and RT did not have an improved outcome compared to historical controls (Chakravarti et al., 2009). Additional studies with these combinations are warranted.

Summary and Future Challenges

Because of the poor responsiveness of MG to conventional therapies, there is a pressing need to identify and implement new treatment approaches to improve patient outcome. Studies have shown that growth factors, growth factor receptors, and their signal transduction pathways normally regulate cell survival, growth, and proliferation, and in tumor cells, alterations of EGFR and its downstream signaling pathways are common. These pathways, therefore, represent a unique opportunity for therapeutic inhibition, and several approaches currently exist for targeting EGFR/HER1, including small molecule TKI, mAb, vaccines, ligand-toxin conjugates, radioimmunoconjugates, RNA-based therapies, such as RNAi, ribozymes, and antisense RNA, and inhibitors of intracellular signaling, such as PI3K and mTOR.

First-generation single-targeted monotherapies with these molecularly targeted therapies, however, have been mostly ineffective in more than a subset of tumors, likely due to the multiple genetic mutations that lead to gliomagenesis and tumor progression. More effective use of these agents will require *combinations* of molecularly targeted therapies and conventional therapies or combinations of several molecularly targeted agents administered as "cocktail" regimens based upon the molecular features specific to the patient's tumor. The number of therapeutic combinations, however, is limitless, and a systematic strategy must be developed to identify promising combinations.

Several strategies are providing novel methods for identifying rational combinations from known drug mechanisms. For instance, genome-wide synthetic lethal screening can be used to identify synergistic drug combinations. A high-throughput RNAi-based screening strategy has offered simultaneous and systematic genome-wide interrogation of the loss-of-function phenotypes associated with protein suppression, and in several pre-clinical studies, this screening strategy has uncovered novel drug combinations in the context of paclitaxel sensitivity, interactions with the Ras oncogene, and PARP inhibition. Furthermore, knowledge of a tumor's mutational profile can be used to determine the most appropriate therapeutic combination.

Targeting other aspects of tumor biology, in combination with conventional therapies or molecularly targeted agents, also holds promise for future therapies. For instance, alterations in a tumor's microenvironment can facilitate cancer growth, progression, recruitment of nonmalignant cells, invasion, and metastasis. Thus, controlling cancer may be achieved indirectly by controlling blood vessels, immune and inflammatory cells, growth factors, and the extracellular matrix, which all constitute the tumor microenvironment. Targeting these aspects of tumor biology in combination with molecularly targeted therapies may provide deeper insight into the interplay between genes and environment in the formation and progression of GBM.

A major ongoing effort is the identification of tumor genotypic and phenotypic features that predict treatment response to EGFR-targeted agents, which holds future promise for selecting patients who are most likely to respond to specific molecularly targeted approaches. The sensitivity of a tumor to a molecularly targeted therapy may be dependent on the specific molecular abnormalities within the tumor, and it is critical to identify markers of response to certain therapies through genomic characterization. For instance, GBM with loss of PTEN and tumors with increased expression of phospho-Akt may be resistant to EGFR inhibitors. However, such tumors may respond to mTOR inhibitors due to activation of the PI3K/Akt pathway. Ultimately, genotyping each patient's tumor through genome-wide characterization studies will enhance our understanding of the molecular changes that drive malignant growth and will guide the rational selection of combination therapies for each patient.

Future studies will also focus on restructuring clinical trials to stratify patients based on tumor genotype. The integration of clinical and molecular information, which is now becoming available through gene expression arrays, proteomics, and molecular imaging, will lead us to a more effective implementation of targeted treatments. Physiological imaging using magnetic resonance spectroscopy, positron emission tomography, and other molecular imaging techniques will provide early insights into treatment efficacy and optimal therapeutic combinations through non-invasive modalities. Future clinical trials utilizing single- and multi-agent molecularly targeted therapies will incorporate tissue analysis to identify the mutations specific to the patient's tumor, making it possible to determine which drug combinations will be most effective for a given tumor.

However, specific challenges remain with respect to the treatment of intracranial tumors. The presence of the blood-brain barrier has complicated the development and implementation of treatment for GBM, since many small-molecule inhibitors and currently available anticancer therapies for GBM poorly penetrate into the CNS and into tumors. Since most current therapies are delivered systemically through oral or intravenous methods, achieving therapeutic concentrations within the brain parenchyma may be challenging. Several methods are being implemented, including convection-enhanced delivery to allow more localized drug delivery to a greater volume of tissue and nanoparticles, which hold promise for improved systemic therapeutic delivery without interfering with normal function of the brain. Improvement in treatment efficacy will rely on future research efforts focusing on these and other avenues of treatment delivery.

Acknowledgment This work was supported in part by NIH grant NSP0140923, the Doris Duke Charitable Foundation, and the American Medical Association.

References

Allen C, Vongpunsawad S, Nakamura T, James CD, Schroeder M, Cattaneo R, Giannini C, Krempski J, Peng KW, Goble JM, Uhm JH, Russell SJ, Galanis E (2006) Retargeted oncolytic measles strains entering via the EGFRvIII receptor maintain significant antitumor activity against gliomas with increased tumor specificity. Cancer Res 66:11840–11850

Ashley D, Sampson J, Archer G, Batra S, Bigner D, Hale L (1997) A genetically modified allogeneic cellular vaccine generates MHC class I-restricted cytotoxic responses against tumor-associated antigens and protects against CNS tumors in vivo. J Neuroimmunol 78:34–46

Brown PD, Krishnan S, Sarkaria JN, Wu W, Jaeckle KA, Uhm JH, Geoffroy FJ, Arusell R, Kitange G, Jenkins RB, Kugler JW, Morton RF, Rowland KM Jr., Mischel P, Yong WH, Scheithauer BW, Schiff D, Giannini C, Buckner JC (2008) Phase I/II trial of erlotinib and temozolomide with radiation therapy in the treatment of newly diagnosed glioblastoma multiforme: north central cancer treatment group study N0177. J Clin Oncol 26:5603–5609

Cao P, Maira SM, Garcia-Echeverria C, Hedley DW (2009) Activity of a novel, dual PI3-kinase/mTor inhibitor NVP-BEZ235 against primary human pancreatic cancers grown as orthotopic xenografts. Br J Cancer 100:1267–1276

Chakravarti A, Berkey B, Robins H, Guha A, Curran W, Brachman D, Shultz C, Mehta M (2009) An update of phase II results from RTOG 0211: A phase I/II study of gefitinib with radiotherapy in newly diagnosed glioblastoma. J Clin Oncol 2006 ASCO Ann Meet Proc 24:1527

Chang SM, Kuhn J, Lamborn K, Cloughesy T, Robins I, Lieberman F, Yung A, Dancey J, Prados M, Wen P (2009) Phase I/II study of erlotinib and temsirolimus for patients with recurrent malignant gliomas (MG) (NABTC 04-02). J Clin Oncol (Meet. Abstr.) 27:2004

Eller JL, Longo SL, Hicklin DJ, Canute GW (2002) Activity of anti-epidermal growth factor receptor monoclonal antibody C225 against glioblastoma multiforme. Neurosurgery 51:1005–1014

Fukuoka M, Yano S, Giaccone G, Tamura T, Nakagawa K, Douillard JY, Nishiwaki Y, Vansteenkiste J, Kudoh S, Rischin D, Eek R, Horai T, Noda K, Takata I, Smit E, Averbuch S, Macleod A, Feyereislova A, Dong RP, Baselga J (2003) Multi-institutional randomized phase II trial of gefitinib for previously treated patients with advanced non-small-cell lung cancer. J Clin Oncol 21:2237–2246

Galanis E, Buckner JC, Maurer MJ, Kreisberg JI, Ballman K, Boni J, Peralba JM, Jenkins RB, Dakhil SR, Morton RF, Jaeckle KA, Scheithauer BW, Dancey J, Hidalgo M, Walsh DJ (2005) Phase II trial of temsirolimus (CCI-779) in recurrent glioblastoma multiforme: a north central cancer treatment group study. J Clin Oncol 23:5294–5304

Hall W, Rustamzadeh E, Asher A (2003) Convection-enhanced delivery in clinical trials. Neurosurg Focus 14:e2

Heimberger AB, Learn CA, Archer GE, McLendon RE, Chewning TA, Tuck FL, Pracyk JB, Friedman AH, Friedman HS, Bigner DD, Sampson JH (2002) Brain tumors in mice are susceptible to blockade of epidermal growth factor receptor (EGFR) with the oral, specific, EGFR-tyrosine kinase inhibitor ZD1839 (iressa). Clin Cancer Res 8:3496–3502

Herbst RS, Giaccone G, Schiller JH, Natale RB, Miller V, Manegold C, Scagliotti G, Rosell R, Oliff I, Reeves JA, Wolf MK, Krebs AD, Averbuch SD, Ochs JS, Grous J, Fandi A, Johnson DH (2004) Gefitinib in combination with paclitaxel and carboplatin in advanced non-small-cell lung cancer: a phase III trial–INTACT 2. J Clin Oncol 22:785–794

Hofer S, Frei K, Rutz HP (2006) Gefitinib accumulation in glioblastoma tissue. Cancer Biol Ther 5:483–484

Kang CS, Zhang ZY, Jia ZF, Wang GX, Qiu MZ, Zhou HX, Yu SZ, Chang J, Jiang H, Pu PY (2006) Suppression of EGFR expression by antisense or small interference RNA inhibits U251 glioma cell growth in vitro and in vivo. Cancer Gene Ther 13:530–538

Lassen U 2007. Cetuximab, bevacizumab and irinotecan for patients with malignant glioblastomas. NIH, Ed Bethesda, MD. http://clinicaltrials.gov/ct2/show/NCT00463073. Accessed 6 Feb 2010

Lieberman FS, Cloughesy T, Fine H, Kuhn J, Lamborn K, Malkin M, Robbins HI, Yung WA, Wen P, Prados M (2004) NABTC phase I/II trial of ZD-1839 for recurrent malignant gliomas and unresectable meningiomas. J Clin Oncol 22:1510

Lynch TJ, Bell DW, Sordella R, Gurubhagavatula S, Okimoto RA, Brannigan BW, Harris PL, Haserlat SM, Supko JG, Haluska FG, Louis DN, Christiani DC, Settleman J, Haber DA (2004) Activating mutations in the epidermal growth factor receptor underlying responsiveness of non-small-cell lung cancer to gefitinib. N Engl J Med. 350:2129–2139

Maira SM, Stauffer F, Brueggen J, Furet P, Schnell C, Fritsch C, Brachmann S, Chene P, De Pover A, Schoemaker K, Fabbro D, Gabriel D, Simonen M, Murphy L, Finan P, Sellers W, Garcia-Echeverria C (2008) Identification and characterization of NVP-BEZ235, a new orally available dual phosphatidylinositol 3-kinase/mammalian target of rapamycin inhibitor with potent in vivo antitumor activity. Mol Cancer Ther 7:1851–1863

Neyns B, Sadones J, Joosens E, Bouttens F, Verbeke L, Baurain JF, D'Hondt L, Strauven T, Chaskis C, In't Veld P, Michotte A, De Greve J (2009) Stratified phase II trial of cetuximab in patients with recurrent high-grade glioma. Ann Oncol 20:1596–1603

Nguyen TD, Lassman AB, Lis E, Rosen N, Shaffer DR, Scher HI, Deangelis LM, Abrey LE (2006) A pilot study to assess the tolerability and efficacy of RAD-001 (everolimus) with gefitinib in patients with recurrent glioblastoma multiforme (GBM). J Clin Oncol (Meet. Abstr) 24:1507

Peereboom DM (2007). Erlotinib and sorafenib in treating patients with progressive or recurrent glioblastoma multiforme. NIH, Ed, Bethesda, MD. http://clinicaltrials.gov/ct2/show/NCT00445588. Accessed 13 Feb 2010

Peereboom DM, Shepard DR, Ahluwalia MS, Brewer CJ, Agarwal N, Stevens GH, Suh JH, Toms SA, Vogelbaum MA, Weil RJ, Elson P, Barnett GH (2010) Phase II trial of erlotinib with temozolomide and radiation in patients with newly diagnosed glioblastoma multiforme. J Neurooncol 2010 May; 98(1):93–99

Perez-Soler R (2004) The role of erlotinib (tarceva, OSI 774) in the treatment of non-small cell lung cancer. Clin Cancer Res 10:4238S–4240

Prados MD, Chang SM, Butowski N, DeBoer R, Parvataneni R, Carliner H, Kabuubi P, Ayers-Ringler J, Rabbitt J, Page M, Fedoroff A, Sneed PK, Berger MS, McDermott MW, Parsa AT, Vandenberg S, James CD, Lamborn KR, Stokoe D, Haas-Kogan DA (2009b) Phase II study of erlotinib plus temozolomide during and after radiation therapy in patients with newly diagnosed glioblastoma multiforme or gliosarcoma. J Clin Oncol 27:579–584

Prados M, Gilbert M, Kuhn J, Lamborn K, Cloughesy T, Lieberman F, Puduvalli V, Robins HI, Lassman A, Wen PY (2009a) Phase I/II study of sorefenib and erlotinib for patients with recurrent glioblastoma (GBM) (NABTC 05-02). J Clin Oncol (Meet. Abstr.) 27:2005

Quang T, Brady L (2004) Radioimmunotherapy as a novel treatment regimen: 125i-labeled monoclonal antibody 425 in the treatment of high-grade brain gliomas. Int J Rad Oncol Biol Phys 58:972–975

Ramos T, Figueredo J, Catala M, González S, Selva J, Cruz T, Toledo C, Silva S, Pestano Y, Ramos M, Leonard I, Torres O, Marinello P, Pérez R, Lage A (2006) Treatment of high-grade glioma patients with the humanized anti-epidermal growth factor receptor (EGFR) antibody h-R3: report from a phase I/II trial. Cancer Biol Ther 5:375–379

Reardon DA, Quinn JA, Vredenburgh JJ, Gururangan S, Friedman AH, Desjardins A, Sathornsumetee S, Herndon JE, Dowell JM, McLendon RE, Provenzale JM, Sampson JH, Smith RP, Swaisland AJ, Ochs JS, Lyons P, Tourt-Uhlig S, Bigner DD, Friedman HS, Rich JN (2006) Phase 1 trial of gefitinib plus sirolimus in adults with recurrent malignant glioma. Clin Cancer Res 12:860–868

Rich JN, Reardon DA, Peery T, Dowell JM, Quinn JA, Penne KL, Wikstrand CJ, Van Duyn LB, Dancey JE, McLendon RE, Kao JC, Stenzel TT, Ahmed Rasheed BK, Tourt-Uhlig SE, Herndon JE, Vredenburgh JJ, Sampson JH, Friedman AH, Bigner DD, Friedman HS (2004) Phase II trial of gefitinib in recurrent glioblastoma. J Clin Oncol 22:133–142

Sampson JH, Akabani G, Archer GE, Bigner DD, Berger MS, Friedman AH, Friedman HS, Herndon Ii JE, Kunwar S, Marcus S, McLendon RE, Paolino A, Penne K, Provenzale J, Quinn J, Reardon DA, Rich J, Stenzel T, Tourt-Uhlig S, Wikstrand C, Wong T, Williams R, Yuan F, Zalutsky MR, Pastan I (2003) Progress report of a phase I study of the intracerebral microinfusion of a recombinant chimeric protein composed of transforming growth factor (TGF)-α and a mutated form of the Pseudomonas exotoxin termed PE-38 (TP-38) for the treatment of malignant brain tumors. J Neurooncol 65:27–35

Sampson JH, Archer GE, Bigner DD, Davis T, Friedman HS, Keler T, Mitchell DA, Reardon DA, Sawaya R, Heimberger AB (2008) Effect of EGFRvIII-targeted vaccine (CDX-110) on immune response and TTP when given with simultaneous standard and continuous temozolomide in patients with GBM. J Clin Oncol 26:2011

Sathornsumetee S, Desjardins A, Vredenburgh JJ, Rich JN, Gururangan S, Friedman AH, Friedman HS, Reardon DA (2009) Phase II study of bevacizumab plus erlotinib for recurrent malignant gliomas. J Clin Oncol (Meet. Abstr.) 27:2045

Stupp R, Mason WP, van den Bent MJ, Weller M, Fisher B, Taphoorn MJB, Belanger K, Brandes AA, Marosi C, Bogdahn U, Curschmann J, Janzer RC, Ludwin SK, Gorlia T, Allgeier A, Lacombe D, Cairncross JG, Eisenhauer E,, Mirimanoff RO (2005) The european organisation for research and treatment of cancer brain tumor and radiotherapy groups, the national cancer institute of canada clinical trials group. Radiotherapy plus concomitant and adjuvant temozolomide for glioblastoma N Engl J Med 352:987–996

Uhm JH, Ballman KV, Giannini C, Krauss JC, Buckner JC, James D, Scheithauer BW, O'Fallon JR, Jaeckle KA (2004) Phase II study of ZD1839 in patients with newly diagnosed grade 4 astrocytoma. J Clin Oncol (Meet. Abstr.) 22:1505

Vollmann A, Vornlocher H, Stempfl T, Brockhoff G, Apfel R, Bogdahn U (2006) Effective silencing of EGFR with RNAi demonstrates non-EGFR dependent proliferation of glioma cells. Int J Oncol 28:1531–1542

Zhang Y, Zhang YF, Bryant J, Charles A, Boado RJ, Pardridge WM (2004) Intravenous RNA interference gene therapy targeting the human epidermal growth factor receptor prolongs survival in intracranial brain cancer. Clin Cancer Res 10:3667–3677

Zhang Y, Zhu C, Pardridge W (2002) Antisense gene therapy of brain cancer with an artificial virus gene delivery system. Mol Ther 6:67–72

Chapter 34

Role of Acyl-CoA Synthetases in Glioma Cell Survival and Its Therapeutic Implication

Tetsuo Mashima and Hiroyuki Seimiya

Abstract Lipid metabolism is frequently up-regulated in cancer cells and is related to tumor growth and malignancy. Particularly, de novo synthesized fatty acids are important in several cellular processes. Acyl-CoA synthetases (ACS) are key enzymes for conversion of the fatty acids to acyl-CoA, an essential step in utilization of the fatty acids. In glioma cells, some of the ACS isozymes are overexpressed and play a critical role in their growth and survival. In addition, inhibition of ACS or lipogenesis induces or enhances glioma cell death. Collectively, these observations suggest that ACS could not only be markers of the cancer but also be potential therapeutic targets.

Keywords Acyl-CoA synthetase · Lipid metabolism · Fatty acid

Introduction

A high rate of lipogenesis is closely linked with cancer pathogenesis since tumor cells require continuous provision of lipids as a source of membrane biosynthesis, as an energy source through β-oxidation, and to produce acylated proteins that are involved in multiple essential processes in signal transduction (Menendez and Lupu, 2007). Cellular fatty acid supply in cancer is largely dependent on de novo biosynthesis (Fig. 34.1). Fatty acid synthase (FASN) plays a key role in the de novo synthesis by generating long-chain fatty acids

from acetyl-coenzyme A (CoA) and malonyl-CoA. In fact, overexpression of FASN or other related mechanisms that cause enhanced lipogenesis are common features in many human cancers, including primary brain cancer (Kuhajda, 2006; Zhao et al., 2006). These observations suggest that the enzymes in the lipid synthesis could be selective markers of tumor and also be potential therapeutic targets (Mashima et al., 2009c).

Acyl-CoA synthetases (ACS) are enzymes that convert long-chain fatty acids to acyl-CoA (Fig. 34.1). This reaction is essential in activation of fatty acid for further metabolism including generation of phospholipid, protein acylation, β-oxidation and other processes (Coleman et al., 2002). Human cells contain 26 genes encoding ACS (Watkins et al., 2007). Depending on the preference of chain length in substrate fatty acid, they are classified into several subfamilies such as short-chain ACS (ACSS), medium-chain ACS (ACSM), long-chain ACS (ACSL), very long-chain ACS (ACSVL) and others, although there are significant overlaps in the chain length specificity between subfamilies. As is described in the following section, some of the ACS isozymes are overexpressed and involved in glioma growth and survival. Moreover, treatments with ACS inhibitor or other lipogenesis inhibitor are shown effective in the suppression of glioma growth.

Expression and Role of ACS Isozymes in Glioma

Among the multiple ACS members, so far, the two isozymes, ACSL5 and ACSVL3, are thought important in gliomagenesis or its malignancy. Therefore, we will focus on these molecules.

H. Seimiya (✉)
Division of Molecular Biotherapy, Cancer Chemotherapy Center, Japanese Foundation for Cancer Research, Tokyo 135-8550, Japan
e-mail: hseimiya@jfcr.or.jp

M.A. Hayat (ed.), *Tumors of the Central Nervous System, Volume 1*,
DOI 10.1007/978-94-007-0344-5_34, © Springer Science+Business Media B.V. 2011

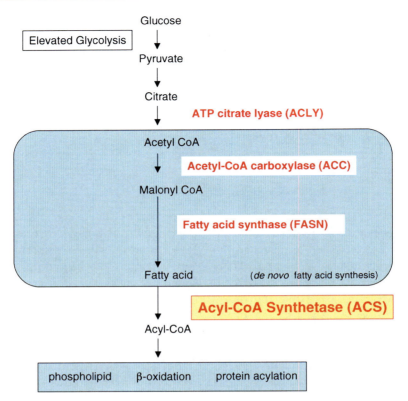

Fig. 34.1 De novo fatty acid synthesis pathway in cancer cells: In cancer cells, increased anaerobic glycolysis is observed (Warburg, 1956). This elevated glucose catabolism produces pyruvate. Pyruvate is converted to citrate and then to acetyl-CoA, which, in turn, is utilized in de novo fatty acid synthesis. ATP citrate lyase (ACLY) is responsible for the conversion of citrate to acetyl-CoA. De novo fatty acid synthesis involves two key enzymes, acetyl-CoA carboxylase (ACC) and fatty acid synthase (FASN). Acyl-CoA synthetases (ACS) act downstream of FASN and convert long-chain fatty acids to acyl-CoA. This reaction is a critical step in several lipid metabolic pathways, including phospholipid production, β-oxidation and protein acylation

(1) ACSL5

ACSL5 is a member of long-chain ACS (ACSL) that activates fatty acid with 12–20 carbons, the major dietary fatty acid. In human, five ACSL genes have been reported (Watkins et al., 2007). The expression in tissues or in organelles and the substrate specificity are different among the isozymes, suggesting distinctive role of each isozyme (Coleman et al., 2002). ACSL5 is a unique enzyme among the long-chain ACS members, since it is the only isozyme that localizes on mitochondria. The human *ACSL5* gene is located on chromosome 10q25.1–q25.2, on which aberrations occur in malignant gliomas (Karlbom et al., 1993; Rasheed et al., 1995; Yamashita et al., 2000). Moreover, it has been reported that the ACSL5 expression is markedly increased in primary glioblastomas of grade IV malignancy

(Yamashita et al., 2000). These observations suggest that ACSL5 plays a role in the pathogenesis of glioma. To test the role of the isozyme, these authors reported the overexpression of the ACSL5 in U87MG glioma cells. They found that the ACSL5 overexpression induced cell growth on exposure to palmitate and increased palmitate uptake (Yamashita et al., 2000). We further analyzed the role of ACSL5 in glioma survival under tumor microenvironment (Mashima et al., 2009b). Extracellular acidosis is one of the tumor microenvironmental stressors that are involved in the malignant progression of tumor (Tannock and Rotin, 1989), while, in order for tumors to survive under the stress conditions, tumor cells have to acquire resistance to the stress-induced cytotoxicity. Gain-of-function (forced overexpression) and loss-of-function (RNAi-mediated knockdown) studies revealed that ACSL5 selectively promotes glioma survival under the extracellular acidosis (Mashima et al., 2009b). We further performed genome-wide gene expression profiling and found that ACSL5 is involved in the expression of some tumor-related factors including midkine, a heparin-binding growth factor overexpressed in multiple cancers. These observations indicate that ACSL5 is a critical factor in glioma growth and survival.

(2) ACSVL3

ACSVL3 is a member of very-long chain ACS subfamily and is also known as SLC27A3 or fatty acid transport protein (FATP)-3. This activates saturated fatty acid of 16-24 carbons. Pei et al. (2009) reported that ACSVL3 was overexpressed in clinical malignant glioma specimens, while it was nearly undetectable in normal glia. This ACSVL3 overexpression was dependent on c-Met and epidermal growth factor receptor (EGFR). More importantly, the inhibition of ACSVL3 expression suppressed both anchorage-dependent and – independent glioma cell growth in vitro and tumor formation in vivo. They further showed that ACSVL3 regulates Akt function. These data show that ACSVL3 is an important factor in the maintenance of the oncogenic properties of malignant glioma cells.

Effect of ACS Inhibitor and Lipogenesis Inhibition on Glioma Growth

Numerous studies have shown that inhibition of lipogenic enzymes causes tumor suppression in several tumor types (Menendez and Lupu, 2007). We previously identified Triacsin c, a selective inhibitor of ACS (Tomoda et al., 1991), as an agent that preferentially induces apoptotic cell death in malignant tumor cells (Mashima and Tsuruo, 2005; Mashima et al., 2005). In human glioma SF268 cells, ACS inhibition by Triacsin c activates mitochondria-mediated intrinsic apoptosis pathway by promoting cytochrome c release from the mitochondria to the cytoplasm and subsequent caspase activation. ACS act as antagonist against the intrinsic cell death pathway and, the combinational treatment with the ACS inhibitor and

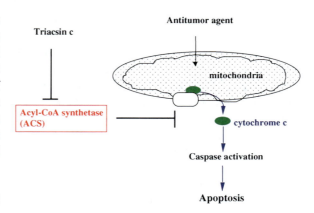

Fig. 34.2 Role of acyl-CoA synthetases (ACS) in cancer cell survival: Several antitumor agents induce apoptosis in cancer cells through mitochondria-mediated intrinsic apoptosis pathway. ACS antagonize this pathway and thereby its inhibition potentiates cell death induction by chemotherapeutic agents (Mashima et al., 2009a)

etoposide, an antitumor agent that induces typical apoptosis, synergistically inhibited glioma cell growth both in vitro and in vivo (Mashima et al., 2009a). These data indicate that ACS is a potential therapeutic target of the cancer (Fig. 34.2). In glioma, it was also reported that the de novo fatty acid synthesis pathway was elevated and FASN inhibition by a selective inhibitor, cerulenin, or by RNAi selectively suppressed glioma cell viability (Zhao et al., 2006). In many cancers including glioma, EGFR/phosphatidylinositol 3'-kinase (PI3K)/Akt/mTOR pathway is elevated and is thought to be selective molecular target of cancer. AMPK regulates this pathway by negatively regulating mTOR. Recently, Guo et al. indicated that an AMPK agonist AICAR inhibits EGFR-overexpressing glioblastoma by inhibiting lipogenesis (Guo et al., 2009). These studies further suggest that lipogenic pathway could play a critical role in the growth factor-mediated cell survival pathway and would be a rational therapeutic target of glioma.

Discussion

As described above, some ACS isozymes are overexpressed in malignant glioma. Moreover, the ACS inhibitor, Triacsin c, induces or enhances cell death in glioma cells, although the specificity of the inhibitor on each ACS isozyme is still open to question. From these observations, we could speculate that ACS would be a critical factor for the tumor development. Among the ACS members, the two enzymes, ACSL5 and ACSVL3, are essential for the maintenance of malignant glioma cells. However, there is still a possibility that other ACS isozymes could also be important as therapeutic targets or diagnostic markers of the cancer. To make sure these points, further studies are required particularly on the expression and the biological role of each ACS isozyme in glioma cells. In addition, identification of more specific compounds that target and inhibit each ACS isozyme would make it more promising the development of ACS-targeted glioma therapy.

References

Coleman RA, Lewin TM, Van Horn CG, Gonzalez-Baro MR (2002) Do long-chain acyl-CoA synthetases regulate fatty acid entry into synthetic versus degradative pathways?. J Nutr 132:2123–2126

Guo D, Hildebrandt IJ, Prins RM, Soto H, Mazzotta MM, Dang J, Czernin J, Shyy JY, Watson AD, Phelps M, Radu CG, Cloughesy TF, Mischel PS (2009) The AMPK agonist AICAR inhibits the growth of EGFRvIII-expressing glioblastomas by inhibiting lipogenesis. Proc Natl Acad Sci USA 106:12932–12937

Karlbom AE, James CD, Boethius J, Cavenee WK, Collins VP, Nordenskjold M, Larsson C (1993) Loss of heterozygosity in malignant gliomas involves at least three distinct regions on chromosome 10. Hum Genet 92:169–174

Kuhajda FP (2006) Fatty acid synthase and cancer: new application of an old pathway. Cancer Res 66:5977–5980

Mashima T, Oh-hara T, Sato S, Mochizuki M, Sugimoto Y, Yamazaki K, Hamada J, Tada M, Moriuchi T, Ishikawa Y, Kato Y, Tomoda H, Yamori T, Tsuruo T (2005) P53-defective tumors with a functional apoptosome-mediated pathway: a new therapeutic target. J Natl Cancer Inst 97:765–777

Mashima T, Sato S, Okabe S, Miyata S, Matsuura M, Sugimoto Y, Tsuruo T, Seimiya H (2009a) Acyl-CoA synthetase as a cancer survival factor: its inhibition enhances the efficacy of etoposide. Cancer Sci 100:1556–1562

Mashima T, Sato S, Sugimoto Y, Tsuruo T, Seimiya H (2009b) Promotion of glioma cell survival by acyl-CoA synthetase 5 under extracellular acidosis conditions. Oncogene 28:9–19

Mashima T, Seimiya H, Tsuruo T (2009c) De novo fatty-acid synthesis and related pathways as molecular targets for cancer therapy. Br J Cancer 100:1369–1372

Mashima T, Tsuruo T (2005) Defects of the apoptotic pathway as therapeutic target against cancer. Drug Resist Updat 8:339–343

Menendez JA, Lupu R (2007) Fatty acid synthase and the lipogenic phenotype in cancer pathogenesis. Nat Rev Cancer 7:763–777

Pei Z, Sun P, Huang P, Lal B, Laterra J, Watkins PA (2009) Acyl-CoA synthetase VL3 knockdown inhibits human glioma cell proliferation and tumorigenicity. Cancer Res 69:9175–9182

Rasheed BK, McLendon RE, Friedman HS, Friedman AH, Fuchs HE, Bigner DD, Bigner SH (1995) Chromosome 10 deletion mapping in human gliomas: a common deletion region in 10q25. Oncogene 10:2243–2246

Tannock IF, Rotin D (1989) Acid pH in tumors and its potential for therapeutic exploitation. Cancer Res 49:4373–4384

Tomoda H, Igarashi K, Cyong JC, Omura S (1991) Evidence for an essential role of long chain acyl-CoA synthetase in animal cell proliferation. Inhibition of long chain acyl-CoA synthetase by triacsins caused inhibition of raji cell proliferation. J Biol Chem 266:4214–4219

Warburg O (1956) On the origin of cancer cells. Science 123:309–314

Watkins PA, Maiguel D, Jia Z, Pevsner J (2007) Evidence for 26 distinct acyl-coenzyme a synthetase genes in the human genome. J Lipid Res 48:2736–2750

Yamashita Y, Kumabe T, Cho YY, Watanabe M, Kawagishi J, Yoshimoto T, Fujino T, Kang MJ, Yamamoto TT (2000) Fatty acid induced glioma cell growth is mediated by the acyl-CoA synthetase 5 gene located on chromosome 10q25.1-Q25.2, a region frequently deleted in malignant gliomas. Oncogene 19:5919–5925

Zhao W, Kridel S, Thorburn A, Kooshki M, Little J, Hebbar S, Robbins M (2006) Fatty acid synthase: a novel target for antiglioma therapy. Br J Cancer 95:869–878

Chapter 35

Malignant Glioma Patients: Combined Treatment with Radiation and Fotemustine

Patrick D. Beauchesne

Abstract Malignant gliomas account for approximately 60% of all primary brain tumours in adults. The prognosis for malignant glioma patients has not significantly changed in recent years. Despite debulking surgery, radiotherapy and cytotoxic chemotherapy, median survival duration is 9–12 months and virtually no patients are cured of their illness. Fotemustine is an alkylating agent characterised by the grafting of a phosphonoalanine group onto the nitrosourea radical with consequent high lipophilia and improved diffusion through the cell membrane and the blood-brain barrier. Fotemustine has been registered for use in two indications: disseminated malignant melanoma including cerebral metastases, and primary brain tumours. Fotemustine can be used for recurrent tumours either after radiotherapy, or in a neo-adjuvant schedule or concomitantly to radiotherapy for de novo malignant gliomas. We now go on to describe all the combinations currently in clinical use.

Keywords Malignant gliomas · Chemotherapy · Nitrosourea · Fotemustine · Neo-adjuvant chemotherapy · Concurrent chemotherapy · Recurrent tumors

Introduction

Malignant gliomas account for approximately 60% of all primary brain tumours in adults (Behin et al., 2003; De Angelis, 2001). There are three distinct histological types: anaplastic astrocytoma (AA), anaplastic oligodendroglioma (AO), and glioblastoma multiforme (GBM). For AA and GBM, the standard of care consists of surgical resection of as much of the tumour as is considered to be safe, followed by radio- and chemotherapy and has been so for many decades (Behin et al., 2003; De Angelis, 2001). A new standard procedure for GBM has recently been defined by the EORTC phase III trial which randomized patients in two groups, receiving either temozolomide (TMZ) concomitant and adjuvant to radiotherapy or radiotherapy alone (Stupp et al., 2005). A significant increase in overall survival was seen in the radiotherapy plus TMZ group than in the radiotherapy alone group. Survival rates were respectively 14.6 and 12.1 months. For AO, the standard treatment is surgical resection followed by radiotherapy. Adjuvant chemotherapy does not provide significant benefits in overall survival (Van den Bent et al., 2006). The median survival for patients with newly diagnosed GBM is 9–12 months, prognosis is slightly better for newly diagnosed AA with a median survival of 24–36 months, and median survival AO is 60 months (Behin et al., 2003; De Angelis, 2001).

The reasons for the poor prognosis of malignant gliomas are due to the ineffectiveness of surgical resection because of the diffuse infiltration of glioma cells into the surrounding brain parenchyma as well as the high degree of chemo-resistance of these tumours giving at best short-lived responses with rapid development of resistance (Stupp et al., 2007). This resistance is due to genetic transformations and the heterogeneity of this type of neoplasm. Another reason for poor prognosis resides in the fact that the anti-neoplastic agents are largely unable to cross the blood-brain barrier to reach the tumour cells intercalated in the normal brain parenchyma (Stupp et al., 2007).

P.D. Beauchesne (✉)
Neuro-Oncologie/Neurologie, CHU de Nancy, CO N°34, Hospital Central, 54035 Nancy, France
e-mail: beaupatt@orange.fr

M.A. Hayat (ed.), *Tumors of the Central Nervous System, Volume 1*,
DOI 10.1007/978-94-007-0344-5_35, © Springer Science+Business Media B.V. 2011

Fotemustine

Two meta-analyses have been published which combine the results of studies randomizing malignant glioma patients to radiotherapy alone or radiation plus chemotherapy (Fine et al., 1993; Stewart, 2002). Most of the chemotherapy schedules used, including nitrosoureas which represent the main class of chemotherapy drugs for these patients, have been tested in the randomized studies analyzed in these meta-analyses. They demonstrate that the addition of adjuvant chemotherapy increases the percentage of long-term survivors by 10.1% over 1 year and 8.6% over 2 years (Fine et al., 1993; Stewart, 2002).

Fotemustine (FTM) is a novel chloroethylnitrosourea characterised by a high liposolubility, a low molecular weight favouring its passage across the blood-brain barrier, and a chemical structure including an alanine phosphonic ester (IRIS, 1999). The anti-tumour activity of FTM is related to its ability to alkylate DNA. Its in vitro or in vivo pharmacological activity is the same as or greater than that of the other nitrosoureas (IRIS, 1999; Deloffre et al., 1990; Filippeschi et al., 1998; Fischel et al., 1990). Significant activity has been found in models of xenografts of human primary cerebral tumours after intra-peritoneal administration (Vassal et al., 1998). FTM rapidly crosses the blood-brain barrier and its plasma pharmacokinetics in animal and human is linear and biphasic, with a terminal half-life of 29 min in human. Metabolism occurs mainly through rapid non-enzymatic chemical decomposition into the carbonium ion, which is responsible for the alkylating activity, and into the isocyanate group, which has carbamoylating properties, and results in the formation of chloroethanol (IRIS, 1999).

FTM has been registered for use in two indications: disseminated malignant melanoma including cerebral metastases, and primary brain tumours. Based on the study of Khayat et al who enrolled 22 recurrent malignant glioma patients, the recommended therapeutic regimen as a monotherapy regimen is an initial treatment of a 1-hour intravenous infusion of 100 mg/m^2/week for 3 consecutive weeks followed by a rest period of 4–5 weeks, and then maintenance treatment at the same dosage every 3 weeks (Khayat et al., 1994). Myelosuppression, leucopenia and thrombocytopenia are the most frequent side effects of treatment by FTM being reported in more than 30% of the subpopulation pre-treated with chemotherapy (Khayat et al., 1994). This myelotoxicity is not a limiting factor but requires postponement of the chemotherapy. FTM is highly photosensitive and it is essential to protect it from the light while preparing and administering the solution (IRIS, 1999).

Fotemustine is an alkylating cytotoxic agent of the lipophilic chloroethyl-nitrosourea group (IRIS, 1999).

Chemical name: Diethyl1-{1-[3-(2-chloroethyl)-3-nitrosoureido]} ethylphosphonate RS

Molecular formula: $C_9 H_{19} Cl N_3 O_5 P$

Structural formula

Molecular weight 315.7

Handling conditions: Fotemustine is an anticancer agent that must be handled according to the general conditions for using cytotoxic agents. Operations must be carried out in suitable premises using clothing kept for this use (long-sleeved overalls, etc...). The wearing of mask, protective glasses and disposable gloves is compulsory. In the case of skin or eyes contact, rinse immediately and abundantly with running water for at least 15 min (IRIS, 1999).

Stability: When packaged in an airtight brown glass bottle, the active substance in powder form is stable for 2 years, between 2°C and 8°C, and for 15 days at room temperature (IRIS, 1999).

Combined Treatment

FTM can be used for recurrent tumours either after radiotherapy, in a neo-adjuvant schedule or concomitantly to radiotherapy. We now go on to describe all the combinations currently in clinical use.

Recurrent Tumours

FTM is clinically administered as a salvage therapy for recurrent malignant gliomas and is currently used in Europe, especially in France and Italy. It was developed by the French pharmaceutical laboratory, SERVIER, and the first clinical trials were French.

The clinical use of FTM, consisting of induction and maintenance phases, was first defined by Khayat et al. (1994). Frenay et al. went on to test FTM as a single agent in 38 recurrent malignant glioma patients; they reported a rate of objective response of 26% and median survival was 10 months (Frenay et al., 1991). Myelotoxicity (thrombocytopenia and leucopenia) was observed in 30% of cases, especially in patients who has previously been treated with chemotherapy. In another phase II study, Malhaire et al. tested induction and maintenance phases of FTM in 21 recurrent malignant gliomas; 18 GBM and 3 AA (Malhaire et al., 1999). Four patients experienced a radiological response and six stabilizations were noted. The overall survival for responder was 9.4 months. Grade 3 and 4 hematologic toxicity was reported in six cases (Malhaire et al., 1999). Mousseau et al found a response rate of 70% and median survival of 10 months in 34 recurrent glioma patients treated with FTM (Mousseau et al., 1996).

The last phase II studies were Italian and analyzed the efficacy and the safety of FTM as a single agent in the treatment of 160 patients with recurrent malignant gliomas (Brandes et al., 2009; Fabi et al., 2009; Fabrini et al., 2009; Scoccianti et al., 2008). As expected, myelotoxicity was the main side effect. Brandes et al. reported a median survival of 6 months in 43 recurrent glioma patients with three partial responses (PR) and 15 stabilization diseases (SD) (Brandes et al., 2009). In the clinical study of Fabi et al., 40 recurrent glioma patients were enrolled; a response rate of 20% was noted and overall survival was 30 months; survival being longer among responders to FTM (Fabi et al., 2009). Fabrini et al. tested FTM in 50 recurrent GBM patients and found one complete response (CR) and eight PR with a median survival time from the first relapse to death of 8.1 months (Fabrini et al., 2009). Scoccianti et al. tested FTM in 27 recurrent GBM patients; eight PR and five cases of SD were observed; median time to progression was 5.7 months, and median survival from the beginning of FTM chemotherapy was 9.1 months (Scoccianti et al., 2008).

Post-radiotherapy FTM Regimen

Ozkan et al. assessed the efficacy and toxicity of FTM administered to 27 malignant glioma patients – including 10 AA and 17 GBM – who had undergone a neurosurgery – radiotherapy sequence (Ozkan et al., 2004). FTM was given at a dose of 100 mg/m2 every 3 weeks for six cycles. Median time from surgery to chemotherapy was 3 months (range 1–6), and radiotherapy was given within a month following the operation (range 11–74 days). Median age was 46 years old (range from 23 to 70), 23 complete resections were reported and 24 patients had performance status (PS) $\leq$ 1. One hundred eleven cycles were administered in all (median cycles 5, range from 1 to 6 cycles). Toxicity was mild, grade 3 neutropenia was observed in two patients, one of whom developed a grade 2 thrombocytopenia, and 14 cycles of FTM were deferred (Ozkan et al., 2004).

The overall survival was 11 months, and PFS was 8 months. The survival rate at 12 and 24 months were respectively 48% and 7%. The completion of six cycles of FTM was found as a significant prognostic factor giving a median survival of 21 months. The median survival was only 9 months for patients who did not complete six cycles and 6.5 months for patients who progressed during chemotherapy (Ozkan et al., 2004). The authors concluded that this sequential chemo-radiotherapy with FTM was feasible and well tolerated. Further prospective studies are required to confirm these findings.

Neo-Adjuvant FTM Regimen

Frenay et al. tested a combination of FTM, Cisplatin and VP16 in a neo-adjuvant setting for non-removable glioblastomas (Frenay et al., 2000). Thirty-three patients were enrolled to receive a total of two to six one monthly cycles of FTM (100 mg/m2/day 1), cisplatin (33 mg/m2/days 1–3) and VP16 (75 mg/m2/days 1–3) followed by and cranial radiotherapy according to standard procedure (60 Gy, 2 Gy/fraction, 30 fractions over 6 weeks). Treatment volumes were calculated on pre-operative CT scan or MRI and included the contrast-enhancing lesion and oedema with a 2–3 cm margin depending on the location. Chemotherapy was discontinued and radiotherapy initiated in cases of proven progressive disease (clinical or radiological progression) (Frenay et al., 2000). The median age of the population was 57.7 years (range from 20 to 73 years), 20 patients were male, and neo-adjuvant chemotherapy began within 4 weeks following stereo-tactic biopsy. All but four patients completed radiotherapy. Chemotherapy was delivered as follows: eight patients received 4 cycles; 10 had 5–6 cycles: all patients completed at least 2 chemotherapy cycles.

Chemotherapy was stopped after two cycles for twelve patients due to hematologic toxicity. Grade 3–4 thrombocytopenia and grade 3–4 leucopenia occured in 20/171 and 25/171 cycles respectively but no platelet transfusion was required and there was no neutropenic fever) (Frenay et al., 2000).

One CR and PR were reported giving an objective response rate of 27%. Seven patients progressed during the chemotherapy regimen; the median survival was 4.8 months and radiatiotherapy was initiated to stabilize them. The overall survival was 10 months, and median survival at 6 and 12 months were 88% and 42% respectively. Seven long-term survivors were reported, four were alive at time of publication and median survival was 34.6 months (Frenay et al., 2000). The authors demonstrated that chemotherapy administered in a neo-adjuvant setting before radiotherapy is feasible and safe. No adverse impact on survival for inoperable GBM was noted, and this regimen seems to produce some responses with a few long-term survivors.

In another study, standard cranial radiatiotherapy was delivered during the 5-weeks rest interval following the induction phase of FTM given at 100 mg/m2 for 3 weeks (Biron et al., 1991). The response rate was 27.1%, and the median survival for responder and stabilized patients was 9.7 months. Thrombocytopenia was reported in 27.1% of patients, and leucopenia in 25.4% of cases and nausea and vomiting in 24.7% (Biron et al., 1991).

Frenay et al. in another study tested a combination of FTM, Cisplatin and VP16 in a neoadjuvant regimen for patients with GBM, in a randomized multicenter phase III study (Frenay et al., 2008a, b). Patients were randomized to neoadjuvant chemotherapy (FTM, Cisplatin and VP16) followed by standard cranial radiotherapy or radiotherapy alone. Fifty patients were included; 26 in chemotherapy arm and 24 in radiotherapy arm. The primary end point was time to progression and secondary end points:

survival time, best response rate, and toxicity. Patients received in chemotherapy group; 4 cycles of short infusion chemotherapy (D1 = D28) during 3 days (FTM 100 mg/m2, Cisplatin 33 mg/m2 D1, and VP 16 75 mg/m2, each drug on day D1, D2, D3), followed by brain radiotherapy over 6 weeks to a total dose of 55–60 Gy (Frenay et al., 2008a, b). For radiotherapy alone arm; 1,8 – 2 Gy per fractions, 5 days a week, for 6 weeks, for a total dose of 55–60 Gy. Median age of population was 59 years old (from 33 to 71), median Performance Status (PS) was 90.4 (from 70 to 100), and 35 were male, and 15 females. Surgery was a partial tumour resection (16 cases) or a stereotactic biopsy (34 patients) (Frenay et al., 2008a, b). Patients of this study were classified as RPA class as RPA V.

Toxicity was hematologic, 65% of patients in chemotherapy group experienced a myelotoxicity; thrombocytopenia in 62% cases, neutropenia in 58% and one sepsis with toxic death. However, 19% of seizure and 8% of motor deficit were noted. For radiotherapy group, 2 toxic deaths were reported (one by sepsis, and one no documented), and 13% of motor deficit were found (Frenay et al., 2008a, b).

The median PFS were 8 months for chemotherapy arm and 4.37 months for radiotherapy alone, respectively, the difference was statistically significant ($p = 0.0085$). The median survival was 12.5 months for chemotherapy group and 10.8 months for radiotherapy alone, respectively, the difference was not significant (Frenay et al., 2008a, b).

The objective response rate, CR and PR, was 23% for chemotherapy group, and 8% only for radiation alone arm.

The results were higher (12.5 months OS) than these of classical RPA V class (8.3 months). These results were encouraging, and this regimen was feasible and well accepted.

Concomitant FTM – Radiotherapy Regimen

Radiation therapy is the most effective treatment modality for malignant gliomas (Behin et al., 2003; De Angelis, 2001) and certain chemotherapy agents may potentiate the effect of the radiation when used concurrently (Brandes et al., 1998; Fountzilas et al., 1999). It was hypothesized that the use of two therapies with a dissimilar toxicity spectrum could enable the eradication of cell lines resistant to a single therapy. Beauchesne et al. thus conducted an in vivo pre-clinical study to test the anti-tumour activity of FTM administered by the intra-peritoneal route either alone or in combination with fractionated low radiation doses on a human malignant glioma xenograft (G152 cell line) subcutaneously implanted in the nude mouse (Beauchesne et al., 2007). The high efficacy of fractionated irradiation with low doses (<1 Gy) (compared to irradiation with an equivalent single dose) had already been demonstrated in this tumour model (Beauchesne et al., 2003). FTM was given intra-peritoneally (IP) either on days 1 and 8 (40 mg/kg/injection) or daily 5 days per week, for 2 consecutive weeks (days 1–5 and days 8–12 at 8 mg/kg/injection). A total of 42 animals were to be distributed in six treatment groups as follows:

- Control group: solvent only, days 1–5 and 8–12, 7 animals,
- FTM alone D1: days 1, 8 ($n = 7$),
- FTM alone D2: days 1–5 and 8–12 IP ($n = 7$),
- Irradiation alone (Ultra-fractionated regimen); mice were exposed to 0.8 Gy per fraction: 3 times a day at 4-hourly intervals, 5 days per week for 2 consecutive weeks ($n = 7$),
- FTM D1 combined with irradiation 0.8 × 3 Gy ($n = 7$),
- FTM D2 combined with irradiation 0.8 × 3 Gy ($n = 7$).

The authors were able to show that the concurrent administration of daily doses of FTM to ultra-fractionated regimen (D2 regimen) dramatically enhanced the effect of ultra-fractionated radiotherapy; the difference was statistically significant, $p = 0.0004$ (Beauchesne et al., 2007). Using univariate linear regression analysis, an inhibition of tumour growth was found with a calculated negative value of 0.62. These results were encouraging, and supported the initiation of a phase II study (Beauchesne et al., 2007).

Beauchesne et al. then tested a concomitant combination of radiotherapy and FTM for de novo malignant gliomas (Beauchesne et al., 2009). Twenty-two patients were enrolled; 16 males and six females, and histology reported 16 GBM, three AA, two AO, and one mixed glioma. Fourteen patients underwent stereotactic biopsy and eight patients tumour resection (with

3 complete tumour resections). Radiotherapy consisted of fractionated cranial irradiation, 2 Gy per fraction, 5 days per week, for 6 consecutive weeks. FTM was concomitantly given at daily dose of 10 mg/m2, 5 days per week, from the first to the last day of radiation therapy, a total of 30 days (Beauchesne et al., 2009).

The main toxicity was hematologic: grade 3 and 4 thrombocytopenias were recorded in three patients, causing the suspension of FTM. Five patients experienced fatigue and two experienced nausea. 86.4% of the patients completed the combined treatment (Beauchesne et al., 2009).

CR was noted in one patient and PR in two patients (Figs. 35.1, 35.2, 35.3, and 35.4). Eight patients experienced a stabilization response. Overall survival was 9.9 months and PFS was 6 months. The survival rate at 18 and 24 months was 13.6% and 9% respectively. Median survival for surgery and stereotactic biopsy was 11 and 9 months, respectively (Beauchesne et al., 2009).

It was concluded that this concurrent radiotherapy and FTM combination was safe and well tolerated. Overall survival was in accordance with the expected results for malignant gliomas.

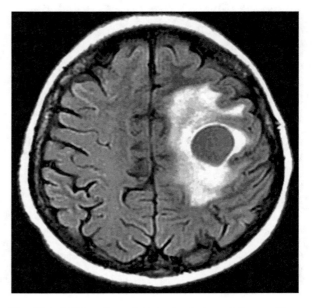

Fig. 35.1 MRI performed at the beginning of the combination radiotherapy – FTM. The patient experienced a complete remission (CR). The lesion is left frontal lobe, and gadolinium enhancement is noted. MRI Flair image

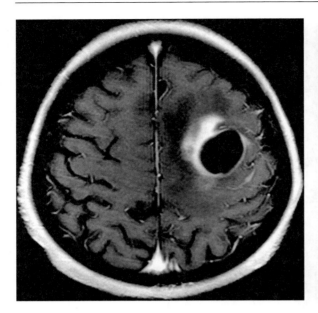

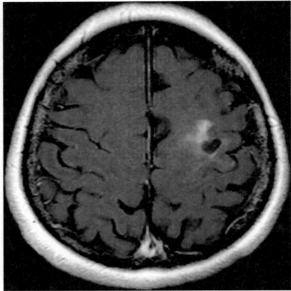

Fig. 35.2 MRI performed at the beginning of the combination radiotherapy – FTM. The patient experienced a complete remission (CR). The lesion is left frontal lobe, and gadolinium enhancement is noted. MRI Gadolinium enhanced sequence

Fig. 35.4 MRI performed at the end of the combination radiotherapy – FTM. The patient experienced a complete remission (CR). The lesion is left frontal lobe, and no recurrent tumour is reported. MRI Gadolinium enhanced sequence

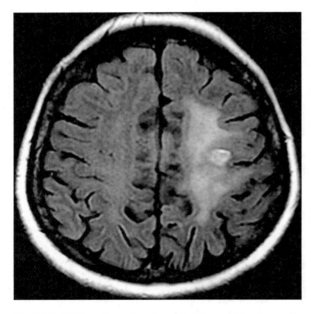

Fig. 35.3 MRI performed at the end of the combination radiotherapy – FTM. The patient experienced a complete remission (CR). The lesion is left frontal lobe, and no recurrent tumour is reported. MRI Flair image

References

Beauchesne P, Bertrand S, Branche R, Linke SP, Revel R, Dore JF, Pedeux R (2003) Human malignant glioma cell lines are sensitive to low radiation doses. Int J Cancer 105:33–40

Beauchesne P, Pourchet J, Dore JF, Branche R, Pedeux R 2007. Effect on human malignant glioma cell lines and glioma xenografts of anti-neoplastic agents combined with low radiation doses. Proceedings AACR 2007: p 5058 (abstract)

Beauchesne P, Taillandier L, Bernier V, Carnin C (2009) Concurrent radiotherapy: fotemustine combination for newly diagnosed malignant glioma patients, a phase II study. Cancer Chemother Pharmacol 64:171–175

Behin A, Hoang-Zuan K, Carpentier A, Delattre JY (2003) Primary brain tumors in adults. Lancet 361:323–331

Biron P, Roux N, Chauvin N, Frenay M, Giroux B (1991) Phase I–II trial of high dose fotemustine followed by autologous bone marrow transfusion in high grade gliomas. Eur J Cancer 27A:S 191 (abstract)

Brandes AA, Rigon A, Zampieri P, Ermani M, Carollo C, Altavilla G, Turazzi S, Chierichetti F, Florentino MV (1998) Carboplatin and teniposide concurrent with radiotherapy in patients with glioblastoma multiforme. Cancer 82:355–361

Brandes AA, Tosoni A, Franceschi E, Blatt V, Santoro A, Faedi M, Amistà P, Gardiman M, Labianca R, Bianchini C, Ermani M, Reni M (2009) Fotemustine as second-line treatment for recurrent or progressive glioblastoma after concomitant and/or adjuvant temozolomide: a phase II trial of gruppo italiano cooperativo di neuro-oncologia (GICNO). Cancer Chemother Pharmacol 64:769–775

De Angelis LM (2001) Brain tumours. N Eng J Med 344:114–123

Deloffre P, Paraire M, Bizzari JP (1990) Muphoran (fotémustine), une nouvelle nitrosourée: études précliniques. Cancer Commun 4:7–16

Fabi A, Metro G, Russillo M, Vidiri A, Carapella CM, Maschio M, Cognetti F, Jandolo B, Mirri MA, Sperduti I, Telera S, Carosi M, Pace A (2009) Treatment of recurrent malignant gliomas with fotemustine monotherapy: impact of dose and correlation with MGMT promoter methylation. BMC Cancer 9:101

Fabrini MG, Silvano G, Lolli I, Perrone F, Marsella A, Scotti V, Cionini L (2009) A multi-institutional phase II study on second-line fotemustine chemotherapy in recurrent glioblastoma. J Neuro Oncol 92:79–86

Filippeschi S, Colombo T, Bassini D (1998) Antitumor activity of the novel nitrosourea S 10036 in rodent tumors. Anticancer Res 8:1351–1354

Fine HA, Dear KB, Loeffler JS, Black PM, Canellos GP (1993) Meta-analysis of radiation with and without chemotherapy for malignant gliomas in adults. Cancer 71:2585–2597

Fischel JL, Formento P, Etienne MC, Gioanni J, Frenay M, Deloffre P, Bizzari JP, Milano G (1990) In vitro chemosensitivity testing of fotemustine (S 10036), a new antitumor nitrosourea. Cancer Chemother Pharmacol 25:337–341

Fountzilas G, Karavelis A, Capizzello A, Kalogera-Fountzila A, Karkavelas G, Zamboglou N, Selviaridis P, Foroglou G, Tourkantonis A (1999) Radiation and concomitant weekly administration of paclitaxel in patients with glioblastoma multiforme. A phase II study. J Neuro Oncol 45:159–165

Frenay M, Giroux B, Khoury S, Derlon JM, Namer M (1991) Phase II study of fotemustine in recurrent supratentorial malignant gliomas. Eur J Cancer 27:852–856

Frenay M, Lebrun C, Lonjon M, Bondiau PY, Chatel M (2000) Up-front chemotherapy with fotemustine/cisplatin/etoposide regimen in the treatment of 33 non-removable glioblastomas. Eur J Cancer 36:1026–1031

Frenay M, Simon J, Benbouker L, Taillandier L, Castera D, Busso A, Lebrun C on behalf of the FOTEGLIO group (2008a) Prospective randomised study comparing first line nitrosourea based chemotherapy/ radiotherapy versus radiotherapy alone in non respectable glioblastomas. Neuro Oncol 10(issue 6): (abstract)

Frenay M, Simon JM, Benbouker L, Taillandier L, Castera D, Lebrun C (2008b) Etude de phase III comparant l'efficacité de la radiothérapie cérébrale à une poly-chimiothérapie + radiothérapie dans les gliomes malins non opérables. Rev Neurol 164(issue 2):(abstract)

I.R.I.S. Cancer Treatment Division. Fotemustine Investigator's Brochure. Version No. 3, September 15, 1999

Khayat D, Giroux B, Berille J, Cour V, Gerard B, Sarkany M, Bertrand P, Bizzari JP (1994) Fotemustine in the treatment of brain primary tumour and metastases. Cancer Invest 12:414–420

Malhaire JP, Lucas B, Simon H, Person H, Dam-Hieu P, Labat JP (1999) Fotemustine (muphoran) in 22 patients with relapses of high-grade cerebral gliomas. Bull Cancer 86:289–294

Mousseau M, Swiercz V, Rougny M, Boutonnat J, Méchin I, Chinal J (1996) Fotemustine in recurrent supratentoriel malignant gliomas. Drugs Today 32:43–50

Ozkan M, Altinbas M, Er O, Kaplan B, Coskun HS, Karahacioglu E, Menku A, Cihan Y, Kontas O, Akdemir H (2004) Post-opertive sequential chemo-radiotherapy in high grade cerebral gliomas with fotemustine. J Chemother 16:298–302

Scoccianti S, Detti B, Sardaro A, Iannalfi A, Meattini I, Leonulli BG, Borghesi S, Martinelli F, Bordi L, Ammannati F, Biti G (2008) Second-line chemotherapy with fotemustine in temozolomide-pretreated patients with relapsing glioblastoma: a single institution experience. Anticancer Drugs 19:613–620

Stewart LA (2002) Chemotherapy in adult high-grade glioma: a systematic review and meta-analysis of individual patient data from 12 randomized trials. Lancet 359: 1011–1018

Stupp R, Hegi ME, Gilbert MR, Chakravarti A (2007) Chemotherapy in malignant glioma: standard of care and future directions. J Clin Oncol 25: 4127–4136

Stupp R, Mason WP, van den Bent MJ, Weller M, Fisher B, Taphoorn MJ, Belanger K, Brandes AA, Marosi C, Bogdahn U, Curschmann J, Janzer RC, Ludwin SK, Gorlia T, Allgeier A, Lacombe D, Cairncross JG, Eisenhauer E, Mirimanoff RO, European Organisation for Research and Treatment of Cancer Brain Tumor and Radiotherapy Groups; National Cancer Institute of Canada Clinical Trials Group (2005) Radiotherapy plus concomitant and adjuvant temozolomide for glioblastoma. N Engl J Med 352: 987–996

Vassal G, Boland I, Terrier-Lacombe MJ, Watson AJ, Margison GP, Vénuat AM, Morizet J, Parker F, Lacroix C, Lellouch-Tubiana A, Pierre-Kahn A, Poullain MG, Gouyette A (1998) Activity of fotemustine in medulloblastoma and malignant glioma xenografts in relation to O6-alkylguanine-DNA alkyltransferase and alkylpurine-DNA N-glycosylase activity. Clin Cancer Res 4:463–468

van den Bent MJ, Carpentier AF, Brandes AA, Sanson M, Taphoorn MJ, Bernsen HJ, Frenay M, Tijssen CC, Grisold W, Sipos L, Haaxma-Reiche H, Kros JM, van Kouwenhoven MC, Vecht CJ, Allgeier A, Lacombe D, Gorlia T (2006) Adjuvant procarbazine, lomustine, and vincristine improves progression-free survival but not overall survival in newly diagnosed anaplastic oligodendrogliomas and oligoastrocytomas: a randomized european organisation for research and treatment of cancer phase III trial. J Clin Oncol 24:2715–2722

Chapter 36

Malignant Glioma Immunotherapy: A Peptide Vaccine from Bench to Bedside

Bryan D. Choi, Kevin S. Chen, and John H. Sampson

Abstract Epidermal growth factor receptor variant III (EGFRvIII) is a constitutively active, mutant form of the wild-type receptor. It is expressed frequently in malignant glioma cells, yet absent in all normal tissues. EGFRvIII arises from an in-frame deletion, the translation of which incidentally alters the extracellular domain of the receptor. This unique motif makes EGFRvIII an especially attractive target for an immunotherapeutic approach. Our laboratory has developed and tested a novel peptide vaccine based on this mutation, and has demonstrated the ability to elicit EGFRvIII-specific immune responses in both preclinical and early clinical models using this vaccine. Furthermore, we have shown that, for patients who bear EGFRvIII-expressing gliomas, vaccination-induced humoral and delayed-type hypersensitivity responses are associated with improved survival, even in the context of concurrent chemotherapy-induced lymphodepletion.

Keywords Antigens · Central nervous system neoplasms · Epidermal growth factor receptor · Immunotherapy

Introduction

Glioblastoma multiforme (GBM) is a devastating illness accounting for more than half of all primary malignant brain tumors diagnosed annually. Although remarkable strides have been made towards improving the management of this lethal disease, the benefit achieved from standard of care surgical resection, radiotherapy, and temozolomide chemotherapy is modest at best, and despite this regimen, patients carry a grim prognosis with an overall median survival of less than 15 months from the time of diagnosis (Stupp et al., 2009). Furthermore, given their nonspecific nature, these conventional treatments are frequently associated with substantial morbidity from collateral toxicity to normal tissue. Thus, the advancement of safer, more effective therapies remains a crucial objective in the field of antitumor research.

Cancer immunotherapy, in contrast to radiotherapy and chemotherapy, offers a highly specific and theoretically potent approach that targets and eradicates neoplastic cells using the effectors of the human immune system. Antitumor efficacy achieved through proper immunological manipulation has been realized in numerous studies, and treatment has led to the dramatic regression of even bulky, invasive tumors (Rosenberg, 2001). To date, promising antitumor immunotherapies have taken multiple forms, including vaccination against tumor antigens as well as adoptive transfer of tumor-specific lymphocytes. While the current understanding is incomplete regarding the degree to which humoral versus cellular mechanisms predominate in an optimal antitumor response, the implications of redirecting the discriminatingly potent nature of the immune system against GBM are undoubtedly far-reaching and thus have an enormous potential impact on the management of patients who are diagnosed with this debilitating disease.

B.D. Choi (✉)
Duke Brain Tumor Immunotherapy Program, Division of Neurosurgery, Department of Surgery, Duke University Medical Center, Durham, NC 27710, USA
e-mail: bryan.choi@duke.edu

M.A. Hayat (ed.), *Tumors of the Central Nervous System, Volume 1,*
DOI 10.1007/978-94-007-0344-5_36, © Springer Science+Business Media B.V. 2011

CNS Immunoprivilege

The concept of a blood-brain barrier (BBB) and CNS immunoprivilege has long been dogma, established first in classical animal work describing the inability to reject allogeneic tissue implanted in the CNS. Therefore, the logic of administering peptide vaccines peripherally for the sake of immunotherapy of gliomas seems self-defeating. Evidence has steadily accumulated, however, for a theory that CNS "immunoprivilege" is not absolute and that intracerebral tumors may be quite accessible to immune surveillance, if in a highly regulated fashion.

Such theories are supported by the fact that drainage of cerebrospinal fluid by the cribriform plate and cervical lymphatics has been shown to permit access of CNS antigens to the periphery. Additionally, in glioma patients, tumor-reactive T-cells have been identified in peripheral blood, and although naïve T-cells do not penetrate the BBB, activated lymphocytes have been shown to infiltrate tumor beds in the CNS. Furthermore, specialized astrocytes and microglia have been shown to function as surrogate professional antigen presenting cells (APCs) in the CNS, thereby facilitating the proliferation and persistence of lymphocytes in the intracerebral tumor microenvironment.

The overall issue of CNS immunoprivilege may be even less critical for patients with malignant glioma, as current state-of-the-art treatments for this disease include irradiation and chemotherapy, both of which have been shown to disrupt the BBB, allowing egress of tumor-associated antigens and entry of immune cells and antibodies. Techniques for further disruption of the BBB at the tumor have also been developed, including osmotic approaches, bradykinin agonists, and focused ultrasound. However, even in the absence of such intervention, evidence suggests that, in the context of intracerebral malignancy and other neuro-inflammatory conditions including multiple sclerosis and neuromyelitis optica, the BBB may be altered or disrupted, which may allow immune effectors to gain CNS entry under certain circumstances.

Despite these data describing putative immune access to the CNS and tumor stroma, the fact remains that endogenous immune responses are insufficient or are neutralized such that CNS malignancies continue to grow. Immunotherapy thus offers a strategy to augment the immune response, thereby overcoming the deficiencies that allow intracerebral tumors to persist. Early animal experiments by Freund suggested that, even in the absence of pathological inflammation, active and passive vaccination could result in detectable antibody titers in the CNS and CSF, albeit at dramatically reduced levels compared to serum. In the same vein, recent outcomes from trials for Alzheimer's disease provide some of the strongest support evidencing the ability to successfully elicit enhanced CNS immune reactivity in humans using a peptide vaccine.

Amyloid-β (Aβ) is a peptide that is characteristically deposited as amyloid plaques in the brain tissue of patients with Alzheimer's disease. Presumed to play a central role in pathogenesis, Aβ thus became an ideal target for peptide vaccine immunotherapy. Preclinical studies of the Aβ vaccine were quite successful, and humoral responses were purported to play a significant role in establishing efficacy. Indeed, in subsequent clinical trials, immune responses were so dramatic that it became necessary to halt the phase II study when a number of patients developed meningoencephalitis after receiving the Aβ vaccine (Orgogozo et al., 2003). Similar to what had been observed in preclinical studies, antibody-mediated immunity was primarily implicated in the human trials, though the involvement of cell-mediated immunity was also hypothesized.

The prospect that therapeutic antibodies can penetrate into the CNS as suggested by the Alzheimer's vaccine literature has great implications for the field of tumor immunotherapy, given that recent evidence supports an important role for humoral immunity in successful anticancer responses. After binding directly to tumor-associated antigens, antibodies on the cell surface can potentially mediate various mechanisms such as complement-mediated and antibody-dependent cellular cytotoxicity (ADCC). Furthermore, when antibodies specifically target surface receptors critical for tumor cell survival and proliferation, binding may lead to receptor internalization, thus decreasing responsiveness of tumor cells to extracellular mitogenic signals; a number of early trials using monoclonal antibodies to target gliomas have taken advantage of this finding.

When administered peripherally, monoclonal antibodies that exhibit exquisite antigen-specificity (e.g. EGFRvIII-targeted mAb ch806) have not only been shown to amass in glioma tissue, but also to have the added benefit of conceivably enhanced tumor localization due to a lack of cross-reactivity with systemic antigens and subsequent antibody sequestration in the periphery (Scott et al., 2007). This ability to localize preferentially to an intracerebral antigen sink may be an important factor for active vaccination approaches as well, and significant humoral responses have indeed been demonstrated in the cerebral spinal fluid of glioma patients after receiving treatment with a peptide vaccine targeting a tumor-specific antigen (Sampson, Heimberger et al., submitted for publication).

Peptide Vaccines Against Tumor Antigens

The peptide vaccine-based strategy for immunotherapy has long held promise and has many advantages when compared to other strategies. Conceptually, peptide vaccines expose the immune system to either over-expression of wild-type gene products or tumor-specific gene mutations that set apart tumor tissue from normal cells. Peptide vaccines are often engineered as nonamer oligopeptides that fit directly in the major histocompatibility complex (MHC) binding cleft. The vaccines hypothetically function via capture of antigen by APCs and subsequent migration of these cells to lymph nodes where lymphocytes can be activated to differentiate and proliferate.

As opposed to DNA or retroviral strategies, peptide vaccines make use of the efficient machinery of the human immune system without the risk of malignant transformation due to inappropriate recombination. Also, when compared to cellular therapies, peptide vaccines have the advantage of logistical simplicity. Bypassing the need for clinical-grade tissue culture facilities and specialized expertise, peptide vaccines are easily synthesized on an industrial scale with minimal risk of contamination, are stably stored for long periods of time, and can be easily transported and administered by providers.

The key to developing peptide-based tumor immunotherapies is thus identifying antigens that will allow the immune system to seek out and eliminate tumor cells while leaving nearby, normal cells intact. Many tumor-associated antigens have been described as proteins that are found over-expressed in tumor tissues. These include melanoma antigen-encoding genes (MAGE), gp240, cancer testis genes, squamous cell carcinoma antigens (SART1 and SART3), SOX genes, Tie2, tenascin-C and others (Yamanaka and Itoh, 2007). To date, peptide-based immunotherapy

has been employed to target many of these antigens, with only a few studies touched on here. The receptor tyrosine kinase erythropoietin-producing hepatocyte (Eph) receptor family has been investigated in this manner; specifically, the variant form EphB6 has been well characterized. Using peripheral blood lymphocytes stimulated with HLA-A*0204 restricted EphB6 variant peptide epitopes, significant cytotoxic T lymphocyte (CTL) responses were observed against the glioma cell line T98G in vitro (Jin et al., 2008). Wilms tumor 1 (WT1), an oncogene expressed in gliomas, has also been targeted with a peptide vaccine in a recent phase II clinical study which showed that WT1 peptide in Montanide ISA51 adjuvant given weekly until tumor progression was comparable to currently approved chemotherapy and radiotherapy regimens (Izumoto et al., 2008). The IL-13 receptor α2 is another example of a tumor-associated target since as it is expressed in glioma cells but not in normal cells of the CNS. Peptide vaccination against this antigen was found to elicit immune responses and, in subcutaneous challenge models, these responses led to complete protection in all challenged mice (Eguchi et al., 2006). Peptide vaccines targeting yet another glioma-associated antigen, survivin, have also been shown to improve survival curves in glioma-bearing mice (Ciesielski et al., 2010).

One possible barrier for immunotherapies designed against tumor-associated antigens such as those listed above is the fact that these proteins are not exclusive to neoplastic tissue. Effector cell tolerance in these cases is possible, in which T-cells raised against a peptide vaccine are rendered anergic or apoptotic when encountering normal tissues expressing the target antigen without appropriate co-stimulation. Furthermore, if T-cells escape mechanisms of tolerance, the opposite extreme, namely autoimmune disease, could be induced by vaccination. The goal, therefore, is to develop targeted immunotherapy against tumor-specific antigens, which are by definition expressed solely in tumor cells yet absent in all other tissues, thereby avoiding concerns for tolerance and autoimmunity. Presently, this approach is limited by the fact that few such tumor-specific targets are known; thus, a major step towards the development of tumor-specific antigen-based therapy includes the characterization of consistent, frequently expressed mutations that are exclusively present in tumor tissue.

EGFRvIII Tumor-Specific Antigen

Among the many tumor antigens that have been found to be over-expressed or overactive in human cancers, the type I epidermal growth factor receptor (EGFR) is perhaps one of the most well described cell-surface targets. In GBM, *EGFR* is amplified in nearly 50% and over-expressed in 95% of tumor specimens; upregulation is considered a poor prognostic indicator for disease progression (Ekstrand et al., 1991; Jaros et al., 1992).

Upon activation via extracellular interactions with stimulatory growth factors including epidermal growth factor and transforming growth factor-α, EGFR dimerizes on the cell surface, resulting in autophosphorylation of intracellular tyrosine residues and subsequent activation of downstream pathways responsible for cellular mitogenesis and survival; these functions, if left unchecked, may promote the uncontrolled proliferation associated with neoplastic processes. Indeed, many tumors, including GBM, not only display enhanced EGFR signaling, but also simultaneously express rearranged, aberrant forms of the receptor that have increased activity and therefore tumorigenic relevance.

Several genomic variants of *EGFR* have been described, though the most common, well-characterized mutant form of the EGFR molecule is the EGFR class III variant (EGFRvIII). EGFRvIII is a 145-kDa transmembrane glycoprotein with an in-frame deletion corresponding to wild-type mRNA exons 2–7. This deletion spans a 267 amino acid region in the extracellular domain, resulting in the translation of a novel glycine residue, flanked by amino acid sequences that are otherwise distant in the wild-type receptor (Bigner et al., 1990). This deletion also renders the receptor constitutively active, yet unable to interact with its cognate ligand. This ligand-independent, prolonged kinase activity of EGFRvIII is at least in part responsible for enhancing tumorgenicity in GBM by increasing proliferation and reducing apoptosis; additionally, the mutant receptor has also been shown to confer malignant cells with resistance to radiation and chemotherapy, while enhancing their ability to migrate, invade surrounding tissues, and promote angiogenesis. Over time, malignant cells have been shown to become somewhat dependent on signaling downstream of EGFRvIII, such that removal of this stimulation leads to reduced cell survival.

EGFRvIII has been implicated in a wide variety of human cancers including those of the lung, breast, colon, and cancers of the head and neck. In GBM, EGFRvIII is present in approximately 20% of tumor specimens (Moscatello et al., 1995), and while the expression tends to be somewhat heterogeneous, some tumors show positive staining for the receptor in over 80% of the cells (Wikstrand et al., 1997). Moreover, recent evidence suggests that cells that do not necessarily translate the receptor variant themselves can gain expression via microvesicular communication with EGFRvIII-positive cells in the surrounding tumor microenvironment.

Given that EGFRvIII contributes functionally to oncogenesis and is expressed consistently yet exclusively in tumor tissue, it has emerged as an obvious target for immunotherapy (Wikstrand et al., 1998). Accordingly, our group has developed and tested a peptide vaccine against the extracellular domain of EGFRvIII, and we have shown that this therapy can be used to successfully elicit EGFRvIII-specific immune responses in both preclinical murine models as well as in early clinical trials.

EGFRvIII Peptide Vaccine

While a number of approaches to antitumor immunotherapy are currently under investigation, the peptide vaccine platform is perhaps the cheapest and most practical, as it bypasses many of the technical limitations and drawbacks associated with other methods such as dendritic cell (DC) vaccines or the adoptive transfer of lymphocytes. Our laboratory has developed and tested a peptide vaccine against the EGFRvIII tumor antigen using a short amino acid sequence spanning the portion of the receptor containing the novel mutation motif. When conjugated to keyhole limpet hemocyanin (KLH), this 14-mer peptide, PEPvIII (H-Leu-Glu-Glu-Lys-Lys-Gln-Asn-Tyr-Val-Val-Thr-Asp-His-Cys-OH) (Sampson et al., 2009) elicits both cellular and humoral EGFRvIII-specific immune responses in both preclinical murine models and early clinical trials, thereby allowing precise targeting of tumor cells expressing the variant receptor in an otherwise healthy milieu.

Preclinical Studies

Our laboratory initially demonstrated that passive administration of EGFRvIII-specific monoclonal antibodies Y10 (IgG$_{2a}$) and L8A4 (IgG$_1$), leads to significant inhibition of tumor growth as well as increases in survival in subcutaneous and intracranial murine melanoma models (Sampson et al., 2000). Furthermore, intraperitoneal injection with Y10 has been shown to achieve lasting tumor-free survival even after treatment is removed. Based on our in vitro observations, the antitumor effect of Y10 is thought to work by multiple mechanisms including inhibition of EGFR-mediated mitogenesis, activation of complement, and ADCC. Another EGFRvIII-specific monoclonal antibody, mAb 806, has also been reported to inhibit growth of EGFRvIII-expressing glioma xenografts in both subcutaneous and intracranial animal models. While mAb 806 exhibits limited reactivity with wild-type EGFR, this interaction is exclusive to settings in which the receptor is over-expressed or associated with dysregulated signaling pathways specific to tumor cells (Johns et al., 2004).

Based on the ability of passively administered monoclonal antibodies to significantly and specifically inhibit EGFRvIII-positive tumors, our group proceeded to examine the potential in vivo efficacy of active vaccination strategies with the unique EGFRvIII junctional peptide vaccine, PEPvIII-KLH. Initially, DCs pulsed with PEPvIII-KLH were injected intraperitoneally into C3H mice bearing intracerebral, EGFRvIII-positive tumors, and this led to significantly increased survival (Heimberger et al., 2002). Following the encouraging results using a DC-based approach, injection with PEPvIII-KLH in complete Freund's adjuvant alone was explored given inherent advantages of the peptide vaccine platform over more labor-intensive approaches. Treatment with the PEPvIII-KLH peptide vaccine similarly increased median survival in C3H mice with well-established intracerebral tumors (Heimberger et al., 2003). Forty percent of the mice receiving the vaccine achieved long-term survival, and upon IHC examination, tumors that appeared to exhibit poor response to the vaccine were found to have either down-regulated or absent EGFRvIII expression after treatment, suggesting that emergence of EGFRvIII-negative escape variants may be responsible for failure to treat a given tumor.

Clinical Studies

Our group has demonstrated in clinical trials that vaccination strategies using PEPvIII-KLH can be used to elicit significant EGFRvIII-specific humoral and delayed-type hypersensitivity (DTH) responses in patients with GBM. In a Phase I clinical trial conducted at Duke University Medical Center (PI: John H. Sampson), patients who received autologous DCs pulsed with PEPvIII-KLH did not suffer any autoimmune side effects beyond Grade II toxicity (National Cancer Institute Common Toxicity Criteria), and almost all patients showed evidence of EGFRvIII-specific T-cell immune responses after three vaccinations (Sampson et al., 2009). While it is unclear whether this treatment led to statistically significant increases in median survival time when compared to an untreated population, this may be due to the fact that EGFRvIII expression in the tumors of treated patients was not used as a criterion for inclusion in this Phase I trial, and any potential therapeutic efficacy was thus presumably underestimated.

These findings, however, when combined with our preclinical results, warranted further study to assess the immunogenicity of PEPvIII-KLH alone when administered as a peptide vaccine. Phase II testing of the KLH-conjugated peptide revealed that intradermal vaccination with PEPvIII-KLH in patients with EGFRvIII-expressing gliomas led to the development of specific humoral and DTH responses that significantly impacted overall survival when compared to a matched control group (Sampson, Heimberger et al., submitted for publication). Symptomatic autoimmune reactions were absent. Additionally, consistent with our preclinical results, the great majority of recurrent tumors were EGFRvIII-negative.

Because myelosuppressive chemotherapies such as temozolomide (TMZ) have been shown to increase survival in patients with GBM, our laboratory extended Phase II investigation of the PEPvIII-KLH vaccine formulation to include concurrent treatment with TMZ at two doses: the standard (200 mg/m^2/5d) and dose-intensified (100 mg/m^2/21d) regimens (Sampson, Aldape et al., submitted for publication). Patients experienced at least transient grade 2 lymphopenia after receiving the standard dose, while the dose-intensified cohort exhibited sustained grade 3 lymphopenia. However, the dose-intensified cohort paradoxically produced greater EGFRvIII-specific immune responses as measured by antibody titer and DTH. Similar to the results of our previous study that did not include concurrent chemotherapy, vaccination with PEPvIII-KLH in the context of TMZ also resulted in increased median progression-free survival and overall survival when compared to historical matched controls. Thus, even in the context of myelodepletive TMZ regimens, our results suggest that EGFRvIII-targeted peptide vaccination therapy successfully eliminates tumors cells expressing the variant receptor without autoimmunity; moreover, it seems that this effect may be enhanced by concurrent TMZ chemotherapy.

Discussion

Despite the potential discovery of additional tumor-specific antigen s and the multitude of published clinical trials, peptide-based vaccines have met with little large-scale clinical success (Rosenberg et al., 2004). This has conferred a reputation on peptides for poor immunogenicity and diminishing promise as a vaccine immunotherapy platform. However, as addressed elsewhere (Choi et al., 2009), the reasons for what may seem to be unimpressive results may not be inherent to the therapeutic platform; indeed, the physiology of the typical glioma patient may hinder the likelihood that any given peptide vaccine will achieve its maximum efficacy. It is widely known that patients with malignancy, particularly those with glioma, have dysfunctional immunity. Although the precise mechanisms for this phenomenon have yet to be elucidated, transforming growth factor-beta (TGFβ) may play a significant role in suppressing immune responses. In an animal model of glioma, systemic inhibition of TGFβ augmented immune responses to a peptide vaccine and improved survival in a mouse model of intracranial glioma (Ueda et al., 2009). New insights into the balance between malignancy and immunosuppression may allow for the dismantling of barriers that keep peptide vaccines from reaching their full potential.

At the interface between glioma cells and immune cells, there are yet additional factors that may be playing a role in promoting immunosuppression in the tumor microenvironment. The B7-H1 costimulatory molecule, for example, has been implicated in the deletion of T-cells via IL-10-mediated signaling and regulation of Fas ligand expression. Glioma cells are frequently found to have lost a key nega-

tive regulator of B7-H1 expression, phosphatase and tensin homolog (PTEN), and in these cases, the normally pro-inflammatory Th1-biasing cytokine, IFNγ, may further upregulate B7-H1, resulting in escalating tumor immune-evasion even in the context of successful anti-tumor immunity (Parsa et al., 2007). Blockage of B7-H1 has shown promising results in mouse models of pancreatic, hepatocellular and ovarian cancer; these findings may eventually prove fruitful in enhancing the immunotherapeutic approach against malignant glioma.

A key mediator of glioma-induced immunosuppression is the signal transducer and activator of transcription-3 (STAT3). STAT3 is a major hub of signaling activity in pathways downstream of EGFR and EGFRvIII; upregulation of STAT3 and loss of STAT3 inhibitors is frequently associated with malignant glioma cells. Besides contributing to malignant proliferation, however, STAT3 may also be relevant to immunosuppression given its association with pathways downstream of the immunosuppressive cytokine IL-10, which is regulated by B7-H1. Experiments inhibiting STAT3 by siRNA seem to restore T-cell function and cytokine production (Wei et al., 2010), and even more promising is work showing that STAT3 inhibition can promote expression of costimulatory molecules on APCs, thus further enhancing T-cell activation (Hussain et al., 2007). Clearly, the pathways by which gliomas evade immune clearance require intense scrutiny, and any headway that can be made in this arena will provide more opportunities to optimize immunotherapy.

Another major suspect mediating immunosuppression in gliomas is the regulatory T-cell (T-reg). T-regs are CD4$^+$CD25$^+$FoxP3$^+$ lymphocytes that dampen the immune response. These cells have been shown to oppose inflammatory and autoimmune pathologies; however, they are also found to be abnormally elevated in patients with high-grade glioma (Fecci et al., 2006a; Learn et al., 2006). Strategies aimed at depleting T-regs by monoclonal antibodies targeting CD25 (high affinity IL-2Rα chain) or the cytotoxic T-lymphocyte antigen 4 (CTLA-4) expressed on T-regs have met with preclinical success (Fecci et al., 2007; Kohm et al., 2006). In a mouse model of malignant glioma, systemic administration of an anti-CD25 monoclonal antibody normalized T-reg fractions and restored cytotoxic T-cell function to normal levels, allowing subsequent immunotherapy to reject tumor in 100% of challenged mice (Fecci et al., 2006b).

Given that state-of-the-art therapy for malignant gliomas includes lymphodepletive doses of temozolomide (TMZ), one might assume that this chemotherapy may present a barrier to the ultimate success of peptide vaccine strategies. However, as accumulating evidence suggests, and as supported by data from our clinical trials, peptide vaccines given during hematopoietic recovery from lymphodepletion may actually augment immune responses (Heimberger et al., 2008). Mechanisms for this phenomenon are unclear and many explanations have been offered, though a combination of factors is likely involved. One theory known as homeostatic proliferation offers a physiologic explanation for the elaboration of post-lymphopenia immune responses; during lymphopenia, there is a surge of supportive cytokines such as IL-7 and IL-15, as the immune system attempts to reconstitute the depleted cellular compartment (Mitchell and Sampson, 2009). When these stimulatory signals in the setting of "room to expand" are combined with favorable selection by vaccine administration, both B- and T-cells specific to the administered antigen may have a competitive advantage and thus proliferate preferentially. With each cycle of depletion and subsequent enrichment, the frequency and potency of tumor-reactive immune cells may reach a level sufficient to overcome what is perceived as global immunosuppression, thus providing a setting in which tumor eradication can occur.

For patients with malignant glioma, treatment alternatives to surgery, radiation and chemotherapy are on the horizon and offer hope. Particularly, peptide vaccines can be a cost-effective yet robust immunotherapeutic strategy. Admittedly, many obstacles have been encountered in the pursuit of a glioma vaccine, yet recent successes with EGFRvIII and daily advances in our understanding of immunity in the context of CNS malignancies provide ample reason to remain optimistic.

References

Bigner SH, Humphrey PA, Wong AJ, Vogelstein B, Mark J, Friedman HS, Bigner DD (1990) Characterization of the epidermal growth factor receptor in human glioma cell lines and xenografts. Cancer Res 50:8017–8022

Choi BD, Archer GE, Mitchell DA, Heimberger AB, McLendon RE, Bigner DD, Sampson JH (2009) EGFRvIII-targeted vaccination therapy of malignant glioma. Brain Pathol 19: 713–723

Ciesielski MJ, Ahluwalia MS, Munich SA, Orton M, Barone T, Chanan-Khan A, Fenstermaker RA (2010) Antitumor cytotoxic T-cell response induced by a survivin peptide mimic. Cancer Immunol Immunother 59:1211–1221

Eguchi J, Hatano M, Nishimura F, Zhu X, Dusak JE, Sato H, Pollack IF, Storkus WJ, Okada H (2006) Identification of interleukin-13 receptor alpha2 peptide analogues capable of inducing improved antiglioma CTL responses. Cancer Res 66:5883–5891

Ekstrand AJ, James CD, Cavenee WK, Seliger B, Pettersson RF, Collins VP (1991) Genes for epidermal growth factor receptor, transforming growth factor alpha, and epidermal growth factor and their expression in human gliomas in vivo. Cancer Res 51:2164–2172

Fecci PE, Mitchell DA, Whitesides JF, Xie W, Friedman AH, Archer GE, Herndon JE 2nd, Bigner DD, Dranoff G, Sampson JH (2006a) Increased regulatory T-cell fraction amidst a diminished CD4 compartment explains cellular immune defects in patients with malignant glioma. Cancer Res 66:3294–3302

Fecci PE, Ochiai H, Mitchell DA, Grossi PM, Sweeney AE, Archer GE, Cummings T, Allison JP, Bigner DD, Sampson JH (2007) Systemic CTLA-4 blockade ameliorates glioma-induced changes to the CD4+ T cell compartment without affecting regulatory T-cell function. Clin Cancer Res 13:2158–2167

Fecci PE, Sweeney AE, Grossi PM, Nair SK, Learn CA, Mitchell DA, Cui X, Cummings TJ, Bigner DD, Gilboa E, Sampson JH (2006b) Systemic anti-CD25 monoclonal antibody administration safely enhances immunity in murine glioma without eliminating regulatory T cells. Clin Cancer Res 12:4294–4305

Heimberger AB, Archer GE, Crotty LE, McLendon RE, Friedman AH, Friedman HS, Bigner DD,, Sampson JH (2002) Dendritic cells pulsed with a tumor-specific peptide induce long-lasting immunity and are effective against murine intracerebral melanoma. Neurosurgery 50:158–164, discussion 164–156

Heimberger AB, Crotty LE, Archer GE, Hess KR, Wikstrand CJ, Friedman AH, Friedman HS, Bigner DD, Sampson JH (2003) Epidermal growth factor receptor VIII peptide vaccination is efficacious against established intracerebral tumors. Clin Cancer Res 9:4247–4254

Heimberger AB, Sun W, Hussain SF, Dey M, Crutcher L, Aldape K, Gilbert M, Hassenbusch SJ, Sawaya R, Schmittling B, Archer GE, Mitchell DA, Bigner DD, Sampson JH (2008) Immunological responses in a patient with glioblastoma multiforme treated with sequential courses of temozolomide and immunotherapy: case study. Neuro Oncol 10:98–103

Hussain SF, Kong LY, Jordan J, Conrad C, Madden T, Fokt I, Priebe W, Heimberger AB (2007) A novel small molecule inhibitor of signal transducers and activators of transcription 3 reverses immune tolerance in malignant glioma patients. Cancer Res 67:9630–9636

Izumoto S, Tsuboi A, Oka Y, Suzuki T, Hashiba T, Kagawa N, Hashimoto N, Maruno M, Elisseeva OA, Shirakata T, Kawakami M, Oji Y, Nishida S, Ohno S, Kawase I, Hatazawa J, Nakatsuka S, Aozasa K, Morita S, Sakamoto J, Sugiyama H, Yoshimine T (2008) Phase II clinical trial of wilms tumor 1 peptide vaccination for patients with recurrent glioblastoma multiforme. J Neurosurg 108:963–971

Jaros E, Perry RH, Adam L, Kelly PJ, Crawford PJ, Kalbag RM, Mendelow AD, Sengupta RP, Pearson AD (1992) Prognostic implications of p53 protein, epidermal growth factor receptor, and ki-67 labelling in brain tumours. Br J Cancer 66:373–385

Jin M, Komohara Y, Shichijo S, Harada M, Yamanaka R, Miyamoto S, Nikawa J, Itoh K, Yamada A (2008) Identification of EphB6 variant-derived epitope peptides recognized by cytotoxic T-lymphocytes from HLA-A24+ malignant glioma patients. Oncol Rep 19:1277–1283

Johns TG, Adams TE, Cochran JR, Hall NE, Hoyne PA, Olsen MJ, Kim YS, Rothacker J, Nice EC, Walker F, Ritter G, Jungbluth AA, Old LJ, Ward CW, Burgess AW, Wittrup KD, Scott AM (2004) Identification of the epitope for the epidermal growth factor receptor-specific monoclonal antibody 806 reveals that it preferentially recognizes an untethered form of the receptor. J Biol Chem 279: 30375–30384

Kohm AP, McMahon JS, Podojil JR, Begolka WS, DeGutes M, Kasprowicz DJ, Ziegler SF, Miller SD (2006) Cutting edge: anti-CD25 monoclonal antibody injection results in the functional inactivation, not depletion, of CD4+CD25+ T regulatory cells. J Immunol 176:3301–3305

Learn CA, Fecci PE, Schmittling RJ, Xie W, Karikari I, Mitchell DA, Archer GE, Wei Z, Dressman H, Sampson JH (2006) Profiling of CD4+, CD8+, and CD4+CD25+CD45RO+FoxP3+ T cells in patients with malignant glioma reveals differential expression of the immunologic transcriptome compared with T cells from healthy volunteers. Clin Cancer Res 12:7306–7315

Mitchell DA, Sampson JH (2009) Toward effective immunotherapy for the treatment of malignant brain tumors. Neurotherapeutics 6:527–538

Moscatello DK, Holgado-Madruga M, Godwin AK, Ramirez G, Gunn G, Zoltick PW, Biegel JA, Hayes RL, Wong AJ (1995) Frequent expression of a mutant epidermal growth factor receptor in multiple human tumors. Cancer Res 55: 5536–5539

Orgogozo JM, Gilman S, Dartigues JF, Laurent B, Puel M, Kirby LC, Jouanny P, Dubois B, Eisner L, Flitman S, Michel BF, Boada M, Frank A, Hock C (2003) Subacute meningoencephalitis in a subset of patients with AD after abeta42 immunization. Neurology 61:46–54

Parsa AT, Waldron JS, Panner A, Crane CA, Parney IF, Barry JJ, Cachola KE, Murray JC, Tihan T, Jensen MC, Mischel PS, Stokoe D, Pieper RO (2007) Loss of tumor suppressor PTEN function increases B7-H1 expression and immunoresistance in glioma. Nat Med 13:84–88

Rosenberg SA (2001) Progress in human tumour immunology and immunotherapy. Nature 411:380–384

Rosenberg SA, Yang JC, Restifo NP (2004) Cancer immunotherapy: moving beyond current vaccines. Nat Med 10: 909–915

Sampson JH, Aldape KD, Archer GE, Coan A, Desjardins A, Friedman AH, Friedman HS, Gilbert MR, Herndon JE 2nd, McLendon RE, Mitchell DA, Reardon DA, Sawaya R, Schmittling R, Shi W, Vrendenburgh JJ, Bigner DD, Heimberger AB (Submitted) Chemotherapy-induced lymphopenia enhances immune responses and eliminates EGFRvIII-expressing tumor cells in patients with glioblastoma. Neuro Oncol

Sampson JH, Archer GE, Mitchell DA, Heimberger AB, Herndon JE 2nd, Lally-Goss D, McGehee-Norman S, Paolino A, Reardon DA, Friedman AH, Friedman HS, Bigner DD (2009) An epidermal growth factor receptor variant III-targeted vaccine is safe and immunogenic in patients with glioblastoma multiforme. Mol Cancer Ther 8:2773–2779

Sampson JH, Crotty LE, Lee S, Archer GE, Ashley DM, Wikstrand CJ, Hale LP, Small C, Dranoff G, Friedman AH, Friedman HS, Bigner DD (2000) Unarmed, tumor-specific monoclonal antibody effectively treats brain tumors. Proc Natl Acad Sci USA 97:7503–7508

Sampson JH, Heimberger AB, Archer GE, Aldape KD, Friedman AH, Friedman HS, Gilbert MR, Herndon JE 2nd, McLendon RE, Mitchell DA, Reardon DA, Sawaya R, Schmittling RJ, Shi W, Vrendenburgh JJ, Bigner DD (Submitted) Immunologic escape after prolonged progression-free survival with epidermal growth factor receptor variant III (EGFRvIII) peptide vaccination in patients with newly diagnosed glioblastoma (GBM). J Clin Oncol

Scott AM, Lee FT, Tebbutt N, Herbertson R, Gill SS, Liu Z, Skrinos E, Murone C, Saunder TH, Chappell B, Papenfuss AT, Poon AM, Hopkins W, Smyth FE, MacGregor D, Cher LM, Jungbluth AA, Ritter G, Brechbiel MW, Murphy R, Burgess AW, Hoffman EW, Johns TG, Old LJ (2007) A phase I clinical trial with monoclonal antibody ch806 targeting transitional state and mutant epidermal growth factor receptors. Proc Natl Acad Sci USA 104:4071–4076

Stupp R, Hegi ME, Mason WP, van den Bent MJ, Taphoorn MJ, Janzer RC, Ludwin SK, Allgeier A, Fisher B, Belanger K, Hau P, Brandes AA, Gijtenbeek J, Marosi C, Vecht CJ, Mokhtari K, Wesseling P, Villa S, Eisenhauer E, Gorlia T, Weller M, Lacombe D, Cairncross JG, Mirimanoff RO (2009) Effects of radiotherapy with concomitant and adjuvant temozolomide versus radiotherapy alone on survival in glioblastoma in a randomised phase III study: 5-year analysis of the EORTC-NCIC trial. Lancet Oncol 10:459–466

Ueda R, Fujita M, Zhu X, Sasaki K, Kastenhuber ER, Kohanbash G, McDonald HA, Harper J, Lonning S, Okada H (2009) Systemic inhibition of transforming growth factor-beta in glioma-bearing mice improves the therapeutic efficacy of glioma-associated antigen peptide vaccines. Clin Cancer Res 15:6551–6559

Wei J, Barr J, Kong LY, Wang Y, Wu A, Sharma AK, Gumin J, Henry V, Colman H, Priebe W, Sawaya R, Lang FF, Heimberger AB (2010) Glioblastoma cancer-initiating cells inhibit T-cell proliferation and effector responses by the signal transducers and activators of transcription 3 pathway. Mol Cancer Ther 9:67–78

Wikstrand CJ, McLendon RE, Friedman AH, Bigner DD (1997) Cell surface localization and density of the tumor-associated variant of the epidermal growth factor receptor, EGFRvIII. Cancer Res 57:4130–4140

Wikstrand CJ, Reist CJ, Archer GE, Zalutsky MR, Bigner DD (1998) The class III variant of the epidermal growth factor receptor (EGFRvIII): characterization and utilization as an immunotherapeutic target. J Neurovirol 4:148–158

Yamanaka R, Itoh K (2007) Peptide-based immunotherapeutic approaches to glioma: a review. Expert Opin Biol Ther 7:645–649

Chapter 37

Malignant Glioma: Chemovirotherapy

Sherise D. Ferguson, Michael J. LaRiviere, Nassir Mansour, and Maciej S. Lesniak

Abstract The most common and aggressive form of glioma is the glioblastoma multiforme (GBM). Despite advances in surgery, chemotherapy, radiotherapy, and cancer biology, patient outcomes remain poor. Limited success in the treatment of these lesions has been attributed to several factors including: diffuse infiltration, micrometastasis, and limited blood brain barrier (BBB) penetration. Due to the poor outcome and limited treatment options, development of novel treatment options has become a priority. Virotherapy is a relatively recent strategy developed to tackle malignant gliomas. Several oncolytic viruses are currently being investigated. This chapter reviews the history of the development of adenoviral-based oncolytic viruses. The authors will discuss the strategies implemented thus far to improve their cytotoxic efficacy and their potential as therapeutic agents in glioma patients. It is well appreciated that the ideal therapeutic agent would be easily combined with conventional treatment modalities. With this in mind, the authors will also highlight the landmark studies examining the therapeutic effects of virotherapy in combination with radiation and chemotherapy. Lastly, we will comment on the challenges facing the advance of virotherapy and how they can be addressed in order to take full advantage of this modality.

Keywords Glioma · Virotherapy · Gene therapy · Oncolytic virus

Introduction

In spite of advances in diagnostics and therapeutics, the prognosis of malignant gliomas remains grim and their outcome uniformly poor. Malignant gliomas are complex, dynamic, and adaptive. The treatment of malignant gliomas remains difficult due to the aggressive nature of the tumors, clonal heterogeneity, acquired resistance to adjuvant treatments, dose limitations of chemotherapeutics due to systemic toxicity, and the presence of the blood brain barrier (BBB). The development of new strategies of treatment is crucial to improve the survival and hence the prognosis of malignant glioma patients. Recently, viral-based therapy has emerged as a therapeutic tool. The combination of viral therapy with conventional chemotherapy and radiotherapy may ultimately lead to rational, tailored treatments for this disease. Viral-based therapies encompass a broad range of topics including suicide gene therapy, immune gene therapy, and oncolytic therapy. In this chapter we will focus on oncolytic virotherapy and its potential in the treatment of malignant gliomas.

History of Oncolytic Virotherapy

The earliest attempt at using viral-based oncolysis in the treatment of malignant gliomas was done by Martuza et al. (1991). At that time it was known that certain herpes simplex virus (HSV) strains, specifically those lacking the gene for thymidine kinase *(tk)*, could only replicate in actively dividing cells. With this in mind, the authors hypothesized that this mutant HSV strain could be used to selectively target and lyse

M.S. Lesniak (✉)
Brain Tumor Center, University of Chicago, Chicago, IL 60637, USA
e-mail: mlesniak@surgery.bsd.uchicago.edu

M.A. Hayat (ed.), *Tumors of the Central Nervous System, Volume 1*,
DOI 10.1007/978-94-007-0344-5_37, © Springer Science+Business Media B.V. 2011

glioma cells. They utilized a thymidine kinase-negative mutant of herpes simplex virus-1 (*dlsptk*) and evaluated the ability of the virus to reduce glioma growth in vitro and vivo. The authors observed a significant decrease in tumor size in virus-treated subcutaneous gliomas in comparison with control tumors. In mice implanted with intracranial tumors, *dlsptk* had a robust impact on survival. By week 7, among animals treated with *dlsptk*, 57% were still alive, whereas all control mice were dead. Even though this study had limitations such as drug toxicity at high levels, these authors were the first to show that a genetically modified virus was capable of glioma cell destruction and hence warranted further investigation (Martuza et al., 1991).

The development of oncolytic virotherapies is advantageous for several reasons. First, they can be used in conjunction with conventional treatment modalities such as surgery, chemotherapy, and radiation (Lamfers et al., 2002). Second, viruses can also be modified to selectively kill actively dividing tumor cells. Third, most of the modern oncolytic viruses are replication competent (Bischoff et al., 1996; Fueyo et al., 2000). Infection of tumor cell by a replicative virus results in viral replication and subsequent release of viral progeny from the tumor cells. This offers the potential to amplify viral vectors in situ and to achieve lateral spread to adjacent cancer cells, thus resulting in efficient tumor penetration. Synthesis of oncolytic viruses that can target and infect tumor cells has become a major challenge in the fight against cancer. Using a virus with high specificity to cancer cells, minimal systemic side effects and ability to spare adjacent normal tissue is the cornerstone of oncolytic virotherapy. During the past decade, many novel oncolytic viruses have come into play and those that are adenovirus based are particularly popular and hence the focus of this chapter.

Biology and Replication Cycle of Adenovirus

Adenovirus is a nonenveloped, double stranded DNA virus. This icosahedral particle consists of an inner nucleoprotein core surrounded by an outer protein shell, and is 70–90 nm in size (McConnell and Imperiale, 2004). The first step in adenoviral replication and production of new viral particles is binding.

At the vertices of the adenoviral capsid, there is a penton base, which acts to anchor a fiber protein. This fiber knob is responsible for the attachment of virions to the coxsackievirus B adenovirus receptor (CAR) on the cell surface. Following binding, an exposed RGD (Arg-Gly-Asp) motif on the penton base interacts with members of the αv integrin family, triggering virus internalization via receptor-mediated endocytosis (Stewart et al., 1997). Once in the endosomes, adenoviral particles are transported to nuclear membrane, and viral DNA is allowed entry to the nucleus. Following viral DNA entry, early (E) genomic transcriptional regions are expressed in a specific sequence starting with E1A. Encoded E1A proteins activate the other adenovirus early transcription unit to allow the cell to enter S phase of the cell cycle. The products of the E2 region function promote replication of the viral genome. E3 proteins allow infected cells to circumvent the host immune system while E4 proteins are involved in cell cycle control. After early gene expression is completed, late genes (L1-5) are expressed and encode proteins necessary for viral assembly. This assembly takes place in the nucleus, followed by packaging, capsid assembly, and ultimately release of new viral particles (McConnell and Imperiale, 2004).

Much of the focus is now on realizing means of targeting different oncolytic viruses to tumor cells and, at the same time, preventing any destruction or toxicity to surrounding normal tissues. Many features of adenovirus make it well suited for virotherapy, particularly its amenability to viral genome manipulation and the ability of recombinant viruses to grow to high titers (Parker et al., 2009). Several adenoviral oncolytic viruses have been proposed and investigated, each with a different strategy of optimizing viral tropism and oncolysis. These include deletion of specific viral genomic regions increased specificity, modifications of viral structure to improve virus-cell interaction, and transcriptional targeting of viral genes using tumor-specific promoters.

ONYX-015

The dl1520 adenovirus (ONYX 015) is the first replication-competent adenovirus (CRAd) developed as an anti-neoplastic agent (Bischoff et al., 1996). The basis of its tumor selectivity is as follows: the adenoviral protein E1B-55 K binds to *p53*, hence inhibiting *p53*-dependent apoptosis and ability to induce expression of proapoptotic genes (Bischoff et al., 1996). This inhibition evades cell cycle control and promotes viral replication and progeny production. ONYX 015 has a deletion in the viral genomic region coding E1B 55 K. Such deletion restricts the replication of this virus to tumor cells with defective *p53* pathway. Loss of function of the *p53* tumor suppressor gene is the most common genetic defect in human malignancies including glioma (Collins, 1995). This virus takes advantage of the *p53* defect in human cancer cells, making this oncolytic virus a potentially powerful tool. In the landmark study confirming the selectivity and oncolytic effect of ONYX-015, the authors performed cytopathic effect assays on a panel of human tumor cells. ONYX failed to have a lytic effect on normal human diploid fibroblasts or on tumor cells with normal *p53* status. In contrast, in tumor lines with confirmed mutant *p53*, ONYX killed these cells with efficiency comparable to that of wild-type adenovirus (Bischoff et al., 1996). This was a promising result and the earliest to show that an adenovirus could be targeted to tumor cells.

Despite the initially promising results, the *p53* selectivity for ONYX has recently been questioned. Geoerger et al. (2002) demonstrated that ONYX replicated and had an oncolytic effect in glioma xenografts independent of *p53* status (Geoerger et al., 2002). Several other studies have shown a similar pattern of results making the specificity of ONYX for *p-53* deficient cells somewhat controversial (Dix et al., 2001). Furthermore, in addition to blocking *p53* binding, E1B 55K has other functions, including selective export and translation of viral mRNAs during infection. It has been suggested that ONYX (where E1B 55 K is deleted) may replicate in tumor cells due to aberrations in cancer cell nuclear mRNA export rather than because of p53 alteration (O'Shea et al., 2004).

Even though its mechanism and selectivity is still ambiguous, ONYX is the first and only oncolytic adenovirus that has had a phase I clinical trial for recurrent glioma (Chiocca et al., 2004). This trial showed that injections of ONYX into resected tumor cavities were tolerable at high doses. Twenty-four patients were enrolled in this trial between January 2000 and May 2002. Ten of these patients experienced an adverse event, (e.g., neuropathy, headache, diarrhea) though none of these were attributed to ONYX treatment. Median time to progression of disease after ONYX for all patients was 46 days (range of 13–452 days) (Chiocca et al., 2004). Thus, while ONYX was shown to be safe, no concrete anti-tumor efficacy could be demonstrated by this trial; thus, suggesting the need for further studies to assess therapeutic potential.

Delta 24

Cancer cells lacking Rb function have been targeted in a similar way. Fueyo et al. (2000) proposed that an adenoviral vector could be developed to exploit Rb deficiency in tumor cells. This system relies on the adenoviral protein E1A. This protein is known to evade cell cycle checkpoints via interference with proteins of the Rb family (McConnell and Imperiale, 2004). E1A-Rb interaction results in the release of E2F from preexisting cellular E2F-Rb complexes. This free E2F subsequently activates both the E2 promoter and several cell cycle-regulatory genes. The transcription of these cellular genes in turn favors viral synthesis (Nevins, 1992). Fueyo et al. (2000) used this mechanism in order to develop Delta 24, a CRAd that encodes an E1A protein with a deletion of amino acids 120–127. This deletion prevents interaction between E1A and Rb; thus, this virus can only replicate in cells with defective Rb protein. These authors found that Delta 24 reliably produced glioma cell lysis within 14 days of infection in vitro. Furthermore, tumor cells with restored Rb were resistant to Delta 24-induced oncolysis. In vivo, subcutaneous D-54 malignant glioma tumors were injected with either Delta 24 or wild-type adenovirus control. Tumors in the Delta 24-treatment group were 66.3% smaller than tumors in the control animals (Fueyo et al., 2000).

Since its conception, the oncolytic effect of Delta 24 has been investigated extensively in vitro and in vivo. This system has served as the backbone for several viral genetic modifications to enhance infectivity, oncolytic potency, and hence efficacy. For example, one of the earliest modifications to Delta 24 was the addition of an RGD (Arg-Gly-Asp) motif. As stated above, CAR is essential for adenovirus entry in cells. It has been demonstrated that gliomas express low levels of this receptor, thereby limiting virulence (Lamfers et al., 2002). In order to address this obstacle, Lamfers et al. (2002) added an RGD motif to the fiber knob of Delta 24 (Delta 24-RGD) to enhance the virus interaction with αv integrins and its subsequent tropism towards gliomas. The antitumor activity of Delta 24-RGD was demonstrated in vivo using subcutaneous human malignant glioma xenografts. Tumors treated with virus for 5 days resulted in significant tumor growth delay (>117 days) compared with untreated controls (Lamfers et al., 2002).

Recently, Piao et al. (2009) offered another proposition to enhance Delta 24 virulence; retargeting the virus to receptors that are expressed in glioma cells. Epidermal growth factor receptor (EGFR) overexpression is the most common genetic alteration in GBMs with a frequency of ~40%. Along with EGFR amplification, there are also mutations; the most common of which is EGFR variant III (EGFRvIII). This variant is observed in 20–30% of patients with malignant glioma and in patients where EGFR gene amplification is confirmed, the proportion of EGFRvIII increases to up to 60% (Frederick et al., 2000). Piao et al. (2009) exploited this tumor-specific expression and constructed Delta-24-RIVER (Retargeted Infectivity Via EGFR). This oncolytic adenovirus, like Delta-24, is restricted to replication in Rb defective cells but has the addition of an EGFRvIII-specific binding peptide to the fiber protein in order to enhance glioma targeting. The authors demonstrated in vitro that Delta-24-RIVER replication and oncolysis was selective for EGFRvIII-expressing glioma cells. Additionally, intracranial glioma xenografts expressing EGFR were treated with Delta-24-RIVER or UV-inactivated Delta-24-RIVER. They found that treatment with Delta-24-RIVER resulted in a statistically significant increase in animal survival (26.1 days versus 14 days in control animals) (Piao et al., 2009). This study was first to successfully target an oncolytic virus using a glioma-specific receptor. In conclusion, oncolytic virotherapy has made significant strides with the development of the Delta-24 paradigm. Although Delta 24-based therapy has not yet been tested in clinical trials, it is clearly effective against gliomas in preclinical evaluations.

Survivin

Another approach used to enhance adenoviral tumor specificity is the manipulation of a tumor-specific promoter, which then responds to the specific cellular cues of tumor cells to mediate its replication. The survivin

gene (encoding the protein survivin) is an example of such a promoter and has become the subject of intense research. Survivin is an anti-apoptotic protein which plays an important role in tumorgenesis and malignancy progression. Its expression has been confirmed in many cancers including gliomas, (Van Houdt et al., 2006), but expression is undetectable in normal adult tissues (Chakravarti et al., 2002). Chakravarti et al. (2002) demonstrated the prognostic significance of survivin in patients with malignant gliomas. The authors prospectively collected and analyzed 92 glioma specimens for this work. Not only did they find that the majority of gliomas (64%) were positive for survivin, but also that GBMs had a higher rate of survivin positivity (80%) compared with non-GBM tumors (39%). Furthermore, patients with survivin-positive gliomas had shorter survival times (median 11 months) compared to their survivin negative counterparts (median 64 months).

Van Houdt et al. (2006) hypothesized that survivin could be used for glioma-specific targeting. They constructed a CRAd incorporating both the survivin promoter (E1 gene regulated by survivin promoter) and a capsid modification RGD-4C to promote infectivity (CRAd-S-RGD). The lytic effect of this virus was examined on a panel of glioma cell lines. After 10 days of incubation, crystal violet staining revealed the profound oncolytic effect of CRAd-S-RGD in all cell lines. In vivo, CRAd-S-RGD significantly inhibited flank tumor growth; the authors demonstrated up to a 67% reduction in volume in tumors treated with CRAd-S-RGD [Van Houdt et al., (2006)]. These data were some of the earliest confirming the utility of survivin in glioma-targeted treatments.

Since its successful incorporation into an oncolytic virus, several studies have made creative modifications to survivin-based viruses to examine anti-tumor effects (Nandi et al., 2009; Ulasov et al., 2007). For example, gliomas are known to over-express CD46, CD80, and CD86, all of which bind adenovirus serotype 3. Nandi et al. (2009) recently demonstrated enhanced cytotoxicity in vivo after the addition of a chimeric fiber consisting of adenoviral serotype 3 knob to a survivin-based CRAd (CRAd-S-5/3). This group also showed that tropism and a subsequent oncolytic effect of CRAd-S could be enhanced with the addition of a pk7 fiber knob modification. In vivo CRAd-S-pk7 suppressed U87glioma growth by > 300% compared to tumors treated with control virus (Ulasov et al., 2007).

Combination Therapies

As mentioned above, one of the advantages of oncolytic virotherapy is that it can be used in conjunction with conventional treatments such as surgery, chemotherapy, and radiation. One of the earliest studies investigating the use of combination therapy was performed by Heise et al. (1997). The authors tested the combined antitumor effect of ONYX-10 and chemotherapy (cisplatin or 5-fluorouracil 5-FU) in nude mouse with HLac (head and neck) tumor xenografts. Tumors that were treated with both ONYX and intraperitoneal cisplatin or 5-FU showed longer survival times compared to treatment with chemotherapy alone (Heise et al., 1997).

Delta 24-based viruses have also been tested in combination with chemotherapy with encouraging results. For example, Gomez-Manzano et al. (2006) looked at the combined effect of Delta-24 with topoisomerase I inhibitor irinotecan (CPT-11). This combination was theorized to be efficacious based on 3 factors. First, adenoviruses induce infected cells to enter the S phase of the cell cycle in order for viral DNA synthesis to occur. Second, Delta-24 specifically induces accumulation of infected cancer cells in the S phase. Third, it is established that the effect of CPT-11 is most marked in cells in the S phase (Fueyo et al., 2000; Gomez-Manzano et al., 2006). Given this evidence, the authors hypothesized that the combination of Delta-24 and CPT-11 may show an increased anti-glioma effect. This effect was tested in vivo in mice with human glioma xenografts implanted intracranially. The combination treatment of Delta-24 followed by CPT-11 resulted in a statistically significant increase in animal survival (median 42 days) when compared to animal treated with virus (median 35 days) or CPT-11 alone (31 days). Furthermore, among the animals receiving a single treatment, there were no long term survivors; however, 22.5% of animals receiving dual treatment survived over 3 months. Microscopic examination of the brains of these long-term survivors showed complete tumor regression (Gomez-Manzano et al., 2006).

Radiation plays a central role in the treatment of malignant gliomas, and it has also been reported to be potentiated by oncolytic adenoviruses. The antitumor effect of ONYX in combination with radiation therapy in vivo was evaluated in the human malignant glioma flank xenografts IGRG121 and IGRG88 by Geoerger et al. (2003). Combined treatment of irradiation given 6–7 h prior to intratumoral ONYX injection yielded an additive antitumor activity with 73% partial tumor regressions (Geoerger et al., 2003). Lamfers et al. (2002) had similarly positive results using Delta-24 RGD. These authors also used IGRG121 subcutaneous xenografts. Animals received either 5 Gy total body irradiation, tumoral injections of Delta-24RGD, or a combination of both treatments for 5 days. In the virus only group, 6 of 9 animals displayed tumor regression (1 with complete regression and 5 with partial regression). However, when Delta-24 RGD was combined with irradiation, all animals experienced tumor regression (5 with partial and 5 with complete regression). Additionally, radiation enhanced Delta-24RGD antitumor activity, such that a 10-fold lower viral dose achieved the same therapeutic response (Lamfers et al., 2002).

Challenges and Future Directions

Uncovering Mechanisms of CRAd-Induced Cell Death

Even though there are several studies confirming the benefit of oncolytic viruses particularly in combination with adjuvant therapy, the mechanisms that govern oncolysis are still the subject of extensive research. Autophagy has been proposed as a potential mechanism. Autophagic cell death is a type of programmed cell death that is an alternative to apoptosis. In addition to studying whether the combination of the Delta-24-RGD and radiation would result in an enhanced an antiglioma effect, Alonso et al. (2008) also investigated whether this dual treatment induced autophagic-cell death. The combination of Delta-24-RGD and radiation did significantly increase the survival of glioma bearing animals. Interestingly, immunofluorescence analyses of glioma xenografts identified high levels of Atg5 (a proautophagic protein) in the virus-treated samples (Alonso et al., 2008). This study emphasized the role of autophagy in the anti-glioma effect of combined therapy and since then, this mechanism been under heavy investigation. In a very recent study, Tyler et al. (2009a) set out to characterize the mechanism of glioma cell death following virotherapy. In vitro, the authors found that treatment of glioma cells CRAd-S-RGD led to formation of autophagic vesicular organelles (AVOs) detected by electron microscopy. Additionally, glioma cells treated with TMZ prior to infection with CRAd-S-pk7, resulted in induction of Atg5 protein and AVOs, further indicating that autophagy, rather than apoptotic mechanisms may play a role in CRAd induced glioma cell death. In vivo, however, they found evidence of both apoptosis and autophagy in CRAd-S-pk7-induced glioma cell death (Tyler et al., 2009a) making the mechanism even more complex than initially described.

Nandi et al. (2008) proposed that glioma stem cells (CD 133+) may also play a role. Glioma stem cells are believed to be responsible for glioma recurrences and decreased survival. CD133+ glioma stem cells are resistant to current modes of therapy, including radiation and TMZ based chemotherapy and are present at a higher fraction in recurrent gliomas. These cells also upregulate anti-apoptotic proteins indicating that they evade normal cellular regulation (Liu et al., 2006). In a recent study, Nandi et al. (2008) found that the survivin-based adenovirus (CRAd-S-pk7) had increased activity in the presence of radiation. In vitro, CRAd-S-pk7 cytotoxicity increased 20–50%. In vivo, mice with flank tumors treated with CRAd-S-pk7 and then exposed to low-dose radiation had significantly smaller tumor size than mice treated with CRAd-S-pk7 alone. More interestingly, the authors were the first to demonstrate that CRAd-S-pk7 also targeted CD133+ glioma stem cells. In vitro, CRAd-S-pk7, showed increased toxicity and viral replication in CD133+ stem cells compared to CD133- cells. In vivo, the authors injected CD133+ U373 cells into the flank of nude mice and found response to radiation; CRAd-S-pk7 treatment group achieved the most significant tumor growth inhibition and this group showed ~a 100 fold increase in viral replication compared to CRAd-S-pk7 alone. In sum, this study showed for the first time that radiation increases the replication of CRAd-S-pk7 and therefore enhances the cytopathic effect in the context of CD133+ glioma stem cells (Nandi et al., 2008). In conclusion, despite preclinical studies confirming the potential therapeutic benefit, the mechanisms of CRAd-mediated killing are not completely deciphered. A more in depth understanding of the mechanisms involved in virus-induced oncolysis is necessary to advance this treatment modality.

Viral Delivery

The issue of virus distribution remains an obstacle in glioma virotherapy (Tyler et al., 2009). Due to dependence on diffusion, after intracranial injection, viral vectors have a limited reach and often do not infect glioma cells that are distant from the injection site (Lang et al., 2003). Due to the infiltrative nature of high-grade gliomas this shortcoming is paramount. In light of these considerations, other delivery methods have been explored to address this limitation, the most notable being convection-enhanced delivery and stem cells.

Convection-enhanced delivery (CED) is a promising emergent neurosurgical technique for intraparenchymal administration of virus. Unlike diffusion following a bolus injection, which relies on a concentration gradient to drive fluid movement, CED relies on a pressure gradient to drive bulk flow of an infusate through parenchyma (Morrison et al., 1994). Because infusion directly into parenchyma circumvents the BBB, blood-tumor barrier (BTB), and the blood-cerebrospinal fluid barrier (BCB), CED has shown great promise as a means to deliver viral vectors that cannot normally cross these barriers. Additionally, because CED allows specific brain regions or structures to be targeted, a much higher level of therapeutic agent can be achieved without toxicity than would be tolerated with systemic administration (Groothuis, 2000). Morrison et al. (1994) developed a mathematical model for CED, or "high-flow microinfusion" of drug into brain tissue. They confirmed their calculations with autoradiography of ^{111}In-transferrin infusions into cat brain and demonstrated a large distribution of infusate beyond what is possible with simple diffusion (Morrison et al., 1994). Bankiewicz et al. (2000) attempted to convect adeno-associated viral vector into parkinsonian monkey brains and concluded that delivery of viral vectors in sufficient quantities to the whole brain could be accomplished with CED. Szerlip et al. (2007) demonstrated the utility of real-time MR imaging of CED to monitor virus distribution indicating an important clinical advantage of CED. Of note, no studies have yet convected an oncolytic adenovirus. The above mentioned study focused on the convection of viral vectors for the delivery of gene therapies for potential treatment of degenerative disease. However, the fact that effective viral infusion and distribution is possible with CED is an accomplishment that can hopefully be utilized by oncolytic CRAd therapies.

Neural and mesenchymal stem cells have also been explored as vehicles for oncolytic viruses, given that they possess an intrinsic tropism for malignant brain tumors (Nakamizo et al., 2005). Tyler et al. (2009b) successfully infected neural stem cells (NSCs) with a modified adenovirus CRAd-S-pk7. They demonstrated that in vivo, NSCs loaded with this oncolytic adenovirus had improved viral distribution compared to injection of the virus alone. Moreover, flank tumors treated with virus loaded NSCs, showed decreased tumor volume (69.4 mm^3 ± 16.5) compared to tumors treated with virus alone (138.22 mm^3 ± 22.7) or saline control (235.9 mm^3 ± 63.3) (Tyler et al., 2009b). Bone marrow derived mesenchymal stem cells (MSCs) have also been reported to transport oncolytic viruses. Sonabend et al. (2008) reported that MSCs could also be utilized to successfully deliver an oncolytic adenovirus to intracranial glioma model.

Conclusion

In conclusion, the treatment of malignant gliomas is currently insufficient. Virotherapy is an exciting, emerging treatment that has undergone significant advances, particularly during the past decade. The construction of tumor-specific CRAds, discovery of survivin, and the potentiation of virus-induced oncolysis by adjuvant treatments are among the highlights of the many accomplishments achieved in this field. Oncolytic adenoviruses have done well in animal models, but more clinical trials are eagerly awaited. However, there is still much unknown regarding the mechanisms governing virotherapy. Additionally, the role of autophagy, glioma stem cells and the issue of viral delivery are important issues that have not yet been completely resolved. Before this modality can progress forward fully, these questions must be answered in order to obtain the full benefit of this potentially powerful oncolytic tool.

References

Alonso MM, Jiang H, Yokoyama T, Xu J, Bekele NB, Lang FF, Kondo S, Gomez-Manzano C, Fueyo J (2008) Delta-24-RGD in combination with RAD001 induces enhanced anti-glioma effect via autophagic cell death. Mol Ther 16: 487–493

Bankiewicz KS, Eberling JL, Kohutnicka M, Jagust W, Pivirotto P, Bringas J, Cunningham J, Budinger TF, Harvey-White J (2000) Convection-enhanced delivery of AAV vector in parkinsonian monkeys; in vivo detection of gene expression and restoration of dopaminergic function using pro-drug approach. Exp Neurol 164:2–14

Bischoff JR, Kirn DH, Williams A, Heise C, Horn S, Muna M, Ng L, Nye JA, Sampson-Johannes A, Fattaey A, McCormick F (1996) An adenovirus mutant that replicates selectively in p53-deficient human tumor cells. Science 274:373–376

Chakravarti A, Noll E, Black PM, Finkelstein DF, Finkelstein DM, Dyson NJ, Loeffler JS (2002) Quantitatively determined survivin expression levels are of prognostic value in human gliomas. J Clin Oncol 20:1063–1068

Chiocca EA, Abbed KM, Tatter S, Louis DN, Hochberg FH, Barker F, Kracher J, Grossman SA, Fisher JD, Carson K, Rosenblum M, Mikkelsen T, Olson J, Markert J, Rosenfeld S, Nabors LB, Brem S, Phuphanich S, Freeman S, Kaplan R, Zwiebel J (2004) A phase I open-label, dose-escalation, multi-institutional trial of injection with an E1B-attenuated adenovirus, ONYX-015, into the peritumoral region of recurrent malignant gliomas, in the adjuvant setting. Mol Ther 10:958–966

Collins VP (1995) Genetic alterations in gliomas. J Neuro-Oncol 24:37–38

Dix BR, Edwards SJ, Braithwaite AW (2001) Does the antitumor adenovirus ONYX-015/dl1520 selectively target cells defective in the p53 pathway?. J Virol 75:5443–5447

Frederick L, Wang XY, Eley G, James CD (2000) Diversity and frequency of epidermal growth factor receptor mutations in human glioblastomas. Cancer Res 60:1383–1387

Fueyo J, Gomez-Manzano C, Alemany R, Lee PS, McDonnell TJ, Mitlianga P, Shi YX, Levin VA, Yung WK, Kyritsis AP (2000) A mutant oncolytic adenovirus targeting the rb pathway produces anti-glioma effect in vivo. Oncogene 19:2–12

Geoerger B, Grill J, Opolon P, Morizet J, Aubert G, Lecluse Y, van Beusechem VW, Gerritsen WR, Kirn DH, Vassal G (2003) Potentiation of radiation therapy by the oncolytic adenovirus dl1520 (ONYX-015) in human malignant glioma xenografts. Br J Cancer 89:577–584

Geoerger B, Grill J, Opolon P, Morizet J, Aubert G, Terrier-Lacombe MJ, Bressac De-Paillerets B, Barrois M, Feunteun J, Kirn DH, Vassal G (2002) Oncolytic activity of the E1B-55 kDa-deleted adenovirus ONYX-015 is independent of cellular p53 status in human malignant glioma xenografts. Cancer Res 62:764–772

Gomez-Manzano C, Alonso MM, Yung WK, McCormick F, Curiel DT, Lang FF, Jiang H, Bekele BN, Zhou X, Alemany R, Fueyo J (2006) Delta-24 increases the expression and activity of topoisomerase I and enhances the antiglioma effect of irinotecan. Clin Cancer Res 12:556–562

Groothuis DR (2000) The blood-brain and blood-tumor barriers: a review of strategies for increasing drug delivery. Neuro-oncology 2:45–59

Heise C, Sampson-Johannes A, Williams A, McCormick F, Von Hoff DD, Kirn DH (1997) ONYX-015, an E1B gene-attenuated adenovirus, causes tumor-specific cytolysis and antitumoral efficacy that can be augmented by standard chemotherapeutic agents. Nat Med 3:639–645

Lamfers ML, Grill J, Dirven CM, Van Beusechem VW, Geoerger B, Van Den Berg J, Alemany R, Fueyo J, Curiel DT, Vassal G, Pinedo HM, Vandertop WP, Gerritsen WR (2002) Potential of the conditionally replicative adenovirus ad5-Delta24RGD in the treatment of malignant gliomas and its enhanced effect with radiotherapy. Cancer Res 62:5736–5742

Lang FF, Bruner JM, Fuller GN, Aldape K, Prados MD, Chang S, Berger MS, McDermott MW, Kunwar SM, Junck LR, Chandler W, Zwiebel JA, Kaplan RS, Yung WK (2003) Phase I trial of adenovirus-mediated p53 gene therapy for recurrent glioma: biological and clinical results. J Clin Oncol 21:2508–2518

Liu G, Yuan X, Zeng Z, Tunici P, Ng H, Abdulkadir IR, Lu L, Irvin D, Black KL, Yu JS (2006) Analysis of gene expression and chemoresistance of CD133+ cancer stem cells in glioblastoma. Mol Cancer 5:67

Martuza RL, Malick A, Markert JM, Ruffner KL, Coen DM (1991) Experimental therapy of human glioma By Means Of a genetically engineered virus mutant. Science 252:854–856

McConnell MJ, Imperiale MJ (2004) Biology of adenovirus and its use as a vector for gene therapy. Hum Gene Ther 15:1022–1033

Morrison PF, Laske DW, Bobo H, Oldfield EH, Dedrick RL (1994) High-flow microinfusion: tissue penetration and pharmacodynamics. Am J Physiol 266:R292–R305

Nakamizo A, Marini F, Amano T, Khan A, Studeny M, Gumin J, Chen J, Hentschel S, Vecil G, Dembinski J, Andreeff M, Lang FF (2005) Human bone marrow-derived mesenchymal stem cells in the treatment of gliomas. Cancer Res 65:3307–3318

Nandi S, Ulasov IV, Rolle CE, Han Y, Lesniak MS (2009) A chimeric adenovirus with an ad 3 fiber knob modification augments glioma virotherapy. J Gene Med 11:1005–1011

Nandi S, Ulasov IV, Tyler MA, Sugihara AQ, Molinero L, Han Y, Zhu ZB, Lesniak MS (2008) Low-dose radiation enhances survivin-mediated virotherapy against malignant glioma stem cells. Cancer Res 68:5778–5784

Nevins JR (1992) E2F: a link between the rb tumor suppressor protein and viral oncoproteins. Science 258:424–429

O'Shea CC, Johnson L, Bagus B, Choi S, Nicholas C, Shen A, Boyle L, Pandey K, Soria C, Kunich J, Shen Y, Habets G, McCormick F (2004) Late viral RNA export, rather than p53 inactivation, determines ONYX-015 tumor selectivity. Cancer Cell 6:611–623

Parker JN, Bauer DF, Cody JJ, Markert JM (2009) Oncolytic viral therapy of malignant glioma. Neurotherapeutics 6:558–569

Piao Y, Jiang H, Alemany R, Krasnykh V, Marini FC, Xu J, Alonso MM, Conrad CA, Aldape KD, Gomez-Manzano C, Fueyo J (2009) Oncolytic adenovirus retargeted to delta-EGFR induces selective antiglioma activity. Cancer Gene Ther 16:256–265

Sonabend AM, Ulasov IV, Tyler MA, Rivera AA, Mathis JM, Lesniak MS (2008) Mesenchymal stem cells effectively deliver an oncolytic adenovirus to intracranial glioma. Stem Cells 26:831–841

Stewart PL, Chiu CY, Huang S, Muir T, Zhao Y, Chait B, Mathias P, Nemerow GR (1997) Cryo-EM visualization of an exposed RGD epitope on adenovirus that escapes antibody neutralization. EMBO J 16:1189–1198

Szerlip NJ, Walbridge S, Yang L, Morrison PF, Degen JW, Jarrell ST, Kouri J, Kerr PB, Kotin R, Oldfield EH, Lonser RR (2007) Real-time imaging of convection-enhanced delivery of viruses and virus-sized particles. J Neurosurg 107:560–567

Tyler MA, Ulasov IV, Lesniak MS (2009a) Cancer cell death by design: apoptosis, autophagy and glioma virotherapy. Autophagy 5:856–857

Tyler MA, Ulasov IV, Sonabend AM, Nandi S, Han Y, Marler S, Roth J, Lesniak MS (2009b) Neural stem cells target intracranial glioma to deliver an oncolytic adenovirus in vivo. Gene Ther 16:262–278

Ulasov IV, Zhu ZB, Tyler MA, Han Y, Rivera AA, Khramtsov A, Curiel DT, Lesniak MS (2007) Survivin-driven and fiber-modified oncolytic adenovirus exhibits potent antitumor activity in established intracranial glioma. Hum Gene Ther 18:589–602

Van Houdt WJ, Haviv YS, Lu B, Wang M, Rivera AA, Ulasov IV, Lamfers ML, Rein D, Lesniak MS, Siegal GP, Dirven CM, Curiel DT, Zhu ZB (2006) The human survivin promoter: a novel transcriptional targeting strategy for treatment of glioma. J Neurosurg 104:583–592

Chapter 38

Intracranial Glioma: Delivery of an Oncolytic Adenovirus

Justin Kranzler, Matthew A. Tyler, Ilya V. Ulasov, and Maciej S. Lesniak

Keywords Glioma · Brain cancer · Oncolytic virus · Adenovirus

Introduction

Intracranial gliomas are the most prevalent form of primary brain tumors. The dynamic biology of these cancers compounded by their elusive location within the brain renders them very difficult to treat by means of conventional therapy. Despite continued advances in surgical and medical therapies, the outcome for patients diagnosed with this form of cancer remains in need of dramatic improvements. Gliomas, like many other forms of cancer, are subject to unpredictable genotypic and phenotypic alterations resulting in treatment resistant clones (Ehtesham et al., 2005). The selective permeability of the blood brain barrier limits the effectiveness of most chemotherapeutic agents, impeding their ability to reach distant tumor cells (Lesniak and Brem, 2004). Surgical treatment also faces many obstacles, as the biological nature of these tumors causes them to infiltrate diffusely within surrounding brain parenchyma (Ehtesham et al., 2005). In light of these challenges, novel techniques and alternative approaches are being explored to treat this terminal condition.

Gene therapy is one method that is being heavily investigated to treat malignant gliomas. With the help of viral vectors, gene therapy allows for the introduction of genetic material into deficient cells to compensate for abnormal genes or to make a beneficial protein. Due to the fact that most brain tumors do not metastasize beyond the walls of the central nervous system, gene therapy and the local delivery of vectors carrying therapeutic genes appears to be a promising frontier in experimental brain tumor treatment. While treating patients with radiation and chemotherapeutic agents, such as temozolomide, following tumor resection provides a survival benefit of several months, the effects are not long lasting (Stupp et al., 2005). The inability of chemotherapy, radiation and gross total resection to cure patients diagnosed with this form of cancer beckons for an alternative pathway to combat this disease.

The use of viruses to specifically kill tumor cells while sparing normal cells is known as virotherapy (Chu et al., 2004). Viruses have evolved to infiltrate host cells and usurp the cellular machinery in order to replicate and package their own genome. Virotherapy, in this sense, involves the targeting of malignant tumor cells in order to infect them with oncolytic viruses. Once internalized, these viruses gain control over the proliferating tumor and induce cell death. The most common viral vectors used in virotherapy include: herpes simplex virus, retrovirus, measles virus, reovirus, and adenovirus (Zheng et al., 2007). The delivery of oncolytic agents to targeted tumor cells can be accomplished using a mélange of different viruses as vessels; however, this chapter will focus on the delivery of an oncolytic adenovirus.

A key component for successful and effective gene therapy resides in the capacity of the gene delivery vectors. Adenoviruses possess many appealing characteristics that render them an excellent

M.S. Lesniak (✉)
Brain Tumor Center, University of Chicago, Chicago,
IL 60637, USA
e-mail: mlesniak@surgery.bsd.uchicago.edu

M.A. Hayat (ed.), *Tumors of the Central Nervous System, Volume 1*,
DOI 10.1007/978-94-007-0344-5_38, © Springer Science+Business Media B.V. 2011

model for developing effective oncolytic therapies for brain tumors. These features, including their intrinsic ability to grow to high titers, large carrying capacity for transgenes, broad tropism, efficient transduction, and mild pathogenicity all favor adenoviruses as significant therapeutic agents (Chu et al., 2004; Pulkkanen and Yla-Herttuala, 2005; Sonabend et al., 2007). Additionally, the viral genome is large enough to incorporate foreign genes and it has been carefully identified and fully sequenced allowing it to be easily manipulated for therapeutic purposes.

Biology of Adenovirus – Molecular Composition

Approximately 50 known human adenovirus serotypes exist and are classified into six subgroups, A-F, with serotypes 2 and 5 of subgroup C being the most extensively characterized in developing therapeutic oncolytic adenoviruses (Palmer and Ng, 2008). The structure and genomic organization is highly conserved amongst all serotypes, with each adenovirus being a non-enveloped virus of approximately 150 μDa (Curiel and Douglas, 2002). An intact virion is composed of multiple copies of 11 different structural proteins, 7 of which form the icosahedral capsid and 4 of which are packaged with the linear double-stranded DNA in the nucleoprotein core. Trimeric hexon proteins comprise the facets of the capsid, and 12 protein fibers protrude from each penton base at the vertices of the icosahedral capsid.

Adenovirus types 2 and 5 bind to host cells via their fiber protein, which recognizes a 46 kDa cell receptor known as CAR (Coxsackie and Adenovirus Receptor). While it has been shown that the transduction efficiency of Ad5-based vectors closely correlates with the cell surface density of CAR (Hemmi et al., 1998), several other proteins and co-receptors are required for successful cell recognition and internalization. Following the initial binding event, the integrin-binding motif (RGD) present on penton base binds αv integrins, triggering viral internalization via clathrin-coated endocytosis. During the intracytoplasmic transport of the virus, disassembly of the viral capsid occurs allowing free viral DNA to enter the nucleus through nuclear pores (Curiel and Douglas, 2002). Viral transcription ensues in a three phase

manner upon entering the nucleus: early, intermediate, and late.

During the early phase of adenoviral transcription, the host cell is transformed into an efficient producer of the viral genome. Viral proteins interact with proteins of the host cell halting normal cellular functions, preventing an anti-viral host response, and making the conditions well suited for viral DNA replication (Curiel and Douglas, 2002). Early genes are expressed in a temporal and coordinated fashion, beginning with the expression of the E1A region (early region 1A) and ending with the E4 region (early region 4). The major function of E1A is to induce the host cell into S-phase, thereby creating an optimal environment for viral DNA replication. The E1B region (early region 1B) is expressed next, and its function is to further enhance the host's intracellular environment for successful DNA synthesis, in addition to preventing cellular apoptosis (Curiel and Douglas, 2002). Regions E2–E4 encode proteins that govern host immune response, apoptosis, and mRNA transport. Following the early phase, viral structure proteins and proteins necessary for the assembly of virulent virions are encoded by genes expressed during the intermediate and late phases of viral replication. Upon completion of viral progeny assembly, approximately 1000 new viral particles are released per cell by cytolysis (Chu et al., 2004).

Adenoviral Therapy

The use of conditionally replicating adenoviruses (CRAds) to treat malignant brain tumors has undergone extensive research and has proven to be a promising mode of cancer therapy. Conditionally-replicating adenoviruses are genetically altered to replicate within tumor cells while exhibiting a high degree of replication, infectivity, cytotoxicity and transgene expression (Chu et al., 2004; Geoerger et al., 2002; Sonabend et al., 2007; Ulasov et al., 2008). With cytotoxic replication as the presumed goal for oncolytic virotherapy, it is imperative that CRAds specifically target tumor cells and spare surrounding normal cells. The precise targeting ability of CRAds has been accomplished by manipulating specific elements residing in the early regions (E1A and E1B) of the adenovirus genome (Ulasov et al., 2008). Vectors of this class that have gained recent attention include ONYX-015, Delta-24-RGD and CRAd-Survivin-pk7.

The conditionally replicating adenoviral vector (CRAd) dl1520, known as ONYX-015, has been engineered to replicate efficiently in neoplastic cells characterized by disruptions in the p53 tumor suppressor pathway (Chiocca et al., 2004). While other mechanisms of replicative selectivity may be operative, it is believed that ONYX-015 attains tumor specificity from an 800 bp deletion in the E1B region encoding the 55 kDa protein, which in infected cells, binds and inactivates cellular p53. Targeting the p53 pathway is important in glioma therapy because approximately 30–50% of gliomas harbor a p53 mutation (Geoerger et al., 2002). The safety of delivering ONYX-015 to treat malignant gliomas lies in the fact that should the virus encounter a non-neoplastic cell bordering the tumor, replication would be aborted because ONYX-015 is incapable of countering the proficient p53 defense mechanism characteristic of non-tumor cells.

While the use of ONYX-015 to combat gliomas is relatively recent, clinical trials have revealed the safety and potential efficacy of using this vector in the treatment of intractable head and neck cancers in both phase I and phase II trials (Lemont et al., 2000; Nemunaitis et al., 2001.). In 2004, Chiocca et al. conducted the first phase I trial consisting of dose-escalating intracerebral injections of ONYX-015 in 24 patients with recurrent malignant gliomas. Following tumor resection, ONYX-015 was injected (volume of 100 μL per injection) at 10 different sites into the wall of the resection cavity at doses varying from 1×10^7 to 1×10^{10} plaque forming units (p.f.u). The median time to progression after treatment was 46 days (range 13–452 + days) and the median survival time was 6.2 months (range 1.3–28.0 + months). None of the 24 patients experienced serious adverse affects related to ONYX-015; on the contrary, the study showed that injections of ONYX-015 into glioma cavities is well tolerated at doses up to 10^{10} p.f.u.

An alternative approach to combat gliomas involves the use of a different CRAd, termed Delta-24-RGD. Delta-24-RGD has been engineered by Fueyo et al. (2007) to selectively replicate in cells harboring a mutation in the retinoblastoma (Rb) protein or its regulatory pathway by a 24 bp deletion in the E1A region. To overcome the paucity of CAR expression on many tumor cells, Delta-24-RGD has been further enhanced to express the RGD motif in its fiber knob H1 loop to increase viral internalization and infectivity (Fueyo et al., 2000; Vecil and Lang, 2003). This modification allows for efficient viral internalization entirely independent of CAR.

Although Delta-24-RGD is currently awaiting clinical trial evaluation, its application has proven to be highly effective against tumors in mice bearing xenografts. A preclinical study conducted by Fueyo et al. (2007) examining the therapeutic potential of Delta-24-RGD to target tumor stem cells revealed that this vector eliminates both brain tumor stem cells as well as gliomal tumor mass cell populations. These findings are of great importance to brain tumor therapy because tumor stem cells are the driving force sustaining tumor growth and recurrence. Tumor stem cells are both chemo-resistant and radio-resistant and are considered to be responsible for tumor progression and recurrence even after conventional methods of glioma therapy have been performed (Altaner, 2008). The results of a recent study indicate that intracranial injection of Delta-24-RGD induces autophagic cell death, and the treatment of xenografts derived from brain tumor stem cells with Delta-24-RGD significantly improved the survival of glioma-bearing mice (means: 38.5 vs. 66.3 days, difference = 27.8 days, 95% confidence interval = 19.5–35.9 days, $p < 0.001$) (Fueyo et al. (2007). Such impressive results have gained Delta-24-RGD much attention in the quest for a better modality of treatment, and this vector is expected to soon undergo phase I clinical trials.

Another approach to treating gliomas utilizes the tumor specific promoter survivin (S), which is a member of the inhibitor of apoptosis protein (IAP) family that acts as a suppressor of apoptosis and plays a vital role in cell division (Ulasov et al., 2007; Van Houdt et al., 2006). Owing to its tremendous up-regulation in tumor cells, defective expression of survivin has been linked with a fundamental role in tumorigenesis, increased rates of tumor recurrence, and resistance to chemo and radiotherapy (Das et al., 2002; Ulasov et al., 2007). Transcriptional targeting by means of exploiting tumor specific promoters allows for adenoviral replication and oncolysis to occur exclusively within tumor tissue because viral replication is mediated by specific internal cellular cues emitted by host tumor cells (Ulasov et al., 2007; Van Houdt et al., 2006).

Since it has been shown that incorporating a survivin promoter into the E1A region of an adenoviral genome enhances viral replication and oncolysis in malignant gliomas, an effort has been put forth to engineer an optimal CRAd possessing this feature (Das et al., 2002; Ulasov et al., 2007; Van Houdt et al., 2006). The adenoviral vector, CRAd-S-pk7, belongs to the class of Ad-5 serotypes that have been carefully crafted with the survivin promotor in addition to having a polylysine residue (pk7) incorporated into its fiber knob enhancing its transduction capability. Ulasov et al. (2007) showed that injecting CRAd-S-pk7 to U87MG glioma xenografts in mice induces strong cytotoxicity in target cells and does not harm surrounding normal cells. In the study, injection of CRAd-S-pk7 inhibited xenograft tumor growth by more than 300% ($p < 0.001$), allowing long-term survivorship to the mice infected with gliomas (> 110 days; $p < 0.005$).

Delivery of an Oncolytic Adenovirus

While the use of various adenoviral vectors has proven safe for intracranial injection in several preclinical trails, a significant therapeutic effect has not been seen in patients thus far. The reason for this shortcoming is largely a result of the limitations involved with local delivery of virolytic agents. Due to the complex biological nature of high grade gliomas, local injection of adenoviral vectors fails to reach scattered infiltrative tumor cells within the brain parenchyma. To remedy this and prevent possible tumor recurrence, stem cells have been explored as vehicles for virotherapy in brain tumors given that they possess an intrinsic tropism for abnormal pathologies (Aboody et al., 2000, 2008). While the exact mechanism for their tumor affinity has yet to be fully elucidated, neural stem cells (NSC) and mesenchymal stem cells (MSC) are currently being explored as viable vehicles for targeting and delivering CRAds to disseminated tumor cells.

Aside from the ethical and technical difficulties associated with isolating NSC, their endogeneity to the central nervous system renders them particularly suitable for vector delivery in the brain. Experiments evaluating the delivery potential of NSC revealed that these cells possess an inherent tropism and unique capacity to target invading glioma cells in vitro as well as in vivo (Khalid et al., 2005; Zhenggang et al., 2004). Furthermore, in terms of delivering an oncolytic

adenovirus, it has been demonstrated that loading NSC cells with CRAds does not compromise their homing abilities (Tyler et al., 2009).

In addition to providing a carrier function, it is also imperative that NSC allow for adequate CRAd genome amplification to achieve optimal infectivity and sustained tumor toxicity upon reaching distant glioma cells. Tyler et al. (2009) proposed that tumor specific promoters (TSP), which control transcription and translation of the viral E1A replication gene, are vital to this process. Qualitative RT-PCR revealed that two tumor specific promoters, survivin and chemokine receptor CXCR4, allow for robust transcriptional activity in most glioma cell lines, while exhibiting relatively modest activity in normal cell lines. As such, Tyler et al. (2009) tested CRAd-S-pk7 and CRAd-CXCR4-5/3, two oncolytic vectors possessing these promoters, in NSC mediated delivery to gliomas. The results indicated relatively attenuated replicative cytotoxicity in NSC, but sufficient replicative cytotoxicity in U87MG tumor cells. In particular, CRAd-S-pk7 displayed limited toxicity to the NSC carrier, superb levels of NSC transduction, potent cytotoxicity to glioma cells, and could be delivered to U87MG cells in vitro.

When comparing the effectiveness of delivering NSC loaded with CRAd-S-pk7 versus CRAd-S-pk7 alone, it would appear the former approach exhibits enhanced efficacy. Moreover, qPCR of laser-captured brain tissue sections from mice receiving injections of NCS-loaded-CRAd-S-pk7 showed greater E1A gene distribution than those of mice injected with CRAd-S-pk7 alone (Tyler et al., 2009). It should be noted that despite these appealing results, the clinical application of NSC may be hampered by the ethical and logistical problems surrounding their isolation and immunologic incompatibility requiring allogenic transplantation with harvesting.

Human mesenchymal stem cells (hMSC) appear to be a more likely candidate for clinical application for a number of reasons. First, MSC can be derived easily from patients, expanded in culture, and genetically manipulated for therapeutic purposes (Sonabend et al., 2008). Additionally, if needed for the same patient, autologous transplantation ensures immunologic compatibility (Nakamizo et al., 2005). In terms of their viability as vessels in virotherapy, MSC can be loaded with CRAds, migrate towards tumors, and deliver CRAds to distant tumor cells (Sonabend et al., 2008).

A recent study conducted by Sonabend et al. (2008) evaluating CRAd delivery in mice bearing intracranial U87GM xenografts revealed that injecting CRAd-CXCR4-5/3 loaded MCS near the tumor site (5 mm away) delivered 46-fold more viral copies than injecting the virus alone without a carrier. In this study, the cell surface C-X-C chemokine receptor 4 (CXCR4) promoter was used to target adenoviral vectors to MSC and glioma cells. The rationale behind using CXCR4 is based on the findings that MSC express CXCR4 and that this promoter is active in human gliomas (Ehtesham et al., 2006; Ponte et al., 2007; Sonabend et al., 2008). While this study produced encouraging results, the delivery of CRAds by MSC still needs to be perfected. Specifically, if viral amplification is too affluent in the carrier vessel, MSC can be exposed to CRAd induced toxicity resulting in suboptimal delivery.

In conclusion, the goal underlying effective and successful treatment of malignant gliomas with oncolytic adenoviruses is based on tumor selectivity by restricting viral replication and infectivity to tumor cells. As discussed, current approaches used to modify adenoviruses for greater tumor specificity include: functional deletions in essential viral genes; tumor specific promoters used to control the expression of these viral genes; and tropism modifications to bestow a greater affinity for tumor cells. While several preclinical trials have yielded hopeful results, others have highlighted the limitations encountered thus far in this mode of therapy. With the overall safety and efficacy of utilizing CRAds being secure, improving their ability to target scattered disseminated tumor cells is the next important step. Perhaps the combination of conventional forms of cancer treatment along with the delivery of oncolytic adenoviruses can successfully combat this resistant malignancy. In the future, continuous progress in elucidating mechanisms of tumor formation and viral replication must persist, and the search for an optimal stem cell carrier to deliver CRAds to scattered glioma cells must advance to improve the overall survival of patients.

References

Aboody KS, Brown A, Rainov NG, Bower KA, Liu S, Yang W, Small JE, Herrlinger U, Ourednik V, Black PM, Breakefield XO, Snyder EY (2000) Neural stem cells display extensive tropism for pathology in adult brain: evidence from intracranial gliomas. Proc Natl Acad Sci USA 97:12846–12851

Aboody KS, Najbauer J, Danks MK (2008) Stem and progenitor cell-mediated tumor selective gene therapy. Gene Ther 15:739–752

Altaner C (2008) Glioblastoma and stem cells. Neoplasma 5:369–374

Chiocca EA, Abbed KM, Tatter S, Louis DN, Hochberg FH, Barker F, Kracher J, Grossman SA, Fisher JD, Carson K, Rosenblum M, Mikkelsen T, Olson J, Markert J, Rosenfeld S, Nabors LB, Brem S, Phuphanich S, Freeman S, Kaplan R, Zwiebel J (2004) A phase iopen-label, dose-escalation, multi-institutional trial of injection with an E1B-attenuated adenovirus, ONYX-015, into the peritumoral region of recurrent malignant gliomas in the adjuvant setting. Mol Ther 10:958–966

Chu RL, Post DE, Khuri FR, Van Meir EG (2004) Use of replicating oncolytic adenoviruses in combination therapy for cancer. Clin Cancer Res 10:5299–5312

Curiel DT, Douglas JT (2002) Adenoviral vectors for gene therapy. Elsevier Science,, San Diego CA

Das A, Tan WL, Teo J, Smith RD (2002) Expression of surviving in primary glioblastomas. J Cancer Res Clin Oncol 128:302–306

Ehtesham M, Stevenson CB, Thompson RB (2005) Stem cell therapies for malignant glioma. Neurosurg Focus 19:E5

Ehtesham M, Winston JA, Kabos P, Thompson RC (2006) CXCR4 expression mediates glioma cell invasiveness. Oncogene 25:2801–2806

Fueyo J, Gomez-Monzano C, Alemany R, Lee PSY, McDonnell TJ, Mitlianga P, Shi YX, Levin VA, Yung WKA, Kyritsis AP (2000) A mutant oncolytic adenovirus targeting the rb pathway produces anti-glioma effect in vivo. Oncogene 19:2–12

Fueyo J, Jiang H, Gomez-Monzano C, Aoki H, Alonso MH, Kondo S, McCormick F, Xu J, Kondo Y, Bekele N, Colman H, Lang FF (2007) Examination of the therapeutic potential of delta-24-RGD in brain tumor stem cells: role of autophagic cell death. J Natl Cancer Inst 99:1410–1414

Geoerger B, Grill J, Opolon P, Morizet J, Aubert G, Terrier-Lacomb MJ, Bressac-de Paillerets B, Barrois M, Feunteun J, Kirn DH, Vassal G (2002) Oncolytic activity of the E1B-55 kDa-deleted adenovirus ONYX-015 is independent of cellular p53 status in human malignant glioma xenografts. Cancer Res 62:764–772

Hemmi S, Geertsen R, Mezzacasa A, Peter I, Dummer R (1998) The presence of human coxsackievirus and adenovirus receptor is associated with efficient adenovirus-mediated transgene expression in human melanoma cell cultures. Hum Gene Ther 16:2363–2373

Khalid S, Emilie B, Kim DE, Atherine Y, Yi T, Ralph W, Xandra OB (2005) Glioma therapy and real-time imaging of neural precursor cell migration and tumor regression. Ann Neurol 57:34–41

Lemont JP, Nemunaitis J, Kuhn JA, Landers SA, McCarthy TM (2000) A prospective phase II trial of ONYX-015 adenovirus and chemotherapy in recurrent squamos cell carcinoma of the head and neck (the baylor experience). Ann Surg Oncol 7:588–592

Lesniak MS, Brem H (2004) Targeted therapy for brain tumours. Nat Rev Drug Discov 3:499–508

Nakamizo A, Marini F, Amano T, Khan A, Studeny M, Gumin J, Chen J, Hentchel S, Vecil G, Dembinski J, Andreeff M, Lang FF (2005) Human bone marrow-derived medenchymal stem cells in the treatment of gliomas. Cancer Res 65: 3307–3318

Nemunaitis J, Khuri F, Ganly I, Arseneau J, Posner M, Vokes E, Kuhn J, McCarty T, Landers S, Blackburn A, Romel L, Randlev B, Kaye S, Kirn D (2001) Phase II trial of intratumoral administration of ONYX-015, a replication-selective adenovirus, in patients with refractory head and neck cancer. J Clin Oncol 19:289–298

Palmer DJ, Ng P (2008) Methods for the production of first generation adenoviral vectors. Methods Mol Bio 433: 55–78

Ponte AL, Marais E, Gallay N, Langonné A, Delorme B, Hérault O, Charbord P, Domenech J (2007) The in vitro migration capacity of human bone marrow mesenchymal stem cells: comparison of chemokine and growth factor chemotactic activities. Stem Cells 25:1737–1745

Pulkkanen KJ, Yla-Herttuala S (2005) Gene therapy for malignant glioma: current clinical status. Mol Ther 12:585–598

Sonabend AM, Ulasov IV, Lesniak MS (2007) Gene therapy trials for the treatment of high grade gliomas. Gene Ther Mol Biol 11:79–92

Sonabend AM, Ulasov IV, Tyler MA, Rivera AA, Mathis JM, Lesniak MS (2008) Mesenchymal stem cells effectively deliver an oncolytic adenovirus to intracranial glioma. Stem Cells 26:831–841

Stupp R, Mason WP, van den Bent MJ, Weller M, Fisher B, Taphoorn MJ, Belanger K, Brandes AA, Marosi C, Bogdahn U, Curschmann J, Janzer RC, Ludwin SK, Gorlia T, Allgeier A, Lacombe D, Cairncross JG, Eisenhauer E, Mirimanoff RO (2005) Radiotherapy plus concomitant and adjuvant temozolomide for glioblastoma. N Engl J Med 10:987–996

Tyler MA, Ulasov IV, Sonabend AM, Nandi S, Marler S, Roth J, Lesniak MS (2009) Neural stemcells target intracranial glioma to deliver an oncolytic adenovirus in vivo. Gene Ther 16(2):262–278

Ulasov IV, Tyler MA, Rivera AA, Nettlebeck DM, Douglas JT, Lesniak MS (2008) Evaluation of E1A double mutant oncolytic adenovectors in anti-glioma gene therapy. Med Virol 80:1595–1603

Ulasov IV, Zhu ZB, Tyler MA, Han Y, Rivera AA, Khramtsov A, Curiel DT, Lesniak MS (2007) Survivin-driven and fiber-modified adenovirus exhibits potent antitumor activity in established intracranial glioma. Hum Gene Ther 18(7): 599–602

Van Houdt WJ, Haviv YS, Lu B, Wang M, Rivera AA, Ulasov IV, Lamfers ML, Rein D, Lesniak MS, Siegal GP, Dirven CM, Curiel DT, Zhu ZB (2006) The human surviving promoter: a novel transcriptional targeting strategy for treatment of glioma. J Neurosurg 104:583–592

Vecil GG, Lang FF (2003) Clinical trials of adenoviruses in brain tumors: a review of ad-p53 and oncolytic adenoviruses. J Neuro-Oncol 65:237–246

Zheng S, Ulasov IV, Han Y, Tyler MA, Zhu ZB,, Lesniak MS (2007) Fiber knob modifications enhance adenoviral tropism and gene transfer in malignant glioma. J Gene Med 9: 151–160

Zhenggang Z, Quan J, Feng J, Guangliang D, Ruilan Z, Lei W, Li Z, Adam MR, Mark K, Michael C (2004) In vivo magnetic resonance imaging tracks adult neural progenitor cell targeting of brain tumor. NeuroImage 23:281–287

Chapter 39

Use of Magnetic Resonance Spectroscopy Imaging (MRSI) in the Treatment Planning of Gliomas

Ashwatha Narayana and Jenghwa Chang

Abstract Radiation therapy of glioma is based on conventional imaging using computerized tomography (CT) and magnetic resonance imaging (MRI). However the results remain poor in part due to uncertainties in delineation of target volume and critical structures. Magnetic resonance spectroscopy imaging (MRSI) can provide additional information on metabolic activity in the selected region of brain tissue that may help in differentiating normal brain from tumor. The information that might be derived from MRSI to better delineate the optimal target volume for radiation therapy of gliomas will be discussed. Technical details of incorporating MRSI into radiation therapy treatment planning process will be presented.

Keywords MRSI · Glioma · Radiation therapy · Treatment planning

Introduction

The combination of surgery, radiation therapy, and chemotherapy represents the standard approach to the treatment of gliomas. However, both local control and survival remain poor with conventional therapy. The median survival time for patients with glioblastoma multiforme is 10–12 months, with a 3-year survival rate of 6–8% (MRC (Medical Research Council Brain Tumour Working Party) 2001). The median survival time for patients with anaplastic astrocytoma is 36 months, and the 3-year survival rate is approximately 50%. The pattern of recurrence in gliomas in spite of therapy is almost always local (Narayana and Liebel, 2002). The inability to resect or deliver adequate radiation to the target volume has been often cited as the cause for local failure. It is also possible that areas of high grade tumor that may need a higher dose of radiation can not be identified separately from areas suspicious for tumor extension that may be treated with a lower dose although to a larger volume.

The approach to defining target volumes for radiation therapy in patients with gliomas at the present time is to deliver a certain dose to the contrast enhancing area, as determined from a contrast enhanced T1-weighted magnetic resonance imaging (MRI) or fluid-attenuated-inversion-recovery (FLAIR) images plus a margin of 2–3 cm (Wallner, 1991; Thornton et al., 1992). The size of this margin is generally chosen since serial biopsies of patients undergoing craniotomy for malignant gliomas have revealed tumor cells up to 3 cm distance from the contrast enhancing margin in a majority of the patients. However, target definition based on MRI information has its limitations. The contrast enhancing lesion on T1-weighted MRI images only reflects areas with a breakdown of the blood–brain barrier. This has been shown to be not always a reliable indicator of high grade tumor due to the presence of both non-enhancing high grade tumor as well as contrast-enhancing necrosis (Byrne, 1994). Similarly, T2 or FLAIR defined volume either over-estimates or underestimates the low grade tumor in a majority of patients (Earnest IV et al., 1988). As a result, new diagnostic tools are being explored that would assist the treating oncologist in better defining the volumes to which dose should be delivered.

A. Narayana (✉)
Department of Radiation Oncology, New York University Medical Center, New York, NY 10016, USA
e-mail: ashwatha.narayana@nyumc.org

M.A. Hayat (ed.), *Tumors of the Central Nervous System, Volume 1*,
DOI 10.1007/978-94-007-0344-5_39, © Springer Science+Business Media B.V. 2011

Magnetic resonance-spectroscopic imaging (MRSI) is one such emerging diagnostic tool that can obtain proton (1H) spectra from selected regions within the brain (Moonen et al., 1989; Duijn et al., 1992). Clinical studies have shown that the degree of changes in metabolite levels may help differentiate normal brain from tumor in patients with suspected glioma (De Stefano et al., 1998; Pirzkall et al., 2001). The MRSI can provide information about tumor activity based upon the levels of cellular metabolites, including choline-containing compounds (Cho), total creatine (Cr), N-acetylaspartate (NAA), and lactate/lipid, as seen in Fig. 39.1. Each of these metabolites acts as biochemical markers. Cho is a membrane component that is increased in viable tumor. Cr is a marker of cellular bioenergetic process. NAA is a neuronal marker that is decreased in tumors due to neuronal loss. Lactate is an end product of anaerobic metabolism. It has been noted that gliomas exhibit a markedly high resonance in the spectral region of Cho and/or a low Cr and NAA resonance, implying increases in the Cho/Cr and/or Cho/NAA ratios. With the advantage of measuring tumor regional variations in abnormalities of metabolite levels, MRSI has recently been used as an in vivo molecular imaging technique that assists in targeting and predicts response to radiation therapy for patients with brain gliomas (Park et al., 2007).

The current standard of care in gliomas for adjuvant radiation therapy has been to use 54–60 Gy using 1.8–2.0 Gy/fraction over 6–6.5 weeks. An improvement in local control and survival has been clearly shown in high-grade gliomas when the radiation dose has been escalated from 0 to 60 Gy (Bleehen and Stenning, 1991). Despite a lack of consistent evidence for a strong dose–response curve beyond 60 Gy when using radiation to treat high grade gliomas, there is interest in employing higher doses, due to the benefit seen in other locations (Nelson et al., 1988; Lee et al., 1999). However, higher radiation dose leads to higher risk of radiation-induced brain injury, which is usually the limiting factor for dose escalation. It is possible that dose escalation may be of greatest clinical value only if all the active disease receives a certain dose and normal tissue is spared as much as possible. One possible approach would be to use IMRT to identify and spare the anatomically and functionally critical structures while performing selective dose escalation to MRSI identified tumor.

Incorporation of the MRSI information into the radiation therapy treatment planning process is difficult since it lacks the essential anatomical features for image registration. The spectroscopic information needs to be co-registered with MR images for radiation treatment planning first which enables more aggressive radiation treatment in the high grade region within a tumor using dose painting technique. We will review the pathological and physiological information that might be derived from MRSI to better delineate the treatment volume for glioma radiation therapy. We will illustrate the feasibility of registering MRSI with

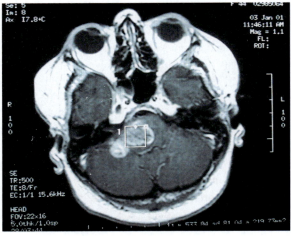
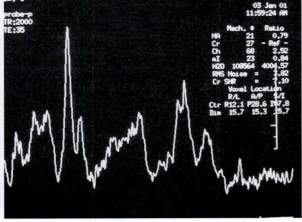
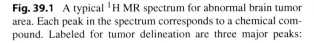

Fig. 39.1 A typical ^{1}H MR spectrum for abnormal brain tumor area. Each peak in the spectrum corresponds to a chemical compound. Labeled for tumor delineation are three major peaks: Choline (Cho), Creatine (Cr), and N-acetyl aspartate (NAA). For an abnormal brain tumor, the Cho intensity is much higher than that of the Cr or NAA intensity

simulation CT in a patient with high grade glioma and the generating a treatment plan.

MRSI Technique and Interpretation of MRSI Data

In diagnostic radiology, ^{1}H MR spectroscopy information is usually acquired as a single voxel using either the point-resolved spectroscopy sequence (PRESS) (Bottomley, 1987) or stimulated-echo acquisition mode pulse sequence (STEAM) (Shimizu et al., 1996; Kaminogo et al., 2001). Here, the data is usually acquired from a large rectangular region of interest positioned on scout MR images and represents the mean of the metabolites. In treatment planning, multidimensional array of voxels that are smaller in size are necessary. For this purpose, the matrix of spectral data is acquired either over a plane (2D MRSI) or a volume (3D MRSI). The choice of localization method depends on the detection efficiency of desired metabolites, voxel resolution, allowable scan time, and areas of coverage with least contamination from outside the volume of interest. Typical acquisition parameters for PRESS sequence are: TE $\geq$ 135 ms to reduce lipid signal contamination and background macromolecular signal and to detect inverted Lac doublet, and TR = 1.0 – 3.0 s. Shorter TE ($\leq$ 30 ms) is usually employed for STEAM sequence to determine the contributions to the characterization of brain tumors of the metabolites inositol/myoinositol and glutamate/glutamine, which are not visible at long TE values with the PRESS sequence. Co-registered MR images for overlaying the MRS voxels such as FLAIR or T1-weighted post contrast images are acquired in the same examination. Commercial MRS data processing packages, such as GE's FuncTool software (GE Medical Systems, Milwaukee, WI), are usually available from vendors.

Due to the subtle variation in metabolite intensity for different tumor types, multiple metabolites should be used to predict brain tumor type and grade. In addition, because the presence of necrosis reduces estimated absolute metabolite concentrations for high-grade tumors, metabolite ratios (e.g., Cho/NAA or Cho/Cr) becomes a more reliable indicator of tumor grade for such tumors (Howe et al., 2003). The group at University of California San Francisco (UCSF) developed an abnormality index (Cho/NAA index or CNI)

using an automated statistic method to analyze the relative Cho and NAA levels (McKnight et al., 2001). They demonstrated that metabolically active (CNI 2 or higher) tumor was observed outside MR defined volumes in a non-uniform manner for both low grade and high grade tumors (Pirzkall et al., 2001, 2002). They also reported that T1 MRI suggested a lesser volume and different location of active disease compared to MRSI (Pirzkall et al., 2001) and other metabolites, such as creatine and lactate, seemed useful for determining less and more radioresistant areas, respectively (Pirzkall et al., 2002).

The histo-pathological validation of MRSI as a predictor of tumor presence has also been described by McKnight et al. from UCSF (McKnight et al., 2002, 2007). They compared the data obtained preoperatively from MRSI with the results of histopathological assays of tissue biopsies obtained during surgery to verify the sensitivity and specificity of a choline-containing compound-N-acetylaspartate index (CNI) used to distinguish tumor from nontumorous tissue within T2-hyperintense and contrast-enhancing lesions of patients with untreated gliomas. Using a CNI threshold of 2.5, they were able to distinguish biopsy samples containing tumor from those containing a mixture of normal, edematous, gliotic and necrotic tissue with 90% sensitivity and 86% specificity (McKnight et al., 2002). The CNIs of nontumorous specimens were significantly different from those of biopsy specimens containing Grade II ($p < 0.03$), Grade III ($p < 0.005$), and Grade IV ($p < 0.01$) tumors. On average, one third to one half of the T2-hyperintense lesion outside the contrast-enhancing lesion contained CNI greater than 2.5 (McKnight et al., 2002).

The Cho/Cr ratio of MRSI is also known to correlate with the pathology grade of glioma. Howe et al. (2003) and Fountas et al. (2004) used single-voxel spectroscopy to examine respectively forty-two and seventy-one patients with brain tumors and concluded that the Cho/Cr ratio is a statistically significant marker for determining the degree of intracranial astrocytoma malignancy. Howe et al. (2003) demonstrated that long-TE (136 ms) Cho/Cr ratio gives the best separation of astrocytoma grade: 1.08 ± 0.11 (mean Cho/Cr ratio ± one standard deviation) for normal parietal white matter, 1.92 ± 0.3 for astrocytoma grade 2, 2.8 ± 0.49 for anaplastic astrocytoma, and 4.66 ± 2.3 for glioblastoma multiforme. They noted that quantified lipid, macromolecule, and lactate levels increased with grade of tumor, consistent with progression from hypoxia to necrosis. Quantification of lipids and macromolecules at short TE provided a good marker for tumor grade, and a scatter plot of the sum of alanine, lactate, and delta 1.3 lipid signals vs. myoinositol/choline provided a simple way to separate most tumors by type and grade. Similar results were obtained by Fountas et al. (2004) with a TE of 135 ms.

Reproducibility of MRSI depends on a couple of factors, including hardware, patient immobilization, baseline irregularities and accuracy of volume position. Li et al. (2002) studied intra- and inter-subject reproducibility of the metabolite levels and report interindividual CVs (coefficients of variation, 100% times the standard deviation divided by the mean) of 15.6, 23.3 and 24.4%, compared with intraindividual CVs of 14.4, 14.8 and 15.3%, for NAA, Cr, and Cho, respectively. They concluded that the measurement uncertainties can be reduced at a cost of either spatial resolution by using larger voxels or time by performing serial follow-ups. Simmons et al. (1998) reported excellent short-term reproducibility of metabolite ratios with CV of NAA/Cho = 5.2%, NAA/Cr = 3.0%, Cho/Cr = 6.6%, for five repeat scans. The long-term reproducibility was slightly worse, with CVs of NAA/Cho = 5.2%, NAA/Cr = 4.8%, Cho/Cr = 7.7% for five repeat scans on eight subjects over 3 months (Simmons et al., 1998). They attributed the precision reported in their series to the use of highly automated techniques for voxel shimming, water suppression and peak area measurements.

scan and the functional scan are intrinsically registered. Geometric uncertainties introduced in the imaging and registration process should be evaluated and included in the margin calculation to assure good PTV coverage.

An approach similar to PET-CT has been adopted for registering MRSI with treatment planning CT using reference MRI images acquired in the same scanning position. For example, Zaider et al. (2000) and DiBiase et al. (2002) used T2-weighted MRI images obtained at the same scanning position to register the MRSI data for prostate implants. Wu et al. (2004) developed a deformable image registration algorithm to overcome the deformation of the prostate by the rectal coil. Graves et al. (2001) used an automatic registration scheme for incorporating the Cho/NAA ratios into glioma treatment planning. In their approach, multiple MRI scans were acquired for each patient and were automatically aligned to the SPGR MRI images acquired immediately before the MRSI data. The SPGR MRI images were then registered to the simulation CT images.

AT UCSF, the CNI images were calculated and interpolated to the resolution of the CT images. Contours of the CNI images were then superimposed on the anatomic images after being transferred using a DICOM protocol to the PACS workstation (Nelson et al., 2002). Chang et al. (2006), on the other hand, developed a registration protocol that successfully overlaid the Cho/Cr ratio on top of the FLAIR MRI in DICOM format and imported the registered images set into the treatment planning system for glioma IMRT.

Co-registration of MRSI with Simulation CT Images

Registration of a functional image set with an anatomical image set has been a major research topic in recent years. One successful approach uses a reference anatomical image set acquired at the same scanning position as the functional image set. The reference scan can be registered with the simulation CT scan using the standard registration methods (e.g., mutual information). The transformation matrix between the reference scan and the simulation CT can then be directly applied to the functional scan since the reference

Incorporation of MRSI into RT Treatment Planning Process: A Case Study

To demonstrate how MRSI information can be incorporated into RT treatment planning process, a glioma patient treated with a standard IMRT plan to the FLAIR MRI defined volume was re-planned to include MRSI information for target delineation. The lesion was located in the left frontal lobe close to the Broca's area. The goal was to device a treatment plan that could provide adequate coverage to the MRSI defined treatment volume and spared the contra-lateral (right) Broca's area and other critical organs.

For MRSI the patient was scanned using a 1.5T GE Excite instrument (GE Medical Systems, Milwaukee, WI). The patient first underwent whole-brain axial FLAIR MRI with 3-mm slice thickness (no spacing), followed by 3D MRSI measurement using a PRESS, TE/TR: 144/1000 ms, 10 mm spacing and $8 \times 8 \times 8$ matrix size on the user-specified MRSI volume using the FLAIR MRI as scout images. The 3D MRSI data were processed using GE's FuncTool software. The Cho/Cr grading system in Table 39.1 was used to convert the Cho/Cr ratios. As illustrated in Fig. 39.2, the FLAIR MRI images and Cho/Cr grades of the same slice location were merged by replacing the image

Table 39.1 The system used to grade the Cho/Cr ratio for each MRS voxel. The first and second columns list the Cho/Cr ratio and grade, which is mapped to the three clinical target volumes in column 3 for dose painting. The dose level in column 4 is for each Cho/Cr grade

Cho/Cr ratio	Grade	Clinical target volume	Dose painting
[0, 1]	0		
[1, 2]	1	CTV1	5400
[2, 3]	2	CTV2	5940
3 and up	3	CTV3	7020

intensity of those voxels inside the MRSI box on the MRI images with the mapped intensity to produce a merged image set. Both the merged MRSI image sets

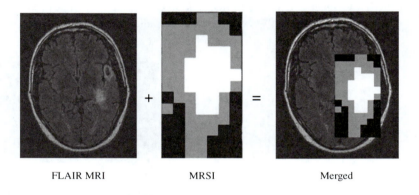

Fig. 39.2 Overlaying MRSI information on a FLAIR MRI image. The pixel values of the MR FLAIR image (*left*) in the MRSI box are replaced by the MRSI image (*middle*) to produce a merged image (*right*)

FLAIR MRI   MRSI   Merged

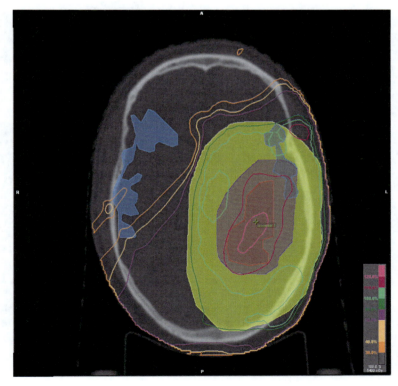

Fig. 39.3 The dose distribution on one CT slice of the IMRT plans using the MRSI defined targets. The *yellow*, *gray* and *orange* structures are MRSIPTV1, MRSIPTV2 and MRSIPTV3, respectively. The *blue* structures are the *right* and *left* Broca's areas

were imported into the treatment planning system and registered with the FLAIR MRI images for contouring the lesion and critical organs. The contoured MRI images were registered with the simulation CT images using a mutual-information algorithm.

Three clinical target volumes (CTVs) were contoured on the MRI images according to their Cho/Cr grades as seen in Column 3 of Table 39.1, and each CTV received a prescription dose as shown in Column 4 of Table 39.1. The enhanced volume on the FLAIR MRI and the spectral data in the registered screen-dumped MRSI were used as reference when the Cho/Cr grades of some MRSI voxels were in doubt. Three PTV's (MRSIPTV1, MRSIPTV2 and MRSIPTV3) were created with margins of 10, 5, and 3 mm added to three CTV's outlined by the radiation

oncologist. Brainstem, cord chiasm, left and right optic nerves, left and right eyes and right Broca's area were designated as organs at risk (OARs).

IMRT plans that simultaneously delivers three different dose levels of 100/110/130% (corresponding to 5400/5940/7020 cGy) to the three PTV's with and without the fMRI information were generated using the dose painting technique. OARs were assigned maximum point dose limits relative to the prescription dose and based on clinically accepted tolerance limits. Dose volume histograms (DVHs) of the treatment plans with and without the fMRI information were compared for PTVs and OARs.

Figure 39.3 illustrates the dose distribution on one CT slice of the IMRT plans using the MRSI defined targets. Figure 39.4 shows the DVHs for (a) the three PTV

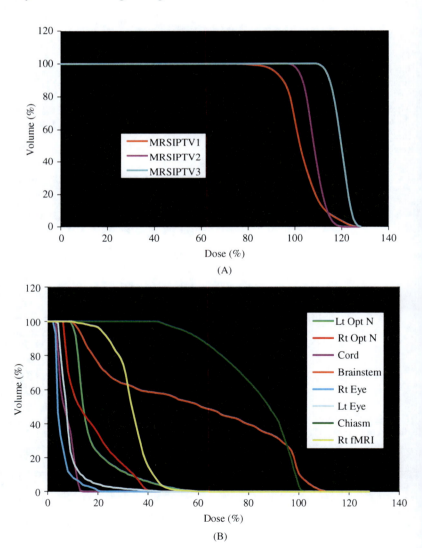

Fig. 39.4 Dose volume histograms for (**a**) the three PTV volumes and (**b**) the critical organs of the IMRT plans using the MRSI defined targets

volumes and (b) the OARs of both plans. It is observed from Fig. 39.4A that minimal doses to the three PTV's (MRSIPTV1, MRSIPTV2 and MRSIPTV3) were lower than the prescription doses for both plans because the doses had to be scaled down to meet the maximal dose constraints on OARs, especially brainstem (5900 cGy, partly involved in MRSIPV2) and chiasm (5400 cGy, partly involved in MRSIPV1). It is also shown in Figs. 39.3 and 39.4B that right Broca's area were spared from high dose area.

A comparison study (Chang et al., 2008) showed that both the PTV would have been 207 cc if only FLAIR MRI is used for contouring the target volume. Although MRSIPTV1 (198 cc) had similar volume, only ~75% (153 cc) of their volumes coincide with each other, indicating that if FLAIR PTV was used for the treatment planning, ~26% (54 cc) of the MRSI defined PTV would be missed. Anther comparison study (Chang et al., 2008) showed that inclusion of that right Broca's area in the optimization reduced the radiation dose to this area considerably but did not significantly alter the dose to other critical organs.

Summary

The variations in glioma cell distribution and the tumor grade makes it difficult to define an adequate target volume for radiation therapy using conventional CT/MR imaging alone. Modern MRSI techniques provide useful pathological information that might be critical to the radiation treatment planning of glioma. Incorporating this information into the radiation therapy treatment planning process is feasible with the image-registration protocols. The location and volume of MRSI defined target can be significantly different from that of the MRI defined target. Further work includes prioritizing the anatomical versus the functional areas for normal tissue sparing as well as defining the dose constraints for the various regions of the brain.

References

Bleehen NM, Stenning SP (1991) A medical research council trial of two radiotherapy doses in the treatment of grades 3 and 4 astrocytoma. Br J Cancer 64:769–774

Bottomley PA (1987) Spatial localization in NMR spectroscopy in vivo. Ann N Y Acad Sci 508:333–348

Byrne TN (1994) Imaging of gliomas. Semin Oncol 21:162–171

Chang J, Thakur SB, Huang W, Narayana A (2008) Magnetic resonance spectroscopy imaging (MRSI) and brain functional magnetic resonance imaging (fMRI) for radiotherapy treatment planning of glioma. Technol Cancer Res Treat 7:349–362

Chang J, Thakur S, Perera G, Kowalski A, Huang W, Karimi S, Hunt M, Koutcher J, Fuks Z, Amols H, Narayana A (2006) Image-fusion of MR spectroscopic images for treatment planning of gliomas. Med Phys 33:32–40

De Stefano N, Caramanos Z, Preul MC, Francis G, Antel JP, Arnold DL (1998) In vivo differentiation of astrocytic brain tumors and isolated demyelinating lesions of the type seen in multiple sclerosis using 1H magnetic resonance spectroscopic imaging. Ann Neurol 44:273–278

DiBiase SJ, Hosseinzadeh K, Gullapalli RP, Jacobs SC, Naslund MJ, Sklar GN, Alexander RB, Yu C (2002) Magnetic resonance spectroscopic imaging-guided brachytherapy for localized prostate cancer. Int J Radiat Oncol Biol Phys 52:429–438

Duijn JH, Matson GB, Maudsley AA, Weiner MW (1992) 3D phase encoding 1H spectroscopic imaging of human brain. Magn Reson Imaging 10:315–319

Earnest IV F, Kelly PJ, Scheithauer BW, Kall BA, Cascino TL, Ehman RL, Forbes GS, Axley PL (1988) Cerebral astrocytomas: histopathologic correlation of MR and CT contrast enhancement with stereotactic biopsy. Radiology 166:823–827

Fountas KN, Kapsalaki EZ, Vogel RL, Fezoulidis I, Robinson JS, Gotsis ED (2004) Noninvasive histologic grading of solid astrocytomas using proton magnetic resonance spectroscopy. Stereotact Funct Neurosurg 82:90–97

Graves EE, Pirzkall A, Nelson SJ, Larson D, Verhey L (2001) Registration of magnetic resonance spectroscopic imaging to computed tomography for radiotherapy treatment planning. Med Phys 28:2489–2496

Howe FA, Barton SJ, Cudlip SA, Stubbs M, Saunders DE, Murphy M, Wilkins P, Opstad KS, Doyle VL, McLean MA, Bell BA, Griffiths JR (2003) Metabolic profiles of human brain tumors using quantitative in vivo 1H magnetic resonance spectroscopy. Magn Reson Med 49:223–232

Kaminogo M, Ishimaru H, Morikawa M, Ochi M, Ushijima R, Tani M, Matsuo Y, Kawakubo J, Shibata S (2001) Diagnostic potential of short echo time MR spectroscopy of gliomas with singlevoxel and point-resolved spatially localised proton spectroscopy of brain. Neuroradiology 43:353–363

Lee SW, Fraass BA, Marsh LH, Herbort K, Gebarski SS, Martel MK, Radany EH, Lichter AS, Sandler HM (1999) Patterns of failure following high-dose 3-D conformal radiotherapy for high-grade astrocytomas: a quantitative dosimetric study. Int J Radiat Oncol Biol Phys 43:79–88

Li BSY, Babb JS, Soher BJ, Maudsley AA, Gonen O (2002) Reproducibility of 3D proton spectroscopy in the human brain. Magn Reson Med 47:439–446

MRC (Medical Research Council Brain Tumour Working Party). (2001) Randomized trial of procarbazine, lomustine, and vincristine in the adjuvant treatment of high-grade astrocytoma: a medical research council trial. J Clin Oncol 19:509–518

McKnight TR, Lamborn KR, Love TD, Berger MS, Chang S, Dillon WP, Bollen A, Nelson SJ (2007) Correlation of magnetic resonance spectroscopic and growth characteristics within grades ii and iii gliomas. J Neurosurg 106: 660–666

McKnight TR, Noworolski SM, Vigneron DB, Nelson SJ (2001) An automated technique for the quantitative assessment of 3D-MRSI data from patients with glioma. J Magn Reson Imag 13:167–177

McKnight TR, Von dem Bussche MH, Vigneron DB, Lu Y, Berger MS, McDermott MW, Dillon WP, Graves EE, Pirzkall A, Nelson SJ (2002) Histopathological validation of a three-dimensional magnetic resonance spectroscopy index as a predictor of tumor presence. J Neurosurg 97:794–802

Moonen CT, von Kienlin M, van Zijl PC, Cohen J, Gillen J, Daly P, Wolf G (1989) Comparison of single-shot localization methods (steam and press) for in vivo proton NMR spectroscopy. NMR Biomed 2:201–208

Narayana A, Leibel SA (2002) Adult brain tumors. In: Leibel SA, Phillips TL (eds) Textbook of radiation oncology. Saunders, Philadelphia, PA, pp 463–495

Nelson DF, Diener-West M, Horton J, Chang CH, Schoenfeld CH, Nelson JS (1988) Combined modality approach to treatment of malignant gliomas – re-evaluation of rtog 7401/ecog 1374 with long-term follow-up: a joint study of the radiation therapy oncology group and the eastern cooperative oncology group. NCI Monogr 279–284

Nelson SJ, Graves E, Pirzkall A, Li X, Chan AA, Vigneron DB, McKnight TR (2002) In vivo molecular imaging for planning radiation therapy of gliomas: an application of 1H MRSI. J Magn Reson Imag 16:464–476

Park I, Tamai G, Lee MC, Chuang CF, Chang SM, Berger MS, Nelson SJ, Pirzkall A (2007) Patterns of recurrence analysis in newly diagnosed glioblastoma multiforme after three-dimensional conformal radiation therapy with respect to pre-radiation therapy magnetic resonance spectroscopic findings. Int J Radiat Oncol Biol Phys 69:381–389

Pirzkall A, McKnight TR, Graves EE, Carol MP, Sneed PK, Wara WW, Nelson SJ, Verhey LJ, Larson DA (2001) MR-spectroscopy guided target delineation for high-grade gliomas. Int J Radiat Oncol Biol Phys 50:915–928

Pirzkall A, Nelson SJ, McKnight TR, Takahashi MM, Li X, Graves EE, Verhey LJ, Wara WW, Larson DA, Sneed PK (2002) Metabolic imaging of low-grade gliomas with three-dimensional magnetic resonance spectroscopy. Int J Radiat Oncol Biol Phys 53:1254–1264

Shimizu H, Kumabe T, Tominaga T, Kayama T, Hara K, Ono Y, Sato K, Arai N, Fujiwara S, Yoshimoto T (1996) Noninvasive evaluation of malignancy of brain tumors with proton MR spectroscopy. Am J Neuroradiol 17:737–747

Simmons A, Smail M, Moore E, Williams SCR (1998) Serial precision of metabolite peak area ratios and water referenced metabolite peak areas in proton MR spectroscopy of the human brain. Magn Reson Imag 16:319–330

Thornton AF Jr., Sandler HM, Ten Haken RK, McShan DL, Fraass BA, La Vigne ML, Yanke BR (1992) The clinical utility of magnetic resonance imaging in 3-dimensional treatment planning of brain neoplasms. Int J Rad Oncol Biol Phys 24:767–775

Wallner KE (1991) Radiation treatment planning for malignant astrocytomas. Semin Radiat Oncol 1:17–22

Wu X, Dibiase SJ, Gullapalli R, Yu CX (2004) Deformable image registration for the use of magnetic resonance spectroscopy in prostate treatment planning. Int J Radiat Oncol Biol Phys 58:1577–1583

Zaider M, Zelefsky MJ, Lee EK, Zakian KL, Amols HI, Dyke J, Cohen G, Hu YC, Endi AK, Chui CS, Koutcher JA (2000) Treatment planning for prostate implants using magnetic-resonance spectroscopy imaging. Int J Radiat Oncol Biol Phys 47:1085–1096

Chapter 40

Malignant Glioma Cells: Role of Trail-Induced Apoptosis

Markus D. Siegelin and Yasemin Siegelin

Abstract Glioblastoma WHO grade IV (GBM) is the most common primary malignant brain tumour with a median survival of approximately 12 months. Current treatment options include surgery, radiation and chemotherapy with only a mild increase in survival times. Therefore new therapeutic agents are highly needed. One promising strategy that may improve prognosis in GBM is induction of apoptosis by activation of the extrinsic apoptotic pathway through Tumor Necrosis Apoptosis Inducing Ligand (TRAIL) which in turn activates membrane bound death receptors. Since 1999 it has been demonstrated and confirmed by many research groups that recombinant human TRAIL induces apoptosis specifically both in glioblastoma cells and in orthotopic glioblastoma xenografts, while producing no effect on most non-transformed cells, including human astrocytes. Unfortunately, GBMs are known to be highly heterogeneous and the majority of GBMs are primary resistance to the pro-apoptotic effects of human recombinant TRAIL. However, TRAIL-resistance can be overcome in glioblastoma cells by combining TRAIL with other therapeutic modalities and reagents, including radiation, chemotherapeutics and small-molecules. Many of these combination therapies are of remarkable efficacy and exhibit only mild effects on non-transformed cells, e.g. human astrocytes and Schwann cells. Despite these recent experimental advances neither TRAIL alone nor a TRAIL-based combination

therapy has been used for the treatment of patients suffering from GBM. This chapter will review some of the progresses and the advances of TRAIL-based therapies for the treatment of experimental models of GBM.

Keywords Glioblastoma · Mechanisms of cell death · Apoptosis-based therapies

Introduction

Apoptosis (programmed cell death) is a physiological cell death mechanism. During tumor development cancer cells acquire mechanisms that provide them the ability to evade from physiological death. Two major cellular pathways are known that initiate programmed cell death (apoptosis). These pathways are distinct, but finally merge into one endpoint, the activation of cysteine-dependent aspartate-directed proteases (caspases). The first pathway is called the intrinsic pathway, which starts in the mitochondria and is executed after chemotherapy and radiation. After induction of the intrinsic pathway, cytochrome-c will be released from the mitochondria into the cytosol, leading to the formation of the apoptosome and subsequent activation of caspase-9. Caspase-9 cleaves effector caspases, such as caspase $-3/-7$ that mediate final cascade of apoptosis.

The extrinsic apoptotic pathway is the second pathway that induces apoptosis through an active process mediated by cell surface death receptors that transmit apoptotic signals after binding by their cognate death ligands, e.g. TRAIL. These death receptors belong to the tumor necrosis factor superfamily and harbor

M.D. Siegelin (✉)
Department of Pathology and Cell Biology, Columbia University College of Physicians and Surgeons, New York, NY 10032, USA
e-mail: msiegelin@t-online.de

M.A. Hayat (ed.), *Tumors of the Central Nervous System, Volume 1*,
DOI 10.1007/978-94-007-0344-5_40, © Springer Science+Business Media B.V. 2011

cysteine-rich extracellular domains. With respect to the intracellular site, all death receptors contain a death domain that serves as a starting point for the apoptotic machinery. For instance, death-receptors can be activated by death-ligands, e.g. Tumor necrosis factor-related apoptosis-inducing ligand (TRAIL). TRAIL was discovered in 1995 and is one of the various member of the TNF-family. Because of its remarkably ability to induce cell death specifically in cancer cells and its specificity (Ashkenazi et al., 1999; Walczak et al., 1999) TRAIL was formulated by pharmaceutical companies and subsequently used in clinical trials. In addition, agonistic antibody towards death-receptor 4 and death-receptor 5 have been developed and reached clinical trials. Despite the tremendous efficacy in several experimental models of GBMs no clinical trial involving TRAIL or its analogues has been initiated in patients suffering from GBM.

Once a death receptors is activated (e.g. through binding of TRAIL to one of its receptors), the initiator caspase-8 is activated within the cytoplasma of the stimulated cell. In turn, Caspase-8 either cleaves effector-caspases or may activate the intrinsic apoptotic pathway. As caspase-8 activation is the starting point of the extrinsic apoptotic pathway, loss of caspase-8 expression in tumor cells is of major significance since death ligands cannot sufficiently activate the apoptotic cascade. Similarly, if cancer cells downregulate death-receptors, apoptosis in tumor cells cannot be induced by death-ligands. In this chapter we will review the structure of TRAIL, TRAIL-receptor signaling and factors that mediate TRAIL-resistance in cancer cells with a particular focus on glioblastoma cells and specimens.

Structure of Trail and the Use of Trail as an Anti-cancer Drug

On the basis of its homology to CD95 Wiley et al. cloned TRAIL cDNA in 1995. In addition, TRAIL has significant homologies to TNF and several lymphotoxins. TRAIL monomers are composed of two anti-parallel beta-pleated sheets that form a beta-sandwich core framework, and the monomers are capable of forming a trimer (Cha et al., 1999a, b). Many studies have clearly demonstrated that the trimer-formation greatly enhances TRAIL activity as compared to monomeric TRAIL (Wiley et al., 1995). For instance, this trimer-formation is facilitated by addition of Zn^{2+} to TRAIL drug formulations. In the late 1990 TRAIL was shown to be an efficient inductor of cell death in tumor cells in vitro and in vivo. This tumor specific profile of TRAIL raised great excitement around the world since this molecule was able to kill tumor cells completely while normal cells were not affected at all. Nevertheless, significant side effects and toxicities associated with TRAIL have been reported since certain formulations of TRAIL (His-tagged TRAIL) induced cell death in human hepatocytes in vitro (Jo et al., 2000). However, recombinant human native TRAIL (aminoacid 114–281) devoid of N-terminal tags exhibited no hepatotoxicity. Consequently, researchers concluded that the detected hepatotoxicity was most likely dependent on the formulation of TRAIL, and the application of untagged TRAIL, e.g. Apo2L/TRAIL.0 (114–281), which is the prototype of native TRAIL, in a therapeutic setting should not be toxic. Many previous studies just deal with the fact that TRAIL is a potent inducer in of apoptosis in tumor. However, TRAIL is important for normal tumor immunosurveillance as TRAIL knockout mice grow tumors at a higher rate compared to normal mice and are more prone to tumor metastasis (Cretney et al., 2002).

Trail-Induced Signaling Cascade

In the late 1990s several TRAIL receptors have been identified and characterized. TRAIL can bind to four known membrane-bound receptors:

1. Death receptor 4 (DR4)/TRAIL receptor-1 (Pan et al., 1997a, b)
2. Death receptor 5 (DR5)/TRAIL receptor-2 (Pan et al., 1997a, b)
3. TRAIL receptor without an intracellular domain (TRID)/decoy receptor 1 (DCR1) TRAIL receptor-3 (Degli-Esposti et al., 1997a, b)
4. TRAIL receptor-4/decoy Receptor 2 (DCR2)/TRAIL receptor with a truncated death domain (TRUNDD) (Degli-Esposti et al., 1997a, b).
5. Osteoprotegerin (OPG), a soluble receptor, that antagonizes the pro-apoptotic functions of TRAIL (Emery et al., 1998).

Importantly, the above-mentioned decoy receptors do not translate TRAIL signaling into the cells (Sheridan et al., 1997).

In sharp contrast, TRAIL receptor-1 (DR4: death-receptor 4) and TRAIL receptor-2 (DR5: death-receptor 5) have a functional cytosolic death domain to initiate the extrinsic apoptotic pathway (Hymowitz et al., 1999). After binding of TRAIL to either DR4 and DR5 a multi-protein structure called the death-inducing signaling complex (DISC) consisting of Fas-associated death domain protein (FADD), procaspase-8 is recruited (Fig. 40.1). At the DISC Procaspase-8 is activated and promotes the activation of effector caspases, e.g. 3, 6 and 7 (Kischkel et al., 2000). In addition, the pro-apoptotic Bcl-2 protein Bid is cleaved by caspase-8 and activates the intrinsic apoptotic pathway (Li et al., 1998).

In some glioblastoma cells, activated caspase-8 triggers directly apoptosis (type I cells), while other cells require activation of the mitochondrial pathway to enhance the apoptotic signal (type II cells). Importantly, in many primary GBM specimens and cell lines caspase-8 expression has shown to be suppressed on the transcriptional level by several epigenetic mechanisms. After activation of the intrinsic pathway the mitochondrial membrane is permeabilized leading to cytochrome-c release from the mitochondria into the cytosol. In turn, cytochrome-c binds to apoptotic peptidase activating factor 1 (Apaf1) and caspase 9 to form the apoptosome resulting in profound activation of effector-caspases that mediate cell death. The TRAIL receptor-signaling pathway is shown in Fig. 40.1.

Trail-Receptor Expression in Normal Human Tissues and Glioblastomas

The expression of TRAIL-receptor is widely distributed on normal human tissue. (Dorr et al., 2002). In the vast majority of glioblastoma cells and GBM specimens TRAIL-R1 (DR4) is suppressed on the level of transcription through hypermethylation of the DR4 promoter region (Elias et al., 2009), whereas in sharp contrast TRAIL-R2 (DR5) is broadly expressed in GBM cells and specimens. There is only weak expression of TRIAL-receptors (DRA and DR5) in vascular brain endothelium. Importantly, human astrocytes only weakly express DR4 and DR5, whereas the majority

of human glioblastoma cells express DR5. Non neoplastic cells like oligodendrocytes and neurons were shown to express the TRAIL-decoy receptors. In summary, the distribution of death-receptors is favorable for a GBM-specific TRAIL-based therapy since most non-transformed cells do not sufficiently express DR4 or DR5, but instead these cells express antagonizing receptors decoy receptors on their surface.

Mediators of Trail-Resistance in GBM and Therapeutic Combinations to Overcome Trail Resistance

Although some glioblastoma cells are highly sensitive to the apoptotic inducing effects of TRAIL, e.g. the glioblastoma cell line LN18, most of established and primary glioblastoma cells reveal an endogenous resistant towards death ligands, including CD95 and TRAIL.

This resistance towards TRAIL-mediated apoptosis is by itself a clear obstacle to clinical efficacy.

On a molecular basis, TRAIL-resistance is mediated by a number of mediated and of course not limited to the below mentioned factors.

1. High expression of decoy receptors that do not engage apoptosis after binding of TRAIL
2. Epigenetically silenced expression of death receptors, in particular DR4
3. Epigenetically silenced expression of caspase-8
4. High expression of the caspase-8 inhibitor, cellular-Flice Inhibitory Protein (cFLIP), including the long and short isoforms (Condorelli et al., 1999)
5. Over-expression of the astrocytic phosphoprotein, PEA15, a death effector domain containing that inhibits caspase-8 in a similar manner as c-FLIP (Eckert et al., 2008).
6. Over-expression of anti-apoptotic bcl-2 family proteins, including Bcl-2, Bcl-xL and Mcl-1
7. Over-expression of the Inhibitor of apoptosis protein (IAPs), including XIAP, Survivin.

With regards to point 2, it was recently discovered that TRAIL-R1 (Death-receptor 4) is an epigenetically regulated gene in low-grade and high-grade gliomas (Elias et al., 2009). The promoter region of DR4

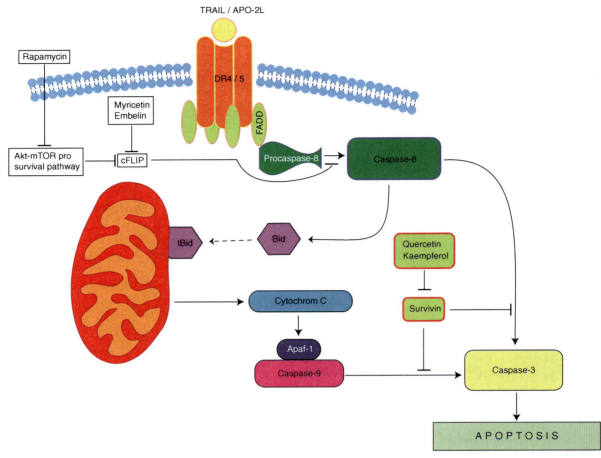

Fig. 40.1 Intrinsic and extrinsic apoptotic pathway: TRAIL binds to its receptors, death-receptors (DR4/5) and thereby induces the binding of adapter protein, FAAD, and caspase-8, leading to the auto-cleavage/activation of caspase-8. An endogenous inhibitor of Caspase-8 is c-FLIP that is over-expressed in many glioblastomas. Some known inhibitors of c-FLIP not limited to are mTOR-inhibitors (Rapamycin), Myricetin and Embelin. Caspase-8 may activate either directly the effector-caspase-3, leading to a straightforward induction of apoptosis in type I cells, or cleave the BH3-only protein, BID. Cleaved BID, tBID, releases cytochrome-c from the inter-mitochondrial membrane space into the cytosol. In the cytosol cytochrome-c builds up a complex, consisting of Apaf-1, Procaspase-9, Apaf-1 and dATP, leading to an activation of Caspase-9. Caspase-9 activates the effector-caspase-3, which is one of the main executor enzymes of apoptosis. Several anti-apoptotic proteins, e.g. survivin, inhibit the active caspase-9. Survivin is over-expressed in glioblastoma cells and flavonoids, e.g. quercetin and kaempferol promote its proteasomal degradation thereby sensitizing glioblastoma cells to the cytotoxic effects of TRAIL

turned out to be frequently hypermethylated, resulting in silenced expression of DR4 in these cell lines or specimens. In particular, 60% ($n = 5$) of diffuse astrocytomas WHO grade 2, 75% ($n = 8$) of anaplastic astrocytomas WHO grade 3 and 70% of glioblastomas WHO grade 4 ($n = 33$) exhibited hypermethylation of the DR4 promoter (Elias et al., 2009). This finding might also implicate therapeutic consequences since agonistic DR4 antibodies, e.g. mapatumumab, will fall short of expectations in glioma with silenced expression of DR4. Established glioma cell lines, such as A172 and U373, also exhibited silenced expression of DR4 and hypermethylation of the DR4 promoter region, respectively. In functional demethylation cell culture experiments with 5-aza-2-deoxycytidine DR4 expression was restored in established glioma cells, suggesting that the DR4 silencing is reversible and therefore demethylating reagents might be promising in combination with TRAIL (Elias et al., 2009).

With respect to Caspase-8 expression, it has been shown that caspase-8 is frequently absent in low-grade and high-grade gliomas. Silencing of caspase-8 might be mediated through an epigenetic mechanism since demethylating-reagents have been shown to restore caspase-8 expression in brain tumor cells (Fulda et al., 2001; Eramo et al., 2005). We also made a recent discovery that functionally linked glioblastoma stem-cell-like cells (SCGs) to caspase-8. Glioblastomas contain a population that reveals stem-cell properties. SCGs are highly tumorigenic and express stem cell markers, e.g. nestin, Oct4 and CD133. Importantly, SCGs exhibit an endogenous resistance to radiotherapy and chemotherapy. We also analysed a limited number of SCGs for TRAIL-resistance and compared them with the sensitivity of the bulk tumor cells, the so called non glioblastoma stem-cell-like cells (NSCGs). We found that SCGs were totally refractory to TRAIL treatment, partly due to selective down-regulation of caspase-8 (Capper et al., 2009). Re-expression of caspase-8 by treating the cells with a demethylating reagent restored Caspase-8 expression but was not sufficient to sensitize SCGs to the cytotoxic effects of TRAIL. Our study illustrates the heterogeneity of GBMs, with defined subpopulations that are more resistant to TRAIL. Therefore, targeting the stem-cell like tumor cell fraction within GBMs is of utmost importance and priority.

One intrinsic inhibitor of caspase-8 is c-FLIP. High expression of c-FLIP has been shown to counteract CD95 and TRAIL-mediated apoptosis, respectively. In particular, the short isoform of c-FLIP, c-FLIP (S), was shown to be very important in mediating TRAIL resistance (Panner et al., 2005). The mammalian target of rapamycin (mTOR) turned out to be a regulator of c-FLIP (S) levels (Fig. 40.1). Importantly, the mTOR inhibitor, rapamycin, which is a downstream inhibitor of the Akt-pathway, that is known to be aberrantly active in primary glioblastomas, sensitizes glioblastoma cells to TRAIL-mediated apoptotic signaling (Panner et al., 2005).

In one of our studies we have found that Myricetin sensitizes GBM cells for TRAIL-mediated apoptosis by down-regulation of c-FLIP and bcl-2 (Siegelin et al., 2009a). Myricetin is a naturally occurring flavonol, a flavonoid found in many grapes, berries, fruits, vegetables, herbs, as well as other plants. Another effective natural compound is Embelin from the Japanese Ardisia herb that has previously been shown to be a XIAP inhibitor and NF-KB inhibitor. We identified Embelin as a potent sensitizer for TRAIL-mediated cell death in malignant glioma cells (Siegelin et al., 2009b). Embelin suppressed protein levels of both the long and short isoform of c-FLIP by a posttranscriptional mechanism. Ectopic-expression of c-FLIP inhibited TRAIL-Embelin mediated apoptosis suggesting that c-FLIP is an important component in TRAIL-Embelin mediated apoptosis in malignant glioma cells (Fig. 40.1).

Another recent example is the combination of TRAIL with Bortezomib, a proteasomal inhibitor that has also been reached clinical trials. This combination turned out to be very powerful and broadly sensitized primary glioma cells (WHO I-IV) by suppression of c-FLIP (Koschny et al., 2007). In conclusion, c-FLIP is an important mediator of TRAIL-resistance in GBM and targeting c-FLIP might prove very powerful to sensitize highly TRAIL-resistant GBMs.

In GBM, anti-apoptotic proteins such as Bcl-2, Bcl-Xl and Mcl-1 are often over-expressed (Tagscherer et al., 2008), thereby promoting resistance to intrinsic apoptotic stimuli. One recent report demonstrates that selective inhibition of these anti-apoptotic proteins has been successfully pursued using the small molecule ABT-737, an inhibitor for Bcl-2 and BcL-xL. ABT-737 significantly increased survival in an orthotopic xenograft GBM model using U251 glioma cells (Tagscherer et al., 2008). However, one critical limitation of this study is that ABT-737 was locally applied. Therefore, it remains to be determined whether a systemic application of ABT-737 might prove to be effective. In this regard, the combination of radiation and/or temezolomide with ABT-737 might be of particular interest. Regarding combinatorial approaches ABT-737 sensitized GBM cells to TRAIL and chemotherapeutics, respectively (in vitro) (Tagscherer et al., 2008). Furthermore the SCG subpopulation of primary glioma specimens was more resistant to treatment with ABT-737 than the non-SCG population since SCGs over-express the anti-apoptotic protein, Mcl-1 (Tagscherer et al., 2008). Over-expression of Mcl-1 is one of the major causes of tumor cell resistance to the apoptotic effects of ABT-737 (Tagscherer et al., 2008). Down-regulation of Mcl-1 by a specific sh-RNA sensitized SCGs to the pro-apoptotic effects of ABT-737. However, it remains to be determined whether ABT-737 has the capability to overcome TRAIL-resistance in SCGs. Since SCGs often exhibit silenced expression of caspase-8 it seems quite unlikely that Bcl-2 inhibitor might be able to sensitize SCGs as Bcl-2 inhibitors act further downstream in the TRAIL-signaling cascade.

With respect to the IAPs, in the past years it has been shown by various groups that IAPs are over-expressed in GBM specimens and cell lines, suggesting that these molecules are suitable druggable targets. In a very elegant study in 2002 it was demonstrated that Smac mimetics that antagonize the anti-apoptotic function of XIAP are powerful anti-cancer reagents when combined with TRAIL. Smac mimetics broadly sensitized glioblastoma cells, other tumor cells cell lines and primary cultures to the cytotoxic effects of TRAIL. The combination of Smac mimetics and TRAIL were proven to be non-toxic for non-transformed cells, such as human Schwann cells. Notably, preclinical combined loco-regional application of TRAIL and Smac mimetics led to long term survival of nude mice in an orthotopic model of malignant glioma (Fulda et al., 2002). This combination was proven to be well tolerated and safe since mice did not exhibit any sign of morphological and clinical neurotoxicity suggesting that this combination might even have potential to enter a clinical trial. However, to this date such a trial has not been initiated. One pitfall and important limitation is that TRAIL was applied intracranially. Therefore it remains to be determined if the combination of TRAIL and Smac mimetics demonstrates similar efficacy when administered systemically. Depending on the formulation the half life of TRAIL is considered to be around 30 min suggesting that for efficient treatment a continuous application is needed. This holds in particular true for GBMs since a report from 2001 demonstrated that the orthotopic GBM xenografts were eradicated upon continuous infusion of TRAIL. A very elegant method to enhance TRAIL delivery to GBMs is the use of neural stem cells delivering soluble TRAIL since neural stem cells are known to enrich in GBMs. By secreting TRAIL neural stem cells might be prove very efficient not only as a single treatment, but also very powerful in TRAIL combination regimens. A recent example for achieved therapeutically synergy in an orthotopic model of GBM is the combination of stem cell delivered TRAIL

and PI3-Kinase inhibitors. The use of TRAIL secreting stem cells is an exciting, tumor-cell specific approach, but further studies are necessary to study particularly the safety of this treatment approach.

Our group also demonstrated that several compounds sensitize both established and primary glioma cells to TRAIL-mediated cell death by antagonizing IAPs. We found that at clinical achievable concentrations of two flavonoids, quercetin and kaempferol, were able to overcome TRAIL-resistance in glioblastoma cells independent of their PTEN or p53 status (Siegelin et al., 2008, 2009c). This combinatorial cell death induced by TRAIL and quercetin/keampferol was partially mediated by an enhanced proteasomal degradation of the IAP, survivin. Over-expression of survivin was shown to protect cells from TRAIL/quercetin mediated cell death (Fig. 40.1). Interestingly, down-regulation of survivin by siRNA was sufficient to restore TRAIL sensitivity in glioblastoma cell lines, suggesting that even survivin small-molecule antagonists might have promising anti-cancer activity when combined with TRAIL. Survivin itself is an anti-apoptotic protein that is over-expressed in almost every tumor whereas it is undetectable in non-transformed human tissues and cells. This makes survivin an ideal druggable target as survivin-antagonists will target almost specifically tumor cells. Thus, the combination of TRAIL and survivin antagonist is expected to be almost tumor cell specific. In line with this contention is the fact that human astrocytes were not affected by the combination of TRAIL and quercetin since astrocytes neither express DR4 or DR5 nor survivin. Another important aspect for the combination of TRAIL and quercetin/kaempferol is that the down-regulation of survivin was not only dependent on the proteasome it also relied on the inhibition of the Akt pathway. Inhibition of the Akt pathway either by LY294002 (an experimental broad inhibitor of the Akt-pathway) or kaempferol significantly suppressed both the levels of phosphorylated-Akt (Ser 473) and survivin levels. Moreover, forced expression of a constitutively active Akt in glioma cells partially inhibited quercetin and kaempferol mediated suppression of survivin, suggesting that the Akt pathway is key regulator of quercetin/kaempferol mediated down-regulation of survivin. Many glioblastomas are dependent on the Akt pro-survival signaling and particularly primary glioblastomas exhibit PTEN mutation leading to a profound activation of the Akt pathway in these specimens or cells. Therefore, therapeutic inhibition of the Akt – signalling pathway is warranted and is expected to render glioblastoma cells sensitive to the cytotoxic effects of TRAIL. Indeed, it has been recently shown that global inhibition of the Phosphatidyl-inositol-3-kinase (PI3K) led to a broad sensitization of GBM cells to several chemotherapeutic drugs and TRAIL, respectively (Opel et al., 2008).

Similar to flavonoids, our group demonstrated that the HSP90 antagonist 17-AAG was capable of sensitizing glioblastoma cells to TRAIL by down-regulation of survivin. We and other groups demonstrated that HSP90 is particularly over-expressed in GBM specimens suggesting that antagonizing HSP90 is a worthwhile strategy to combat GBM. We also found that the down-regulation of survivin mediated by 17-AAG was a critical factor in TRAIL-17-AAG mediated apoptosis since ectopic over-expression of survivin partially restored loss of cellular viability in glioma cells treated with TRAIL and 17-AAG. Mechanistically, 17-AAG mediated down-regulation of survivin was most likely to be mediated post-translational by a mechanism involving the proteasome.

The mainstay of GBM treatment remains radiation and/or chemotherapy with Temezolomide (TMZ). TMZ is an oral chemotherapeutic drug that is generally well tolerated by patients. Although some patients respond to this treatment, the gain in survival time even when combined with radiation is moderate. As TRAIL shows tremendous activity in combination with various reagents, including radiation (Gong and Almasan, 2000), researchers studied the combinatorial approach of TMZ and TRAIL. Since the combination of TRAIL and TMZ was efficient in cell culture experiments, the combination of both was studied in an intracranial model of glioblastoma. It turned out that the efficacy of intracerebral infused TRAIL was significantly enhanced by co-treatment with TMZ in a U87MG intracranial xenograft model (Saito et al., 2004). Although this group used an intracranial delivery approach of TRAIL, which in the case of glioblastoma is a viable option since many 90% of GBMs recur at their initial location, these results might hold significant promise for patients suffering from GBM. However one important limitation in this study is that the combinatorial approach of TRAIL and TMZ was analysed in an orthotopic glioblastoma model utilizing the U87 glioblastoma cell line. The U87 GBM cell line is known to be sensitive to TMZ since it harbors a hypermethylated O-6-methylguanine-DNA methyltransferase (MGMT) promoter leading to suppressed expression of MGMT rendering U87 cells in particular sensitive to the effects of TMZ. Therefore, it remains to be determined whether this combination might also work in the background of cells (in vivo) that do not exhibit silenced expression of MGMT.

Another important treatment modality for GBMs in patients remains radiation. Recently, it was shown that human glioblastoma cells can be effectively sensitized to TRAIL by genotoxic ionizing radiation (Nagane et al., 2007). Mechanistically, the combination of TRAIL and radiation were dependent on DR5 expression, FADD protein and caspase-8, suggesting that cells that do not or only weakly express caspase-8 might not respond to this combinatorial treatment as compared to cells that highly express caspase-8. Furthermore, over-expression of the anti-apoptotic bcl-2 family protein, bcl-X(L), attenuated the cytotoxic effect of combined TRAIL and radiation treatment (Nagane et al., 2007).

Conclusion

In summary, the combinatorial drug approaches might prove very powerful in the treatment of recalcitrant, highly resistant glioblastomas. TRAIL might be a welcome contribution for several future combinatorial drug regimens since it has been shown to induce apoptosis specifically in tumor cells while having minor effects on non-cancerous cells. In a number of recent studies TRAIL, either alone or in combinatorial approaches, has been shown to exert anti-tumor effects in many experimental xenograft models (including challenging models such as the orthotopic glioblastoma xenograft model). The evidence from these preclinical data might lead to new promising drug regimens for the treatment of GBM.

References

Ashkenazi A, Pai RC, Fong S, Leung S, Lawrence DA, Marsters SA, Blackie C, Chang L, McMurtrey AE, Hebert A, DeForge L, Koumenis IL, Lewis D, Harris L, Bussiere J, Koeppen H, Shahrokh Z, Schwall RH (1999) Safety and antitumor activity of recombinant soluble Apo2 ligand. J Clin Invest 104:155–162

Capper D, Gaiser T, Hartmann C, Habel A, Mueller W, Herold-Mende C, von Deimling A, Siegelin MD (2009) Stem-cell-like glioma cells are resistant to TRAIL/Apo2L and exhibit down-regulation of caspase-8 by promoter methylation. Acta Neuropathol 117:445–456

Cha SS, Kim MS, Choi YH, Sung BJ, Shin NK, Shin HC, Sung YC, Oh BH (1999a) 2.8 A resolution crystal structure of human TRAIL, a cytokine with selective antitumor activity. Immunity 11:253–261

Cha SS, Shin HC, Choi KY, Oh BH (1999b) Expression, purification and crystallization of recombinant human TRAIL. Acta Crystallogr D Biol Crystallogr 55:1101–1104

Condorelli G, Vigliotta G, Cafieri A, Trencia A, Andalo P, Oriente F, Miele C, Caruso M, Formisano P, Beguinot F (1999) PED/PEA-15: an anti-apoptotic molecule that regulates FAS/TNFR1-induced apoptosis. Oncogene 18:4409–4415

Cretney E, Takeda K, Yagita H, Glaccum M, Peschon JJ, Smyth MJ (2002) Increased susceptibility to tumor initiation and metastasis in TNF-related apoptosis-inducing ligand-deficient mice. J Immunol 168:1356–1361

Degli-Esposti MA, Dougall WC, Smolak PJ, Waugh JY, Smith CA, Goodwin RG (1997a) The novel receptor TRAIL-R4 induces NF-kappaB and protects against TRAIL-mediated apoptosis, yet retains an incomplete death domain. Immunity 7:813–820

Degli-Esposti MA, Smolak PJ, Walczak H, Waugh J, Huang CP, DuBose RF, Goodwin RG, Smith CA (1997b) Cloning and characterization of TRAIL-R3, a novel member of the emerging TRAIL receptor family. J Exp Med 186:1165–1170

Dorr J, Bechmann I, Waiczies S, Aktas O, Walczak H, Krammer PH, Nitsch R, Zipp F (2002) Lack of tumor necrosis factor-related apoptosis-inducing ligand but presence of its receptors in the human brain. J Neurosci 22:RC209

Eckert A, Bock BC, Tagscherer KE, Haas TL, Grund K, Sykora J, Herold-Mende C, Ehemann V, Hollstein M, Chneiweiss H, Wiestler OD, Walczak H, Roth W (2008) The PEA-15/PED protein protects glioblastoma cells from glucose deprivation-induced apoptosis via the ERK/MAP kinase pathway. Oncogene 27:1155–1166

Elias A, Siegelin MD, Steinmuller A, von Deimling A, Lass U, Korn B, Mueller W (2009) Epigenetic silencing of death receptor 4 mediates tumor necrosis factor-related apoptosis-inducing ligand resistance in gliomas. Clin Cancer Res 15:5457–5465

Emery JG, McDonnell P, Burke MB, Deen KC, Lyn S, Silverman C, Dul E, Appelbaum ER, Eichman C, DiPrinzio R, Dodds RA, James IE, Rosenberg M, Lee JC, Young PR (1998) Osteoprotegerin is a receptor for the cytotoxic ligand TRAIL. J Biol Chem 273:14363–14367

Eramo A, Pallini R, Lotti F, Sette G, Patti M, Bartucci M, Ricci-Vitiani L, Signore M, Stassi G, Larocca LM, Crino L, Peschle C, De Maria R (2005) Inhibition of DNA methylation sensitizes glioblastoma for tumor necrosis factor-related apoptosis-inducing ligand-mediated destruction. Cancer Res 65:11469–11477

Fulda S, Kufer MU, Meyer E, van Valen F, Dockhorn-Dworniczak B, Debatin KM (2001) Sensitization for death receptor- or drug-induced apoptosis by re-expression of caspase-8 through demethylation or gene transfer. Oncogene 20:5865–5877

Fulda S, Wick W, Weller M, Debatin KM (2002) Smac agonists sensitize for Apo2L/TRAIL- or anticancer drug-induced apoptosis and induce regression of malignant glioma in vivo. Nat Med 8:808–815

Gong B, Almasan A (2000) Apo2 ligand/TNF-related apoptosis-inducing ligand and death receptor 5 mediate the apoptotic signaling induced by ionizing radiation in leukemic cells. Cancer Res 60:5754–5760

Hymowitz SG, Christinger HW, Fuh G, Ultsch M, O'Connell M, Kelley RF, Ashkenazi A, de Vos AM (1999) Triggering cell death: the crystal structure of Apo2L/TRAIL in a complex with death receptor 5. Mol Cell 4:563–571

Jo M, Kim TH, Seol DW, Esplen JE, Dorko K, Billiar TR, Strom SC (2000) Apoptosis induced in normal human hepatocytes by tumor necrosis factor-related apoptosis-inducing ligand. Nat Med 6:564–567

Kischkel FC, Lawrence DA, Chuntharapai A, Schow P, Kim KJ, Ashkenazi A (2000) Apo2L/TRAIL-dependent recruitment of endogenous FADD and caspase-8 to death receptors 4 and 5. Immunity 12:611–620

Koschny R, Holland H, Sykora J, Haas TL, Sprick MR, Ganten TM, Krupp W, Bauer M, Ahnert P, Meixensberger J, Walczak H (2007) Bortezomib sensitizes primary human astrocytoma cells of WHO grades I to IV for tumor necrosis factor-related apoptosis-inducing ligand-induced apoptosis. Clin Cancer Res 13:3403–3412

Li L, Ma R, Cheng H, Ni H, Cheng J (1998) Application of time-frequency filter of wavelet to single-trail ERP extracting. Sheng Wu Yi Xue Gong Cheng Xue Za Zhi 15:116–119

Nagane M, Cavenee WK, Shiokawa Y (2007) Synergistic cytotoxicity through the activation of multiple apoptosis pathways in human glioma cells induced by combined treatment with ionizing radiation and tumor necrosis factor-related apoptosis-inducing ligand. J Neurosurg 106:407–416

Opel D, Westhoff MA, Bender A, Braun V, Debatin KM, Fulda S (2008) Phosphatidylinositol 3-kinase inhibition broadly sensitizes glioblastoma cells to death receptor- and drug-induced apoptosis. Cancer Res 68:6271–6280

Pan G, Ni J, Wei YF, Yu G, Gentz R, Dixit VM (1997a) An antagonist decoy receptor and a death domain-containing receptor for TRAIL. Science 277:815–818

Pan G, O'Rourke K, Chinnaiyan AM, Gentz R, Ebner R, Ni J, Dixit VM (1997b) The receptor for the cytotoxic ligand TRAIL. Science 276:111–113

Panner A, James CD, Berger MS, Pieper RO (2005) mTOR controls FLIPS translation and TRAIL sensitivity in glioblastoma multiforme cells. Mol Cell Biol 25:8809–8823

Saito R, Bringas JR, Panner A, Tamas M, Pieper RO, Berger MS, Bankiewicz KS (2004) Convection-enhanced delivery of tumor necrosis factor-related apoptosis-inducing ligand with systemic administration of temozolomide prolongs survival in an intracranial glioblastoma xenograft model. Cancer Res 64:6858–6862

Sheridan JP, Marsters SA, Pitti RM, Gurney A, Skubatch M, Baldwin D, Ramakrishnan L, Gray CL, Baker K, Wood WI, Goddard AD, Godowski P, Ashkenazi A (1997) Control of TRAIL-induced apoptosis by a family of signaling and decoy receptors. Science 277:818–821

Siegelin MD, Gaiser T, Habel A, Siegelin Y (2009a) Myricetin sensitizes malignant glioma cells to TRAIL-mediated apoptosis by down-regulation of the short isoform of FLIP and bcl-2. Cancer Lett 283:230–238

Siegelin MD, Gaiser T, Siegelin Y (2009b) The XIAP inhibitor Embelin enhances TRAIL-mediated apoptosis in malignant glioma cells by down-regulation of the short isoform of FLIP. Neurochem Int 55:423–430

Siegelin MD, Reuss DE, Habel A, Herold-Mende C, von Deimling A (2008) The flavonoid kaempferol sensitizes human glioma cells to TRAIL-mediated apoptosis by proteasomal degradation of survivin. Mol Cancer Ther 7: 3566–3574

Siegelin MD, Reuss DE, Habel A, Rami A, von Deimling A (2009c) Quercetin promotes degradation of survivin and thereby enhances death-receptor-mediated apoptosis in glioma cells. Neuro Oncol 11:122–131

Tagscherer KE, Fassl A, Campos B, Farhadi M, Kraemer A, Bock BC, Macher-Goeppinger S, Radlwimmer B, Wiestler OD, Herold-Mende C, Roth W (2008) Apoptosis-based treatment of glioblastomas with ABT-737, a novel small molecule inhibitor of Bcl-2 family proteins. Oncogene 27: 6646–6656

Walczak H, Miller RE, Ariail K, Gliniak B, Griffith TS, Kubin M, Chin W, Jones J, Woodward A, Le T, Smith C, Smolak P, Goodwin RG, Rauch CT, Schuh JC, Lynch DH (1999) Tumoricidal activity of tumor necrosis factor-related apoptosis-inducing ligand in vivo. Nat Med 5: 157–163

Wiley SR, Schooley K, Smolak PJ, Din WS, Huang CP, Nicholl JK, Sutherland GR, Smith TD, Rauch C, Smith CA et al (1995) Identification and characterization of a new member of the TNF family that induces apoptosis. Immunity 3:673–682

Part V
Prognosis

Chapter 41

Long-Term Survivors of Glioblastoma

Oliver Bähr and Joachim P. Steinbach

Abstract Population-wide, only a disappointingly small number of patients with glioblastoma survives for more than 5 years. Hopefully, these figures will improve in the coming years as a result of improved neurosurgical techniques and the use of radiochemotherapy according to the EORTC 26981 protocol also outside of clinical studies. Additionally, new and innovative therapies are hoped to contribute to better outcomes. In this review, we summarize current knowledge about prognosticators of long-term survival in glioblastoma patients. In addition, we address the functional status of long-term survivors including neurological deficits, neuropsychological impairment and quality of life. Younger age and higher Karnofsky performance score are known independent clinical factors associated with longer overall survival (OS). Extent of surgery and chemotherapy are also favorable factors supporting long-term survival. An abundance of molecular markers has been repeatedly screened for their influence on survival of glioblastoma patients. To date, only a methylated MGMT promoter status and more recently the presence of IDH1 mutations, have been shown to be associated with better survival rates in glioblastoma. Clinical outcome has special significance for long-term survivors. The reviewed data show that neurological deficits are common in these patients, and many patients additionally suffer from seizures and fatigue. Cognitive deficits are commonly underestimated if not carefully examined. Neuropsychological testing reveals deficits in one or several domains in the majority of long-term surviving patients, even in those with normal Mini-Mental status score. Nonetheless, only little reduction in overall quality of life and global health status were reported for the population of long-term survivors. With some patients in full remission for more than 10 years, the question arises, whether a glioblastoma can ever be considered to be cured. However, the occurrence of late and very late relapses after more than 5 and even more than 10 years in full remission rather argues for the maintenance of a tight control schedule for this remarkable population.

Keywords Glioblastoma · Long term survival · Prognosis · Outcome

Introduction

Long-term survival of patients with glioblastoma is a very rare event. In this regard, the available survival data should be interpreted cautiously, since clinical data and histopathological results must be carefully reviewed. Scott et al. (1999) accurately analyzed a Canadian tumor registry for gliobastoma patients and reported a 3 year survival rate of 2.2%, whereas the Central Brain Tumor Registry of the United States (CBTRUS, www.cbtrus.org) identifies a rate of 6.82% of all glioblastoma patients. The figures on patients surviving for more than 5 years range from 1.2% (Ohgaki and Kleihues, 2005) to 2% (McLendon and Halperin, 2003) to 4.46% (CBTRUS). These numbers are far below the 5 year survival rates of many other common malignancies, emphasizing the particularly malignant phenotype of glioblastoma.

O. Bähr (✉)
Dr. Senckenberg Institute of Neurooncology, University Cancer Center, Goethe University Hospital Frankfurt, Frankfurt, Germany
e-mail: Oliver.baehr@med.uni-frankfurt.de

M.A. Hayat (ed.), *Tumors of the Central Nervous System, Volume 1,*
DOI 10.1007/978-94-007-0344-5_41, © Springer Science+Business Media B.V. 2011

Several studies in the last decades have addressed different aspects of long-term survival in glioblastoma. Population based studies, as mentioned above, tried to identify the real-life proportion of long-term survivors. Others examined the necessary prerequisites which might support long-term survival. The influences of clinical and treatment-related factors as well as those of histological features have been studied for a long time. With new techniques emerging, the analysis of molecular markers in glioblastoma started two decades ago. Robust studies examining the influence of molecular alterations on the outcome of glioblastoma patients have been conducted in the last 10–15 years. Despite recent advancement in understanding these molecular changes, only a few markers have reached general relevance in glioblastomas and only the methylation status of the O^6-methylguanine methyltransferase (MGMT) has established as a predictive marker with regard to therapy with alkylating agents so far. Hypermethylation of the MGMT promoter leads to a transcriptional silencing of the DNA repair protein MGMT and is associated with a prolonged progression-free survival (PFS) and overall survival (OS) in patients with glioblastoma treated with alkylating agents such as temozolomide or nitrosoureas. As the patient's perspective in oncology gained more significance in the last years, some studies followed, dealing with the clinical outcome of long-term survivors. Especially neurological and cognitive outcome is relevant in glioblastoma patients, since the tumor itself or the applied therapies may cause a number of deficits. Particularly for the group of long-term survivors clinical outcome is crucial in terms of quality of life. Finally, the question has been discussed, whether there is a possibility of a definite cure for some of these patients surviving for 5 years or even longer.

Prognostic and Predictive Factors

Characteristics of the patient or the tumor at the time of diagnosis that can be used to estimate the risk of recurrence of the disease without any therapy are called prognostic factors. Predictive factors, on the other hand, are characteristics that are associated with the response or the lack of response to a particular therapy.

The population of long-term survivors differs in some respects from the entire population of glioblastoma patients. When these characteristics can be used to estimate the chance to become a long-term survivor they might have prognostic significance. As the proportion of long-term survivors is small, statistical considerations are somewhat limited.

Clinical Factors

At the time of diagnosis long-term survivors are significantly younger than the group of all glioblastoma patients. The mean age of all glioblastoma patients at diagnosis is just above 60 years (Krex et al., 2007; Ohgaki and Kleihues, 2005; www.cbtrus.org). Whereas the three largest cohorts of published long-term survivors show a median age of 38 years/39 cases (Burton et al., 2002), 47 years/39 cases (Hottinger et al., 2009) and 51 years/55 cases (Krex et al., 2007). In an extended list of Shinojima et al. (2004) and Krex et al. (2007) show all published patients with glioblastoma who survived longer than 3 years. The result is a number of 281 published cases with a mean age at diagnosis of 36.9 years. As this list starts with published patients in the year 1950, the data have to be interpreted cautiously, because the older studies might be contaminated with low-grade or anaplastic tumors. Despite the fact, that age is a significant prognostic factor for survival, some long-term survivors are older than 65 years (Burton et al., 2002; Krex et al., 2007), indicating that older age at least does not prohibit long-term survival.

Another important clinical factor is the Karnofsky performance score (KPS), an indicator for the general health status of cancer patients. Long-term survivors have a significantly higher KPS than the average of all glioblastoma patients. The median KPS in long-term survivors ranges between 80 and 90% (Hottinger et al., 2009; Krex et al., 2007; Scott et al., 1999; Shinojima et al., 2004; Sonoda et al., 2009) and in the population of all glioblastoma patients ∼76.7% (Scott et al., 1999). A recent study of the German Glioma Network corroborated the influence of the KPS on survival. For patients with a KPS below 80% (208 cases) Weller et al. (2009) reported a median PFS of 5.4 months and a median OS of 7.6 months, whereas for the 72 patients with a KPS of at least 80% the PFS was 7.2 months and the OS was 14.9 months.

Usually glioblastomas are more frequent in males, with a male/female ratio of ~1.34 (Ohgaki and Kleihues, 2005). In contrast, the male/female ratio in the group of long-term survivors is rather 1:1 (Krex et al., 2007; Shinojima et al., 2004), suggesting that female gender might be a somewhat favorable prognostic factor. The only study regarding environmental, occupational and socioeconomic risk factors in glioblastoma long-term survivors by Krex et al. (2007) did not identify any of these factors to be under- or overrepresented in the examined group of long-term survivors.

Treatment Related Factors

Despite the fact that randomized trials have been missing, the extent of resection has always been thought to strongly influence the prognosis of glioblastoma patients. A randomized trial studying fluorescence-guided surgery with 5-aminolevulinic acid provided strong data on a correlation between extent of surgery and progression-free survival (Stummer et al., 2006). In patients resected with fluorescence-guidance a complete resection of contrast-enhancing tumor was achieved in 65%, and this was only the case in 36% of the patients resected without this support. This difference resulted in a significantly higher 6-month progression-free survival (41.0%) for patients after fluorescence-guided resection compared with the group of patients resected under white light (21.1%). Follow-up of this study has also demonstrated that gross-total resection is an important prognostic factor for OS (Pichlmeier et al., 2008; Stummer et al., 2008).

Because standard therapy for glioblastomas in patients with a KPS of at least 60% includes radiotherapy, it is not possible to determine whether it is a prognostic factor in the group of long-term surviving glioblastoma patients, although the efficacy of radiotherapy has been clearly demonstrated in randomized trials. In all studies specifically examining long-term survival in glioblastoma all patients received postoperative radiotherapy (Hottinger et al., 2009; Krex et al., 2007; Scott et al., 1999).

Concomitant and adjuvant temozolomide chemotherapy has a significant benefit on survival of glioblastoma patients (Stupp et al., 2009) in the study population. Temozolomide not only positively influences median PFS and median OS, but also enhances long-term survival rates. Patients in the combined therapy group reached a 3 year survival rate of 16.0% and a 5 year survival rate of 9.8%, compared to the radiotherapy group reaching only 4.4 and 1.9%, respectively. Because patients in clinical trials underlie strict inclusion and exclusion criteria, these figures should not be compared with the figures from population based studies. Nonetheless not all of the long-term survivors have received any kind of chemotherapy. Hottinger et al. (2009) report a proportion of 10% and Krex et al. (2007) of 33% of their long-term survivors that have not received any kind of chemotherapy. However, recent data on long-term survival of patients treated with radiotherapy, temozolomide, and lomustine (Glas et al., 2009) underline the significance of chemotherapy for survival. Patients treated with an intensive regimen of two chemotherapeutic drugs reached promising 2, 3, 4, and 5 year survival rates of 47.4, 26.4, 18.5 and 15.8%, respectively. In conclusion, additional chemotherapy is a favorable factor but long-term survival is possible without chemotherapy.

Histological Features

Some histopathological subtypes of glioblastoma might have a better prognosis. Giant cell glioblastomas, for example, are overrepresented in the group of long-term survivors. Krex et al. (2007) report on a proportion of 9.1% in their cohort compared to 2.1% in a control group. Supporting these data, Shinojima et al. (2004) found a giant cell glioblastoma in 3 of their 6 long-term survivors and none in their control group consisting of 107 short-term survivors. But one has to consider that patients with giant cell glioblastoma seem to be younger than the average glioblastoma patient, and therefore this may not be an independent progonosticator that reflects a different biological behavior (Louis et al., 2007). Gliosarcoma and glioblastoma with oligodendroglial component might also have a slightly favorable prognosis, but due to the low incidence detailed studies are missing (Louis et al., 2007). Regardless of the specific histology, the presence and extent of necrosis is an unfavorable factor for survival (Louis et al., 2007), but studies on long-term survivors are not available.

Molecular Factors

Hypermethylation of the MGMT promoter has been reported to confer better PFS and OS (Stupp et al., 2009) without being associated with age, KPS, extent of surgery or with the first-line treatment (Weller et al., 2009). Therefore, it is not surprising that a methylated MGMT promoter status is more common in glioblastoma long-term survivors. Krex et al. (2007) found a promoter methylation in 74% of their long-term survivors compared to 43% in the control group. Martinez et al. (2007) found comparable figures with a promoter methylation in 7 out of 9 (77.8%) long-term survivors and 73 out of their entire population of 186 glioblastoma patients (39.2%). A third study by Sonoda et al. (2009) confirmed these data with a promoter methylation in 11 out of 14 (79%) long-term survivors and 4 out of 16 (25%) control patients. These results are corroborated by the 5 year analysis of the EORTC-NCIC trial (Stupp et al., 2009), which reported that MGMT promoter methylation status was the strongest predictor for outcome. In the combined treatment group an unmethylated MGMT promoter resulted in a 3 year OS of 11.1% and of 27.6% for the group with a methylated promoter status. However, not all long-term survivors exhibit a methylated MGMT promoter status. Therefore, factors other than MGMT may in some cases support long-term survival.

Two studies on long-term survival report on a lower Ki-67 labeling index in long-term survivors. Scott et al. (1999) describe a Ki-67 labeling of 10.4% of the tumor nuclei in long-term survivors and 20.6% in the control group ($p = 0.0064$). In the second study by Sonoda et al. (2009) 25% of the nuclei were positive for Ki-67 in long-term survivors and 35% in the short-term survivors, whereas this difference was not significant due to the small number of patients.

Efforts have been made to evaluate several other molecular markers, such as TP53, EGFR, PTEN, CDK4, CDKN2A, MDM2, LOH 1p, LOH 9p, LOH 10q, and LOH 19q for their prognostic significance. In most of the studies no robust influence on outcome could be detected for any of these markers. The most recent and detailed work was presented by the German Glioma Network (Weller et al., 2009).

This study confirmed younger age, higher performance score, MGMT promoter methylation and temozolomide radiochemotherapy as independent factors associated with longer OS. Additionally, isocitrate dehydrogenase 1 (IDH1) mutations were identified as a strong favorable prognostic factor on PFS and were associated with a trend towards prolonged OS. However, these mutations are rare in glioblastoma, with only 16 of 286 patients showing an IDH1 mutation (Weller et al., 2009). They again found the other markers mentioned above not to be significant factors for outcome of glioblastoma patients.

Clinical Outcome

As the prognosis of patients with glioblastoma has improved with the development of effective multimodal therapy and the proportion of long-term survivors has considerably grown (Stupp et al., 2009), the functional clinical outcome of these patients and their quality of life has become the subject of increasing interest. Neurological sequelae in this population can be due to both, the direct effects of the tumor itself and side effects of therapy. Only very few studies have carefully examined the clinical outcome of glioblastoma long-term survivors. Most studies looked for the clinical status at the time of diagnosis only, so data on the follow-up of these patients are rare.

Neurological Deficits

Focal neurological deficits are common in brain tumor patients. Seizure is another typical symptom at initial presentation and during the course of the disease. In a cohort of 39 long-term survivors examined by Hottinger et al. (2009) 85% of the patients showed a significant neurological deficit. These data match with the results of a smaller cohort study by Steinbach et al. (2006) where 7 out of 10 patients had a neurological deficit. In both studies motor deficits followed by aphasia and visual field deficits were the most common sequelae. Steinbach et al. (2006) reported on mild to moderate deficits in their patients, whereas Hottinger et al. (2009) report on 8 (20.5%) patients being wheel chair-bound. The rather good general condition of this population is reflected in a relatively high KPS. The cohort of Steinbach et al. (2006) showed a median KPS of 70% (60–100) which equates the results of Hottinger et al. (2009) with a median KPS of 70% (40–100). Steinbach et al. (2006) additionally examined their cohort for seizures and antiepileptic medication. At least one seizure after completion of primary therapy was found in 5 of the 10 patients, with one patient having generalized seizures. Five patients were on long-term antiepileptic medication.

Regarding the occupational situation, 10 (9 full-time) of the 39 patients in the work of Hottinger et al. (2009) and 4 (1 full-time) of the 10 patients in the cohort of Steinbach et al. (2006) were employed. In this cohort quality of life was assessed via the EORTC-QLQ C30 version 3.0 questionnaire. The most prominent mean reductions in functioning were observed with the physical functioning scale and the role functioning scale. The role functioning scale assesses the ability to work, perform activities of daily life, and participate in leisure activities. Fatigue was also a common complaint. In contrast, little reduction in mean global health status and overall quality of life was perceived.

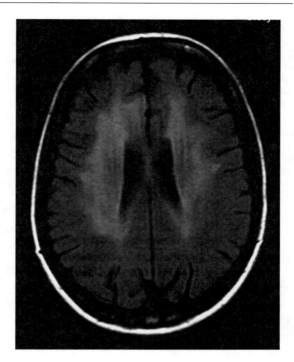

Fig. 41.1 MRI scan (FLAIR sequence) showing a severe leukoencephalopathy after involved field irradiation

Cognitive Deficits

Radiation-induced leukoencephalopathy (Fig. 41.1) is the main established cause of cognitive impairment. The risk is higher in patients who had received whole brain radiotherapy and is time-dependent. However, multimodal insult to the brain caused by the tumor itself (Savaskan et al., 2008), surgical procedures, seizures and possibly chemotherapy may add to the deleterious effects of radiotherapy. All 49 patients in the already mentioned cohorts (Steinbach et al., 2006; Hottinger et al., 2009) developed a leukoencephalopathy during the course of their disease. But not all patients developed related clinical symptoms attributed to leukoencephalopathy. Hottinger et al. (2009) report on 11 patients (23%) with cognitive impairment or slowing, difficulties with recent memory, distractibility and fatigue being the most common complaints. These symptoms developed a median of 3.5 years (1.25–11.57 years) after the initial diagnosis of the glioblastoma. Those patients described their symptoms as mild in 5 and severe in 6 cases. Steinbach et al. (2006) performed a detailed neuropsychological testing in 8 of their 10 patients. Deficits in at least one area were uncovered even in clinically asymptomatic patients with normal scores on the Mini-Mental State Examination. In particular, attention was severely impaired in almost every patient, in both the d2 test and the test for attention functions. Constructional and arithmetic abilities were also reduced in the majority of patients. Noteworthy, memory was well conserved in many patients.

Late Relapses

With some patients in full remission for >10 years, the question arises, whether a glioblastoma can ever be considered to be cured. A study by Salvati et al. (1998) suggested that death from recurrent tumor was unusual in glioblastoma patients who had survived for >5 years. Therefore, one could consider to reduce the frequency of follow-up MRI scans after 5 years of progression free survival.

However, Bähr et al. (2009) report on an extended follow-up of the cohort earlier published by Steinbach et al. (2006), showing that 3 of the 10 patients

Fig. 41.2 Individual progression-free survival curves in long-term surviving glioblastoma patients. Recurrences are indicated by a step downward in the individual curve. The *numbers* correspond to the patient numbers in the original report. *Patient alive, †patient deceased, #patient died from leukoencephalopathy without evidence of tumor progression

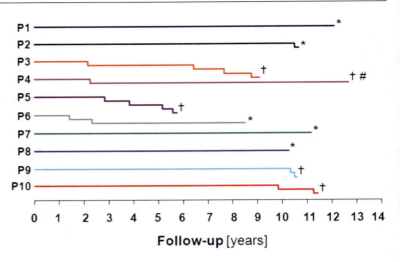

had their first tumor progression 9–10 years after initial diagnosis (Fig. 41.2). Additionally, only 3 patients remained free from recurrence after >10 years. One patient died from leukoencephalopathy-associated complications >12 years after diagnosis and 10 years after his only tumor progression. Four patients died from tumor progression more than 5, 9, 10, and 11 years after diagnosis of glioblastoma undergoing 2–4 recurrences. Although uncommon, in this small cohort of 10 patients there might be 3 patients that appear to be cured of their disease. On the other hand, late relapses occurred in 3 patients even after 10 years of progression-free survival since initial diagnosis (Fig. 41.2). Hottinger et al. (2009) support these data with at least one quarter of their patients dying from tumor progression between 5 and 10 years after diagnosis. In our opinion this illustrates, that one can never be sure that a recurrence will not occur and that the maintenance of a tight control schedule even 5–10 years after diagnosis should be considered.

Discussion

For glioblastoma patients surviving >5 years the clinical outcome and quality of life is of particular importance. If examined in-depth, virtually all of these patients have focal neurological and also cognitive deficits. The neurological deficits are primarily caused by the tumor or the neurosurgical procedures and are mild to moderate in the majority of the patients. However, a relevant proportion has severe deficits that

may result in a reduced independence of the patients. In general, the physical condition of long-term survivors is unexpectedly high, which is reflected by a high median KPS of 70% in at least two current studies (Hottinger et al., 2009; Steinbach et al., 2006). In the future these figures might be expected to improve as neurosurgical interventions advance and become safer.

Although nearly every long-term survivor develops some degree of cognitive impairment that can be detected by formal testing, by far not every patient displays impairment in the activities of daily life. In daily routine cognitive deficits are often measured by the MMSE. Long-term survivors infrequently have pathologic results in this superficial test, but demonstrate deficits when a detailed neuropsychological testing is done. The main established cause of these cognitive deficits is a radiation-induced leukoencephalopathy. The risk for developing a leukoencephalopathy is higher in patients who had received radiotherapy and is time-dependent. However, the tumor itself, surgical procedures, seizures, and chemotherapy may add to the detrimental effects of radiotherapy.

Taken together the clinical deficits often result in an impaired working capacity. In the two studies mentioned above, ~75% of all patients were not employed at the long-term follow-up. This matches with the fact that the most prominent mean reductions in quality of life evaluation were observed with the physical functioning scale and the role functioning scale, which assesses the ability to work, perform activities of daily life, and participate in leisure activities. But noteworthy, only little reductions in mean global health status and overall quality of life were perceived.

For the future, it will be of high importance to include rigorous assessments of therapy-induced neurotoxicity in clinical trials of novel therapeutic regimens in order to establish therapies that not only prolong survival, but also maintain independence and quality of life. For the daily care of glioblastoma patients awareness of the prognosis is indispensable for the information of our patients and for decisions about appropriate treatment options.

Patient factors definitely influencing the overall survival rates are young age at diagnosis, high KPS, methylated MGMT promoter status, and the presence of IDH1 mutations. The influences of female gender, histological subtype, and the extent of necrosis are less well established. Therapeutic relevance has been demonstrated for extent of resection, radiotherapy, and, in patients younger than 70 years of age with a KPS of at least 70%, for temozolomide radiochemotherapy.

However, the chances of long-term survival are very modest even for patients that have all favorable patient factors who receive optimal therapy. It is somewhat consoling, on the other hand, that there are some long-term surviving patients without obviously favorable prognosticators. If long-term survival is achieved, however, we recommend to avoid considering a patient cured from glioblastoma even when he or she is free from progression for >5 or 10 years, since late and very late relapses seem to be common. Therefore, a continuous control schedule should be maintained even after 10 years of progression-free survival.

Acknowledgment The Dr. Senckenberg Institute of Neurooncology is supported by the Dr. Senckenberg Foundation and the Hertie Foundation. J.P.S. is "Hertie Professor of Neurooncology."

References

Burton EC, Lamborn KR, Feuerstein BG, Prados M, Scott J, Forsyth P, Passe S, Jenkins RB, Aldape KD (2002) Genetic aberrations defined by comparative genomic hybridization distinguish long-term from typical survivors of glioblastoma. Cancer Res 62:6205–6210

Bähr O, Herrlinger U, Weller M, Steinbach JP (2009) Very late relapses in glioblastoma long-term survivors. J Neurol 256:1756–1758

Glas M, Happold C, Rieger J, Wiewrodt D, Bähr O, Steinbach JP, Wick W, Kortmann RD, Reifenberger G, Weller M, Herrlinger U (2009) Long-term survival of patients with glioblastoma treated with radiotherapy and lomustine plus temozolomide. J Clin Oncol 27:1257–1261

Hottinger AF, Yoon H, DeAngelis LM, Abrey LE (2009) Neurological outcome of long-term glioblastoma survivors. J Neuro-oncol 95:301–305

Krex D, Klink B, Hartmann C, von Deimling A, Pietsch T, Simon M, Sabel M, Steinbach JP, Heese O, Reifenberger G, Weller M, Schackert G (2007) German glioma network. Long-term survival with glioblastoma multiforme Brain 130:2596–2606

Louis DN, Ohgaki H, Wiestler OD, Cavenee WK, Burger PC, Jouvet A, Scheithauer BW, Kleihues P (2007) The 2007 WHO classification of tumours of the central nervous system. Acta Neuropathol 114:97–109

Martinez R, Schackert G, Yaya-Tur R, Rojas-Marcos I, Herman JG, Esteller M (2007) Frequent hypermethylation of the DNA repair gene MGMT in long-term survivors of glioblastoma multiforme. J Neuro-oncol 83:91–93

McLendon RE, Halperin EC (2003) Is the long-term survival of patients with intracranial glioblastoma multiforme overstated?. Cancer 98:1745–1748

Ohgaki H, Kleihues P (2005) Genetic pathways to primary and secondary glioblastoma. Am J Pathol 170:1445–1453

Pichlmeier U, Bink A, Schackert G, Stummer W; and ALA Glioma Study Group (2008) Resection and survival in glioblastoma multiforme: an RTOG recursive partitioning analysis of ALA study patients. Neuro Oncol 10:1025–1034

Salvati M, Cervoni L, Artico M, Caruso R, Gagliardi FM (1998) Long-term survival in patients with supratentorial glioblastoma. J Neuro-oncol 36:61–64

Savaskan NE, Heckel A, Hahnen E, Engelhorn T, Doerfler A, Ganslandt O, Nimsky C, Buchfelder M, Eyüpoglu IY (2008) Small interfering RNA-mediated xCT silencing in gliomas inhibits neurodegeneration and alleviates brain edema. Nat Med 14:629–632

Scott JN, Rewcastle NB, Brasher PM, Fulton D, MacKinnon JA, Hamilton M, Cairncross JG, Forsyth P (1999) Which glioblastoma multiforme patient will become a long-term survivor? A population-based study. Ann Neurol 46:183–188

Shinojima N, Kochi M, Hamada J, Nakamura H, Yano S, Makino K, Tsuiki H, Tada K, Kuratsu J, Ishimaru Y, Ushio Y (2004) The influence of sex and the presence of giant cells on postoperative long-term survival in adult patients with supratentorial glioblastoma multiforme. J Neurosurg 101:219–226

Sonoda Y, Kumabe T, Watanabe M, Nakazato Y, Inoue T, Kanamori M, Tominaga T (2009) Long-term survivors of glioblastoma: clinical features and molecular analysis. Acta Neurochir 151:1349–1358

Steinbach JP, Blaicher HP, Herrlinger U, Wick W, Nägele T, Meyermann R, Tatagiba M, Bamberg M, Dichgans J, Karnath HO, Weller M (2006) Surviving glioblastoma for more than 5 years: the patient's perspective. Neurology 66:239–242

Stummer W, Pichlmeier U, Meinel T, Wiestler OD, Zanella F, Reulen HJ (2006) Fluorescence-guided surgery with 5-aminolevulinic acid for resection of malignant glioma: a randomised controlled multicentre phase III trial. Lancet Oncol 7:392–401

Stummer W, Reulen HJ, Meinel T, Pichlmeier U, Schumacher W, Tonn JC, Rohde V, Oppel F, Turowski B, Woiciechowsky

C, Franz K, Pietsch T and ALA-Glioma Study Group (2008) Extent of resection and survival in glioblastoma multiforme: identification of and adjustment for bias. Neurosurgery 62:564–576

Stupp R, Hegi ME, Mason WP, van den Bent MJ, Taphoorn MJ, Janzer RC, Ludwin SK, Allgeier A, Fisher B, Belanger K, Hau P, Brandes AA, Gijtenbeek J, Marosi C, Vecht CJ, Mokhtari K, Wesseling P, Villa S, Eisenhauer E, Gorlia T, Weller M, Lacombe D, Cairncross JG,, Mirimanoff RO European Organisation for Research and Treatment of Cancer Brain Tumour and Radiation Oncology Groups, and National Cancer Institute of Canada Clinical Trials Group (2009) Effects of radiotherapy with concomitant and adjuvant temozolomide versus radiotherapy alone on survival in glioblastoma in a randomised phase III study: 5-year analysis of the EORTC-NCIC trial. Lancet Oncol 10:459–466

Weller M, Felsberg J, Hartmann C, Berger H, Steinbach JP, Schramm J, Westphal M, Schackert G, Simon M, Tonn JC, Heese O, Krex D, Nikkhah G, Pietsch T, Wiestler O, Reifenberger G, von Deimling A, Loeffler M (2009) Molecular predictors of progression-free and overall survival in patients with newly diagnosed glioblastoma: a prospective translational study of the german glioma network. J Clin Oncol 27:5743–5750

Chapter 42

Glioblastoma Patients: p15 Methylation as a Prognostic Factor

Steffi Urbschat, Silke Wemmert, and Ralf Ketter

Abstract Glioblastomas are the most frequent and malignant brain tumors in adults. Surgical cure is virtually impossible and despite of radiation and chemotherapy the clinical course is very poor. Epigenetic silencing of MGMT has been associated with a better response to temozolomide-chemotherapy. We previously showed that temozolomide increases the median survival time of patients with tumors harbouring deletions on 9p within the region for p15(INK4b), p16(INK4a), and 10q (MGMT). The aim of this study was to investigate the methylation status of p15, p16, 14^{ARF} and MGMT in glioblastomas and to correlate the results with the clinical data. Only patients with KPS >70, radical tumor resection, radiation and temozolomide-chemotherapy after recurrence were included. We observed promoter methylation of MGMT in 56% (15/27) and of p15 in 37% (10/27) of the tumors, whereas methylation of p16 and p14^{ARF} were rare. Interestingly, methylation of p15 emerged as a significant predictor of shorter overall survival (16.9 vs. 23.8 months, $p = 0.025$), whereas MGMT promoter methylation had no significant effect on median overall survival under this treatment regimen (22.5 vs. 22.1 months, $p = 0.49$). In the presence of other clinically relevant factors, p15 methylation remains the only significant predictor ($p = 0.021$; Cox regression). Although these results need to be confirmed in larger series and under different treatment conditions, our retrospective study shows clear evidence that p15 methylation can act as an additional prognostic factor for survival. This tumor suppressor gene, involved in cell cycle control, can act as an attractive candidate for therapeutic approaches in glioblastomas.

Keywords Methylation · MGMT · p15 · p16

Introduction

Glioblastomas [World Health Organization (WHO) grade IV] are the most frequent and the most malignant brain tumors in adults. They arise either de novo without recognizable precursor lesions (primary glioblastomas) or develop from lower grade astrocytomas (secondary glioblastomas). Despite of multimodal therapy approaches, the prognosis is generally poor. According to Stupp et al. (2005) the average survival time is 12.1 months with standard therapy (surgery and radiation) and 14.6 months with the application of multimodal therapy concepts. Besides radical surgery, a higher preoperative Karnofsky Performance Score and younger age are predictors of a more favourable clinical course (Burger and Green, 1987; Lacroix et al., 2001; Stummer et al., 2008). In the search for efficient therapeutic procedures, the oncological biological understanding of these aggressive tumor diseases is of fundamental significance. The difficulties of analysis of these complex genetic alterations are not only to identify the tumor-relevant aberrations, but also to access the chronological order of these genetic changes in terms of initiation- and progression phenomena. In addition, Glioblastomas are tumors with an unusual large intratumoral and intertumoral genetic heterogeneity, which is in the histological findings only conditionally expressed, but obviously exercises substantial influence on – passing therapy success.

By means of chromosome analysis as well as established cell lines and primary tumor cell culture,

S. Urbschat (✉)
Department of Neurosurgery/Neurooncology, Saarland University, 66421 Homburg, Germany
e-mail: Steffi.Urbschat@uks.eu

M.A. Hayat (ed.), *Tumors of the Central Nervous System, Volume 1*,
DOI 10.1007/978-94-007-0344-5_42, © Springer Science+Business Media B.V. 2011

complex cytogenetic changes in gliomas have been revealed. The investigations of native tumor material brought a significant methodical advantage using comparative genomic hybridisation (CGH). A lot of further quantitative genomic alterations have been found in the last few years which contributed to a broader characterisation of these tumors. More and more molecular genetic investigations have been and are being carried out, e.g. searching for loss of heterozygosity (LOH) and microsatellite polymorphism for a detailed mapping of these alterations. Due to these extensive analyses a high number of numerical chromosomal changes in gliomas are known, in particular in glioblastoma multiforme (GBM). In the meantime the following chromosomal alterations and changes in the therein located genes are being looked for and are characteristic: gains of chromosome 7 (and/or EGFR amplification), as well as partial or complete losses on/of 9p (CDKN2A, CDKN2B), of 10q (PTEN, DMBT1, MGMT), of 17p (EGFR) and on 12q13-q15 (MDM2, CDK4, GLI, SAS), of 13q14 (RB) (Brunner et al., 1999; Thiel et al., 1992). Several alterations were also shown to be correlated with prognosis. Glioblastomas with EGFR amplification were characterized by a short patient survival (Idbaih et al., 2008). Patients with a deletion of 13q14 or 17p13.1 show also a significantly shortened survival time (Yin et al., 2009). Brat et al., 2004 found that 9p and 10q deletions were slightly more frequent in short-term survivors, though none of the comparisons achieved statistical significance. These and other molecular markers for progression-free and overall survival in patients with high grade gliomas were still discussed controversially in the current literature. However, some studies underlines the association of glioblastoma long-term survival with prognostic favourable clinical factors, in particular young age, good initial performance score, as well as MGMT promoter hypermethylation (Krex et al., 2007; Weller et al., 2009).

In novel investigations Microarrays improve our understanding of tumor biology considerably, whose assistance allows us not only to analyse structural rearrangements of the genome, but also complex gene expression patterns. For example Yin et al. (2009) examined glioblastoma tissues and cell lines using single nucleotide polymorphism DNA microarray (SNP-Chip) and found abnormalities in the p16(INK4A)/p15(INK4B)-CDK4/6-pRb or p14 (ARF)-MDM2/4-p53 pathways in 89%.

Deletion or mutation of the p16(INK4a)/ARF/p15(INK4b) locus on chromosome 9p21 is among the most common alterations seen in human cancer and also in human gliomas (Jen et al., 1994; Rasheed et al., 2002). The INK4a locus encodes two gene products that are involved in cell cycle regulation through inhibition of CDK4-mediated RB phosphorylation (p16) and binding to MDM2 leading to p53 stabilization (p14^{ARF}). The tumor suppressor gene products p16 and p15 are both capable of binding to CDK4 and CDK6, these kinases associate with D-type cyclines and these binary complexes are responsible for phosphorylation of RB-protein at mid G1 of the cell cycle. The phosphorylation of RB is assumed to be critical for progression through G1 and entry into S-phase of the cell cycle. Binding of INK4 to CDK4/6 inhibits its kinase activity and thereby arrests progression through the cell cycle in mid-late G1 (Gil and Peters, 2006).

Over half of the high grade gliomas lack a functional INK4a/ARF locus. Gliomas with intact INK4a/ARF carry mutations in other components of the RB and p53 pathways implicating these two pathways as being absolutely critical in cell growth and death control (Fulci et al., 2000; Ichimura et al., 2000). Previous studies showed that deletion of 9p including the INK4a/b locus is a significant unfavorable prognostic factor for survival of glioblastoma patients (Kamiryo et al., 2002; Wemmert et al., 2005). Further on, this alteration has been reported to be inversely correlated with the chemosensitivity of malignant gliomas (Simon et al., 2006).

Over the past years aberrant DNA methylation was shown to be a common molecular lesion in human tumors as well, which had also impact on patient prognosis and treatment response. Epigenetic silencing of p16 and p15 was shown in a variety of human neoplasms, in glioma patients hypermethylation is reported in about 30% of the cases (Esteller et al., 2001; Herman et al., 1996; Uhlmann et al., 2003). Whereas in other tumors inactivation of both tumor suppressor genes was associated with prognosis and response to chemotherapy, a prognostic and predictive role in gliomas is not shown (Kudoh et al., 2002; Lee et al., 2006; Rasheed et al., 2002).

In our previous study we identified the negative prognostic impact for deletions on 9p and 10q

(Wemmert et al., 2005). In our further setting, we investigate the methylation status of p15, p16, p14^{ARF} and MGMT, and correlate the results with the clinical data of the glioblastoma patients.

Methylation-Specific Polymerase Chain Reaction: Methodology

Methylation-specific polymerase chain reaction (MS-PCR) is a sensitive method to discriminately amplify and detect a methylated region of interest using methylated – or unmethylated specific primers on bisulfite-converted genomic DNA. Such primers will only anneal to sequences that are methylated and thus containing 5-methylcytosines that are resistant to conversion by bisulfite. The great sensitivity of this technique allows qualitative methylation analysis from DNA obtained not only from fresh frozen tissues, peripheral blood, bone marrow, or body fluids but also from paraffin-embedded samples. It is a rapid and cost-effective method that does not require radioactive reagents and can be used for the analysis of a large number of clinical samples.

DNA of the tumor samples was isolated following standard protocols with chloroforme followed by sodium bisulfite modification. Promoter hypermethylation of the MGMT, p15, p16 and p14^{ARF} genes were determined by MS-PCR as described previously (Herman et al., 1996; Paz et al., 2004; Sato et al., 2002). The amplified products were electrophoresed on 3.5% agarose gels and visualized with ethidium bromide. Methylated blood DNA was included in each PCR set as methylated and unmethylated controls, respectively.

Statistical Analyses

Comparison of survival times between groups defined by methylation status was performed by Kaplan-Meier curves and with two-sided log rank tests. Multivariate Cox regression analysis was performed to identify significant predictors for survival. Effects in these models were quantified by hazard ratio estimates with 95% confidence intervals. Median survival rates were calculated using the Kaplan-Meier method.

Tumor Samples

The retrospective study included 27 tumor specimens of gliomas classified as WHO grade IV: 23 primary and 4 secondary glioblastomas. After radical tumor surgery, all patients received standard radiation therapy (RT) (1.8-2 Gy, total dose of 60 Gy) and adjuvant temozolomide chemotherapy in case of recurrence. The doses were 150 mg/m^2 for 5 days in 4 week cycles. Specimens of resected tumor were immediately shock frozen in liquid nitrogen and stored at –80°C or fixed in formalin and embedded in paraffin.

Prognostic Impact of the Methylation Status of p15, p16, p14^{ARF} and MGMT

Clinical Data

Median age at surgery was 49 years (range 26–70), the sex ratio was 2.375 (19 men/8 women) and median post operative Karnofsky Performance Score (KPS) was 100 (range 80–100, 18 patients with KPS 100).

Methylation Analyses

The MGMT promoter was methylated in 15/27 cases (55.6%), the p15 promoter was methylated in 10/27 (37%) glioblastomas. All secondary GBM (4/4) showed a methylated MGMT promoter and an unmethylated p15 promoter. Methylation of p14^{ARF} was absent in all (27/27) investigated GBM. Methylation status of p16 was available for 23/27 glioblastomas. Hypermethylation of p16 was detected in only 1/23 cases (4.3%).

Clinical Outcome

Overall median survival was 22.5 months with a 2-year survival rate of 35.0%.

In univariate analyses, MGMT methylation had no impact on overall survival (22.5 vs. 22.1 months, $p = 0.49$, log-rank test), whereas p15 methylation was associated significantly with a shorter overall survival (16.9 vs. 23.8 months; $p = 0.0252$, log-rank test).

We also performed a multivariate analysis including parameters previously identified as significant. Only p15 methylation emerged as a significant prognostic factor after adjusting for KPS, sex, age and MGMT. In the first analysis, the predictors KPS and age enter as numerical variables in the model, in the second analysis KPS and age are dichotomized with cutoffs 90 and 50 in order to reduce model complexity. The gender variable sex is set to 1 for females and 0 for males. Both analyses yield very similar results, identifying p15 methylation as the only significant predictor in these analyzed cases.

Discussion

A better understanding of the genetic alterations predicting disease outcome and therapy response in patients with high grade gliomas will help to optimize both treatment and overall outcome. In our study setting, MGMT promoter methylation had no significant impact on survival, in contrast with other studies that observed a strong effect on patient response and on survival in larger cohorts treated with radio- and temozolomide-chemotherapy (Hegi et al., 2005; Paz et al., 2004). This discrepancy might result, besides our smaller patient cohort, from the different treatment schedules. Actually, comparing various treatment modalities in glioblastomas, the prognostic effect of MGMT methylation was observed only when simultaneous chemoirradiation was administered (Crinière et al., 2007; Paz et al., 2004).

Further on, our PCR-results showed besides the methylated band also unmethylated bands in a large number of tumors. Taking into account this heterogeneity and that we are dealing with diffusely growing gliomas (Hegi et al., 2008; Jung et al., 1999; Loeper et al., 2001), this observation arises most likely from a different tumor cell population and from normal cells contaminating the tumor sample. Nevertheless, this heterogeneous methylation pattern may also result in different amounts of MGMT and therefore affect chemotherapy response.

All evidence collected to date implicates that the INK4a/ARF gene products are critically important in control of growth arrest and senescence. Loss of p16 and ARF expression is associated with many human cancers, particularly gliomas (Esteller et al.,

2001). A number of studies have shown that reconstitution of INK4a/ARF expression in glioma cells altered growth characteristics, reduced tumorigenicity and decreased invasive potential. These studies demonstrate the importance of the INK4a/ARF pathway in suppression of the neoplastic phenotype and suggest that restoration of a functional INK4a/ARF locus will be an important means of controlling the growth of gliomas (Inoue et al., 2004; Komata et al., 2003).

A striking observation of our study is the significant correlation of p15 methylation with a poorer clinical course. Loss of p15 had not been widely investigated previously as a potential determinant of chemo- and radiosensitivity or as a prognostic factor. We were able to show that an inactivation of p15 by promoter hypermethylation acts as a predictor for an unfavorable clinical course. (Wemmert et al., 2009). Cyclin dependent kinase inhibitors (p16, p21, p27) were shown to exhibit an antitumor effect in malignant gliomas inducing growth arrest and apoptosis in cell culture (Inoue et al., 2004; Komata et al., 2003). Further on, retrovirus mediated transfer of INK4a halts glioma formation in a rat model (Strauss et al., 2002). This corroborates the idea that retrovirus mediated gene transfer of INK4a/b may also be an effective means to arrest human gliomas. Therefore, restoring the normal function of p15 by gene therapy is an attractive goal in the treatment of human gliomas.

Furthermore, our finding that glioblastomas have not simultaneously hypermethylated the investigated tumor suppressor genes on 9p implicates that these tumors carry no general defect in their pattern of CpG island methylation. Interestingly, all secondary GBM (4/4) showed a methylated MGMT promoter and an unmethylated p15 promoter which indicates that distinct molecular pathways constitute for primary and for secondary glioblastomas and let them differ both in biological behavior and in clinical outcome. This corresponds to the finding that methylation of p14^{ARF} is associated with a shorter patient survival and is mutually exclusive of MGMT promoter methylation except of one case in low grade astrocytoma who underwent progression or recurrence (Watanabe et al., 2007). In our patient cohort that mainly consists of primary glioblastoma, p14^{ARF} was not observed, supporting that this alteration is mainly restricted to secondary glioblastoma and therefore in the pathway of astrocytoma progression.

Although these results need to be confirmed in larger series, our retrospective study suggests that p15 hypermethylation can act as an additional important prognostic factor for survival in glioblastomas. Further investigations have to clarify if p15 methylation is a predictive factor for temozolomide treatment response and can act as a prognostic parameter for survival, independent of therapy.

References

Brat DJ, Seiferheld WF, Perry A, Hammond EH, Murray KJ, Schulsinger AR, Mehta MP, Curran WJ (2004) Analysis of 1p, 19q, 9p, and 10q as prognostic markers for high-grade astrocytomas using fluorescence in situ hybridization on tissue microarrays from radiation therapy oncology group trials. Neuro-Oncol 6:96–103

Brunner C, Jung V, Henn W, Zang KD, Urbschat S (1999) Comparative genomic hybridization reveals recurrent enhancements on chromosome 20 and in one case combined amplification sites on chromosome 15q24q26 and 20p11p12 in glioblastomas. Cancer Genet Cytogenet 121:124–127

Burger PC, Green SB (1987) Patient age, histologic features, and length of survival in patients with glioblastoma multiforme. Cancer 59:1617–1625

Crinière E, Kaloshi G, Laigle-Donadey F, Lejeune J, Auger N, Benouaich-Amiel A, Everhard S, Mokhtari K, Polivka M, Delattre JY, Hoang-Xuan K, Thillet J, Sanson M (2007) MGMT prognostic impact on glioblastoma is dependent on therapeutic modalities. J Neuro-oncol 83:173–179

Esteller M, Corn PG, Baylin SB, Herman JG (2001) A gene hypermethylation profile of human cancer. Cancer Res 61:3225–3229

Fulci G, Labuhn M, Maier D, Lachat Y, Hausmann O, Hegi ME, Janzer RC, Merlo A, Van Meir EG (2000) P53 gene mutation and ink4a-arf deletion appear to be two mutually exclusive events in human glioblastoma. Oncogene 19:3816–3822

Gil J, Peters G (2006) Regulation of the INK4b-ARF-INK4a tumour suppressor locus: all for one or one for all. Nat Rev Mol Cell Biol 7:667–677

Hegi ME, Diserens AC, Gorlia T, Hamou MF, de Tribolet N, Weller M, Kros JM, Hainfellner JA, Mason W, Mariani L, Bromberg JE, Hau P, Mirimanoff RO, Cairncross JG, Janzer RC, Stupp R (2005) MGMT gene silencing and benefit from temozolomide in glioblastoma. N Engl J Med 352:997–1003

Hegi M, Liu L, Herman JG, Stupp R, Wick W, Weller M, Mehta MP, Gilbert MR (2008) Correlation of O6-methylguanin methyltransferase (MGMT) promotor methylation with clinical outcomes in glioblastoma and clinical strategies to modulate MGMT activity. J Clin Oncol 26:4189–4199

Herman JG, Graff JR, Myöhänen S, Nelkin BD, Baylin SB (1996) Methylation-specific PCR: a novel PCR assay for methylation status of CpG islands. Proc Natl Acad Sci USA 93:9821–9826

Ichimura K, Bolin MB, Goike HM, Schmidt EE, Moshref A, Collins VP (2000) Deregulation of the p14ARF/MDM2/p53 pathway is a prerequisite for human astrocytic gliomas

with G1-S transition control gene abnormalities. Cancer Res 60:417–424

Idbaih A, Marie Y, Lucchesi C, Pierron G, Manié E, Raynal V, Mosseri V, Hoang-Xuan K, Kujas M, Brito I, Mokhtari K, Sanson M, Barillot E, Aurias A, Delattre JY, Delattre O (2008) BAC array CGH distinguishes mutually exclusive alterations that define clinicogenetic subtypes of gliomas. Int J Cancer 122:1778–1786

Inoue R, Moghaddam KA, Ranasinghe M, Saeki Y, Chiocca EA, Wade-Martins R (2004) Infectious delivery of the 132 kb CDKN2A/CDKN2B genomic DNA region results in correctly spiced gene expression and growth suppression in glioma cells. Gene Ther 11:1195–1204

Jen J, Harper JW, Bigner SH, Bigner DD, Papadopoulos N, Markowitz S, Willson JK, Kinzler KW, Vogelstein B (1994) Deletion of p16 and p15 genes in brain tumors. Cancer Res 54:6353–6358

Jung V, Romeike BF, Henn W, Feiden W, Moringlane JR, Zang KD, Urbschat S (1999) Evidence of focal genetic micro-heterogeneity in glioblastoma multiforme by area-specific CGH on microdissected tumor cells. J Neuropathol Exp Neurol 58:993–999

Kamiryo T, Tada K, Shiraishi S, Shinojima N, Nakamura H, Kochi M, Kuratsu J, Saya H, Ushio Y (2002) Analysis of homozygous deletion of the p16 gene and correlation with survival in patients with glioblastoma multiforme. J Neurosurg 96:815–822

Komata T, Kanzawa T, Takeuchi H, Germano IM, Schreiber M, Kondo Y, Kondo S (2003) Antitumor effect of cyclin-dependent kinase inhibitors (p16(INK4A), p18(INK4C), p19(INK4D). P21 (WAF1/CIP1) and p27 (KIP1)) on malignant glioma cells. Br J Cancer 88:1277–1280

Krex D, Klink B, Hartmann C, von Deimling A, Pietsch T, Simon M, Sabel M, Steinbach JP, Heese O, Reifenberger G, Weller M, Schackert G (2007) Long-term survival with glioblastoma multiforme. Brain 130:2596–2606

Kudoh K, Ichikawa Y, Yoshida S, Hirai M, Kikuchi Y, Nagata I, Miwa M, Uchida K (2002) Inactivation of p16/CDKN2 and p15/MTS2 is associated with prognosis and response to chemotherapy in ovarian cancer. Int J Cancer 99:579–582

Lacroix M, Abi-Said D, Fourney DR, Gokaslan ZL, Shi W, DeMonte F, Lang FF, McCutcheon IE, Hassenbusch SJ, Holland E, Hess K, Michael C, Miller D, Sawaya R (2001) A multivariate analysis of 416 patients with glioblastoma multiforme: prognosis, extent of resection, and survival. J Neurosurg 95:190–198

Lee M, Sup Han W, Kyoung Kim O, Hee Sung S, Sun Cho M, Lee SN, Koo H (2006) Prognostic value of p16INK4a and p14ARF gene hypermethylation in human colon cancer. Pathol Res Pract 202:415–424

Loeper S, Romeike BF, Heckmann N, Jung V, Henn W, Feiden W, Zang KD, Urbschat S (2001) Frequent mitotic errors in tumor cells of genetically micro-heterogeneous glioblastomas. Cytogenet Cell Genet 94:1–8

Paz MF, Yaya-Tur R, Rojas-Marcos I, Reynes G, Pollan M, Aguirre-Cruz L, García-Lopez JL, Piquer J, Safont MJ, Balaña C, Sanchez-Cespedes M, García-Villanueva M, Arribas L, Esteller M (2004) CpG island hypermethylation of the DNA repair enzyme methyltransferase predicts response to temozolomide in primary gliomas. Clin Cancer Res 10:4933–4938

Rasheed A, Herndon JE, Stenzel TT, Raetz JG, Kendelhardt J, Friedman HS, Friedman AH, Bigner DD, Bigner SH, McLendon RE (2002) Molecular markers of prognosis in astrocytic tumors. Cancer 94:2688–2697

Sato F, Harpaz N, Shibata D, Xu Y, Yin J, Mori Y, Zou TT, Wang S, Desai K, Leytin A, Selaru FM, Abraham JM, Meltzer SJ (2002) Hypermethylation of the p14 (ARF) gene in ulcerative colitis-associated colorectal carcinogenesis. Cancer Res 62:1148–1151

Simon M, Voss D, Park-Simon TW, Mahlberg R, Köster G (2006) Role of p16 and p14ARF in radio-and chemosensitivity of malignant gliomas. Oncol Rep 16:127–132

Strauss BE, Fontes RB, Lotfi CF, Skorupa A, Bartol I, Cipolla-Neot J, Costanzi-Strauss E (2002) Retroviral transfer of the p16INK4a cDNA inhibits C6 glioma formation in Wistar rats. Cancer Cell Int 2:1–9

Stummer W, Reulen HJ, Meinel T, Pichlmeier U, Schumacker W, Tonn JC, Rohde V, Oppel F, Turowski B, Woiciechowsky C, Franz K, Pietsch T (2008) Extent of resection and survival in glioblastoma multiforme: Identification of and adjustment for bias. Neurosurgery 62:564–576

Stupp R, Mason WP, van den Bent MJ, Weller M, Fisher B, Taphoom MJ, Belanger K, Brandes AA, Marosi C, Bogdahn U, Curschmann J, Janzer RC, Ludwin SK, Gorlia T, Allgeier A, Lacombe D, Cairncross JG, Eisenhauer E, Mirimanoff RO (2005) Radiotherapy plus concomitant and adjuvant temozolomide for glioblastoma. N Engl J Med 352:987–996

Thiel G, Losanowa T, Kintzel D, Nisch G, Martin H, Vorpahl K, Witkowski R (1992) Karyotypes in 90 human gliomas. Cancer Genet Cytogenet 58:109–120

Uhlmann K, Rohde K, Zeller C, Szymas J, Vogel S, Marczinek K, Thiel G, Nürnberg P, Laird PW (2003) Distinct methylation profiles of glioma subtypes. Int J Cancer 106:52–59

Watanabe T, Katayama Y, Yoshino A, Yachi K, Ohta T, Ogino A, Komine C, Fukushima T (2007) Aberrant hypermethylation of p14ARF and O6-methylguanine-DNA methyltransferase genes in astrocytoma progression. Brain Pathol 17:5–10

Weller M, Felsberg J, Hartmann C, Berger H, Steinbach JP, Schramm J, Westphal M, Schackert G, Simon M, Tonn JC, Heese O, Krex D, Nikkhah G, Pietsch T, Wiestler O, Reifenberger G, von Deimling A, Loeffler M (2009) Molecular predictors of progression-free and overall survival in patients with newly diagnosed glioblastoma: A prospective translational study of the German glioma network. J Clin Oncol 27:5743–5750

Wemmert S, Bettscheider M, Alt S, Ketter R, Kammers K, Feiden W, Steudel WI, Rahnenführer J, Urbschat S (2009) p15 promotor methylation – a novel prognostic marker in glioblastoma patients . Int J Oncol 34:1743–1748

Wemmert S, Ketter R, Rahnenführer J, Beerenwinkel N, Strowitzki M, Feiden W, Hartmann C, Lengauer T, Stockhammer F, Zang KD, Meese E, Steudel WI, von Deimling A,, Urbschat S (2005) Patients with high-grade gliomas harboring deletions of chromosomes 9p and 10q benefit from temozolomide treatment. Neoplasia 7:883–893

Yin D, Ogawa S, Kawamata N, Tunici P, Finocchiaro G, Eoli M, Ruckert C, Huynh T, Liu G, Kato M, Sanada M, Jauch A, Dugas M, Black KL, Koeffler HP (2009) High-resolution genomic copy number profiling of glioblastoma multiforma by single nucleotide polymorphism DNA microarray. Mol Cancer Res 7:665–677

Index

Notes: The letters 'f' and 't' following the locators refer to figures and tables respectively.